INTRAVENOUS MEDICATIONS

a handbook for nurses
and allied health professionals

INTRAVENOUS MEDICATIONS

a handbook for nurses and allied health professionals

BETTY L. GAHART, RN

Nurse Consultant in Education
Formerly Director, Education and Training
Queen of the Valley Hospital
Napa, California

EIGHTH EDITION

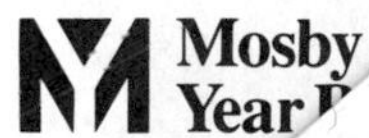

St. Louis Baltimore Boston Chicago

osby
Year Book

to Publishing Excellence

ecutive editor: Don Ladig
anaging editor: Robin Carter
Project manager: Lin A. Dempsey
Manuscript editor: Suzanne Aboulfadl
Designer: Gail Morey Hudson

EIGHTH EDITION

Previous editions copyrighted 19, 1977, 1981, 1985, 198, 1990, 1991

Printed in the United States of America

Mosby–Year Book, Inc.
11830 Westline Industrial Drive, St. Louis, Missouri 63146

Library of Congress Cataloging in Publication Data

Gahart, Betty L.
Intravenous medications: a handbook for nurses and other allied health personnel / Betty L. Gahart.—8th ed.
p. cm.
Bibliography: p.
Includes index.
ISBN 0-8016-1792-8
Intravenous therapy—Handbooks, manuals, etc.
Nursing—
ks, manuals, etc. I. Title.
; 1, Injections, Intravenous—handbook
1991

ress

4 3 2

INTRAVENOUS MEDICATIONS

a handbook for nurses and allied health professionals

BETTY L. GAHART, RN

Nurse Consultant in Education
Formerly Director, Education and Training
Queen of the Valley Hospital
Napa, California

EIGHTH EDITION

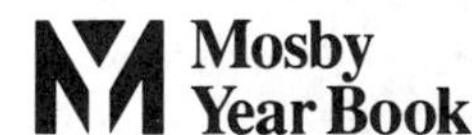

St. Louis Baltimore Boston Chicago London Philadelphia Sydney Toronto

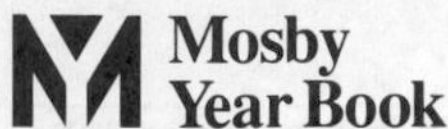

Dedicated to Publishing Excellence

Executive editor: Don Ladig
Managing editor: Robin Carter
Project manager: Lin A. Dempsey
Manuscript editor: Suzanne Aboulfadl
Designer: Gail Morey Hudson

EIGHTH EDITION

Printed in the United States of America

Mosby–Year Book, Inc.
11830 West line Industrial Drive, St. Louis, Missouri 63146

Library of Congress Cataloging in Publication Data

Gahart, Betty L.
Intravenous medications: a handbook for nurses and other allied health personnel / Betty L. Gahart.—8th ed.
p. cm.
Bibliography: p.
Includes index.
ISBN 0-8016-1792-8
1. Intravenous therapy—Handbook, manuals, etc.
2. Nursing—
Handbooks, manuals, etc. I. Title.
[DNLM: 1. Injections, Intravenous—handbooks. WB 39 G133i]
RM170.G33 1991
615.8'55—dc20
DNLM/DLC
for Library of Congress 90-6595
CIP

CL/DC 9 8 7 6 5 4 3 2

To

ALL NURSES, PHYSICIANS, AND OTHER HEALTH CARE PROFESSIONALS

who care enough to quickly review
every intravenous medication
before administration

NURSING CONSULTANTS

CYNTHIA CUSACK, RN, BSN
Nurse Clinician
University of Maryland Hospital
Baltimore, Maryland

DONNA IGNATAVICIUS, RN, MS
Health Care Consultant
DI Associates
Easton, Maryland

JACQUELINE MURPHY, RN, MSc
Instructor and Staff Nurse
Foothills Hospital School of Nursing
Calgary, Alberta

REGINA SHANNON-BODNAR, RN, MS, MSN, OCN
Clinical Nurse Specialist
University of Maryland Cancer Center
Baltimore, Maryland

RENEE SEMONIN-HOLLERAN, RN, MSN, CEN, CCRN, CS
Chief Flight Nurse, University Air Care
Center for Emergency Care, University of Cincinnati
Cincinnati, Ohio

BRENDA SHELTON, RN, BS, CCRN, OCN
Critical Care Instructor
The Johns Hopkins Oncology Center
Baltimore, Maryland

JANE C. SHIVNAN, RN, BSc, CCRN
Head Nurse
Johns Hopkins Hospital
Baltimore, Maryland

RICHARD WATTERS, RN, BSc, BEd
Nursing Consultant
Ottawa, Ontario

SHEILA RANKIN ZERR, RN, MEd
Assistant Professor
University of Victoria
Victoria, British Columbia

PHARMACOLOGY CONSULTANTS

DAVID DOMANN, MS, RPh
Professional Services Manager
E.R. Squibb and Sons, U.S.
Princeton, New Jersey

BOZENA MICHNIAK, PhD, MPS
Assistant Professor
University of South Carolina
Columbia, South Carolina

ADRIENNE R. NAZARENO, PharmD
Clinical Pharmacy Coordinator
Queen of the Valley
Napa, California

PREFACE

The 1990s are here! Our knowledge of pharmacology is compounding almost daily. Many new drugs are being approved for clinical use and additional research finds new, sometimes previously contraindicated, uses for many approved drugs. We therefore felt that annual publication was an imperative step to provide health professionals with the most up-to-date information as quickly as possible.

Intravenous injection has rapidly become the route of choice in most health care settings. The inconvenience and discomfort associated with repeated intramuscular injections are markedly reduced and drug absorption is consistent, as contrasted with unreliable intramuscular absorption in the patient with compromised peripheral perfusion. Intravenous drugs are instantly absorbed into the bloodstream, hopefully leading to a prompt therapeutic action, but the risk of an inappropriate reaction is a constant threat that can easily become a frightening reality.

In such an intense environment, health professionals expected to administer intravenous medications must have an accurate, accessible, complete, and concise reference tool available to them. This eighth edition of *Intravenous Medications* is that tool. All drugs presently approved for intravenous use are included. In addition to new drugs, all information has been thoroughly revised to incorporate the most current documented knowledge available.

The nurse is with the acutely ill, hospitalized patient 24 hours a day and is frequently placed in a variety of difficult situations. While the physician verbally requests or writes an order, the nurse must evaluate it for appropriateness, prepare it, administer it, and observe the effects. It will be the nurse who must initiate emergency measures should adverse effects occur. This is an awesome responsibility.

If after reviewing the information in *Intravenous Medications,* you should have any questions about any order you are given or have conflict with a physician, clarify it with the physician, consult with the pharmacist, and consult with your supervisor. The circumstances will determine whom you approach first. If the physician feels it is imperative that an order be carried out even though you have unanswered questions or concerns, never hesitate to request that the physician administer the drug, drug combination, or dose himself or herself. The physician should be very willing to supply you, your supervisor, and the Pharmacy and Therapeutics Committee with current studies documenting the validity and appropriateness of orders.

All information presented is pertinent only to the intravenous use of the drug and not necessarily to intramuscular, subcutaneous, oral, or other means of administration. Before preparing any intravenous medication, check all labels carefully to confirm use as an intravenous injection.

At all times the patency of the vein must be determined to avoid extravasation into the surrounding tissue. Accidental arterial injection can cause gangrene and must be avoided.

Knowledgeable health professionals need more than dose and dilution; here is what you can expect from *Intravenous Medications:*

The generic name of the drug is in capital letters and boldface type.

Associated trade names are in parentheses under the generic name. Boldface type and alphabetical order enable you to verify correct drug names easily. The use of a Canadian maple leaf symbol (✹) preceding a trade name indicates trade names available in Canada only, as shown below.

BRETYLIUM TOSYLATE **pH 5 to 7**

(**✹Bretylate, Bretylol**)

In this example, Bretylate is the Canadian trade name. The pH is listed in the upper right-hand corner of the monograph. Information on drug pH is not consistently available; however, the pH is provided whenever possible.

It represents either the pH of the undiluted drug, the drug after the addition of diluents supplied by the manufacturer, or after initial dilution required for administration.

Usual dose: Doses recommended are the usual range for adults unless specifically stated otherwise. Doses calculated on body weight are usually based on pretreatment weight and not on edematous weight. Impaired renal function may increase the blood levels of circulating drugs, and dose reductions are frequently required.

Pediatric dose: Pediatric doses are specifically stated if they vary from mg/kg of body weight or M^2 dose recommended for adults. Not all drugs are recommended for use in children.

Dilution: All diluents and solutions mentioned must be suitable for intravenous use. Sterile technique is imperative in all phases of preparation. Specific directions for dilution are given for all drugs if dilution is necessary or permissible. Ensure adequate mixing of all drugs when added to a solution. Do not hang plastic containers in a series; this may cause an air embolism.

Rate of administration: Accepted rates of administration are clearly stated. As a general rule, slow is better. A 25-gauge needle aids in giving a small amount of medication over a stretch of time. Life-threatening reactions (time-related overdose or allergy) are frequently precipitated by a too-rapid rate of injection.

Actions: Clear, concise statements outline the origin of each drug, how it affects body systems, length of action, and method of excretion.

Indications and uses: Uses recommended by the manufacturer are listed. An experimental or research use is stated as such.

Precautions: The section on precautions includes the balance of information needed before injecting any drug. All necessary nursing considerations are listed here. Number 15 is as important as number 1.

Contraindications: All contraindications are those specifically listed by the manufacturer. Consultation with the physician is necessary if an ordered drug is contraindicated for your patient. The physician may have additional historical information that alters the situation or may decide that use of the drug is indicated in a critical situation.

Incompatible with: Incompatible drugs are alphabetized by generic name for ease in locating the drugs you are working with. Not all incompatibilities are absolute. They are intended to alert the nurse to a problem requiring consultation with a pharmacist or the physician. It may be that a specific order of mixing is required or that particular drugs are compatible only in a specific solution. The brand of intravenous fluids or additives, concentrations, containers, rate of mixing, pH, and temperature all affect solubility and compatibility. Knowledge is growing daily in this field. After receiving specific directions from the pharmacist on correctly mixing two drugs that have a compatibility problem, write the directions on the patient's medication record or nursing care plan so others will not have to retrace your research steps when the medication is to be given again.

Side effects: Alphabetical order simplifies your confirmation that a patient's symptom could be associated with specific drug use. Where there is a distinct line of tolerance for side effects, they are listed as minor or major and alphabetized after each of these subheadings. Reactions may be caused by a side effect of the drug itself, allergic response, or overdose. Allergic response and overdose are frequently related to the rate of injection.

Antidote: Specific antidotes are listed in this section. In addition, specific nursing actions to reverse undesirable side effects are clearly stated, an instant refresher course for critical situations.

Intravenous Medications is designed for use in critical care areas, at the nursing station, in the office, in the public health field, and by students and the armed services. Pertinent information can be found in a few seconds. Take advantage of its availability and quickly review every intravenous medication before administration.

My sincere appreciation is extended to Adrienne Nazareno for her thorough review of all new drugs, to Merrilee Newton and Linda Grant for their assistance with research, and to my husband Bill for his patience and assistance during the preparation of this manuscript.

Betty L. Gahart

INTRAVENOUS MEDICATIONS

a handbook for nurses and allied health professionals

ACETAZOLAMIDE SODIUM pH 9.2

(Diamox)

Usual dose: 5 mg/kg of body weight/24 hr, or 250 mg to 1 Gm/24 hr. Given in divided doses over 250 mg. Dose in epilepsy may range from 8 to 30 mg/kg of body weight/24 hr in divided doses.

Dilution: Each 500 mg should be diluted in 5 ml sterile water for injection. May then be given directly IV or added to standard IV fluids.

Rate of administration: 500 mg or fraction thereof over at least 1 minute or added to IV fluids to be given over 4 to 8 hours.

Actions: A potent carbonic anhydrase inhibitor and non-bacteriostatic sulfonamide, acetazolamide depresses the tubular reabsorption of sodium, potassium, and bicarbonate. Excreted unchanged in the urine, producing diuresis, alkalinization of the urine, and a mild degree of metabolic acidosis.

Indications and uses: (1) Glaucoma; (2) congestive heart failure; (3) intracranial pressure; (4) epilepsy (petit mal seizures); (5) acute mountain sickness; (6) drug-induced edema (e.g., steroids).

Investigational use: Treatment of paralysis of hypokalemia or hyperkalemia.

Precautions: (1) Chemically related to sulfonamides. (2) May be alternated with other diuretics to achieve maximum effect. (3) Greater diuretic action is achieved by skipping a day of treatment rather than increasing dose. (4) Direct IV administration is preferred. (5) Use with caution in severe respiratory acidosis. (6) Potassium excretion is proportional to diuresis. Hypokalemia may result from diuresis, severe cirrhosis, or concurrent use of steroids. Toxicity may occur with digitalis. (7) Use within 24 hours of dilution. (8) Potentiates amphetamines, ephedrine, procainamide, and quinidine. Inhibits lithium, methotrexate, phenobarbital, primidone, salicylates, tricyclic antidepressants, and urinary antiinfectives. (9) Salicylates may cause metabolic acidosis and salicylate toxicity.

Contraindications: Depressed sodium and potassium levels, first trimester of pregnancy, hyperchloremic acidosis, marked kidney or liver disease, sensitivity to sulfonamides, adrenocortical insufficiency.

Incompatible with: Specific information not available. Note precautions.

Side effects: Minimal with short-term therapy. Respond to symptomatic treatment or withdrawal of drug: acidosis, anorexia, bone marrow depression, confusion, crystalluria, drowsiness, fever, hemolytic anemia, paresthesias, photosensitivity, polyuria, rash, renal calculus, thrombocytopenic purpura.

Antidote: Notify physician of any adverse effects and discontinue drug if necessary. Treat allergic reactions as indicated.

ACYCLOVIR

pH 10.5 to 11.6

(Acycloguanosine, Zovirax)

Usual dose: *Mucosal and cutaneous HSV infections in immunocompromised patients:* 5 mg/kg of body weight every 8 hours for 7 days.

Severe initial clinical episodes of herpes genitalis: 5 mg/kg every 8 hours for 5 days.

Varicella zoster infections (shingles) in immunocompromised patients: 10 mg/kg every 8 hours for 7 days. Calculate dose by ideal body weight in obese individuals. Do not exceed 500 mg/M^2 every 8 hours.

Herpes simplex encephalitis: 10 mg/kg every 8 hours for 10 days.

Normal renal function required; reduce dose in impaired renal function based on creatinine clearance. Specific calculation required (see literature).

Pediatric dose: ***Children under 12 years of age:***

Mucosal and cutaneous HSV infections in immunocompromised patients: 250 mg/M^2 every 8 hours for 7 days.

Severe initial clinical episodes of herpes genitalis: 250 mg/M^2 every 8 hours for 5 days.

Varicella zoster infections (shingles) in immunocompromised patients: 500 mg/M^2 every 8 hours for 7 days. Do not exceed this dose.

Children over 6 months of age:

Herpes simplex encephalitis: 500 mg/M^2 every 8 hours for 10 days.

Normal renal function required (see comments in Usual dose).

Dilution: Initially dissolve each 500 mg vial with 10 ml sterile water for injection (50 mg/1 ml). Do not use bacteriostatic water containing parabens; will cause precipitation. Shake well to dissolve completely. Withdraw the desired dose and further dilute in an amount of solution to provide a concentration less than 7 mg/ml (70 kg adult at 5 mg/kg equals 350 mg dissolved in a total of 100 ml of solution equals 3.5 mg/ml). Compatible with most infusion solutions.

Rate of administration: A single dose must be administered at a constant rate over 1 hour as an infusion. Renal tubular damage will occur with too rapid rate of injection. Acyclovir crystals will occlude renal tubules. Use of an infusion pump or microdrip (60 gtt/ml) recommended.

Actions: An antiviral agent with in vitro inhibitory action against herpes simplex virus, varicella zoster virus, Epstein-Barr virus, and cytomegalovirus. Onset of action is prompt and therapeutic levels maintained for 8 hours. Widely distributed in tissues and body fluids. Excreted in the urine.

Indications and uses: (1) Treatment of initial and recurrent mucosal and cutaneous herpes simplex infections in immunosuppressed patients. (2) Severe initial clinical episodes of herpes genitalis in patients who are not immunocompromised. (3) Varicella zoster infections (shingles) in immunocompromised patients. (4) Herpes simplex encephalitis in patients over 6 months of age.

Unlabeled uses: Cytomegalovirus and HSV infection after bone marrow or renal transplantation; disseminated primary eczema herpeticum; varicella pneumonia; various herpes simplex infections (e.g., erythema multiforme, ocular, proctitis).

Precautions: (1) Confirm diagnosis of herpes simplex virus (HSV-1 or HSV-2) through laboratory culture. Initiate therapy as quickly as possible after symptoms identified. (2) Maintain adequate hydration and urine flow before and during infusion. (3) Use caution in patients with underlying neurological abnormalities, in patients receiving intrathecal methotrexate or interferon, or with patients who have had previous neurological reactions to cytotoxic drugs. (4) Use extreme caution in pregnancy and lactation. Adequate studies not available. (5) Caution patients to avoid sexual intercourse when visible herpes lesions are present. (6) May cause severe drowsiness and lethargy with zidovudine. (7) Side effects increased by other nephrotoxic drugs. (8) Potentiated by probenecid. (9) Confirm patency of vein; will cause thrombophlebitis. Rotate site of infusion. (10) Use reconstituted solution within 12 hours. Use solution fully diluted for administration within 24 hours.

Contraindications: Hypersensitivity to acyclovir or ganciclovir.

Incompatible with: Blood products, dobutamine (Dobutrex), dopamine (Intropin), protein solutions.

Side effects: Acute renal failure, agitation, coma, confusion, diaphoresis, hallucinations, headache, hematuria, hives, hypotension, lethargy, nausea, obtundation, phlebitis, rash, seizures, transient increased serum creatinine levels, tremors, vomiting. Some patients (fewer than 1%) may have abdominal pain, anemia, anorexia, anuria, chest pain, edema, fever, hemoglobinemia, hypokalemia, ischemia of digits, leukocytosis, lightheadedness, neutropenia, neutrophilia, pulmonary edema with cardiac tamponade, rigors, thirst, thrombocytosis, thrombocytopenia.

Antidote: Notify physician of all side effects. Discontinue drug with onset of CNS side effects. Treatment will be symptomatic and supportive. Removed by hemodialysis. Treat anaphylaxis and resuscitate as necessary.

ADENOSINE

(Adenocard, ATP)

Usual dose: 6 mg loading dose. If supraventricular tachycardia not eliminated in 1 to 2 minutes, give 12 mg. An additional 12 mg dose may be repeated once if required. Do not exceed the 12 mg dose.

Do not administer a repeat dose to patients who develop a high-level block on one dose of adenosine.

Metabolism of adenosine is independent of hepatic or renal function. No dose adjustment indicated.

Dilution: Give undiluted directly into a vein. If given into an IV line, use the closest port to the insertion site and follow with a rapid normal saline flush (± 50 ml) to be certain the solution reaches the systemic circulation.

Rate of administration: Must be given as a rapid bolus IV injection over 1 to 2 seconds.

Actions: A naturally occurring nucleoside present in all cells of the body. Has many functions, but use as an antiarrhythmic drug results from the ability to slow directly electrical conduction through the AV node of the heart. It interrupts the reentry circuit that perpetuates most cases of supraventricular tachycardia and reestablishes a normal sinus rhythm. Effective within 1 minute. Half-life is estimated to be less than 10 seconds. Adenosine is salvaged immediately by erythrocytes and blood vessel endothelial cells and metabolized for natural uses throughout the body (regulation of coronary and systemic vascular tone, platelet function, lipolysis in fat cells, intracardiac conduction).

Indications and uses: To convert acute paroxysmal supraventricular tachycardia (PSVT) to normal sinus rhythm. Includes PSVT associated with accessory bypass tracts (Wolff-Parkinson-White syndrome). Effective in up to 92% of patients.

Investigational uses: Studies of the use of adenosine as an adjuvant to treatment of brain tumors; in the prevention of myocardial reperfusion damage; and as a substitute for exercise stress testing in diagnosis of coronary artery disease are underway.

Precautions: (1) Absolutely confirm labeling for IV use. Do not use adenosine phosphate, which is for IM use in the symptomatic relief of varicose vein complications. (2) ECG monitoring during administration recommended. Monitor blood pressure. (3) At the time of conversion to normal sinus rhythm, PVCs, PACs, sinus bradycardia, sinus tachycardia, skipped beats, and varying degrees of atrioventricular nodal block are seen on the ECG in many patients. Usually last only a few seconds and resolve without intervention. (4) Adenosine is not blocked by atropine. Digitalis; quinidine; beta-adrenergic blocking agents (e.g., atenolol, esmolol); calcium channel blocking agents (verapamil [Isoptin]); angiotensin-converting enzyme inhibitors (e.g., enalapril [Vasotec]); and other cardiac drugs can be administered without delay if indicated because of the short half-life of adenosine. (5) Valsalva maneuver may be used before use of adenosine in PSVTs if clinically appropriate. (6) Emergency resuscitation drugs and equipment must always be available. (7) Effects antagonized by methylxanthines (e.g., caffeine, theophylline); larger doses may be required or adenosine may not be effective. (8) Potentiated by dipyridamole (Persantine); smaller doses of adenosine may be indicated. (9) May produce a higher degree of heart block with carbamazepine (Tegretol). (10) Has not to date, but could produce bronchoconstriction in patients with asthma. (11) Use in pregnancy only if clearly needed. (12) Controlled studies have not been conducted in pediatric patients, but preliminary trials indicate similar response rate and side effects. (13) Considered the emerging drug of choice by many investigators; others limit use to hemodynamically stable patients who do not require direct-current cardioversion but do require rapid conversion to a normal sinus rhythm; patients who have not responded to cumulative doses of verapamil, 10 mg IV, or those with congestive heart failure, concomitant beta blockade, hypotension, or left ventricular dysfunction when verapamil is relatively contraindicated. (14) Store at room temperature; refrigeration will cause crystallization. If crystals do form, dissolve by warming to room temperature. Solution must be clear; do not use if discolored or particulate matter present. Discard unused portion.

Contraindications: Atrial flutter or fibrillation and ventricular tachycardia (not effective in converting these dysrhythmias to normal sinus rhythm). Known hypersensitivity to adenosine, sick sinus syndrome, and second- or third-degree atrioventricular block unless a functioning artificial pacemaker is in place.

Incompatible with: Any other drug in syringe or solution due to pharmacologic actions and specific use.

Side effects: Generally predictable, short lived, and easily tolerated. Most will appear immediately and last less than 1 minute. Chest pressure, dizziness, dyspnea, facial flushing, headache, lightheadedness, nausea, PACs, PVCs, sinus bradycardia, sinus tachycardia, skipped beats, varying degrees of atrioventricular nodal block. Less than 1% of patients complain of apprehension, blurred vision, burning, chest pain, head pressure, heavy arms, hyperventilation, hypotension, metallic taste, neck and back pain, palpitations, tight throat, and tingling in arms.

Antidote: Notify physician of any side effect that lasts more than 1 minute. Treat symptomatically if indicated. Bradycardia may be refractory to atropine. Short half-life generally precludes overdose problems but caffeine and theophylline are competitive antagonists. Resuscitate as necessary.

ALPHA$_1$-PROTEINASE INHIBITOR (HUMAN) pH 6.6 to 7.4

(Alpha$_1$-PI, Prolastin)

Usual dose: 60 mg/kg once a week.

Dilution: Sterile water for injection supplied by manufacturer. Should yield approximately 20 mg/ml alpha$_1$-PI when reconstituted. Must be given within 3 hours of reconstitution.

Rate of administration: 0.08 ml/kg/minute is recommended. May be given at a faster rate. A 50 kg (110 lb) woman would receive 3,000 mg (150 ml reconstituted solution) over no more than 37 minutes (4 ml/min).

Actions: A sterile, stable, lyophilized preparation obtained from human plasma. Increases and maintains functional levels of alpha$_1$-PI in the epithelial lining of the lower respiratory tract. Provides adequate anti-elastase activity in the lungs of individuals with alpha$_1$-antitrypsin deficiency.

Indications and uses: Treatment of congenital alpha$_1$-antitrypsin deficiency, a potentially fatal disease. Used for chronic replacement only in individuals with clinically demonstrated panacinar emphysema.

Precautions: (1) Confirm diagnosis of congenital alpha$_1$-antitrypsin deficiency with clinically demonstrated panacinar emphysema. (2) Each unit of plasma tested and found nonreactive to HIV antibody and hepatitis B surface antigen. Transmission of these viruses is still possible. (3) Every patient should be immunized against hepatitis B before administration. If immediate treatment is required, give a single dose of hepatitis B immune globulin (human) at the same time as the initial dose of hepatitis B vaccine. (4) Blood levels of alpha$_1$-PI have been maintained above the functional level of 80 mg/dl with this replacement therapy. Serum levels determined by commercial immunologic assays may not reflect actual functional alpha$_1$-PI levels. (5) Store in refrigerator before reconstitution, at room temperature after reconstitution, and give within 3 hours. (6) Safety for use in children not yet established. (7) Use in pregnancy only when clearly needed. Potential hazard to fetus.

Contraindications: None known when used for the specific indication listed.

Incompatible with: Sufficient information not available. Do not mix with other drugs.

Side effects: Mild transient leukocytosis several hours after transfusion. Dizziness, fever, or lightheadedness may occur. Consider risk potential of contracting AIDS or hepatitis.

Antidote: All side effects except AIDS and hepatitis usually subside spontaneously. Keep the physician informed. Treat anaphylaxis (antihistamines, epinephrine, corticosteroids) and resuscitate as necessary.

ALPROSTADIL

(PGE$_1$, Prostaglandin E$_1$, Prostin VR Pediatric)

Usual dose: Begin with 0.05 to 0.1 mcg/kg of body weight/min. When therapeutic response is achieved, reduce infusion rate to lowest dose that maintains the response (0.1 mg to 0.05 to 0.025 to 0.01 mcg/min). If necessary, dose may be increased gradually to a maximum of 0.4 mcg/kg/min. Generally, these higher rates do not produce greater effects. May be given through infusion into a large vein or if necessary through an umbilical artery catheter placed at the ductal opening.

Dilution: Each 500 mcg must be further diluted with normal saline or dextrose for infusion. Various volumes may be used depending on infusion pump capabilities and desired infusion rate. 250 ml provides 2 mcg/ml. To deliver 0.1 mcg/kg/min requires an infusion rate of 0.05 ml/min/kg. 25 ml provides 20 mcg/ml and requires an infusion rate of 0.005 ml/min/kg to deliver the same dose.

Rate of administration: See Usual dose. Infusion pump capable of delivering 0.005, 0.01, 0.02, or 0.05 ml/min/kg required. Use for the shortest time possible at the lowest rate therapeutically effective.

Actions: A naturally occurring acidic lipid. Smooth muscle of the ductus arteriosus is susceptible to its relaxing effect, reducing blood pressure and peripheral resistance and increasing cardiac output and rate. Metabolized by oxidation almost instantly (80% in one pass through the lungs). Remainder excreted as metabolites in the urine.

Indications and uses: Temporarily maintain the patency of the ductus arteriosus until corrective or palliative surgery can be performed on infants with pulmonary atresia, pulmonary stenosis, tricuspid atresia, tetralogy of Fallot, interruption of the aortic arch, coarctation of the aorta, or transposition of the great vessels.

Investigational uses: To promote vasodilation in severe peripheral vascular disease; and to reduce ischemic damage in the treatment of acute myocardial infarction.

Precautions: (1) Usually administered by trained personnel in pediatric intensive care facilities. (2) Monitor respiratory status continuously. Ventilatory assistance must be immediately available. Will cause apnea, especially in infants under 2 kg. (3) Measure effectiveness with increase of Po_2 in infants with restricted pulmonary blood flow and increase of blood pressure and blood pH in infants with restricted systemic blood flow. (4) Monitor arterial pressure intermittently by umbilical artery catheter, auscultation, or Doppler transducer. Decrease rate of infusion stat if a significant fall in arterial pressure occurs. (5) Refrigerate until dilution. Prepare fresh solution for administration every 24 hours. (6) Response is poor in infants with Po_2 values of 40 mm Hg or more than 4 days old. More effective with lower Po_2. (7) Use caution in neonates with bleeding tendencies.

Contraindications: None known. Not indicated for respiratory distress syndrome (hyaline membrane disease).

Incompatible with: Specific information not available.

Side effects: Cardiac arrest, cerebral bleeding, cortical proliferation of long bones, diarrhea, DIC, hyperextension of the neck, hyperirritability, hypothermia, seizures, sepsis, tachycardia. Many other side effects have occurred in 1% or less of infants receiving alprostadil. *Overdose:* Apnea, bradycardia, flushing, hypotension, pyrexia.

Antidote: Notify physician of all side effects. Discontinue immediately if apnea or bradycardia occurs. Institute emergency measures. If infusion is restarted use extreme caution. Decrease rate if pyrexia or hypotension occurs. Flushing is usually caused by incorrect intraarterial catheter placement. Reposition.

ALTEPLASE, RECOMBINANT pH 7.3

(Activase, Tissue Plasminogen Activator, tPA)

Usual dose: *Acute myocardial infarction:* 100 mg titrated over 3 hours as an IV infusion. Give a bolus of 6 to 10 mg initially, followed by 50 to 54 mg (total 60 mg dose) over the first hour. Follow with 20 mg/hr for 2 hours. For patients under 65 kg calculate total dose using 1.25 mg/kg of body weight. Give three fifths of this total calculated dose divided as above into a bolus and first hour dose. Give one fifth of this total calculated dose/hr for 2 hours. Most effective administered within 4 to 6 hours of onset of symptoms of acute myocardial infarction.

Pulmonary embolism: 100 mg titrated over 2 hours as an IV infusion.

In all situations follow total dose with at least 30 ml of normal saline or 5% dextrose in water through the IV tubing to ensure administration of total dose.

A 150 mg dose has caused increased intracranial bleeding; do not use.

Dilution: Must be diluted with sterile water for injection without preservatives (provided by manufacturer). Use 20 ml for the 20 mg vial and 50 ml for the 50 mg vial (1 mg/ml). Use a large-bore (18-gauge) needle and direct the stream of diluent into the lyophilized cake. A vacuum must be present when the diluent is added to the powder for injection. Do not use if vacuum not present. Slight foaming is expected; let stand for several minutes to dissipate large bubbles. May be further diluted to 0.5 mg/ml immediately before administration with an equal volume of normal saline or 5% dextrose for injection. Mix by swirling or slow inversion; avoid agitation during dilution. Use balance (at least 30 ml) of 250 ml bottle of normal saline or 5% dextrose in water to clear tubing after infusion and assure delivery of total dose.

Connect normal saline or 5% dextrose in water to metriset and pump tubing. Clamp between solution and metriset. Add alteplase to metriset. Prime tubing with alteplase. Bolus dose can be given when indicated by direct IV through a med port or by IV pump. Administer balance of dose as outlined in usual dose section, adjusting pump rate of delivery as required. Complete by flushing tubing with IV solution.

Rate of administration: *Acute myocardial infarction:* Initial bolus dose evenly distributed over 2 minutes. Give balance of first hour dose evenly distributed over 1 hour. Each succeeding dose evenly distributed over 1 hour.

*Pulmonary embolism:*Total dose equally distributed over 2 hours.

In all situations use a metriset with microdrip (60 gtt/ml), or an infusion pump and IV tubing without a filter to facilitate accurate administration. Do not use any filters.

Distribute final flush over 30 minutes.

Actions: A tissue plasminogen activator and enzyme produced by recombinant DNA. It binds to fibrin in a thrombus and converts plasminogen to plasmin. Some conversion may take place in the absence of fibrin. The result is local fibrinolysis with limited systemic proteolysis. With therapeutic doses, a decrease in circulating fibrinogen makes the patient susceptible to bleeding. Onset of action is prompt, effecting patency of the vessel within 1 to 2 hours in most patients. Cleared from the plasma by the liver within 5 (50%) to 10 (80%) minutes after the infusion is discontinued. Some effects may linger for 45 minutes to several hours.

Indications and uses: (1) Management of acute myocardial infarction in adults for the lysis of thrombi obstructing coronary arteries, the improvement of ventricular function, and the reduction of the incidence of congestive heart failure. (2) Management of acute massive pulmonary embolism in adults for the lysis of acute pulmonary emboli either obstructing blood flow to a lobe or multiple segments of the lung or accompanied by unstable hemodynamics (e.g., failure to maintain blood pressure).

Unlabeled uses: Treatment of unstable angina pectoris and deep vein thrombosis.

Precautions: (1) Administered under the direction of a physician knowledgeable in its use and with appropriate diagnostic and laboratory facilities available. (2) Baseline ECG, CPK, and clotting studies (PT, PTT,

CBC, fibrinogen level, platelets) and baseline assessment (patient condition, pain, hematomas, petechiae, or recent wounds) should be completed before administration. Type and cross-match may also be ordered. (3) Monitor ECG continuously, and record strips with greatest ST segment elevation initially and every 15 minutes for at least 4 hours. A 12-lead ECG is indicated when therapy is complete. (4) Start IV if indicated (not previously established, other medications being administered through current IV, to have a line available for additional treatment). (5) Reperfusion arrhythmias occur frequently (e.g., sinus bradycardia, accelerated idioventricular rhythm, PVCs, ventricular tachycardia); have antiarrhythmic meds available at bedside. (6) A greater alteration of hemostatic status than with heparin, use extreme care with the patient, avoid any excessive or rough handling or pressure (including too frequent BPs), avoid invasive procedures (e.g., arterial puncture, venipuncture, IM injection). If these procedures are absolutely necessary, use extreme precautionary methods (use radial artery instead of femoral; small-gauge catheters and needles, and sites that are easily observed and compressible where bleeding can be controlled; avoid handling of catheter sites; and use extended pressure application of up to 30 minutes). Minor bleeding occurs often at catheter insertion sites. Avoid use of razors and toothbrushes. (7) In *myocaridal infarction* Simultaneous therapy with continuous infusion of heparin (without a loading dose) is frequently used to reduce the risk of rethrombosis. Markedly increases risk of bleeding. In *pulmonary emboli* begin heparin at end of infusion or immediately after it is complete. PT or PTT should be twice normal or less. (8) Monitor the patient carefully and frequently for anginal pain and signs of bleeding; observe catheter sites at least every 15 minutes; watch for hematuria, hematemesis, bloody stool, petechiae, hematoma, flank pain, muscle weakness; and do neuro checks every hour. Continue until normal clotting function returns. (9) Use caution with drugs that may alter platelet function (e.g., aspirin, dipyridamole (Persantin), indomethacin, phenylbutazone). Risk of bleeding will be increased if used concomitantly. (10) Use extreme caution in the following situations: major surgery, trauma, GI or GU bleeding, or puncture of noncompressible vessels (e.g., spinal puncture, thoracentesis), within the previous 10 days; cerebrovascular disease; hypertension (systolic above 180 or diastolic above 110); mitral stenosis with atrial fibrillation (likelihood of left heart thrombus); acute pericarditis; coagulation disorders, including those secondary to severe hepatic or renal disease; severe liver dysfunction; pregnancy and first 10 days postpartum; hemorrhagic ophthalmic conditions (e.g., diabetic hemorrhagic retinopathy); septic thrombophlebitis; patients on anticoagulants; patients over 75 years of age; any situation where bleeding might be hazardous or difficult to manage because of location. (11) Standard treatment for myocardial infarction continues simultaneously with alteplase therapy except if temporarily contraindicated (arterial blood gases, etc., unless absolutely necessary). (12) Coagulation tests will be unreliable; specific procedures can be used; notify the lab of alteplase use. (13) Safety for use in children not established. (14) Refrigerate before dilution. Discard unused solution.

Contraindications: Active internal bleeding, arteriovenous malformation or aneurysm, bleeding diathesis, cerebral vascular accident, intracranial or intraspinal surgery or trauma within 2 months, intracranial neoplasm, severe uncontrolled hypertension, subacute bacterial endocarditis.

Incompatible with: Manufacturer states "do not add other medications to infusion solution."

Side effects: Bleeding is most common: internal (GI tract, GU tract, retroperitoneal, or intracranial sites), epistaxis, gingival, and superficial or surface bleeding (venous cutdowns, arterial punctures, sites of recent surgical intervention). Mild allergic reactions (urticaria) have occurred. Fever, hypotension, nausea, and vomiting have occurred but may be due to the myocardial infarction itself.

Antidote: Notify physician of all side effects. Note even the minutest bleeding tendency. Oozing at IV sites is expected. Control minor bleeding by local pressure. For severe bleeding in a critical location discontinue alteplase and any heparin therapy immediately. Whole blood, packed red blood cells, cryoprecipitate, fresh-frozen plasma, and aminocaproic acid may all be indicated. Treat reperfusion arrhythmias with specific appropriate protocols (e.g., bradycardia with atropine, ventricular tachycardia with lidocaine). Treat minor allergic reactions symptomatically. Discontinue drug and treat anaphylaxis as indicated; resuscitate as necessary.

AMIKACIN SULFATE pH 4.5

(Amikin)

Usual dose: Up to 15 mg/kg of body weight/24 hr equally divided into 2 or 3 doses at equally divided intervals. Dosage based on ideal weight of lean body mass. Do not exceed a total adult dose of 15 mg/kg/24 hr in average weight patient or 1.5 Gm in heavier patients by all routes in 24 hours. Normal renal function necessary.

Newborn dose: 10 mg/kg of body weight as a loading dose, then 7.5 mg/kg every 12 hours. Lower doses may be appropriate because of immature kidney function.

Dilution: Each 500 mg or fraction thereof must be diluted with 100 to 200 ml IV 5% dextrose in water, 5% dextrose in normal saline, or normal saline. Amount of diluent may be decreased proportionately with dosage for children and infants.

Rate of administration: A single dose over at least 30 to 60 minutes. Infants should receive a 1- to 2-hour infusion.

Actions: An aminoglycoside antibiotic with neuromuscular blocking action. Bactericidal against many gram-negative organisms resistant to other antibiotics including other aminoglycosides such as gentamicin (Garamycin), kanamycin (Kantrex), and tobramycin (Nebcin). Well distributed through all body fluids. Usual half-life is 2 to 3 hours. Half-life is prolonged in infants, postpartum females, fever, liver disease and ascites, spinal cord injury, cystic fibrosis, and the elderly; shorter in severe burns. Crosses the placental barrier.

Excreted in the kidneys. Cross-allergenicity does occur between aminoglycosides.

Indications and uses: Short-term treatment of serious infections caused by susceptible organisms resistant to alternate drugs that have less potential toxicity.

Precautions: (1) Use extreme caution if therapy is required over 7 to 10 days. (2) Sensitivity studies indicated to determine susceptibility of causative organism to amikacin. (3) Reduce daily dose commensurate with amount of renal impairment. Increase intervals between injections. (4) Maintain good hydration. (5) Narrow range between toxic and therapeutic levels. Monitor peak and trough concentrations to avoid peak serum concentrations above 35 mcg/ml and trough concentrations above 5 mcg/ml. Therapeutic level is between 8 and 16 mcg/ml. (6) Watch for decrease in urine output, rising BUN and serum creatinine, and declining creatinine clearance levels. Dosage may require decreasing. Routine serum levels and evaluations of hearing are recommended. (7) Response should occur in 24 to 48 hours. (8) Use during pregnancy and lactation only when absolutely necessary. (9) Concurrent use topically or systemically with any other ototoxic or nephrotoxic agents should be avoided. May have dangerous additive effects with anesthetics, other neuromuscular blocking antibiotics (e.g., kanamycin, streptomycin), diuretics (e.g., furosemide [Lasix]), cephalosporins, vancomycin, and many others. All aminoglycosides are also potentiated by anticholinesterases (e.g., edrophonium), antineoplastics (e.g., nitrogen mustard, cisplatin), barbiturates, muscle relaxants (e.g., tubocurarine), phenothiazines (e.g., promethazine [Phenergan]), procainamide, quinidine, and sodium citrate (citrate-anticoagulated blood). *Apnea can occur.* (10) Superinfection may occur from overgrowth of nonsusceptible organisms. (11) Synergistic when used in combination with penicillins and cephalosporins. Dose adjustment and appropriate spacing required due to physical incompatibilities and interactions.

Contraindications: Known amikacin or aminoglycoside sensitivity.

Incompatible with: Administer separately as recommended by manufacturer. Note precautions. Amphotericin B, cephalothin (Keflin), chlorothiazide (Diuril), heparin, phenytoin (Dilantin), thiopental (Pentothal), vitamin B complex with C, warfarin (Coumadin). Inactivated by carbenicillin, ticarcillin, and other penicillins.

Side effects: Occur more frequently with impaired renal function, higher doses, or prolonged administration.

Minor: Fever, headache, hypotension, nausea, paresthesias, skin rash, tremor, vomiting.

Major: Albuminuria, anemia, arthralgia, azotemia, neuromuscular blockade, oliguria, ototoxicity, respiratory arrest.

Antidote: Notify physician of all side effects. If minor side effects persist or any major symptom appears, discontinue drug and notify the physician. Treatment is symptomatic, or a reduction in dose may be required. In overdose, hemodialysis may be indicated. Complexation with ticarcillin or carbenicillin may be as effective as hemodialysis. Consider exchange transfusion in the newborn. Calcium salts or neostigmine may reverse neuromuscular blockade. Resuscitate as necessary.

AMINOCAPROIC ACID — pH 6.8

(Amicar)

Usual dose: 5 Gm initially. Follow with 1 to 1.25 Gm/hr for 6 to 8 hours. Maximum dose is 30 Gm/24 hr.

Prevent recurrence of subarachnoid hemorrhage: 36 Gm/24 hr equally divided into 6 doses.

Reduce need for platelet transfusion in management of amegakaryocytic thrombocytopenia: 8 to 24 Gm/24 hr for 3 days to 13 months.

Dilution: 1 Gm equals 4 ml of prepared solution. Further dilute with compatible infusion solutions (normal saline, dextrose in saline or distilled water, or Ringer's solution). 50 ml of diluent may be used for each 1 Gm.

Rate of administration: 5 Gm or fraction thereof over first hour in 250 ml of solution, then administer each succeeding 1 Gm over 1 hour in 50 to 100 ml of solution.

Actions: A monaminocarboxylic acid with the specific action of inhibiting plasminogen activator substances; to a lesser degree inhibits plasmin activity. Increases fibrinogen activity in clot formation by inhibiting the enzyme required for destruction of formed fibrin. Onset of action is prompt, but will last less than 3 hours. Readily excreted in the urine. Easily penetrates red blood cells and tissue cells after prolonged administration.

Indications and uses: (1) Hemorrhage caused by overactivity of the fibrinolytic system; (2) systemic hyperfibrinolysis (pathological), which may result from heart surgery, portacaval shunt, aplastic anemia, abruptio placentae, hepatic cirrhosis, or carcinoma of the prostate, lung, stomach, and cervix; (3) urinary fibrinolysis (normal physiological phenomenon), which may result from severe trauma, anoxia, shock, surgery on the genitourinary system, or carcinoma of the genitourinary system.

Investigational uses: To prevent recurrence of subarachnoid hemorrhage; and to reduce need for platelet transfusions in management of amegakaryocytic thrombocytopenia.

Precautions: (1) Use extreme care in cardiac, hepatic, or renal diseases. Endocardial hemorrhage, myocardial fat degeneration, teratogenicity, and kidney stones have resulted in animals. (2) Use only in conjunction with general and specific tests to determine the amount of fibrinolysis present. (3) Rapid administration or insufficient dilution may cause hypotension, bradycardia, and/or dysrhythmia. (4) Whole blood transfusions may be given if necessary. (5) Large doses in the presence of anticoagulants may induce incoagulability. (6) Safety for use in pregnancy not established.

Contraindications: Disseminated intravascular coagulation, evidence of thrombosis, first and second trimester of pregnancy.

Incompatible with: Sodium lactate.

Side effects: Cramps, diarrhea, dizziness, headache, grand mal seizure, malaise, nausea, skin rash, stuffy nose, tearing, thrombophlebitis, tinnitus.

Antidote: Treat side effects symptomatically. Discontinue use of drug if any suspicion of thrombophlebitis.

AMMONIUM CHLORIDE pH 4.5 to 6.0

Usual dose: Dependent on patient condition and tolerance. Monitor serum bicarbonate repeatedly to determine individualized dosage. Begin with contents of 1 or 2 vials (100 to 200 mEq). Use minimal effective dose initially. Maximum effect of a single dose not fully apparent for several days.

26.75% solution: contains 5 mEq NH_4 and 5 mEq Cl/ml.

Dilution: Each 100 mEq (20 ml) of 26.75% solution must be diluted with 500 ml normal saline for infusion to achieve the desired 1% to 2% solution. Potassium chloride, 20 to 40 mEq/L, may be added to the ammonium infusion (serum potassium usually low). For infants dilute each 1 ml of ammonium chloride in a minimum of 5 to 10 ml diluent.

Rate of administration: Up to 5 ml diluted solution/min for adults. Reduce rate significantly for infants.

Actions: Acidifying agent. Ammonium chloride dissociates into an ammonium cation and a chloride anion. Ammonium ions are converted to urea by the liver, freeing hydrogen ions and chloride ions. Hydrogen ion reacts with bicarbonate to form water and carbon dioxide (excreted by the lungs). Chloride ion combines with fixed bases (mostly sodium) to produce diuresis. Combined process reduces the alkaline reserve of the body. A compensatory action occurs within the body to halt this process within 3 days.

Indications and uses: Treatment of hypochloremic states and metabolic alkalosis, which may be due to chloride loss from vomiting (including vomiting due to pyloric stenosis in infants); gastric fistula drainage; gastric suction; or excessive alkalinizing medication to prevent tetany or renal damage due to persistent severe alkalemia.

Precautions: (1) Accurate blood chemistry data required before, during, and after therapy to avoid serious metabolic acidosis and deficiencies. Replacement of sodium or potassium ions may be required. (2) Observe respirations closely (increased ventilation at rest and exertional dyspnea indicate acidosis). Record intake and output. (3) Use caution in impaired renal function, pulmonary insufficiency, or cardiac edema. (4) Inhibits or potentiates many drugs as an acidifying agent. (5) Slow infusion rate for pain along venipuncture site. (6) If crystals form, warm in a water bath to room temperature before administration. (7) Safety for use during pregnancy not established; use only if clearly needed.

Contraindications: Severe hepatic impairment, sodium loss resulting in excretion of sodium bicarbonate in the urine in a patient with renal dysfunction, primary respiratory acidosis with high total CO_2 and buffer base.

Incompatible with: Chlortetracycline (Aureomycin), codeine, dimenhydrinate (Dramamine), levorphanol (Levo-Dromoran), methadone hydrochloride, warfarin (Coumadin). All alkalis.

Side effects: Most side effects are caused by ammonia toxicity. Bradycardia, calcium-deficient tetany, coma, depression, disorientation, EEG abnormalities, excitability, glycosuria, headache, hyperglycemia, hypokalemia, increased rate and depth of breathing (Kussmaul), irregular respiration, metabolic acidosis, nausea, pallor, skin rash, stupor, twitching, vomiting, weakness.

Antidote: For all side effects reduce rate of administration or discontinue drug and notify the physician. Treat hypokalemia with potassium and tetany with calcium. Sodium lactate or sodium bicarbonate IV may be used to treat acidosis. Resuscitate as necessary.

AMOBARBITAL SODIUM **pH 9.6 to 10.4**

(Amytal sodium)

Usual dose: 65 to 500 mg (gr 1 to 7½). 1 Gm (gr 15) is the maximum single adult dose.

Pediatric dose: *Children over 6 years:* 65 mg (gr 1) to 250 mg (gr 3¾); 500 mg (gr 7½) is the maximum dose.
Convulsions: 5 to 8 mg/kg of body weight is usually required.

Dilution: Each 125 mg (gr 2) must be diluted with a minimum of 1.25 ml of sterile water for injection to make a 10% solution. Inject diluent slowly and rotate vial to dissolve powder. Do not shake.

Rate of administration: Each 100 mg or fraction thereof over 1 minute for adults and 60 mg/min for children. Titrate slowly to desired effect. Do not exceed 1 ml of a 10% solution/min.

Actions: A sedative, hypnotic barbiturate of intermediate duration with anticonvulsant effects. Amobarbital is a CNS depressant. Onset of action is prompt by the IV route and lasts about 4 to 6 hours. Pain perception is unimpaired. Rapidly absorbed by all body tissues and excreted fairly quickly in changed form in the urine. Crosses the placental barrier. Secreted in breast milk.

Indications and uses: (1) Control of convulsive seizures due to disease, eclampsia, psychiatric management, and drug poisoning; (2) sedation; (3) narcoanalysis and narcotherapy.

Precautions: (1) IV route for emergency use only. Use of large veins preferred to prevent thrombosis. Intraarterial injection causes gangrene. (2) Hydrolyzes in dry or solution form when exposed to air. Use only absolutely clear solutions and discard powder or solution that has been exposed to air for 30 minutes. (3) Use only enough medication to achieve desired effect. Rapid injection may cause symptoms of overdose. (4) Record blood pressure, pulse, and respiration every 3 to 5 minutes. Keep patient under constant observation. (5) Keep equipment for artificial ventilation available. Maintain a patent airway. (6) Treat the cause of a convulsion. (7) Use caution in asthma, cardiovascular diseases, hypertension, hypotension, pulmonary diseases, depressive states after convulsions, shock, uremia, and in the elderly. (8) May be habit forming. Status epilepticus can occur from too rapid withdrawal. (9) Use with extreme caution if any other CNS depressants have been given, such as alcohol, narcotic analgesics, anesthetics, antidepressants, antihistamines, hypnotics, MAO inhibitors, phenothiazines, sedatives, neuromuscular blocking antibiotics, and tranquilizers. Potentiation with respiratory depression may occur. (10) Inhibits corticosteroids, doxycycline (Vibramycin), griseofulvin, oral anticoagulants, oral contraceptives, quinidine, theophylline, and β-adrenergic blockers (e.g., propranolol [Inderal]). Capable of innumerable interactions with many drugs. (11) May increase orthostatic hypotension with furosemide (Lasix). (12) Monitor phenytoin and barbiturate levels when both drugs are used concurrently. (13) Will cause birth defects; use in pregnancy is not recommended. (14) May cause paradoxical excitement in children or the elderly.

Contraindications: History of porphyria, impaired liver function, known hypersensitivity to barbiturates, severe respiratory depression.

Incompatible with: Cefazolin (Kefzol), cephalothin (Keflin), chlorpromazine (Thorazine), cimetidine (Tagamet), clindamycin (Cleocin), codeine, dimenhydrinate (Dramamine), diphenhydramine (Benadryl), droperidol (Inapsine), hydrocortisone sodium succinate (Solu-Cortef), hydroxyzine (Vistaril), insulin (aqueous), levarterenol (Levophed), levorphanol (Levo-Dromoran), meperidine (Demerol), methadone, morphine, pentazocine (Talwin), penicillin G potassium, phytonadione (Aquamephyton), procaine, prochlorperazine (Compazine), streptomycin, tetracycline (Achromycin), thiamine (Betalin S), trifluoperazine (Stelazine), vancomycin (Vancocin).

Side effects: *Average dose:* Asthma, bronchospasm, depression, dermatitis, facial edema, fever, hypotension, neonatal apnea, respiratory depression (slight), thrombocytopenic purpura.

Overdose: Apnea, coma, cough reflex depression, flat EEG (reversible unless hypoxic damage has occurred), hypotension, hypothermia, laryngospasm, pulmonary edema, reflexes (sluggish or absent), renal shutdown, respiratory depression.

Antidote: Notify the physician of any side effect. Symptomatic and supportive treatment is most important in overdose. Maintain an adequate airway with artificial ventilation if indicated. Keep the patient warm. IV volume expanders (dextran) and other IV fluids will help maintain adequate circulation. Osmotic diuretics (mannitol) or hemodialysis will promote elimination of the drug. Vasopressors (e.g., dopamine [Intropin]) will maintain blood pressure.

AMPHOTERICIN B pH 5.7 to 8.0

(Fungizone)

Usual dose: Begin with a test dose of 1 mg in 20 ml 5% dextrose. Infuse over 10 to 30 minutes. Determine size of therapeutic dose by intensity of reaction over a 4-hour period. Usual is 0.25 mg/kg of body weight/24 hr, gradually increased to 1 mg/kg/24 hr as tolerance permits. Up to 1.5 mg/kg/24 hr may be given on alternate-day therapy. Several months of therapy are usually required and recommended for cure. Dosage must be adjusted to each specific patient. In some instances higher doses can be used.

Dilution: A 50 mg vial is initially diluted with 10 ml of distilled water for injection (without a bacteriostatic agent); 5 mg equals 1 ml. Shake well until solution is clear. Further dilute each 1 mg in at least 10 ml of 5% dextrose in water for injection. Dextrose must have a pH above 4.2. Do not use any other diluent. Do not wipe vials with alcohol sponges. Use a sterile 20-gauge or larger needle at each step of the dilution. Maintain aseptic technique. Larger pore 1 micron filters may be used.

Rate of administration: Daily dose over 6 hours by slow IV infusion. Concentration of solution must not be greater than 0.1 mg/ml.

Actions: Antifungal antibiotic agent. It injures the membrane of the fungi. Not effective against other organisms. Remains in the body at a therapeutic level up to 20 hours after each infusion. Excreted very slowly in the urine.

Indications and uses: Treatment of fungal infections that are progressive in nature and potentially fatal, such as cryptococcosis, blastomycosis, and disseminated forms of candidiasis, coccidioidomycosis, and histoplasmosis, mucormycosis, sporotrichosis, and aspergillosis. These infections must be caused by specific organisms. Diagnosis must be positively established by culture or histological study.

Precautions: (1) Use only fresh solutions without evidence of precipitate or foreign matter. (2) Light sensitive but protection from light not required unless solution exposed over 8 hours. (3) Preserve concentrate in refrigerator up to 7 days. (4) Should be used only on hospitalized patients. (5) Monitor vital signs and intake and output. (6) Use caution in concomitant use of corticosteroids (unless required for drug reaction), nephrotoxic antibiotics, and antineoplastic agents (e.g., nitrogen mustard). (7) Potentiates antifungal effects of flucytosine and other antibiotics. May increase toxicity. (8) Synergistic with rifampin or tetracycline. (9) During therapy, frequent renal and liver function tests, blood counts, and electrolyte panels are necessary. (10) Mannitol 12.5 Gm immediately before and after each dose of amphotericin B may reduce nephrotoxic effects. (11) A small amount of heparin added to the infusion may reduce the incidence of thrombophlebitis. (12) Whenever medicine is not given for 7 days or longer, restart treatment at lowest dosage level. (13) Hydrocortisone 0.7 mg/kg of body weight added to the infusion may prevent chills; corticosteroids not recommended for concomitant use in other situations. (14) May potentiate digitalis and skeletal muscle relaxants (e.g., succinylcholine [Anectine], diazepam [Valium]). (15) Use extreme caution with other nephrotoxic antibiotics (e.g., gentamicin [Garamycin]) and antineoplastics (e.g., nitrogen mustard).

Contraindications: Known amphotericin B sensitivity and pregnancy, unless a life-threatening situation is present.

Incompatible with: Do not mix with any drug unless absolutely necessary. Amikacin (Amikin); calcium chloride; calcium gluconate; calcium disodium edetate; carbenicillin (Geopen); chlorpromazine (Thorazine); chlortetracycline (Aureomycin); cimetidine (Tagamet); diphenhydramine (Benadryl); dopamine (Intropin); gentamicin (Garamycin); heparin; kanamycin (Kantrex); electrolyte solutions; metaraminol (Aramine); normal saline; penicillin G, potassium, or sodium; polymyxin B (Aero-sporin); potassium chloride; preservatives such as benzyl alcohol; prochlorperazine (Compazine); ranitidine (Zantac); saline solutions; tetracycline (Achromycin); vitamin B with C. Not compatible in any solution with a pH below 4.2.

Side effects: Common even at doses below therapeutic levels: anorexia, chills, convulsions, diarrhea, fever, headache, phlebitis, vomiting. Anaphylactoid reactions, anemia, cardiac disturbances (including fibrillation and arrest), coagulation defects, hypertension, hypokalemia, hypotension, and numerous other side effects occur fairly frequently. Renal function impaired in 80% of patients. May reverse after treatment ends.

Antidote: Notify the physician of all side effects. Many are reversible if the drug is discontinued. Some will respond to symptomatic treatment. Administration of this drug on alternate days may decrease the incidence of some side effects. Urinary alkalinizers may minimize renal tubular acidosis. Reduce dose or discontinue drug if BUN above 40 mg/100 ml or serum creatinine above 3 mg/100 ml. Treat allergic reactions and resuscitate as necessary.

AMPICILLIN SODIUM — pH 8.5 to 10

(✤ Ampicin, ✤ Ampilean, Omnipen-N, ✤ Penbritin, Polycillin N, Totacillin-N)

Usual dose: 1 to 12 Gm/24 hr in equally divided doses every 6 hours. Increase interval to 12 hours in severe renal impairment.

Pediatric dose: 50 to 200 mg/kg of body weight/24 hr in equally divided doses at 6- to 8-hour intervals. Do not exceed adult dose.

Neonatal dose: *Over 2,000 Gm; age up to 7 days:* 75 mg/kg of body weight/24 hr in divided doses every 8 hours. 150 mg/kg/24 hr for meningitis. *Over 7 days of age:* 100 mg/kg/24 hr in divided doses every 6 hours. 200 mg/kg/24 hr for meningitis.

Under 2,000 Gm; age up to 7 days: 50 mg/kg/24 hr in divided doses every 12 hours. 100 mg/kg/24 hr for meningitis. *Over 7 days of age:* 75 mg/kg/24 hr in divided doses every 8 hours. 150 mg/kg/24 hr for meningitis.

Dilution: Each 500 mg or fraction thereof must be diluted with at least 5 ml of sterile water for injection. If necessary, this may be further diluted in 50 ml or more of one of the following solutions and given as an IV infusion over not more than 4 hours: 5% dextrose in water, 5% dextrose in 0.45 sodium chloride solution, 10% invert sugar in water, and 1/6 sodium lactate solution. In isotonic sodium chloride, potency is maintained over 8 hours. After initial dilution, may also be added to the last 100 ml of a compatible IV solution.

Rate of administration: A single dose over 10 to 15 minutes when given direct IV. In 100 ml or more of solution, administer at prescribed infusion rate but never exceed direct IV rate. Too rapid injection may cause seizures.

Actions: A semisynthetic penicillin. Bactericidal against many gram-positive and some gram-negative organisms. Appears in all body fluids. Appears in cerebrospinal fluid only if inflammation is present. Crosses the placental barrier. Excreted in the urine. Secreted in breast milk.

Indications and uses: Highly effective against severe infections caused by gram-positive and some gram-negative organisms, except penicillinase-producing staphylococci.

Precautions: (1) Sensitivity studies indicated to determine susceptibility of the causative organism to ampicillin. (2) Individuals with a history of allergic problems are more susceptible to untoward reactions. Watch for early symptoms of allergic reaction. (3) Avoid prolonged use of this drug; superinfection caused by overgrowth of nonsusceptible organisms may result. (4) Use within 1 hour of reconstitution unless diluted in aforementioned solutions. (5) Streptomycin potentiates bactericidal activity against enterococci. (6) SGOT may be increased. Renal, hepatic, and hematopoietic function should be checked during prolonged therapy. (7) May be used concurrently with aminoglycosides (e.g., gentamicin [Garamycin]) but must be administered in separate infusions; inactivates aminoglycosides. (8) Inactivated by chloramphenicol, erythromycin, and tetracyclines. Bactericidal action is actually negated by these drugs. (9) Concomitant use with β-adrenergic blockers (e.g., propranolol [Inderal]) may increase risk of anaphylaxis and inhibit treatment. (10) False positive glucose reaction with Clinitest and Benedict's or Fehling's solution. (11) Potentiated by probenecid (Benemid); toxicity may result. (12) May potentiate heparin. (13) Neuromuscular excitability or convulsions may be caused by higher than normal doses. (14) Elimination rate markedly reduced in neonates. (15) Decreases effectiveness of oral contraceptives; breakthrough bleeding or pregnancy could result.

Contraindications: Known penicillin or cephalothin sensitivity. Infectious mononucleosis because of increased incidence of rash.

Incompatible with: Do not use as an additive with any other drug. Do not mix in any solutions other than those specifically recommended. Some drugs may be administered through the Y-tubing in small amounts. Consult with the pharmacist.

Side effects: Primarily hypersensitivity reactions such as anaphylaxis, exfoliative dermatitis, rashes, and urticaria. Anemia, leukopenia, and thrombocytopenia have been reported. Thrombophlebitis will occur with long-term use. Incidence of side effects increased in patients with viral infections or those taking allopurinol (Zyloprim).

Antidote: Notify the physician of any side effect. For severe symptoms, discontinue the drug, treat allergic reaction (antihistamines, epinephrine, corticosteroids), and resuscitate as necessary. Hemodialysis or peritoneal dialysis is effective in overdose.

AMPICILLIN SODIUM AND SULBACTAM SODIUM — pH 8.0 to 10.0

(Unasyn)

Usual dose: 1.5 Gm (1 Gm ampicillin plus 0.5 Gm sulbactam) to 3 Gm (2 Gm ampicillin plus 1 Gm sulbactam) every 6 hours. Do not exceed 4 Gm sulbactam/24 hr. Normal renal function required.

Dilution: Each 1.5 Gm or fraction thereof must be initially diluted with at least 4 ml of sterile water for injection (375 mg/ml). Allow to stand to dissipate foaming. Solution should be clear. Must be further diluted in 50 ml or more of one of the following solutions and given as an intermittent IV infusion: dextrose in water, 5% dextrose in 0.45 sodium chloride solution, 10% invert sugar in water, lactated Ringer's injection, ⅙ sodium lactate solution, and isotonic sodium chloride. Desired concentration for administration is 3 mg/ml to 45 mg/ml. 3 Gm/L equals 3 mg/ml, 3 Gm/125 ml equals 24 mg/ml. Also available in piggyback vials.

Rate of administration: A single dose over 15 to 30 minutes or longer depending on amount of solution. Too rapid injection may cause seizures.

Actions: A semisynthetic penicillin. The addition of sulbactam improves ampicillin's bactericidal activity against β-lactamase–producing strains resistant to penicillins and cephalosporins. A broad-spectrum antibiotic and β-lactamase inhibitor effective against selected gram-positive, gram-negative, and anaerobic organisms (see literature). Appears in all body fluids. Crosses the placental barrier. Excreted in the urine. Secreted in breast milk.

Indications and uses: Treatment of skin and skin structure, intraabdominal and gynecologic infections due to susceptible strains of specific organisms.

Precautions: (1) Studies indicated to determine the causative organism and susceptibility to ampicillin/sulbactam. (2) Individuals with a history of allergic problems are more susceptible to untoward reactions. Watch for early symptoms of allergic reaction. (3) Avoid prolonged use of this drug; superinfection caused by overgrowth of nonsusceptible organisms may result. (4) Stable in all specifically listed solutions in any dilution for at least 2 hours. Stability in each solution varies (see literature). (5) Streptomycin potentiates bactericidal activity against enterococci. (6) SGOT may be increased. Renal, hepatic, and hematopoietic function should be checked during prolonged therapy. (7) May be used concurrently with aminoglycosides (e.g., gentamicin [Garamycin]) but must be administered in separate infusions; inactivates aminoglycosides. (8) Inactivated by chloramphenicol, erythromycin, and tetracyclines. Bactericidal action can be negated by these drugs. (9) Concomitant use with β-adrenergic blockers (e.g., propranolol [Inderal]) may increase risk of anaphylaxis and inhibit treatment. (10) False positive glucose reaction with Clinitest and Benedict's or Fehling's solution. (11) Potentiated by probenecid (Benemid); higher blood levels may be a positive interaction. (12) May potentiate heparin. (13) Neuromuscular excitability or convulsions may be caused by higher than normal doses. (14) Safety for use in infants and children not established. Elimination rate markedly reduced in neonates. (15) This combination is indicated only in specific infections; however, mixed infections caused by ampicillin-susceptible organisms should not require an additional antibiotic. (16) May cause thrombophlebitis. Observe carefully and rotate infusion sites.

Contraindications: Known penicillin or cephalothin sensitivity.

Incompatible with: Do not use as an additive with any other drug. Do not mix in any solutions other than those specifically recommended. Some drugs may be administered through the Y-tubing in small amounts. Consult with the pharmacist.

Side effects: Full scope of allergic reactions including anaphylaxis are possible. Burning, discomfort, and pain at injection site; diarrhea; rash; and thrombophlebitis occur most frequently. Abdominal distention; candidiasis; chest pain; chills; decreased hemoglobin, hematocrit, RBC, WBC, lymphocytes, neutrophils, and platelets; decreased serum albumin and total protein; dysuria; edema; epistaxis; erythema; facial swelling; fatigue; flatulence; glossitis; headache; increased alkaline phosphatase, BUN, creatinine, LDH, SGOT, SGPT; increased basophils, eosinophils, lymphocytes, monocytes and platelets; itching; malaise; mucosal bleeding; nausea and vomiting; RBCs and hyaline casts in urine; substernal pain; tightness in throat; and urine retention can occur.

Antidote: Notify the physician of any side effect. For severe symptoms, discontinue the drug, treat allergic reaction (antihistamines, epinephrine, corticosteroids), resuscitate as necessary. Hemodialysis or peritoneal dialysis may be effective in overdose.

AMRINONE LACTATE pH 3.2 to 4.0

(Inocor)

Usual dose: 0.75 mg/kg of body weight as the initial dose (52.5 mg [10.5 ml] for a 70 kg person). Follow with a maintenance infusion of 5 to 10 mcg/kg/min (350 to 700 mcg/min for a 70 kg person). The initial dose (0.75 mg/kg) may be repeated once in 30 minutes if indicated. Do not exceed a total dose of 10 mg/kg/24 hr including boluses.

Dilution: May be given undiluted, or each 5 mg (1 ml) may be diluted in 1 ml normal saline or 0.45% saline for injection. For infusion dilute 250 mg (50 ml) in 50 ml normal saline or 0.45% saline (2.5 mg/ml). 1 ml will deliver 2,500 mcg/min. May be given through Y-tube or three-way stopcock of IV infusion set. Use diluted solution within 24 hours.

Rate of administration: *Bolus dose:* A single dose over 2 to 3 minutes.

Infusion: Using a microdrip (60 gtt/ml) or an infusion pump deliver amrinone in recommended doses. Manufacturer supplies an individualized dosage chart defining selected dose in mcg/min/body weight in ml/hr. Adjust as indicated by physician's orders and progress in patient's condition.

Actions: A new class of cardiac inotropic agent different in chemical structure and mode of action from digitalis glycosides and catecholamines. With a bolus dose, peak effect occurs within 10 minutes. Continuous administration is required to maintain serum levels. It has positive inotropic action with vasodilator activity. Reduces afterload and preload by direct relaxant effect on vascular smooth muscle. Cardiac output is increased without measurable increase in myocardial oxygen consumption or changes in arteriovenous oxygen difference. Pulmonary capillary wedge pressure, total peripheral resistance, diastolic blood pressure, and mean arterial pressure are decreased. Heart rate generally remains the same. Metabolized by conjugated pathways, it is primarily excreted in the urine.

Indications and uses: Short-term management of congestive heart failure in patients who have not responded adequately to digitalis, diuretics, or vasodilators.

Precautions: (1) Observe patient continuously; monitoring of ECG, cardiac index, pulmonary capillary wedge pressure, central venous pressure, and plasma concentration are recommended. Also monitor blood pressure, urine output, and body weight. Observe for orthopnea, dyspnea, and fatigue. Reduce rate or stop infusion for excessive drop in blood pressure. (2) Use caution in impaired renal or liver function; serum levels may increase considerably. (3) May be given to digitalized patients without causing signs of digitalis toxicity. (4) May increase ventricular response in atrial flutter/ fibrillation. Pretreat with digitalis. (5) Additional fluids and electrolytes may be required to facilitate appropriate response in patients who have been vigorously diuresed and may have insufficient cardiac filling pressure. Use caution. (6) Not recommended for use in the acute phase of myocardial infarction due to lack of clinical trials to this date. (7) Monitor electrolytes; hypokalemia due to diuretics may cause arrhythmias. (8) May cause excessive hypotension with disopyramide (Norpace). (9) Safety for use during pregnancy, lactation, and in children not established. Use during pregnancy only if potential benefit justifies potential risk. (10) May aggravate outflow tract obstruction in hypertrophic subaortic stenosis.

Contraindications: Hypersensitivity to amrinone or bisulfites, severe aortic or pulmonic valvular disease instead of surgical relief of the obstruction.

Incompatible with: Dextrose solutions (direct dilution only), furosemide (Lasix).

Side effects: Abdominal pain, anorexia, burning at site of injection, chest pain, dysrhythmias, fever, hepatotoxicity, hypotension, nausea and vomiting, thrombocytopenia. Hypersensitivity reactions manifested by ascites, myositis with interstitial shadowing on chest x-ray and elevated sedimentation rate, pericarditis, pleuritis, vasculitis with nodular pulmonary densities, hypoxemia, and jaundice have been reported.

Antidote: Notify the physician of any side effect. Based on degree of severity and condition of the patient, may be treated symptomatically, and dose may remain the same, be decreased, or the amrinone may be discontinued. Reduce rate or discontinue the drug at the first sign of marked hypotension and notify the physician. May be resolved by these measures alone or vasopressors (e.g., dopamine [Intropin]) may be required. Treat dysrhythmias with the appropriate drug. Resuscitate as necessary.

ANISTREPLASE

(APSAC, Eminase)

Usual dose: 30 units direct IV as soon as possible after onset of symptoms of acute myocardial infarction. Most effective when given within 4 to 6 hours.

Dilution: Each single-dose vial must be diluted with 5 ml sterile water for injection. Add diluent slowly, direct to sides of vial, and roll and tilt gently to mix. Do not shake. No further dilution recommended. Should be clear to pale yellow with no particulate matter. May be given through Y-tube or three-way stopcock of infusion set. Discard if not administered within 30 minutes of dilution.

Rate of administration: A single dose evenly distributed over 2 to 5 minutes (4 to 5 minutes is usual).

Actions: A thrombolytic agent. An inactive derivative of a fibrinolytic enzyme (p-anisoylated lys-plasminogen streptokinase activator complex). Made from streptokinase and human plasminogen. Activation begins with dilution; on injection activation continues in a progressive and controlled manner. The process converts plasminogen to plasmin, which degrades fibrin clots, fibrinogen, and other plasma proteins. This activation takes place within a thrombus as well as on the surface. Onset of action is prompt. It has a slow rate of degradation and an active half-life up to 2 hours. Anistreplase is 10 times more potent than streptokinase as a thrombolytic. Fibrin binding compares favorably to alteplase.

Indications and uses: Management of acute myocardial infarction in adults for the lysis of thrombi obstructing coronary arteries, the reduction of infarct size, the improvement of ventricular function, and the reduction of mortality.

Precautions: (1) Administered under the direction of a physician knowledgeable in its use and with appropriate diagnostic and laboratory facilities available. (2) Baseline ECG, CPK, and clotting studies (PT, PTT, CBC, fibrinogen level, platelets) and baseline assessment (patient condition, blood pressure, pain, hematomas, petechiae, or recent wounds) should be completed before administration. Type and cross-match may also be ordered. (3) Monitor ECG continuously, and record strips with greatest ST segment elevation initially and every 15 minutes for at least 4 hours. May cause severe hypotension; monitor blood pressure with caution to prevent bruising or bleeding. A 12-lead ECG is indicated when therapy is complete. (4) Start IV if indicated (not previously established, other medications being administered through current IV, to have a line available for additional treatment). (5) Reperfusion arrhythmias occur frequently (e.g., sinus bradycardia, accelerated idioventricular rhythm, PVCs, ventricular tachycardia); have antiarrhythmic medications available at bedside. (6) A greater alteration of hemostatic status than with heparin; use extreme care with the patient, avoid any excessive or rough handling or pressure (including too frequent BPs), avoid invasive procedures (e.g., arterial puncture, venipuncture, IM injection). If these procedures are absolutely necessary, use extreme precautionary methods (use radial artery instead of femoral, small-gauge catheters and needles, and sites that are easily observed and compressible where bleeding can be controlled; avoid handling of catheter sites; use extended pressure application of up to 30 minutes). Minor bleeding occurs often at catheter insertion sites. Avoid use of razors and toothbrushes. (7) Follow-up therapy with continuous infusion of heparin (without a loading dose) is frequently used to reduce the risk of rethrombosis. Increases risk of bleeding. (8) Monitor the patient carefully and frequently for anginal pain and any signs of bleeding; observe catheter sites at least every 15 minutes; watch for hematuria, hematemesis, bloody stool, petechiae, hematoma, flank pain, muscle weakness; and do neuro checks every hour. Continue until normal clotting function returns. (9) Use caution with drugs that may alter platelet function (e.g., aspirin, dipyridamole [Persantin], indomethacin, phenylbutazone). Risk of bleeding will be increased if used concomitantly. (10) Use extreme caution in the following situations: major surgery, trauma, GI or GU bleeding, or puncture of noncompressible vessels (e.g., spinal puncture, thoracentesis) within the previous 10 days; cerebrovascular disease; hypertension (systolic above 180 or diastolic above 110); mitral stenosis with atrial fibrillation (likelihood of left heart thrombus); acute pericarditis; subacute bacterial endocarditis; coagulation disorders, including those secondary to severe hepatic or renal disease; severe liver dysfunction; pregnancy and first 10 days postpartum; hemorrhagic ophthalmic conditions (e.g., diabetic hemorrhagic retinopathy); septic thrombophlebitis; patients taking anticoagulants; patients over 75 years of age; any situation where bleeding might be hazardous or difficult to manage because of location. (11) Standard treatment for myocardial infarction continues simultaneously with anistreplase therapy except if temporarily contraindicated (arterial blood gases, etc., unless absolutely necessary). (12) Coagulation tests will be unreliable; specific procedures can be used; notify the laboratory of anistreplase use. (13) Use during pregnancy only if clearly needed. Discontinue breast feeding temporarily. (14) Safety for use in children and patients over 75 years of age not established. (15) Repeat injections of anistreplase or streptokinase 5 days to 6 months after first injection or after streptococcal infection may not be effective (increased antistreptokinase antibodies) or may increase incidence of allergic reactions. (16) Refrigerate before dilution. Discard any solution not used within 30 minutes.

Contraindications: Known hypersensitivity to anistreplase or streptokinase. Active internal bleeding, arteriovenous malformation or aneurysm, bleeding diathesis, cerebrovascular accident, intracranial or intraspinal surgery or trauma within 2 months, intracranial neoplasm, severe uncontrolled hypertension.

Incompatible with: Manufacturer states "do not add to any infusion fluid. Do not add any other medication to vial or syringe."

Side effects: Bleeding is most common: internal (GI tract, GU tract, retroperitoneal, ocular, or intracranial sites), epistaxis, gingival, and superficial or surface bleeding (venous cutdowns, arterial punctures, sites of recent surgical intervention). Delayed purpuric rash, fever, eosinophilia, flushing, hypotension (severe and not secondary to bleeding or anaphylaxis), itching, nausea and vomiting, rashes. Anaphylactic reactions such as angioedema and bronchospasm are rare but have occurred. No cases of hepatitis or AIDS have been reported. Manufacturing process includes a vapor heat treatment to inactivate viruses. Other side effects have occurred but may be due to the myocardial infarction itself.

Antidote: Notify physician of all side effects. Note even the minutest bleeding tendency. Oozing at IV sites is expected. Control minor bleeding by local pressure. For severe bleeding in a critical location, discontinue anistreplase and any heparin therapy immediately. Whole blood, packed red blood cells, cryoprecipitate, fresh frozen plasma, and aminocaproic acid may all be indicated. Treat hypotension with vasopressors (e.g., dopamine [Intropin]). Treat reperfusion arrhythmias with specific appropriate protocols (e.g., bradycardia with atropine, ventricular tachycardia with lidocaine). Treat minor allergic reactions symptomatically. Discontinue drug and treat anaphylaxis with epinephrine, diphenhydramine (Benadryl), and corticosteroids. Resuscitate as necessary.

ANTIHEMOPHILIC FACTOR (HUMAN)

(AHF, Hemofil M, Factor VIII, Humate P, Koate HP, Koate HS, Monoclate, Profilate HP)

Usual dose: Completely individualized. Suggested doses are as follows:

Prophylaxis of spontaneous hemorrhage: 10 AHF IU/kg of body weight to increase factor VIII by 20%. Minimum of 30% of normal indicated. If early hemarthrosis is treated promptly, smaller doses may be adequate.

Mild hemorrhage: Above dosage may be repeated only if further bleeding occurs.

Moderate hemorrhage and minor surgery: 15 to 25 AHF IU/kg to increase factor VIII by 30% to 50% of normal. Maintain with 10 to 15 AHF IU/kg every 8 to 12 hours for 3 to 4 days as necessary.

Severe hemorrhage: 40 to 50 AHF IU/kg to increase factor VIII to 80% to 100% of normal. Maintain with 20 to 25 AHF IU/kg every 8 to 12 hours.

Major surgery: Sufficient dose to increase factor VIII to 80% to 100% of normal given 1 hour before surgery. Confirm with AHF level assays just before surgery. Give a second dose one half of the first in 5 hours. Maintain factor VIII at 30% of normal for 10 to 14 days. Some clinicians recommend 26 to 30 AHF IU/kg before surgery followed by 15 AHF IU/kg every 8 hours after surgery. Increase dose if level falls below 30%.

Dilution: All preparations provide diluent and administration equipment. Actual number of AHF units shown on each vial. Use only the diluent provided, and maintain strict aseptic technique.

Rate of administration: Preparations with less than 34 AHF IU/ml infuse each 10 to 20 ml over 3 minutes. Preparations with more than 34 AHF IU/ml should infuse at a maximum rate of 2 ml/min. Reduce rate of infusion if a significant increase in pulse rate occurs.

Actions: A lyophilized or dried (depending on specific preparation) concentrate of coagulation factor VIII (antihemophilic factor). Obtained from fresh (less than

3 hours old) human plasma and prepared, irradiated, and dried by a specific process.

Indications and uses: (1) Treatment of the congenital deficiency of factor VIII (classical hemophilia A); (2) used to control unexpected hemorrhagic episodes, during emergency or elective surgery, and prophylactically to maintain known hemophiliac patients as necessary to prevent hemorrhage.

Precautions: (1) Identification of factor VIII deficiency with level assays mandatory before administration and during treatment. Adjust dosage as indicated. (2) Must be refrigerated. Give within 3 hours of reconstitution. (3) Use a new sterile needle and syringe or administration set for each vial. (Use a plastic syringe to prevent binding to glass surfaces.) (4) Can transmit AIDS and hepatitis. Risk markedly reduced with newer highly purified products. (5) If AHF does not significantly improve the partial thromboplastin time, increase the dose; factor VIII antibodies are probable. (6) Intravascular hemolysis can occur when large volumes are given to individuals with blood groups A, B, or AB. (7) Type-specific cryoprecipitate has been used to maintain adequate factor VIII levels.

Contraindications: None when used for the specific indications listed. Not effective for bleeding of patients with von Willebrand's disease. Hypersensitivity to mouse protein (monoclonal-antibody-derived factor VIII).

Incompatible with: Sufficient information not available. Do not mix with other drugs.

Side effects: Occur infrequently; backache, erythema, fever, hepatitis, hives. Consider risk potential of contracting AIDS or hepatitis. Massive doses may cause acute hemolytic anemia, hyperfibrinogenemia, or increased bleeding tendency.

Antidote: All side effects except AIDS and hepatitis usually subside spontaneously in 15 to 20 minutes. Keep the physician informed. Treat anaphylaxis (antihistamines, epinephrine, corticosteroids) and resuscitate as necessary.

ANTI-INHIBITOR COAGULANT COMPLEX

(Autoplex T, Feiba VH Immuno)

Usual dose: Range is 25 to 100 factor VIII correctional units/kg. May be repeated in 6 to 12 hours. Do not exceed 200 units/kg/24 hr. Completely individualized and adjusted according to patient response.

Dilution: All preparations provide diluent for IV infusion. Actual number of factor VIII inhibitor bypassing activity units shown on each vial. Use only the diluent provided and maintain strict aseptic technique. May be given through Y-tube or three-way stopcock of infusion set.

Rate of administration: 10 ml or less per minute. If symptoms of too rapid infusion (headache, flushing, changes in blood pressure or pulse rate) occur, discontinue until symptoms subside. Restart at 2 ml/min.

Actions: A 1-unit volume of factor VIII correctional activity (quantity of activated prothrombin complex) will correct clotting time to normal (35 seconds) when added to an equal volume of factor VIII deficient or inhibitor plasma. A dried or freeze-dried concentrate prepared from human plasma by a specific process.

Indications and uses: To control hemorrhagic episodes in hemophiliacs (hemophilia A) with factor VIII inhibitors who are bleeding or will undergo elective or emergency surgery. Most frequently indicated if factor VIII inhibitor levels are above 2 to 10 Bethesda units or rise to that level following treatment with AHF.

Precautions: (1) Identification of factor VIII inhibitor levels mandatory previous to administration. (2) Monitor PT before and after treatment. Only accurate means of treatment evaluation. Must be two thirds of preinfusion value after treatment if patient is to receive any additional doses. (3) APTT, WBCT, and other clotting factor tests do not correlate with actual results and may lead to overdose and DIC. (4) Could transmit AIDS and hepatitis. (5) Refrigerate before reconstitution. (6) Not recommended for use with antifibrinolytic products (aminocaproic acid, tranexamic acid). (7) Use extreme caution in newborns and patients with liver disease. (8) Safety for use in pregnancy not established.

Contraindications: DIC, symptoms (signs) of fibrinolysis, known hypersensitivity.

Incompatible with: Specific information not available. Do not mix directly with other drugs.

Side effects: Anaphylaxis, bradycardia, chest pain, chills, cough, decreased fibrinogen concentration, decreased platelet count, fever, flushing, headache, hypertension, hypotension, prolonged PTT, prolonged thrombin time, prolonged PT, respiratory distress, tachycardia, urticaria. Consider risk potential of contracting AIDS or hepatitis.

Antidote: If side effects occur, discontinue the infusion and notify the physician. May be resumed at a slower rate or an alternate product may be used. Symptoms of DIC (blood pressure and pulse rate changes, respiratory discomfort, chest pain, cough, prolonged clotting tests) require immediate treatment. Treat anaphylaxis (antihistamines, epinephrine, corticosteroids) and resuscitate as necessary.

ANTITHROMBIN III pH 6.5 to 7.5

(AT-III, ATnativ)

Usual dose: Loading dose, maintenance dose, and dosing intervals are completely individualized based on patient weight, clinical condition, degree of deficiency, type of surgery or procedure involved, physician judgment, desired level of antithrombin III (AT-III), and actual plasma levels achieved as verified by appropriate lab tests. 1 Unit/kg should raise the level of AT-III by 1% to 2.1%. The desired antithrombin-III level after the first dose should be about 120% of normal (normal is 0.1 to 0.2 Gm/L). AT-III levels must be maintained at normal or at least above 80% of normal for 2 to 8 days depending on individual patient factors. Usually achieved by administration of a maintenance dose once daily. Concomitant administration of heparin usually indicated. (See Precautions).

Calculate the initial loading dose using the following formula (assumes a plasma volume of 40 ml/kg):

$$\text{Dosage units} = \frac{(\text{desired AT-III level [\%]} - \text{baseline AT-III [\%]} \times \text{body weight (kg)}}{1\% \text{ (1 International Unit/kg)}}$$

For a 70 kg patient with a baseline AT-III level of 57% the initial dose would be (120%–57%) × 70 ÷ 1 = 4410 IU. Plasma AT-III levels should be measured preceding the initial dose and 30 minutes later to calculate the in vivo recovery. If recovery differs from the anticipated rise of 1% for each IU/kg, modify the formula accordingly. If the above patient has a 30 minute AT-III level of 147%, the increase in AT-III measured for each 1 IU/kg administered is (147%–57%) × 70 kg ÷ 4410 Units = 1.43% rise for each IU/kg administered. This in vivo recovery would be used to calculate future doses.

Dilution: Each 500 IU must be diluted with 10 ml of sterile water for injection (preferred), normal saline or 5% dextrose in water. Swirl to dissolve. Do not shake. Bring solution to room temperature and use within 3 hours of reconstitution. May be further diluted with additional amounts of the same infusion solutions if desired.

Rate of administration: Each 50 IU or fraction thereof should be given over 1 minute. Do not exceed a rate of 100 IU/min. Too rapid injection may cause dyspnea.

Actions: Manufactured from human plasma, purified and heat-treated through specific processes, antithrombin III is a plasma-based protein produced by the body to inactivate specific clotting proteins and control clot formation. Identical to heparin cofactor I, a factor in plasma necessary for heparin to exert its anticoagulant effect. It inactivates thrombin and the activated forms of factors IX, X, XI, and XII (all coagulation enzymes except factors VIIa and XIIIa). Increases antithrombin III levels within 30 minutes and has a half-life of up to 3 days.

Indications and uses: Treatment of patients with hereditary antithrombin III deficiency to prevent thrombosis during surgical or obstetric procedures (replacement therapy) or during acute thrombotic episodes.

Precautions: (1) Confirm diagnosis of hereditary antithrombin III deficiency based on a clear family history of venous thrombosis as well as decreased plasma antithrombin III levels and the exclusion of acquired deficiency. Present lab tests may not be able to identify all cases of congenital AT-III deficiency. (2) Half-life of AT-III decreases with concurrent heparin treatment. The anticoagulant effect of heparin is enhanced and a reduced dose of heparin is indicated to avoid bleeding. (3) Every unit of plasma used to manufacture antithrombin III is tested and found nonreactive for HBsAg and negative for antibody to HIV by FDA-approved tests; then heat-treated by a special process. Even with these precautions, individuals who receive multiple infusions may develop viral infection, particularly non-A non-B hepatitis. HIV infection remains a remote possibility. (4) AT-III levels should be measured twice daily initially, monitored until the patient is stabilized, then measured daily. All blood work should be drawn immediately before the next infusion of AT-III. (5) Patient should be informed about risks of thrombosis in connection with pregnancy and surgery and the fact that it is inherited. (6) Neonatal AT-III levels should be measured immediately after birth if parents are known to have AT-III deficiency. Treatment of the neonate should be under the direction of a physician knowledgeable about coagulation disorders. Safety and efficacy for use in children not established. (7) Safety for use during pregnancy not established, use only if clearly indicated. Fetal abnormalities not noted when administered in the third trimester.

Contraindications: None when used as indicated.

Incompatible with: Specific information not available.

Side effects: None noted in patients with hereditary AT-III deficiency. Some patients with acquired AT-III deficiency diagnosed with desseminated intravascular coagulopathy (DIC) have had diuretic and vasodilatory effects. Rapid infusion may cause dyspnea.

Antidote: Levels of 150% to 210% found in a few patients have not caused any apparent complications. Observe for bleeding. Reduce rate of infusion immediately for dyspnea. Keep physician informed of patient's lab values and condition.

ANTIVENIN (CROTALIDAE) POLYVALENT

Usual dose: Testing for sensitivity to horse serum required before use (see Precautions). Dosage based on severity of envenomation when patient is initially assessed.
No envenomation: None.
Minimal envenomation: 2 to 4 vials (20 to 40 ml).
Moderate envenomation: 5 to 9 vials (50 to 90 ml).
Severe envenomation: 10 to 15 vials (100 to 150 ml). Additional antivenin need based on clinical response and progression of symptoms. If condition deteriorates, 1 to 5 additional vials (10 to 50 ml) may be given. Most effective within 4 hours of the bite; less effective after 8 hours, but in the presence of envenomation is to be given even after 24 hours have elapsed.

Pediatric dose: Not based on weight. Small children bitten by large snakes may require larger doses of antivenin.

Dilution: Each single vial must be diluted with 10 ml sterile water for injection (supplied). Must be further diluted with normal saline or 5% dextrose for infusion to a 1:1 to 1:10 solution (1 ml antivenin to 10 ml infusion solution preferred unless patient's condition limits fluid intake). Avoid foaming by gently swirling to mix thoroughly.

Rate of administration: Infuse 5 to 10 ml over a minimum of 3 to 5 minutes. If no adverse reaction occurs give remaining initial dose at maximum rate of administration based on severity of envenomation and fluid tolerance appropriate for this patient's body weight and condition.

Actions: Prepared from the blood serum of horses immunized against the venom of crotalids (pit vipers) found in North, Central, and South America. Will neutralize the venom of rattlesnakes, copperheads, and cottonmouth moccasins. (See literature for specific species.)

Indications and uses: Treatment of patients with symptoms of envenomation sustained from the bite of a rattlesnake, copperhead, cottonmouth moccasin, or other specific pit viper species of snake.

Precautions: (1) Read drug literature supplied with antivenin completely before use. Essential to evaluate symptoms and individual status of each patient. (2) Determine patient response to any previous injections of serum of any type and history of any allergic-type reactions. (3) Hospitalize patient. (4) Test every patient without exception for sensitivity to horse serum (1 ml vial of 1:10 dilution horse serum supplied). Conjunctival test and skin test recommended for maximum safety. Always begin with the conjunctival test.

Conjunctival test: Instill 1 drop 1:10 horse serum into conjunctival sac for adults (1 drop 1:100 dilution for children). Itching, redness, burning, and/or lacrimation within 30 minutes is a positive reaction. A drop of normal saline in the opposite eye is used as a control and should be asymptomatic. Reverse adverse effects of positive reaction with 1 drop epinephrine ophthalmic solution.

Scratch test: Make a ¼ inch skin scratch through a drop of 1:100 dilution in normal saline. Make a similar scratch through a drop of normal saline on a comparable skin site as a control. Compare sites in 20 minutes. An urticarial wheal surrounded by a zone of erythema is a positive reaction.

Skin test: Inject 0.02 to 0.1 ml of 1:100 horse serum intradermally. In patients with a history of allergies use a 1:1,000 solution. A similar injection of normal saline can be used as a control. Compare in 20 minutes. An urticarial wheal surrounded by a zone of erythema is a positive reaction.

Other testing methods may be used. Use at least two. (5) A systemic reaction may occur even when both sensitivity tests are negative. Concomitant use of antihistamines may interfere with sensitivity tests. (6) In most cases, the sooner a sensitivity reaction occurs, the greater the sensitivity. Observe patient continuously. (7) Monitor all vital signs at frequent intervals. Before antivenin administered draw adequate blood for baseline studies (type and cross-match, CBC, hematocrit, platelet count, PT, clot retraction, bleeding and coagulation times, BUN, electrolytes, bilirubin). Have urine specimens tested frequently for microscopic erythrocytes. (8) Initiate two IV lines as soon as possible; one to be used for supportive therapy, the other for antivenin and electrolytes. (9) Keep emergency equipment available at all times including oxygen, epinephrine, antihistamines (e.g., diphenhydramine [Benadryl]), vasopressors (e.g., dopamine [Intropin]), corticosteroids, and ventilation equipment. (10) Tetanus prophylaxis is indicated. (11) Corticosteroids are the drugs of choice if antivenin is not available until 24 hours after the snake bite but are not recommended for concomitant administration. (12) Consider use of broad-spectrum antibiotic. (13) Check with poison control center; many authorities do not recommend packing the bitten extremity in ice.

Contraindications: Hypersensitivity to horse serum unless only treatment available for life-threatening situation. Several techniques including preload of antihistamines and/or desensitization may be considered (see literature).

Incompatible with: Specific information not available. Do not mix with any other drug in syringe or solution because of specific use.

Side effects: Acute anaphylaxis with urticaria, respiratory distress, and vascular collapse. Serum sickness may occur. Usually appears in 7 to 12 days. Local pain, local erythema, and urticaria without systemic reaction can occur.

Antidote: Discontinue the drug and notify the physician of all side effects. Treat anaphylaxis immediately. Epinephrine (Adrenalin) and diphenhydramine (Benadryl), oxygen, vasopressors (dopamine), corticosteroids, and ventilation equipment must always be available. Resuscitate as necessary.

ANTIVENIN *(LATRODECTUS MACTANS)*

(Black Widow Spider Species Antivenin)

Usual dose: Testing for sensitivity to horse serum required before use (see Precautions). Entire contents of 1 vial of antivenin (2.5 ml) is recommended for adults and children. One vial is usually enough, but a second dose may be necessary in rare instances.

Dilution: Each single dose (6,000 antivenin units) must be initially diluted with 2.5 ml sterile water for injection (supplied). Keep needle in rubber stopper of antivenin and shake vial to dissolve contents completely. Must be further diluted in 10 to 50 ml normal saline for IV injection.

Rate of administration: A single dose over a minimum of 15 minutes.

Actions: Prepared from the blood serum of horses immunized against the venom of the black widow spider. One unit will neutralize one average mouse-lethal dose of black widow spider venom when both are injected simultaneously under laboratory conditions.

Indications and uses: Treatment of patients with symptoms resulting from black widow spider bites *(Latrodectus mactans)*.

Precautions: (1) Read drug literature supplied with antivenin completely before use. Essential to evaluate symptoms and individual status of each patient. (2) Determine patient response to any previous injections of serum of any type and history of any allergic-type reactions. (3) Hospitalize patient if possible. (4) Test every patient without exception for sensitivity to horse serum (1 ml vial of 1:10 dilution horse serum supplied). Conjunctival test and skin test recommended for maximum safety. Always begin with the conjunctival test.

Conjunctival test: Instill 1 drop 1:10 horse serum into conjunctival sac for adults (1 drop 1:100 dilution for children). Itching, redness, burning, and/or lacrimation within 30 minutes is a positive reaction. A drop of normal saline in the opposite eye is used as a control and should be asymptomatic. Reverse adverse effects of positive reaction with 1 drop epinephrine ophthalmic solution.

Scratch test: Make a ¼ inch skin scratch through a drop of 1:100 dilution in normal saline. Make a similar scratch through a drop of normal saline on a comparable skin site as a control. Compare sites in 20 minutes. An urticarial wheal surrounded by a zone of erythema is a positive reaction.

Skin test: Inject 0.02 to 0.1 ml of 1:100 horse serum intradermally. In patients with a history of allergies use a 1:1,000 solution. A similar injection of normal saline can be used as a control. Compare in 20 minutes. An urticarial wheal surrounded by a zone of erythema is a positive reaction.

Other testing methods may be used. Use at least two. (5) A systemic reaction may occur even when both sensitivity tests are negative. Concomitant use of antihistamines may interfere with sensitivity tests. (6) Supportive therapy is indicated. 10 ml of 10% calcium gluconate IV may control muscle pain. Morphine may be needed. Barbiturates or diazepam may be used for restlessness. Prolonged warm baths are helpful; corticosteroids have been used. (7) Observe patient constantly for respiratory paralysis. Can occur from toxin alone, and narcotics and sedatives may precipitate respiratory depression. (8) Muscle relaxants may be the initial treatment of choice in healthy individuals between 16 and 60. Antivenin use may be deferred while patient is observed. (9) May be given IM. IV preferred in severe cases, if patient is in shock, or in children under 12 years of age. (10) Safety for use in pregnancy and lactation not established.

Contraindications: Hypersensitivity to horse serum unless only treatment available for a life-threatening situation. Several techniques including preload of antihistamine and/or desensitization may be considered (see literature).

Incompatible with: Specific information not available. Do not mix with any other drug in syringe or solution because of specific use.

Side effects: Acute anaphylaxis with urticaria, respiratory distress, and vascular collapse. Serum sickness may occur. Usually appears in 7 to 12 days. Local pain, local erythema, and urticaria without systemic reaction can occur.

Antidote: Discontinue the drug and notify the physician of all side effects. Treat anaphylaxis immediately. Epinephrine (Adrenalin), diphenhydramine (Benadryl), oxygen, vasopressors (dopamine), corticosteroids, and ventilation equipment must always be available. Resuscitate as necessary.

ANTIVENIN *(MICRURUS FULVIUS)* pH 6.5 to 7.5

(North American Coral Snake Antivenin)

Usual dose: Testing for sensitivity to horse serum required before use (see Precautions). Entire contents of 3 to 5 vials (30 to 50 ml) are recommended depending on the nature and severity of envenomation. Up to 10 vials may be required if the snake's entire venom load was delivered by the bite.

Dilution: Each single vial must be diluted with 10 ml sterile water for injection (supplied). Start an IV infusion of 250 to 500 ml normal saline. May be administered through the tubing of the free-flowing IV or added to the infusion solution after initial 2 ml given without adverse reaction.

Rate of administration: Inject the first 1 to 2 ml over a minimum of 3 to 5 minutes. If no adverse reaction, give remaining initial dose at maximum rate of administration based on severity of envenomation and fluid tolerance appropriate for patient's body weight and condition.

Actions: Prepared from the blood serum of horses immunized against the venom of specific coral snakes. Will neutralize the venom of *M. fulvius fulvius* (eastern coral snake) and *M. fulvius tenere* (Texas coral snake). Response should be rapid and dramatic.

Indications and uses: Treatment of patients with symptoms resulting from the venom of *M. fulvius fulvius* (eastern coral snake) and *M. fulvius tenere* (Texas coral snake). Not effective for *M. euryxanthus* (Arizona or Sonoran coral snake).

Precautions: (1) Read drug literature supplied with antivenin completely before use. Essential to evaluate symptoms and individual status of each patient. (2) Determine patient response to any previous injections of serum of any type and history of any allergic-type reactions. (3) Immobilize victim. At a minimum, splint bitten extremity. Hospitalize patient if possible. (4) Test every patient without exception for sensitivity to horse serum (1 ml vial of 1:10 dilution horse serum supplied). Conjunctival test and scratch test recommended for maximum safety. Always begin with the conjunctival test.

Conjunctival test: Instill 1 drop 1:10 horse serum into conjunctival sac for adults (1 drop 1:100 dilution for children). Itching, redness, burning, and/or lacrimation within 30 minutes is a positive reaction. A drop of normal saline in the opposite eye is used as a control and should be asymptomatic. Reverse adverse effects of positive reaction with 1 drop epinephrine ophthalmic solution.

Scratch test: Place 1 drop of 1:100 solution on the skin. Make a ¼ inch scratch through this drop. Establish a normal saline control in the same manner on a similar skin surface. Compare in 20 minutes. An urticarial wheal surrounded by a zone of erythema is a positive reaction.

Other testing methods may be used. Use at least two. Concomitant use of antihistamines may interfere with sensitivity tests. (5) A systemic reaction may occur even when both sensitivity tests are negative. (6) Observe patient constantly. Additional antivenin may be needed. Paralysis can occur within 2 to 2 ½ hours. Local tissue reaction does not reflect the amount of envenomation. Observe signs and symptoms to assess amount of toxin injected. Symptoms may begin in 1 hour or be delayed up to 18 hours. (7) Supportive therapy is indicated. Respiratory depressants (e.g., narcotics, sedatives) are contraindicated or used with extreme caution. Keep equipment for artificial ventilation immediately available. (8) Tetanus prophylaxis indicated.

Contraindications: Hypersensitivity to horse serum unless only treatment available for a life-threatening situation.

Several techniques including preload of antihistamines and/or desensitization may be considered (see literature).

Incompatible with: Specific information not available. Do not mix with any other drug in syringe or solution because of specific use.

Side effects: Acute anaphylaxis with urticaria, respiratory distress, and vascular collapse. Serum sickness may occur. Usually appears in 7 to 12 days. Local pain, local erythema, and urticaria without systemic reaction can occur.

Antidote: Discontinue the drug and notify the physician of all side effects. Treat anaphylaxis immediately. Epinephrine (Adrenalin) and diphenhydramine (Benadryl), oxygen, vasopressors (dopamine), corticosteroids, and ventilation equipment must always be available. Resuscitate as necessary.

ARGININE HYDROCHLORIDE pH 5.0 to 6.5

(R-Gene 10)

Usual dose: 300 ml as a single test dose under specific clinical conditions and procedures.

Pediatric dose: 5 ml/kg of body weight.

Dilution: Available as 10% solution in 500 ml bottles ready for use as an IV infusion.

Rate of administration: A single dose evenly distributed over 30 minutes. Recommended dose must be infused in 30 minutes to ensure accurate test results.

Actions: A diagnostic aid, it is an IV stimulant to the pituitary that often induces a pronounced rise in plasma level of human growth hormone (HGH) in normal individuals. This rise does not occur if pituitary function is diminished or absent.

Indications and uses: IV stimulant to pituitary as a diagnostic aid. May be useful in panhypopituitarism, pituitary dwarfism, chromophobe adenoma, postsurgical craniopharyngioma, hypophysectomy, pituitary trauma, acromegaly, gigantism, and problems of growth or stature.

Investigational use: Reverse ammonium intoxication.

Precautions: (1) Inspect each bottle. Discard if not clear or vacuum is not present. (2) Confirm absolute patency of vein; infiltration may cause necrosis of tissue. (3) Specific test procedure must be observed. Schedule in morning; patient must be fasting overnight and have had a normal night's rest. Maintain bed rest and calming atmosphere from 30 minutes before infusion to completion of test process. Draw blood samples from opposite arm of infusion 30 minutes before, at time infusion is begun, and every 30 minutes times five. Technician should promptly centrifuge and store all samples at −20° C until processed. (4) False positive or negative results 30% of time. Cross-check or confirm result with insulin hypoglycemia test and a second arginine test. Allow 1 day between each test. (5) Confirm serum electrolyte balance before administration; high chloride content. May cause bicarbonate deficit and/or potassium excess. (6) Use caution in renal impairment; high nitrogen content. (7) False positive results will be obtained during pregnancy or with oral contraceptives.

Contraindications: Individuals with known severe allergic tendencies.

Incompatible with: Specific information not available. Should be considered incompatible with any other drug or solution because of specific use.

Side effects: Usually result from rate or hypertonicity of solution. Flushing, headache, local venous irritation, nausea, numbness, rash, tissue necrosis at site of infiltration, vomiting.

Antidote: Slow infusion to reduce side effects, but must be infused in 30 minutes for accurate results. Notify physician of all side effects. Discontinue drug and treat allergic reaction with diphenhydramine (Benadryl) or epinephrine. Resuscitate as necessary.

ASCORBIC ACID pH 5.5 to 7.0

(Cenolate, Cevalin, ✦ Redoxon, sodium ascorbate, vitamin C)

Usual dose: 200 mg to 2 Gm/24 hr. Up to 6 Gm/24 hr has been given without toxicity.

Infant dose: 100 to 300 mg/24 hr is the curative dose recommended.

Premature infant dose: 75 to 100 mg/24 hr.

Dilution: May be given undiluted or may be administered diluted in IV infusion solutions. Soluble in the more commonly used solutions, such as 5% dextrose in water or saline, normal saline, lactated Ringer's injection, Ringer's injection, or sodium lactate injection.

Rate of administration: 100 mg or fraction thereof over 1 minute by direct IV administration.

Actions: This water-soluble vitamin is necessary to the formation of collagen in all fibrous tissue, carbohydrate metabolism, connective tissue repair, maintenance of intracellular stability of blood vessels, and many other body functions. Not stored in the body. Daily requirements must be met. Completcly utilized; excess is excreted unchanged in the urine. Crosses placental barrier. Secreted in breast milk.

Indications and uses: (1) Preoperative and postoperative maintenance of optimum health; (2) prolonged IV therapy; (3) increased vitamin requirements or replacement therapy in severe burns, extensive injuries, and severe infections; (4) prematurity; (5) deficient intestinal absorption of water-soluble vitamins; (6) prolonged or wasting diseases; (7) hemovascular disorders and delayed fracture and wound healing require increased intake; (8) specific for the treatment of scurvy.

Precautions: (1) Vitamin C is better absorbed and utilized by IM injection. (2) Increased urinary excretion is diagnostic for vitamin C saturation. (3) Slight coloration does not affect the medication. Protect from freezing and from light. (4) Potentiates barbiturates, dicumarol, ferrous iron absorption, salicylates, and sulfonamides. (5) Antagonizes anticoagulants. (6) Use caution in pregnancy; high dosage may adversely affect fetus. (7) 2 Gm/day will lower urine pH and will cause reabsorption of acidic drugs and crystallization with sulfonamides. (8) Use caution in cardiac patients. Sodium or calcium content may antagonize other drugs or overall condition. Use caution in diabetics and patients prone to recurrent renal calculi or undergoing stool occult-blood tests. (9) Inhibits amphetamines and tricyclic antidepressants. (10) Inhibited by smoking.

Contraindications: There are no absolute contraindications.

Incompatible with: Aminophylline, bleomycin (Blenoxane), chloramphenicol (Chloromycetin), chlordiazepoxide (Librium), chlorothiazide (Diuril), conjugated estrogens (Premarin), dextran, erythromycin (Erythrocin), hydrocortisone, nafcillin (Unipen), phytonadione (Aquamephyton), sodium bicarbonate, sulfisoxazole, triflupromazine (Vesprin), vitamin B_{12} (e.g., Redisol), warfarin (Coumadin).

Side effects: Occur only with too rapid injection: temporary dizziness or faintness. Diarrhea or renal calculi may occur with large doses.

Antidote: Discontinue administration temporarily. Resume administration at a decreased rate. If side effects persist, discontinue drug and notify the physician.

ASPARAGINASE pH 7.4

(Elspar, ✦ Kidrolase)

Usual dose: *Skin test:* Required before initial dose and whenever 7 days or more elapse between doses. Give 0.1 ml containing 2.0 IU intradermally and observe for 1 hour for the appearance of a wheal or erythema.

Direct IV: Very specific amount to be given on a specific day or days in a specific regimen of other chemotherapeutic agents; i.e., 1,000 IU/kg of body weight/day for 10 successive days beginning on day 22 of regimen with specific prednisone and vincristine doses. When used as a single agent, the usual dose for adults and children is 200 IU/kg/day for 28 days.

Desensitization process for administration: Extensive process. See drug literature.

Dilution: *Specific techniques required, see Precautions.* Initially dilute each 10 ml vial (10,000 IU) with 5 ml of sterile water or sodium chloride for injection. 2,000 IU/ml.

Skin test: Withdraw 0.1 ml from the above solution and further dilute with 9.9 ml sodium chloride for injection (20 IU/ml). 0.1 ml of this solution equals 2 IU.

Direct IV: Use 2,000 IU/ml solution. Must be further diluted by administering through Y-tube or three-way stopcock of a free-flowing infusion of 5% dextrose in water or normal saline.

Rate of administration: *Direct IV:* Each dose evenly distributed over at least 30 minutes.

Actions: An enzyme derived from *Escherichia coli* that rapidly depletes asparagine from cells. Some malignant cells have a metabolic defect that makes them dependent on exogenous asparagine for survival, but they are unable to synthesize asparagine as normal cells do.

Indications and uses: Induces remissions in acute lymphocytic leukemia. Primarily used in specific combinations with other chemotherapeutic agents.

Precautions: (1) Follow guidelines for handling cytotoxic agents recommended. See Appendix, page 677. (2) A lethal drug; administered by or under the direction of the physician specialist. Toxicity and short-term effectiveness limit use. More toxic in adults than in children. Observe patient carefully during and after infusion. (3) Appropriate treatment for anaphylaxis must always be available. Risk increased if patient has received asparaginase before. (4) Rarely used as a single agent; not recommended for maintenance therapy. (5) Impairs liver function; may increase toxicity of other drugs. (6) Increases toxicity of vincristine and prednisone if given before or concurrently. (7) Inhibits methotrexate. (8) Allopurinol, increased fluid intake, and alkalinization of the urine may be required to reduce uric acid levels. (9) Frequent blood counts, bone marrow evaluation, serum amylase, blood sugar, and evaluation of liver and kidney function are necessary. (10) Will produce teratogenic effects on the fetus. Has a mutagenic potential. Discontinue breast feeding. (11)

Nausea and vomiting can be severe. Prophylactic administration of antiemetics recommended to increase patient comfort. (12) Predisposition to infection probable. (13) Refrigerate before and after dilution. Discard after 8 hours or any time solution is cloudy. Use only clear solutions. (14) May contain fiber-like particles; use of 5.0 micron filter recommended. (15) Do not administer any vaccine or chloroquine to patients receiving antineoplastic drugs.

Contraindications: Hypersensitivity to asparaginase, pancreatitis, or past history of pancreatitis.

Incompatible with: Specific information not available. Consider incompatible in syringe or solution because of toxicity and specific use.

Side effects: Occur frequently even with the initial dose and may cause death. Allergic reactions including anaphylaxis (even if skin test negative and/or allergic symptoms have not occurred with previous doses), agitation, azotemia, bleeding, bone marrow depression, coma, confusion, depression, fatigue, hallucinations, hyperglycemia, hyperthermia (fatal), hypofibrinogenemia and depression of other clotting factors, nausea and vomiting, fulminating pancreatitis (fatal).

Antidote: Notify physician of all side effects. Asparaginase may have to be discontinued until recovery or permanently discontinued. Symptomatic and supportive treatment is indicated. Treat anaphylaxis with epinephrine, corticosteroids, oxygen, and antihistamines. There is no specific antidote.

ATENOLOL

pH 5.5 to 6.5

(Tenormin)

Usual dose: 5 mg. Initiate as soon as the patient's hemodynamic condition has stabilized and eligibility has been established. If initial dose well tolerated, repeat in 10 minutes. If full IV dose well tolerated, give 50 mg orally 10 minutes after last bolus. Repeat in 12 hours. Follow with an oral maintenance dose of 100 mg daily or 50 mg twice a day for 6 to 9 days or until discharged from hospital. Discontinue if bradycardia or hypotension requiring treatment occurs.

Dilution: May be given undiluted by direct IV or diluted in 10 ml to 50 ml 5% dextrose in water, 0.45% normal saline, or normal saline and given as an infusion.

Rate of administration: Distribute a single dose evenly over 5 minutes. Monitor ECG, heart rate, and blood pressure and discontinue atenolol if adverse symptoms occur (bradycardia less than 45 beats/min, heart block greater than first degree, systolic blood pressure less than 90 mm Hg, or moderate to severe cardiac failure).

Actions: Atenolol is a cardioselective (β_1) adrenergic blocking agent. Its mechanism of action in patients with suspected or definite myocardial infarction is not known. Reduces heart rate, cardiac output, blood pressure, and myocardial oxygen consumption. Promotes redistribution of blood flow from adequately supplied areas of the heart to ischemic areas. May also reduce chest pain. It reduces the incidence of recurrent myocardial infarctions and reduces the size of the infarct and the incidence of fatal arrhythmias. Inhibits isoproterenol-induced tachycardia and reduces reflex orthostatic tachycardia. Well distributed throughout the body, it acts within 1 to 2 minutes and lasts about 3 to 4 hours. Undergoes little or no metabolism by the liver. Excreted in urine. Secreted in breast milk.

Indications and uses: (1) To reduce cardiac mortality in hemodynamically stable individuals with suspected or definite myocardial infarction; (2) oral form also used to treat hypertension and angina pectoris.

Precautions: (1) Continuous ECG, heart rate, and blood pressure monitoring are mandatory during administration of IV atenolol. (2) Use caution in the presence of heart failure. (3) Use caution in heart failure controlled by digitalis; both drugs slow AV conduction. (4) May mask tachycardia occurring with hypoglycemia in diabetes and tachycardia of hyperthyroidism. Abrupt withdrawal in patients with thyroid disease may precipitate a thyroid storm. (5) β-Adrenergic blocking agents may be inhibited by nonsteroidal antiinflammatory agents, sympathomimetics (e.g., epinephrine, norepinephrine, isoproterenol [Isuprel], dopamine [Intropin], dobutamine [Dobutrex]), and ritodrine. (6) May potentiate catecholamine-depleting drugs (e.g., reserpine), lidocaine, prazosin (Minipress), disopyramide (Norpace), and verapamil (Isoptin). (7) Use with verapamil may potentiate both drugs and result in severe depression of myocardium and AV conduction. (8) May cause severe hypotension and/or bradycardia with catecholamine-depleting drugs (e.g., reserpine); observe patient closely. (9) Used concurrently with digitalis, alpha-adrenergic blockers (e.g., phentolamine [Regitine]), vasodilators (e.g., nitroglycerine), and clot-dissolving drugs (e.g., alteplase recombinant [tPA], anistreplase [Eminase]), as indicated. (10) May be potentiated by atropine. (11) Use with caution and reduce dose by one half in patients with asthma or other bronchospastic disease. Isoproterenol (Isuprel) should be available. (12) Reduced dose may be indicated in patients already taking a beta blocker (e.g., propranolol [Inderal]). Titrate by clinical observations. (13) Use with clonidine may precipitate acute hypertension. May aggravate rebound hypertension if clonidine stopped abruptly; discontinue atenolol several days before gradual withdrawal of clonidine. (14) Reduce dose by one half in renal impairment with a creatinine clearance less than 35 ml/min (see literature). (15) Some authorities recommend that β-adrenergic blockers be discontinued 48 hours before major surgery (beta blockade interferes with cardiac response to reflex stimuli). If continued, use caution administering general anesthetics that depress the myocardium (e.g., cyclopropane, trichlorethylene). (16) Reduce oral dose gradually to avoid rebound angina, myocardial infarction, or ventricular dysrhythmias. (17) Use with caution and only when specifically indicated in pregnancy and lactation. May have to postpone breast feeding. (18) Safety for use in children not established. (19) Stable for 48 hours after dilution.

Contraindications: Sinus bradycardia, heart block greater than first degree, cardiogenic shock, overt cardiac failure.

Incompatible with: Any other drug in syringe or solution because of specific use.

Side effects: Bradycardia, bronchospasm, cardiac arrest, cardiac failure, cold extremities, depression, diarrhea, dizziness, dreaming, drowsiness, dyspnea, fatigue, heart block, hypotension, lightheadedness, nausea, postural hypotension, pulmonary emboli, supraventricular tachycardia, ventricular tachycardia, vertigo, wheezing.

Antidote: For any side effect, discontinue the drug and notify the physician immediately. Physician may elect to continue atenolol at a reduced dose. Patients with myocardial infarction may be more hemodynamically unstable; treat with caution. Bradycardia and hypotension may respond spontaneously after atenolol discontinued. If indicated, use atropine for bradycardia; use isoproterenol with caution if atropine is not effective. Glucagon, 5 to 10 mg IV, may be effective if atropine and isoproterenol are not (investigational use). Transvenous cardiac pacing may be needed. Treat hypotension with IV fluids if indicated or vasopressors (epinephrine rather than norepinephrine [Levarterenol] or isoproterenol [Isuprel]); treat cause of hypotension (e.g., bradycardia). Use all vasopressors with extreme caution; severe hypotension can result. Use digitalis and diuretics at first signs of cardiac failure; dobutamine, isoproterenol, or glucagon may be required. Use aminophylline or isoproterenol with extreme care for bronchospasm. Use IV glucose for hypoglycemia. Treat other side effects symptomatically and resuscitate as necessary. Hemodialysis is effective in overdose.

ATRACURIUM BESYLATE pH 3.25 to 3.65

(Tracrium)

Usual dose: Must be individualized, depending on previous drugs administered and degree and length of muscle relaxation required. 0.4 to 0.5 mg/kg of body weight initially as an IV bolus. Patient should be unconscious before administration. Reduce dose by one third (0.25 to 0.35 mg/kg) if isoflurane or enflurane are used as general anesthetics. Reduce dose to 0.3 to 0.4 mg/kg if using halothane anesthetic or following succinylcholine administration. Determine need for maintenance dose based on beginning symptoms of neuromuscular blockade reversal determined by a peripheral nerve stimulator. A maintenance dose of 0.08 to 0.10 mg/kg is required in approximately 25 to 40 minutes and every 15 to 25 minutes. This is accomplished with 2 to 15 mcg/kg/min as a continuous IV infusion to maintain muscle relaxation.

Infant dose: *1 month to 2 years of age:* 0.3 to 0.4 mg/kg for infants and children under halothane anesthesia. Maintenance dose may be required on a more frequent basis.

Dilution: Initial IV bolus may be given undiluted. Maintenance dose must be further diluted in normal saline or 5% dextrose in water or normal saline, and given as a continuous infusion titrated to symptoms of neuromuscular blockade reversal. 20 mg (2 ml) diluted in 98 ml yields 200 mcg/ml. 50 mg (5 ml) diluted in 95 ml yields 500 mcg/ml.

Rate of administration: Initial IV bolus over 30 to 60 seconds. Maintenance dose: In the 200 mcg/ml dilution, 5 mcg/kg/min will be delivered by a rate of 0.025 ml/kg/min or 1.75 ml/min for a 70 kg man. Adjust rate to specific dose desired. Drug literature has additional rate calculations.

Actions: A nondepolarizing skeletal muscle relaxant with a duration of blockade one third to one half that of tubocurarine chloride (curare). A less potent histamine releaser than tubocurarine or metocurine. Causes paralysis by interfering with neural transmission at the myoneural junction. Onset of action is dose dependent.

Produces maximum neuromuscular blockade within 3 to 5 minutes and lasts about 25 minutes. It may take another 30 minutes or up to several hours before complete recovery occurs. Excreted as metabolites in bile and urine. Crosses the placental barrier.

Indications and uses: (1) Adjunctive to general anesthesia; (2) facilitate endotracheal intubation; (3) management of patients undergoing mechanical ventilation.

Precautions: (1) For IV use only. (2) Administered only by or under the direct observation of the anesthesiologist. (3) This drug produces apnea. Controlled artificial ventilation with oxygen must be continuous and under direct observation at all times. Maintain a patent airway. (4) Use a peripheral nerve stimulator to monitor response to atracurium and avoid overdosage. (5) Repeated doses have no cumulative effect if recovery is allowed to begin prior to administration. (6) Use extreme caution in patients with significant cardiovascular disease, a history of allergies or allergic reactions. (7) Myasthenia gravis and other neuromuscular diseases increase sensitivity to drug. Can cause critical reactions. (8) Potentiated by hypokalemia, some carcinomas, general anesthetics (e.g., enflurane, isoflurane, halothane), neuromuscular blocking antibiotics (e.g., clindamycin [Cleocin], kanamycin [Kantrex], gentamicin [Garamycin]), polypeptide antibiotics (e.g., bacitracin, colistimethate), diuretics, diazepam (Valium) and other muscle relaxants, magnesium sulfate, quinidine, morphine, meperidine, procainamide (Pronestyl), succinylcholine, verapamil, and others. Reduced dose of atracurium must be used with caution. (9) Antagonized by acetylcholine, anticholinesterases, azathioprine, carbamazepine, phenytoin, and theophylline. (10) Succinylcholine must show signs of wearing off before atracurium is given. Use caution. (11) Patient may be conscious and completely unable to communicate by any means. Has no analgesic properties. Respiratory depression with morphine may be preferred in some patients requiring mechanical ventilation. (12) Action is altered by dehydration, electrolyte imbalance, body temperatures, and acid-base imbalance. (13) Bradycardia fairly common since atracurium will not counteract the bradycardia produced by many anesthetic agents or vagal stimulation. (14) Use in pregnancy only if use justifies potential risk to fetus. Has been used during cesarean section; monitor infant carefully. Use caution during lactation. (15) Safety for use in infants under 1 month of age not established. (16) Store under refrigeration.

Contraindications: Known hypersensitivity to atracurium.

Incompatible with: Alkaline solutions, barbiturates. Do not mix in the same syringe or simultaneously through the same needle. A precipitate will form.

Side effects: Prolonged action resulting in respiratory insufficiency or apnea. Airway closure caused by relaxation of epiglottis, pharynx, and tongue muscles. Hypersensitivity reactions including anaphylaxis are possible. Bradycardia, bronchospasm, dyspnea, flushing, histamine release, hypotension, laryngospasm, reaction at injection site, shock, and tachycardia may occur.

Antidote: All side effects are medical emergencies. Treat symptomatically. Controlled artificial ventilation must be continuous. Pyridostigmine (Mestinon) or neostigmine (Prostigmin) given with atropine will probably reverse the muscle relaxation. Not effective in all situations; may aggravate severe overdosage. Resuscitate as necessary.

ATROPINE SULFATE

pH 3.5 to 6.5

Usual dose: *Bradyarrhythmias:* 0.5 to 1.0 mg bolus repeated every 5 minutes up to a total dose of 2 mg can be used to achieve a desired pulse rate above 60. Subsequent doses of 0.3 to 1.0 mg may be given at 4- to 6-hour intervals.

Smooth muscle relaxation and suppression of secretions: 0.4 to 0.6 mg every 3 to 4 hours.

During surgery: Above doses appropriate except during cyclopropane anesthesia. Start with 0.4 mg or less. Administer very slowly to avoid ventricular dysrhythmias.

Cardiac asystole: 1.0 mg bolus recommended in asystole with specific protocol. May be repeated in 5 minutes.

Antidote for acute poisoning: Up to 3 mg may be given in a single dose.

Pediatric dose: *Bradyarrhythmias:* 0.02 mg/kg of body weight can be used to achieve a pulse rate above 80 in a distressed infant under 6 months or above 60 in a child. May be repeated in 5 minutes. Maximum total dose for a child is 1 mg; for an adolescent 2 mg.

Smooth muscle relaxation and suppression of secretions: 0.1 mg in the newborn; up to 0.6 mg for a 12 year old. Usually given SC.

Dilution: May be given undiluted, but many prefer to dilute desired dose in at least 10 ml of sterile water for injection. Do not add to IV solutions. Inject through Y-tube or three-way stopcock of infusion set.

Rate of administration: 1.0 mg or fraction thereof over 1 minute.

Actions: Atropine is an anticholinergic drug and a potent belladonna alkaloid. It produces local, central, and peripheral effects on the body. The main therapeutic uses of atropine are peripheral, affecting smooth muscle, cardiac muscle, and gland cells. This drug can interfere with vagal stimuli. It is widely distributed in all body fluids. Excretion is through all body fluids, but chiefly through urine and bile. Crosses placental barrier. Secreted in breast milk.

Indications and uses: (1) Treatment of sinus bradycardia, syncope from Stokes-Adams syndrome, and high-degree atrioventricular block with profound bradycardia; (2) cardiac asystole; (3) suppression of salivary, gastric, pancreatic, and respiratory secretions; (4) to relieve pylorospasm, hypertonicity of the small intestine, and hypermotility of the colon; (5) to relieve biliary and ureteral colic; (6) antidote for overdose of choline ester; (7) antidote for specific poisons such as organophosphorous insecticides, nerve gases, and mushroom poisoning *(Amanita muscaria);* (8) used in combination with many other drugs to produce a desired effect.

Precautions: (1) Use caution in prostatic hypertrophy, chronic lung disease, infants and small children, the elderly and debilitated, in urinary retention, and during cyclopropane anesthesia. (2) Potentiated by amantadine, antidepressants (e.g., amitriptyline [Elavil]), antihistamines, antiparkinson agents, benzodiazepines (e.g., diazepam [Valium]), buclizine, isoniazid, MAO inhibitors (e.g., pargyline [Eutonyl]), meperidine (Demerol), orphenadrine, phenothiazines (e.g., prochlorperazine [Compazine]), procainamide (Pronestyl), and quinidine. Reduced dose of either or both drugs may be indicated. (3) Antagonistic to many drugs, such as acetylcholine, echothiophate (Phospholine), edrophonium (Tensilon), methacholine (Mecholyl), metoclopramide, morphine, and pyridostigmine (Mestilon). (4) Use caution with cholinergics, digitalis, digoxin, diphenhydramine, levodopa, and neostigmine. May cause adverse effects. (5) Antagonized by guanethidine, histamine, and reserpine. (6) Potentiates atenolol (Tenormin), sympathomimetics (e.g., terbutaline), nitrofurantoin, and thiazide diuretics. (7) Safety for use in pregnancy, lactation, and children not established. Toxicity to nursing infants probable. When used for bradycardia or asystole in infants and small children, vagolytic doses are required. Smaller doses may cause paradoxical bradycardia. (8) May produce excitement, agitation, or drowsiness in the elderly.

Contraindications: Hypersensitivity to atropine, acute glaucoma, acute hemorrhage with unstable cardiovascular status, asthma, hepatic disease, intestinal atony of the elderly or debilitated, myasthenia gravis, myocardial ischemia, obstructive disease of the GI or GU tracts, paralytic ileus, renal disease, pyloric stenosis, severe ulcerative colitis, tachycardia, toxic megacolon.

Incompatible with: Amobarbital (Amytal), ampicillin (Omnipen), chloramphenicol (Chloromycetin), chlortetracycline (Aureomycin), cimetidine (Tagamet), epinephrine (Adrenalin), heparin, isoproterenol (Isuprel), levarterenol (Levophed), metaraminol (Aramine), methicillin (Staphcillin), methohexital (Brevital), nitrofurantoin (Ivadantin), pentobarbital (Nembutal), promazine (Sparine), sodium bicarbonate, sodium iodide, thiopental (Pentothal), warfarin (Coumadin).

Side effects: *Average dose:* Anhidrosis, anticholinergic psychosis, blurred vision, bradycardia (temporary), dilation of the pupils, dryness of the mouth, flushing, gastroesophageal reflux, heat prostration from decreased sweating, nausea, paralytic ileus, postural hypotension, urinary hesitancy and retention, and vomiting may occur.

Overdose: Coma, death, delirium-elevated blood pressure, fever, paralytic ileus, rash, respiratory failure, stupor, tachycardia.

Antidote: Use standard treatments to manage cardiac dysrhythmias. Physostigmine salicylate (Antilirium) reverses most cardiovascular and CNS effects; however, it may cause profound bradycardia, seizures, or asystole. Administer pilocarpine, 10 mg (H), until the mouth is moist. Sustain physiological functions at a normal level. Use diazepam (Valium), short-acting barbiturates (amobarbital), or chloral hydrate to relieve excitement. Neostigmine methylsulfate (Prostigmin) is an alternate antidote.

AZATHIOPRINE SODIUM pH 9.6

(Imuran)

Usual dose: 3 to 5 mg/kg of body weight/24 hr. Begin treatment within 24 hours of renal homotransplantation. Some authorities recommend doses of 1 to 5 mg/kg for several days previous to transplant. Maintenance dose is 1 to 2 mg/kg/24 hr. Individualized adjustment is imperative and may be required on a daily basis.

Dilution: Each 100 mg should be diluted initially with 10 ml of sterile water for injection. Swirl the vial gently until completely in solution. May be further diluted in a minimum of 50 ml of sterile saline or glucose in saline and given as an infusion. Mixing with alkaline solutions may result in conversion to 6-mercaptopurine.

Rate of administration: A single dose properly diluted over 30 to 60 minutes. Actual range may be 5 minutes to 8 hours.

Actions: An immunosuppressive drug. It is a derivative of the antineoplastic preparation mercaptopurine. Maximum response occurs if administered when antibody response begins. Has a selective action but achieves good response in many situations. Metabolized readily with small amounts excreted in the urine.

Indications and uses: Adjunct to prevent rejection in renal homotransplantation.

Precautions: (1) Oral dosage preferred; begin as soon as feasible. (2) Diluted IV solution must be used within 24 hours. (3) Monitor frequently bone marrow function, red and white blood cell counts, platelet count, and BUN. Drug should be withdrawn or dosage reduced at first sign of abnormally large fall in the leukocyte count or other evidence of persistent bone marrow depression. (4) May increase possibility of malignant tumor growth. (5) Potentiated by allopurinol (Zyloprim). Reduce dose to one third or one fourth of usual. (6) Use caution with other myelosuppressive drugs or radiation therapy. (7) Reduce dosage in impaired kidney function (especially immediately after transplant or with cadaveric kidneys) and in persistent negative nitrogen balance. (8) Observe constantly for signs of infection. (9) Safety for use in pregnancy, lactation, and men and women capable of conception not established. Has mutagenic and teratogenic potential. (10) Toxic hepatitis or biliary stasis may necessitate discontinuing drug. (11) Inhibits nondepolarizing muscle relaxants (e.g., tubocurarine).

Contraindications: Anuria, known hypersensitivity, severe rejection.

Incompatible with: Sufficient information not available. Administer separately. Converts to 6-mercaptopurine in alkaline solutions and sulfhydryl compounds (e.g., cysteine).

Side effects: Alopecia, anemia, anorexia, arthralgia, bleeding, diarrhea, fever, jaundice, leukopenia, nausea, oral lesions, pancreatitis, skin rash, thrombocytopenia, vomiting.

Antidote: Notify the physician of all side effects. Most can be treated symptomatically. Drug may be decreased or discontinued or other immunosuppressive agents utilized. Hematopoietic depression may require temporary or permanent withholding of treatment.

AZLOCILLIN SODIUM pH 6.0 to 8.0

(Azlin)

Usual dose: 100 to 300 mg/kg of body weight/day equally divided in 4 to 6 doses (3 Gm every 4 hours equals 18 Gm/day). Do not exceed 24 Gm/day.

Pediatric dose: *Infants 1 month to children 12 years:* 75 mg/kg of body weight every 4 hours (450 mg/kg/day). Limited data available on use in children.

Dilution: Each 1 Gm or fraction thereof should be diluted with at least 10 ml of sterile water, 5% dextrose, or 0.9% sodium chloride for injection. Shake vigorously to dissolve. Must be further diluted to desired volume (50 to 100 ml) with 5% dextrose in water, 0.45 normal saline, or other compatible infusion solution (see literature) and given as an intermittent infusion. For direct IV administration dilute to a 10% solution.

Rate of administration: *Direct IV:* A single dose properly diluted over 3 to 5 minutes.

Intermittent infusion: A single dose properly diluted over 30 minutes. Discontinue primary IV infusion during administration. Pediatric dose must be given over 30 minutes.

Actions: An extended-spectrum penicillin. Bactericidal against a variety of gram-negative and gram-positive bacteria including aerobic and anaerobic strains. Especially effective against *Pseudomonas.* Well distributed in all body fluids, tissue, bone, and through inflamed meninges. Onset of action is prompt. Crosses placental barrier. Some excretion in urine and breast milk.

Indications and uses: (1) Serious infections of the lower respiratory tract, urinary tract, skin and skin structure, bone and joint infections, and bacterial septicemia caused by susceptible organisms; (2) acute pulmonary exacerbation of cystic fibrosis in children.

Precautions: (1) Stable at room temperature for only 24 hours. (2) Warm to 37° C (98.6° F) in a water bath for 20 minutes if precipitation occurs on refrigeration. Shake vigorously. (3) Slightly darkened color does not affect potency. (4) Frequently used concurrently with aminoglycosides (e.g., gentamicin [Garamycin]), but must be administered in separate infusions; inactivates aminoglycosides. (5) Sensitivity studies indicated to determine susceptibility of the causative organism to azlocillin. (6) Oral probenecid will achieve higher and more prolonged blood levels. May be desirable or may cause toxicity. (7) Watch for early symptoms of allergic reaction. (8) Avoid prolonged use of drug; superinfection caused by overgrowth of nonsusceptible organisms may result. (9) Periodic evaluation of renal, hepatic, and hematopoietic systems and serum potassium is recommended in prolonged therapy. (10) Electrolyte imbalance and cardiac irregularities resulting from high sodium content are very possible. Contains 2.17 mEq sodium per gram. (11) Confirm patency of vein; avoid extravasation or intraarterial injection. Slow infusion rate for pain along venipuncture site. (12) Usual duration of therapy is 7 to 10 days. Continue at least 2 days after symptoms of infection disappear. (13) Reduce dose only in severe renal impairment with creatinine clearance temporarily below 30 ml/min. May be given to patients undergoing hemodialysis and peritoneal dialysis (see literature for dose). (14) Test for syphilis also before treating gonorrhea. (15) Elimination rate markedly reduced in neonates. (16) Concomitant use with beta-adrenergic blockers (e.g., propranolol [Inderal]) may increase risk of anaphylaxis and inhibit treatment. (17) Risk of bleeding with anticoagulants (e.g., heparin) is increased. (18) Inactivated by chloramphenicol, erythromycin, and tetracyclines. Bactericidal action is actually negated by these drugs. (19) Potentiates cefotaxime. (20) Neuromuscular excitability or convulsions may be caused by higher than normal doses. (21) May decrease effectiveness of oral contraceptives; breakthrough bleeding or pregnancy could result.

Contraindications: History of sensitivity to multiple allergens, neonates, penicillin sensitivity.

Incompatible with: Aminoglycosides (e.g., amikacin, colistimethate, gentamicin, kanamycin, streptomycin, tobramycin), amphotericin B (Fungizone), chloramphenicol, lincomycin, oxytetracycline, polymyxin B, promethazine (Phenergan), tetracycline (Achromycin), vitamin B with C.

Side effects: Anaphylaxis; bleeding; convulsions; decreased hemoglobin or hematocrit; decreased uric acid level; diarrhea; eosinophilia; elevated SGOT, SGPT, and BUN; fever; hypokalemia; interstitial nephritis; leukopenia; nausea; neuromuscular excitability; neutropenia; pruritus; pseudoproteinuria; skin rash; taste sensation (abnormal); thrombocytopenia; thrombophlebitis; urticaria; vomiting.

Antidote: Notify the physician immediately of any adverse symptoms. For severe symptoms, discontinue the drug, treat allergic reaction (antihistamines, epinephrine, corticosteroids), and resuscitate as necessary. Hemodialysis is effective in overdose.

AZTREONAM pH 4.5 to 7.5

(Azactam)

Usual dose: Range is from 500 mg to 2 Gm every 6, 8, or 12 hours. Dosage based on severity of infection. Use the full suggested dose. Normal renal function required. Continue for at least 2 days after all symptoms of infection subside. Do not exceed 8 Gm/24 hr.

Dilution: *Direct IV:* Dilute a single dose with 6 to 10 ml of sterile water for injection. Shake immediately and vigorously.

Intermittent IV: Initially dilute each single dose with a minimum of 3 ml of sterile water for injection. Shake immediately and vigorously. Must be further diluted in at least 50 ml of 5% dextrose in water, 0.9% sodium chloride, or other compatible infusion solutions for injection for each 1 Gm of aztreonam (see literature). Solution desired is not greater than 20 mg/ml. Available in 15 ml vials and 100 ml infusion bottles.

Rate of administration: *Direct IV:* A single dose equally distributed over 3 to 5 minutes.

Intermittent IV: A single dose over 20 to 60 minutes. May be given through Y-tube or three-way stopcock of infusion set. Do not infuse simultaneously with other drugs or solutions except in proven compatibility. Flush common IV tubing before and after administration.

Actions: A new class of antibiotic called monobactam. Bactericidal through inhibition of bacterial cell wall synthesis to a wide spectrum of specific gram-negative aerobic organisms including *Pseudomonas aeruginosa*. Effective against many otherwise resistant organisms. Therapeutic levels absorbed into many body fluids and tissues. Primarily excreted in the urine with some excretion through feces. Crosses placental barrier. Secreted in breast milk.

Indications and uses: (1) Treatment of serious lower respiratory tract, urinary tract, skin and skin structure, gynecological, and intraabdominal infections and bacterial septicemia. Most effective against specific organisms (see literature); (2) adjunctive therapy to surgery for the management of infections.

Precautions: (1) Specific studies are indicated to identify the causative organism and susceptibility to aztreonam. (2) Reduce total daily dose in the elderly and if renal function impaired. Calculated according to degree of impairment (see literature). (3) Avoid prolonged use of drug; superinfection caused by overgrowth of nonsusceptible organisms may result. (4) Use concentrated solution for direct IV immediately and discard any unused solution. Solution diluted for infusion is stable for 48 hours at room temperature or refrigerated for up to 7 days. When specific diluents are used, solution diluted for infusion may be frozen for up to 3 months. Thaw at room temperature (see instructions); do not refreeze. Usually light yellow, may become slightly pink on standing, does not affect potency. (5) Watch for early symptoms of allergic reaction. Use extreme caution in the penicillin-sensitive patient. (6) Monitor renal and hepatic function, especially in the elderly. (7) Adverse interaction may occur with β-lactamase–inducing antibiotics (e.g., cefoxitin, imipenem); do not use concurrently. (8) May be used concomitantly with aminoglycosides in severe infections. Nephrotoxicity and ototoxicity can be markedly increased when both drugs utilized. (9) Use only if absolutely necessary in pregnancy and lactation. Consider discontinuation of breast feeding. (10) Safety for use in infants and children not established. (11) Probenecid and furosemide do increase blood levels; not clinically significant. (12) May cause thrombophlebitis. Use small needles and large veins, and rotate infusion sites. (13) Can produce therapeutic serum levels given intraperitoneally in dialysis fluid. (14) Compatible and stable for 48 hours with clindamycin, gentamicin, tobramycin, or cefazolin in normal saline or 5% dextrose in water. Compatible and stable for 24 hours with ampicillin in normal saline or for 2 hours in 5% dextrose in water. Mixing of these drugs is not suggested by manufacturers of the other drugs at this time.

Contraindications: Known sensitivity to aztreonam.

Incompatible with: Ampicillin, cephradine (Velosef), metronidazole (Flagyl IV), nafcillin.

Side effects: Full scope of allergic reactions including anaphylaxis. Burning, discomfort, and pain at injection site; diarrhea; nausea and vomiting; pseudomembranous colitis; and rash occur most frequently. Abdominal cramps; altered taste; confusion; diaphoresis; diplopia; dizziness; dyspnea; elevated alkaline phosphatase, SGOT, SGPT, and serum creatinine; eosinophilia; erythema multiforme; exfoliative dermatitis; fever; halitosis; headache; hematologic changes; hepatitis; hypotension; insomnia; jaundice; mouth ulcer; nasal congestion; numb tongue; paresthesia; petechiae; positive Coombs' test; prolonged PT and PTT; pruritus; purpura; transient ECG changes (ventricular bigeminy and PVCs); seizures; sneezing; tinnitus; urticaria; vaginitis; and vertigo can occur.

Antidote: Notify physician of any side effects. Discontinue the drug if indicated. Treat allergic reaction as indicated and resuscitate as necessary. Mild cases of colitis may respond to discontinuation of drug. Oral vancomycin is the treatment of choice for antibiotic-related pseudomembranous colitis. Hemodialysis or peritoneal dialysis may be useful in overdose.

BENZQUINAMIDE HYDROCHLORIDE pH 3.0 to 4.0

(Emete-Con)

Usual dose: 25 mg (0.2 to 0.4 mg/kg of body weight) as initial dose, one time only. If additional doses indicated, give IM.

Dilution: Each 50 mg must be diluted with 2.2 ml of sterile water for injection (25 mg/ml). May be administered direct IV through Y-tube or three-way stopcock of infusion tubing. Further dilution is not recommended.

Rate of administration: A single dose over a minimum of 30 to 60 seconds.

Actions: Chemically unrelated to phenothiazines and other antiemetics. Exhibits antiemetic, antihistaminic, mild anticholinergic, and sedative actions. Mechanism of action unknown. Effective within minutes and lasts about 1 hour. Metabolized in the liver. Some excretion in the urine.

Indications and uses: Prevention and treatment of nausea and vomiting during anesthesia and surgery.

Precautions: (1) Prophylactic use restricted to specific situations under direction of the anesthesiologist. (2) Monitor blood pressure closely. (3) Markedly reduce dose of benzquinamide in patients receiving pressor agents (e.g., epinephrine). (4) Sudden hypertension, PVCs, and PACs (transient) may result with IV injection. Limit use to patients without cardiovascular disease, not receiving preanesthetic or concomitant cardiovascular drugs. (5) Antiemetic action may mask signs of drug overdose or may obscure diagnosis of conditions such as intestinal obstruction or brain tumor. (6) Safety for use in pregnancy and children is not established. (7) Discard diluted solution after 14 days at room temperature.

Contraindications: Cardiovascular disease, hypersensitivity to benzquinamide hydrochloride.

Incompatible with: Chlordiazepoxide (Librium), diazepam (Valium), pentobarbital (Nembutal), phenobarbital (Luminal), secobarbital (Seconal), sodium chloride, thiopental (Pentothal).

Side effects: Allergic reactions, atrial fibrillation, blurred vision, diaphoresis, dizziness, dry mouth, excitement, fever, flushing, hiccups, hypertension, hypotension, nervousness, PACs, PVCs, salivation, tremors, weakness.

Antidote: Notify the physician of side effects. Depending on severity, physician may discontinue the drug. For overdose treatment will be symptomatic and supportive. Atropine may be helpful. Resuscitate as necessary.

BENZTROPINE MESYLATE pH 5.0 to 8.0

(Cogentin)

Usual dose: 1 to 2 mg. May be increased gradually to 4 to 6 mg/24 hr if required.

Dilution: 1 ml of prepared solution equals 1 mg. May be given undiluted.

Rate of administration: 1 mg or fraction thereof over 1 minute.

Actions: Anticholinergic and antihistaminic agent. Effectively relieves tremor, rigidity, drooling, dysphagia, gait disturbances, pain caused by muscle spasm, and other annoying symptoms of parkinsonism. Provides excellent relief in combination with levodopa. Onset of action is prompt by IV or IM route. Primarily excreted in the urine.

Indications and uses: Parkinsonism: drug-induced (especially phenothiazines and reserpine), postencephalitic, idiopathic, or arteriosclerotic.

Precautions: (1) IV route seldom used except in acute drug reactions or psychotic patients. (2) IM and oral routes are satisfactory. (3) Has a potent cumulative action; the patient must be under close observation. (4) Observe carefully in patients with hypotension, narrow angle glaucoma, myasthenia gravis, tachycardia, prostatic hypertrophy, in children over 3 years, and in the elderly. (5) Dosage adjustment is required if an inability to move particular muscle groups persists. (6) Treatment of drug-induced parkinsonism can precipitate toxic psychosis. (7) Side effects may be potentiated by alcohol, antihistamines, barbiturates, narcotic analgesics, phenothiazines, quinidine, and tricyclic antidepressants. (8) May reduce amount of levodopa absorbed in the GI tract. (9) Inhibits haloperidol and phenothiazines. (10) May potentiate oral digoxin. (11) Potentiated by isoniazid, MAO inhibitors. (12) Do not discontinue other antiparkinsonian drugs abruptly; reduce gradually. (13) May inhibit lactation.

Contraindications: Known hypersensitivity, pregnancy, children under 3 years. Ineffective in tardive dyskinesia.

Incompatible with: No specific incompatibilities are known.

Side effects: *Average dose:* Allergic reactions including skin rash, blurred vision, constipation, depression, dizziness, dry mouth, listlessness, nausea, nervousness, numbness of the fingers, vomiting.

Overdose: Anhidrosis, circulatory collapse, coma, dilation of the pupils, dry mucous membranes, flushed skin, hyperpyrexia, incipient glaucoma, paralytic ileus, respiratory depression, tachycardia, urinary retention.

Antidote: Notify the physician of all side effects. Symptoms of an average dose may be relieved by reducing the dose or discontinuing for a day or so and then resuming at a lesser dose. Treat overdose symptomatically, including respiratory support. Physostigmine salicylate (Antilirium) will reverse symptoms of anticholinergic intoxication. Observe for relapses up to 12 hours. Diazepam (Valium) reduces CNS excitation. Resuscitate as necessary.

BIPERIDEN LACTATE pH 4.8 to 5.8

(Akineton)

Usual dose: 2 mg. Repeat every 30 minutes until symptoms are relieved. Do not exceed 4 doses of 2 mg in 24 hours.

Dilution: May be given undiluted.

Rate of administration: 2 mg or fraction thereof over 1 minute.

Actions: An anticholinergic agent with atropine-like effects. Inhibits the parasympathetic nervous system. Effectively relieves tremor, rigidity, drooling, dysphagia, gait disturbances, and pain caused by muscle spasm. Primarily excreted in the urine.

Indications and uses: (1) Control of drug-induced extrapyramidal disorders (reserpine, phenothiazines); (2) parkinsonism: postencephalitic, arteriosclerotic, and idiopathic.

Precautions: (1) IV route seldom used except in acute drug reactions or psychotic patients; use IM route for children. (2) Has a potent cumulative action; the patient must be under close observation. (3) Use caution in hypotension, hypertension, and tachycardia; cardiac, liver, and kidney disorders; narrow-angle glaucoma; myasthenia gravis; obstructive disease of GI or GU tracts; prostatic hypertrophy; pregnancy and lactation; in children; and in the elderly. (4) Treatment of drug-induced parkinsonism can precipitate toxic psychosis. (5) Side effects may be potentiated by alcohol, antihistamines, barbiturates, narcotic analgesics, phenothiazines, quinidine, and tricyclic antidepressants. (6) May reduce amount of levodopa absorbed in the GI tract. (7) Potentiated by isoniazid, MAO inhibitors (e.g., pargyline [Eutonyl]). (8) Inhibits haloperidol and phenothiazines. (9) May potentiate oral digoxin. (10) May inhibit lactation.

Contraindications: Known hypersensitivity. Ineffective in tardive dyskinesia.

Incompatible with: No specific information available. Consider atropine similarities.

Side effects: *Average doses:* Allergic reactions including skin rash, blurred vision, constipation, depression, dizziness, dry mouth, listlessness, nausea, nervousness, numbness of the fingers, vomiting.

Overdose: Anhidrosis, circulatory collapse, coma, dilation of the pupils, dry mucous membranes, flushed skin, hyperpyrexia, incipient glaucoma, paralytic ileus, respiratory depression, tachycardia, urinary retention.

Antidote: Notify the physician of all side effects. Symptoms of an average dose may be relieved by reducing the dose or discontinuing for a day or so and then resuming at a lesser dose. Treat overdose symptomatically, including respiratory support. Physostigmine salicylate (Antilirium) will reverse symptoms of anticholinergic intoxication. Observe for relapses up to 12 hours. Diazepam (Valium) reduces CNS excitation. Resuscitate as necessary.

BLEOMYCIN SULFATE pH 4.5 to 6.0

(Blenoxane)

Usual dose: 0.25 to 0.5 unit/kg of body weight/24 hr (10 to 20 units/M^2), once or twice weekly. The first 2 doses in lymphoma patients should not exceed 2 units in order to rule out hypersensitivity.

Hodgkin's disease: Dosage as above. After a 50% response, a maintenance dose of 1 unit/24 hr or 5 units weekly is recommended.

Dilution: *Specific techniques required, see Precautions.* Each 15 units or fraction thereof must be diluted with 5 ml or more of sterile water for injection, 5% dextrose, or sodium chloride for injection. Further dilution with 50 to 100 ml of same solution is recommended. May be given through Y-tube or three-way stopcock of a free-flowing IV.

Rate of administration: Each 15 units or fraction thereof over 10 minutes.

Actions: An antibiotic antineoplastic agent, cell cycle phase specific, that seems to act by splitting and fragmentation of double-stranded DNA, leading to chromosomal damage. It localizes in tumors. Improvement usually noted within 2 weeks. Well distributed in skin, lungs, kidneys, peritoneum, and lymphatics. About 40% excreted in the urine.

Indications and uses: (1) Testicular carcinoma; may induce complete remission with vinblastine and cisplatin; (2) a palliative treatment, adjunct to surgery or radiation, in patients not responsive to other chemotherapeutic agents, or those with squamous cell carcinoma of the skin; head; esophagus; neck; GU tract including the cervix, vulva, scrotum, and penis; in Hodgkin's disease; and other lymphomas.

Precautions: (1) Follow guidelines for handling cytotoxic agents recommended. See Appendix p. 677. (2) Administered by or under the direction of the physician specialist. (3) Determine patency of vein; avoid extravasation. (4) Obtain a baseline chest x-ray, and recheck every 1 to 2 weeks to detect pulmonary changes. (5) Monitor renal, hepatic, and central nervous systems and skin for symptoms of toxicity. (6) Dosage based on average weight in presence of edema or ascites. (7) Safety for use in pregnancy or lactation not established. (8) Do not administer vaccines or chloroquine to patients receiving antineoplastic drugs. (9) May be used with other antineoplastic drugs to achieve tumor remission. (10) May cause severe anaphylaxis with lymphomas; use a test dose. (11) Pulmonary toxicity increases markedly with advancing age or larger doses; will occur at lower doses when bleomycin is used in combination with other antineoplastic agents. To identify subclinical pulmonary toxicity, monitor pulmonary diffusion capacity for carbon monoxide monthly. Should remain 30% to 35% above pretreatment value. Most toxic when total cumulative dose exceeds 350 to 450 units. (12) Vascular toxicities (e.g., myocardial infarction, CVA, thrombotic microangiopathy, cerebral arteritis) or Raynaud's phenomenon have occurred rarely when bleomycin is used in combination with other antineoplastic agents. (13) May decrease GI absorption of digoxin and hydantoins (e.g., phenytoin). (14) Maintain adequate hydration. (15) Prophylactic antiemetics may reduce nausea and vomiting and increase patient comfort. (16) Observe closely for all signs of infection.

(17) Aspirin and diphenhydramine (Benadryl) may be used prophylactically to reduce incidence of fever and anaphylaxis. (18) Diluted solution stable at room temperature for 24 hours.

Contraindications: Known hypersensitivity to bleomycin, elderly patients with pulmonary disease.

Incompatible with: Amino acids, aminophylline, ascorbic acid, diazepam (Valium), furosemide (Lasix), riboflavin, and sulfhydryl groups (e.g., cysteine). Consider toxicity and specific use.

Side effects: *Minor:* Alopecia, anorexia, chills, dyspnea, fever, hypotension, nausea, phlebitis (infrequent), rales, tenderness of the skin, tumor site pain, vomiting, weight loss.

Major: Anaphylaxis (up to 6 hours after test dose), chest pain (acute with sudden onset suggestive of pleuropericarditis), pneumonitis, pulmonary fibrosis, skin toxicity (including nodules on hands, desquamation of skin, hyperpigmentation, and gangrene).

Antidote: Notify the physician of all side effects. Minor side effects will be treated symptomatically. Discontinue the drug immediately and notify the physician of any symptom of major side effects. Provide immediate treatment (epinephrine [Adrenalin] and diphenhydramine [Benadryl] for anaphylaxis, antibiotics and steroids for pneumonitis) or supportive therapy as indicated.

BRETYLIUM TOSYLATE pH 4.2 to 7.0

(✦ Bretylate, Bretylol)

Usual dose: *Ventricular fibrillation:* 5 mg/kg of body weight. Increase to 10 mg/kg and repeat at 15- to 30-minute intervals if dysrhythmia persists. A total dose of 40 mg/kg/24 hr has been given without ill effects.

Other ventricular dysrhythmias: 5 to 10 mg/kg by IV infusion. Repeat in 1 to 2 hours if dysrhythmia persists.

Maintenance dose: 5 to 10 mg/kg by infusion every 6 hours or a continuous infusion at 1 to 2 mg/min. Replace with oral antiarrhythmic therapy as soon as practical, usually within 24 hours.

Dilution: May be given undiluted in ventricular fibrillation. For other ventricular dysrhythmias each dose must be diluted with 50 ml or more of 5% dextrose in water or normal saline to be given as an intermittent infusion. Larger amounts may be further diluted in any amount of the above solutions and given as a continuous infusion (1 Gm in 1,000 ml equals 1 mg/ml).

Rate of administration: *Ventricular fibrillation:* A single dose over 15 to 30 seconds.

Intermittent infusion: A single dose over a minimum of 10 to 30 minutes.

Continuous infusion: 1 to 2 mg diluted solution/min. Use an infusion pump or microdrip (60 gtt/ml). Adjust as indicated by progress in patient's condition.

Actions: A quaternary ammonium compound with antiarrhythmic effects. It increases the ventricular fibrillation threshold, suppresses ventricular dysrhythmias and aberrant impulses, and increases the refractory period without increasing heart rate. Probably effective through its adrenergic blocking action. Antifibrillatory effects occur within 15 to 20 minutes; suppression of premature beats requires constant plasma levels. Half-life ranges from 4 to 17 hours. Excreted in the urine.

Indications and uses: Prophylaxis and treatment of ventricular fibrillation and treatment of life-threatening ventricular dysrhythmias that have failed to respond to adequate doses of lidocaine or procainamide.

Precautions: (1) Monitor the patient's ECG and BP continuously. (2) Keep patient in supine position; postural hypotension is almost always present. Tolerance to hypotensive effect may develop after several days. (3) Correct dehydration or hypovolemia. (4) May aggravate digitalis toxicity; use with caution if patient receiving digitalis. (5) May cause severe hypotension if fixed cardiac output present (aortic stenosis, pulmonary hypertension). (6) May cause transient hypertension and increased frequency of dysrhythmias. (7) Used during pregnancy or in children only in life-threatening situations. (8) Use caution if renal function impaired. (9) Will potentiate catecholamines (e.g., dopamine [Intropin]); use diluted solution and monitor BP closely when indicated. (10) Reduce dose under ECG monitoring after 3 to 5 days; then discontinue. (11) Observe for increased anginal pain in susceptible patients.

Contraindications: None when used as indicated.

Incompatible with: Phenytoin (Dilantin). Is physically compatible with calcium chloride, dopamine, lidocaine, nitroglycerin, potassium chloride, procainamide, and verapamil; however, therapeutic rates of administration may differ.

Side effects: Anginal attacks, bradycardia, dizziness, hypotension and postural hypotension, increased frequency of PVCs, lightheadedness, nausea and vomiting, substernal pressure, syncope, transitory hypertension, vertigo.

Antidote: Notify the physician of all side effects. Nausea and vomiting may subside with reduction in rate of administration. Use dopamine to correct hypotension. Resuscitate as necessary.

BROMPHENIRAMINE MALEATE pH 6.8 to 7.0

(Codimal-A, Cophene-B, Dehist, Histaject, Nasahist B, ND Stat Revised, Oraminic II)

Usual dose: 10 mg initially. 5 to 20 mg may be given. Repeat every 3 to 12 hours as indicated. Do not exceed 40 mg/24 hr.

Pedriatric dose: Under 12 years, 0.5 mg/kg of body weight/24 hr or 15 mg/M^2/24 hr divided into 3 or 4 doses.

Dilution: May be given undiluted, but further dilution of each ml with 10 ml normal saline for injection is preferred to reduce incidence of side effects. May be added to normal saline or 5% dextrose in water and given as an infusion. May be added to whole blood.

Rate of administration: A single dose over 1 minute. A single dose in an IV infusion may be given at the desired or ordered rate.

Actions: An antihistamine with anticholinergic and sedative effects. Acts by blocking the effects of histamine at various receptor sites. Either eliminates allergic reaction or greatly modifies it. Readily absorbed, widely distributed, and excreted in changed form in the urine.

Indications and uses: (1) Prevention or reduction of allergic reactions to blood or plasma; (2) treatment of anaphylactic reactions; (3) treatment of other allergic conditions if IV route indicated.

Precautions: (1) IM or SC use is generally preferred after an initial IV dose. (2) Note label; only the 10 mg/ml brompheniramine may be used IV. (3) Often used in conjunction with epinephrine. (4) Use caution in patients with a history of bronchial asthma, cardiovascular disease, renal disease, diabetes, hypertension, hyperthyroidism, increased intravascular pressure, and the elderly. (5) Potentiates CNS depressants (alcohol, analgesics, antianxiety agents, hypnotics, sedatives, tranquilizers). Reduced dosage of CNS depressant is indicated. (6) Keep patient in recumbent position. (7) Protect from light to prevent discoloration in ampoule. (8) If necessary, warm to dissolve any crystals that may have formed.

Contraindications: Hypersensitivity to antihistamines; pregnancy; lactation; newborn or premature infants; patients on MAO inhibitors (e.g., pargyline [Eutonyl]); narrow-angle glaucoma; stenosing peptic ulcer; symptomatic prostatic hypertrophy; asthmatic attack; bladder neck obstruction; pyloroduodenal obstruction.

Incompatible with: Aminophylline, insulin, iodipamide meglumine (Cholografin), pentobarbital (Nembutal).

Side effects: Anaphylaxis; confusion; convulsions; death; dizziness; dryness of mouth, nose, and throat; hallucinations; headache; hypertension; hypotension; hysteria; nausea; palpitations; paresthesias; sedation; tachycardia; thickening of bronchial secretions; urinary retention; vomiting; wheezing.

Antidote: Notify the physician of all side effects. Most will subside after the drug is discontinued or will respond to symptomatic treatment. Anticonvulsant barbiturates or analeptics (e.g., doxapram [Dopram]) may increase toxicity. Treat hypotension promptly to avoid cardiovascular collapse. Use dopamine (Intropin), norepinephrine, or phenylephrine. Epinephrine will cause further hypotension. Propranolol (Inderal) is indicated for ventricular dysrhythmias. Treat convulsions with diazepam (Valium). Avoid analeptics (e.g., caffeine); will cause convulsions. Resuscitate as necessary.

BUMETANIDE — pH 7.0

(Bumex)

Usual dose: 0.5 to 1.0 mg. May be repeated at 2- to 3-hour intervals. Do not exceed 10 mg/24 hr.

Dilution: May be given undiluted. Not usually added to IV solutions but compatible with 5% dextrose in water, 0.9% sodium chloride, and lactated Ringer's infusion solutions. Usually given through Y-tube or three-way stopcock of infusion set.

Rate of administration: A single dose direct IV over 1 to 2 minutes.

Actions: A sulfonamide diuretic, antihypertensive, and antihypercalcemic agent related to the thiazides. A loop diuretic agent. Extremely potent and has a rapid onset of action. Effectiveness is noted within 5 minutes and may last for 4 hours. Apparently acts on the proximal and distal ends of the tubule and the ascending limb of the loop of Henle to excrete water, sodium, chlorides, and potassium. Will produce diuresis in alkalosis or acidosis. Rapidly absorbed and distributed, it is excreted unchanged in the urine.

Indications and uses: (1) Congestive heart failure; (2) acute pulmonary edema; (3) cirrhosis of the liver with ascites; (4) renal diseases including the nephrotic syndrome; (5) edema unresponsive to other diuretic agents; (6) diuresis in patients allergic to furosemide.

Precautions: (1) Can be used for patients allergic to furosemide. 1 mg to 40 mg ratio (bumetanide to furosemide) is used to determine dose. (2) Use only freshly prepared solutions for infusion. Discard after 24 hours. (3) Do not give concurrently with indomethacin (Indocin), probenecid, or lithium. (4) May precipitate excessive diuresis with water and electrolyte depletion. Routine checks on electrolyte panel, CO_2, and BUN are necessary during therapy. Potassium chloride replacement may be required. (5) May be used concurrently with aldosterone antagonists (e.g., spironolactone [Aldactone]) for more effective diuresis and to prevent excessive potassium loss. (6) Potentiates antihypertensive drugs, salicylates, muscle relaxants (e.g., tubocurarine [Curare]), and hypotensive effect of other diuretics and MAO inhibitors (e.g., pargyline [Eutonyl]). (7) May cause transient deafness in doses exceeding the usual or in conjunction with ototoxic drugs (e.g., cisplatin, dihydrostreptomycin, kanamycin). (8) May increase blood glucose; has precipitated diabetes mellitus. May lower serum calcium level, causing tetany; and in rare instances precipitates an acute attack of gout. (9) May cause cardiac dysrhythmias with digitalis, ethacrynic acid (Edecrin), or any condition causing hypokalemia; increased toxicity with tetracycline.

Contraindications: Anuria, known hypersensitivity to bumetanide. Use caution and improve basic condition first in hepatic coma, electrolyte depletion, and advanced cirrhosis of the liver.

Incompatible with: Dobutamine (Dobutrex), milrinone (Primacor). Note Precautions.

Side effects: Usually occur in prolonged therapy, seriously ill patients, or following large doses.

Minor: Abdominal pain, arthritic pain, azotemia, dizziness, ECG changes, elevated serum creatinine, encephalopathy, headache, hyperglycemia, hyperuricemia, hypochloremia, hyponatremia, hypotension, impaired hearing, muscle cramps, nausea, pruritus, rash.

Major: Anaphylactic shock, blood volume reduction, circulatory collapse, dehydration, excessive diuresis, hypokalemia, metabolic acidosis, vascular thrombosis and embolism.

Antidote: If minor side effects are noted, discontinue the drug and notify the physician, who may treat the side effects symptomatically and continue the drug. If side effects are progressive or any major side effect occurs, discontinue the drug immediately and notify the physician. Treatment of major side effects is symptomatic and aggressive and includes fluid and electrolyte replacement. Resuscitate as necessary.

BUPRENORPHINE HYDROCHLORIDE

pH 3.5 to 5.5

(Buprenex)

Usual dose: 0.3 mg (1 ml). Repeat every 6 hours as necessary. May be repeated in 30 to 60 minutes, if indicated. Reduce dose by one half in high-risk patients (e.g., elderly or debilitated, respiratory disease), when other CNS depressants have been given, and in the immediate postoperative period (see precautions). These dose recommendations have been lowered because of excessive respiratory depression with doses up to 0.6 mg.

Dilution: May be given undiluted.

Rate of administration: A single dose over 3 to 5 minutes. May be titrated according to symptom relief and respiratory rate.

Actions: A synthetic narcotic agonist-antagonist analgesic. Thirty times as potent as morphine in analgesic effect (0.3 mg equivalent to 10 mg morphine) and has the antagonist effect of naloxone in larger doses. Does produce respiratory depression. Pain relief is effected in 2 to 3 minutes and lasts up to 6 hours. Metabolized in the liver. Primarily excreted through feces. Crosses the placental barrier. May be secreted in breast milk.

Indications and uses: Relief of moderate to severe pain.

Precautions: (1) IM use preferred. (2) May precipitate withdrawal symptoms if stopped too quickly after prolonged use or if patient has been on opiates. (3) Oxygen and controlled respiratory equipment must be available. Naloxone is only partially effective in reversing respiratory depression. (4) Observe patient frequently and monitor vital signs. (5) Physical dependence can develop with abuse. (6) Potentiated by phenothiazines (e.g., chlorpromazine [Thorazine]) and by other CNS depressants such as narcotic analgesics, general anesthetics, alcohol, anticholinergics, antihistamines, barbiturates, cimetidine (Tagamet), hypnotics, MAO inhibitors, neuromuscular blocking agents (e.g., tubocurarine), psychotropic agents, and sedatives. Reduced doses of both drugs may be indicated. (7) Use caution in asthma, respiratory depression or difficulty from any source, impaired renal or hepatic function, the elderly or debilitated, myxedema or hypothyroidism, adrenocortical insufficiency, CNS depression or coma, toxic psychoses, prostatic hypertrophy or urethral stricture, acute alcoholism, delirium tremens, or kyphoscoliosis. (8) May elevate cerebrospinal fluid pressure; use caution in head injury, intracranial lesions, and other situations with increased intracranial pressure. (9) Safety for use during pregnancy and lactation not established. Use only when clearly needed. Safety for use during labor and delivery not established.

Contraindications: Children 12 years of age and younger, hypersensitivity to buprenorphine.

Incompatible with: Alcohol solutions, diazepam (Valium), lorazepam (Ativan).

Side effects: Excessive sedation is a major side effect. Has caused death from respiratory depression. Anaphylaxis, bradycardia, clammy skin, constipation, cyanosis, dizziness, dyspnea, headache, hypertension, hypotension, nausea, pruritus, tachycardia, vertigo, visual disturbances, vomiting.

Antidote: With increasing severity of any side effect or onset of symptoms of overdose, discontinue the drug and notify the physician. Naloxone hydrochloride (Narcan) will help to reverse respiratory depression, but is not as effective as with other narcotics. A patent airway, artificial ventilation, oxygen therapy, and other symptomatic treatment must be instituted promptly. Treat anaphylaxis and resuscitate as necessary.

BUTORPHANOL TARTRATE **pH 3.0 to 5.5**

(Stadol)

Usual dose: 1 mg. Repeat every 3 to 4 hours as necessary. Range is 0.5 to 2 mg. Reduced dose may be required in hepatic or renal disease.

Dilution: May be given undiluted.

Rate of administration: Each 2 mg or fraction thereof over 3 to 5 minutes. Frequently titrated according to symptom relief and respiratory rate.

Actions: A potent narcotic analgesic with some narcotic agonist-antagonist effects. Exact mechanism of action is unknown. Analgesia similar to morphine is produced. Does produce respiratory depression, but this does not increase markedly with larger doses. Pain relief is effected almost immediately, peaks at 30 minutes, and lasts about 3 hours. Causes some hemodynamic changes that increase the workload of the heart. Metabolized in the liver. Excreted in urine. Crosses the placental barrier. Secreted in breast milk.

Indications and uses: (1) Relief of moderate to severe pain; (2) preoperative medication.

Precautions: (1) Not used for narcotic-dependent patients because of antagonist activity. (2) Can produce dependency; monitor dosage carefully. (3) Oxygen and controlled respiratory equipment must be available. (4)

Observe patient frequently and monitor vital signs. (5) Use in myocardial infarction, ventricular dysfunction, and coronary insufficiency only if the patient is hypersensitive to morphine or meperidine. (6) Use caution in respiratory depression or difficulty from any source, obstructive respiratory conditions, head injury, and impaired liver or kidney function. (7) Potentiated by barbiturates (e.g., secobarbital [Seconal]), phenothiazines (e.g., Compazine), cimetidine (Tagamet), droperidol (Inapsine), and other tranquilizers. Reduced doses of both drugs may be indicated. (8) Will cause an increase in conjunctival changes with pancuronium (Pavulon). (9) Safety for use in pregnancy not established, could result in neonatal withdrawal. Has been used safely during labor and delivery of term infants, but use caution during labor and delivery of premature infants. Discontinue breastfeeding. (10) Not recommended for children under 18 years.

Contraindications: Hypersensitivity to butorphanol. Biliary surgery is a probable contraindication.

Incompatible with: Barbiturates (e.g., pentobarbital [Nembutal]).

Side effects: Anaphylaxis, clammy skin, confusion, diplopia, dizziness, dry mouth, floating feeling, flushing, hallucinations, headache, lethargy, lightheadedness, nausea, respiratory depression, sedation, sensitivity to cold, sweating, unusual dreams, vertigo, vomiting, warmth. May cause increased pulmonary artery pressure, pulmonary wedge pressure, left ventricular end-diastolic pressure, systemic arterial pressure, pulmonary vascular resistance, and cardiac workload.

Antidote: With increasing severity of any side effect or onset of symptoms of overdose, discontinue the drug and notify the physician. Treat side effects symptomatically. Naloxone hydrochloride (Narcan) will reverse respiratory depression. A patent airway, artificial ventilation, oxygen therapy, and other symptomatic treatment must be instituted promptly.

CAFFEINE AND SODIUM BENZOATE

pH 6.5 to 8.5

Usual dose: 500 mg to 1 Gm. Maximum dose is 2.5 Gm/24 hr.

Pediatric dose: 8 mg/kg of body weight up to 500 mg every 4 hours.

Neonatal apnea: Caffeine citrate or caffeine without sodium benzoate is preferred for IV dosage in neonates. Sodium benzoate can displace bilirubin from its protein binding sites. An initial dose of up to 10 mg/kg of body weight (20 mg/kg if caffeine citrate is used) is given. Follow with a maintenance dose of 2.5 mg/kg/day (5 mg/kg caffeine citrate). Plasma concentrations of 5 to 20 mcg/ml have controlled apnea. Oral therapy with caffeine only is preferred.

Dilution: May be given undiluted.

Rate of administration: 250 mg or fraction thereof over 1 minute. Extend rate of administration in neonate.

Actions: A xanthine derivative and descending analeptic CNS stimulant. Small doses cause wakefulness and mental alertness. Larger doses stimulate the respiratory center and increase heart action. It is believed to constrict the intracranial blood vessels and lower intracranial pressure. Widely distributed throughout the body and excreted in the urine. Crosses the placental barrier. Secreted in breast milk.

Indications and uses: Rarely used. (1) To alleviate headaches after spinal cord puncture; (2) alcoholic stupor/excitement; (3) barbiturate poisoning antidote; (4) narcotic poisoning antidote if naloxone (Narcan) is not available.

Unlabeled use: Treatment of neonatal apnea.

Precautions: (1) Usually given IM; IV route is for emergencies only. (2) Most people have developed a tolerance level for caffeine because of daily ingestion of coffee or tea. (3) MAO inhibitors (e.g., isocarboxazid [Marplan]) potentiate caffeine and can cause an acute hypertensive crisis. (4) May produce convulsions with overdose of propoxyphene (Darvon). (5) Metabolism inhibited by oral contraceptives and cimetidine (Tagamet); a lower dose of caffeine may be indicated. (6) Smoking promotes elimination of caffeine, may inhibit effectiveness. (7) Death has occurred with IV administration.

Contraindications: Acute myocardial infarction.

Incompatible with: Chlorpromazine (Thorazine).

Side effects: Generally only occur with very large doses; cardiac irregularities, death, diuresis, excessive irritability, hypertension (transient), insomnia, muscle twitching, nausea and vomiting, palpitations, and tachycardia.

Neonatal: Bradycardia, coarse tremors, hypertonicity alternating with hypotonicity, hypotension, intracranial hemorrhage, opisthotonic posturing, and severe acidosis.

Antidote: For major symptoms, discontinue drug and notify the physician. Short-acting sedatives (e.g., pentobarbital [Nembutal]) or diazepam (Valium) will quiet CNS stimulation. Resuscitate as necessary.

CALCIUM CHLORIDE pH 5.5 to 7.5

Usual dose: *Hypocalcemia:* 5 to 10 ml (500 mg to 1 Gm) at intervals of 1 to 3 days.

Magnesium intoxication: 5 ml (500 mg). Observe for signs of recovery before giving any additional calcium.

Hyperkalemia ECG disturbances of cardiac function: 1 to 10 ml (100 mg to 1 Gm); titrate dose by monitoring ECG changes.

Cardiac resuscitation: (See Indications) 2 ml (200 mg); repeat in 10 minutes if indicated by measured serum deficits of calcium. Consider need for calcium (usually gluconate or gluceptate) for every 500 ml of whole blood if arrest occurs in a situation requiring copious blood replacement. *1 Gm (10 ml) contains 13.6 mEq (272 mg) of calcium.*

Infant dose: 0.2 ml of a 10% solution/kg of body weight (20 mg/kg) for cardiac resuscitation (see Indications).

Dilution: May be given undiluted, but preferably diluted with an equal amount of distilled water or normal saline for injection to make a 5% solution.

Rate of administration: 0.5 to 1 ml of solution over 1 minute. Stop or slow infusion rate if patient complains of discomfort.

Actions: Calcium is a basic element prevalent in the human body. It affects bones, nerves, muscles, glands, cardiac and vascular tone, and normal coagulation of the blood. It is excreted in the urine and feces.

Indications and uses: Calcium preparations other than calcium chloride are often preferred except in cardiac resuscitation or verapamil toxicity. (1) Hypocalcemia tetany (e.g., neonatal, parathyroid deficiency); (2) antidote for magnesium sulfate; (3) ECG disturbances caused by hyperkalemia or verapamil-induced hypotension; (4) cardiac resuscitation only to treat hypocalcemia, hyperkalemia, or calcium channel block toxicity (verapamil), or after open heart surgery if epinephrine does not produce effective myocardial contractions; (5) adjunctive therapy in sensitivity reactions, insect bites or stings, or acute symptoms of lead colic.

Precautions: (1) Three times more potent than calcium gluconate. (2) For IV use only. Confirm patency of vein, select a large vein, and use a small needle to reduce vein irritation. Necrosis and sloughing will occur with IM or SC injection or extravasation. (3) Solution should be warmed to body temperature. (4) Will increase digitalis toxicity. Use with extreme care in patients receiving digitalis. (5) Can reduce neuromuscular paralysis and respiratory depression produced by antibiotics such as kanamycin (Kantrex). (6) Inhibits tetracycline absorption. (7) Vitamin D aids absorption. (8) Keep patient recumbent after injection to prevent postural hypotension. Monitor vital signs carefully. (9) Antagonizes effects of verapamil. (10) Usual doses will produce peripheral vasodilation, local burning sensation, and a moderate drop in blood pressure.

Contraindications: Ventricular fibrillation, potential for existing digitalis toxicity.

Incompatible with: Amphotericin B (Fungizone), cephalothin (Keflin), chlorpheniramine (Chlortrimeton), chlortetracycline (Aureomycin), digitalis (e.g., digitoxin), epinephrine (Adrenalin), sodium bicarbonate, tetracycline (Achromycin), warfarin (Coumadin). Calcium salts not generally mixed with carbonates, phosphates, sulfates, or tartrates.

Side effects: Rare when given as recommended; bradycardia, calcium taste, cardiac arrest, depression, heat waves, prolonged state of cardiac contraction, tingling sensation.

Overdose: Coma, intractable nausea and vomiting, lethargy, markedly elevated plasma calcium level, weakness, and sudden death.

Antidote: If side effects occur, discontinue the drug and notify the physician. Further dilution and decrease in the rate of administration may be necessary. Resuscitate as necessary. Disodium edetate may be used with extreme caution as a calcium-chelating agent if overdose is critical. For extravasation inject affected area with 1% procaine hydrochloride and hyaluronidase to reduce venospasm and dilute calcium. Use a 27- or 25-gauge needle. Warm moist compresses may be helpful.

CALCIUM DISODIUM EDETATE pH 6.5 to 8.0

(Calcium Disodium Versenate, Calcium EDTA, Edetate Calcium Disodium)

Usual dose: 1 Gm (5 ml) twice in 24 hours for 3 to 5 days. Give second dose after 6 hours. Repeat after several days if indicated. Do not exceed 50 mg/kg/24 hr.

Pediatric dose: Should not exceed 70 mg/kg of body weight/24 hr in 2 or 3 equal doses. *Do not exceed recommended dosage.*

Dilution: Each dose must be diluted in 250 to 500 ml of 5% dextrose in water or isotonic saline for IV infusion.

Rate of administration: Each dose must be given over at least 1 hour; 2 hours in the symptomatic patient. Physician will order a specific rate.

Actions: A chelating agent that helps to remove metals, especially lead, from the body. Forms stable compounds, which are then excreted in the urine; up to 50% in 1 hour and 95% in 24 hours. Mostly chelates from bone.

Indications and uses: (1) Acute and chronic lead poisoning and lead encephalopathy; (2) heavy metal poisoning; (3) removal of radioactive and nuclear fission products.

Precautions: (1) Establish urine flow before drug is administered. (2) Monitor vital signs, ECG, BUN, and urine output. (3) Daily urine specimens are recommended to determine status of renal function. (4) Obtain specific fluid orders from the physician. Increased fluid intake is desirable except in the presence of cerebral edema or lead encephalopathy. (5) IM injection preferred in presence of increased intracranial pressure. (6) May produce toxic and fatal effects. (7) Use with caution in active or healed tuberculosis and mild renal disease. Use only if clearly indicated in pregnancy. (8) Do not confuse with disodium edetate (Endrate), which does not chelate lead but actually removes calcium from the body and can be very dangerous. (9) Not effective in mercury poisoning. (10) Usually given IM in children. May be given concurrently with dimercaprol (BAL). (11) May cause hypocalcemic tetany with too rapid injection.

Contraindications: Anuria, severe renal disease.

Incompatible with: Must be diluted in specific IV solutions. *Do not mix with any other IV medication.*

Side effects: Acute renal tubular necrosis, hematuria, hypotension, leg and other muscle cramps, malaise, proteinuria, tetany, weakness.

Antidote: Notify the physician of any side effects. Most will improve with a decrease in rate of the infusion or will be treated symptomatically. Evidence of increasing renal damage will require temporary discontinuation of the drug.

CALCIUM GLUCEPTATE pH 5.6 to 7.0

Usual dose: 5 to 20 ml (5 ml is equal in calcium content [0.09 Gm] to 10 ml of 10% calcium gluconate). May be repeated if indicated.

Cardiac resuscitation: (See Indications) 5 to 7 ml; repeat in 10 minutes if indicated by measured serum deficits of calcium.

Newborn exchange transfusion: The average dose is 0.5 ml after each 100 ml of blood exchanged.

Dilution: May be given undiluted.

Rate of administration: 1 ml or fraction thereof over 1 minute. Stop or slow infusion rate if patient complains of discomfort.

Actions: Calcium is a basic element prevalent in the human body. It affects bones, nerves, muscles, glands, cardiac and vascular tone, and normal coagulation of the blood. It is excreted in the urine and feces.

Indications and uses: (1) Hypocalcemia caused by neonatal tetany, parathyroid deficiency tetany, vitamin D deficiency tetany, alkalosis; (2) prevention of hypocalcemia during exchange transfusions; (3) cardiac resuscitation only to treat hypocalcemia and hyperkalemia; (4) antidote for magnesium sulfate; (5) adjunctive therapy in sensitivity reactions, insect bites or stings, or acute symptoms of lead colic.

Precautions: (1) IV use is preferred in adults, infants, and young children. Necrosis and sloughing can occur with IM or SC injection or extravasation. Confirm patency of vein. (2) Will increase digitalis toxicity. Use with extreme care in patients receiving digitalis. (3) Solution should be warmed to body temperature. (4) Keep patient lying down after injection to prevent postural hypotension.

Contraindications: According to some authorities IM use is contraindicated in infants and small children. Potential for existing digitalis toxicity.

Incompatible with: Cefamandole (Mandol), cefazolin (Kefzol), cephalothin (Keflin), magnesium sulfate, prednisolone sodium phosphate (Hydeltrasol), prochlorperazine (Compazine), tetracyclines. Calcium salts are not generally mixed with carbonates, phosphates, sulfates, or tartrates.

Side effects: Usually occur only with rapid administration and may include tingling sensations, calcium taste, and heat waves.

Overdose: Coma, intractable nausea and vomiting, lethargy, markedly elevated plasma calcium level, weakness, and sudden death.

Antidote: Decrease rate of administration. If side effects persist, discontinue the drug and notify the physician. Further dilution and decrease in the rate of administration may be necessary. Resuscitate as necessary. Disodium edetate may be used with extreme caution as a calcium-chelating agent if overdosage is critical. For extravasation inject affected area with 1% procaine hydrochloride and hyaluronidase to reduce venospasm and dilute calcium. Use a 27- or 25-gauge needle. Warm moist compresses may be helpful.

CALCIUM GLUCONATE pH 6.0 to 8.2

Usual dose: 0.5 to 2.0 Gm (5 to 20 ml). Repeat as required. Daily dosage ranges from 1 to 15 Gm. 10 ml of 10% solution equals 0.09 Gm of calcium. Up to 30 ml may be given if indicated. Up to 60 ml may be given in an IV infusion.

Cardiac resuscitation: (See Indications) 5 to 8 ml. Repeat in 10 minutes if indicated by measured serum deficits of calcium.

Hypocalcemia: 4.5 to 16 mEq (10 to 35 ml).

Magnesium intoxication: 4.5 to 9 mEq (10 to 20 ml). Observe for signs of recovery before giving any additional calcium.

Exchange transfusion: Approximately 1.35 mEq (2.9 ml) with each 100 ml of citrated blood.

Pediatric dose: 2 to 5 ml/24 hr, every other day, or every third day. Up to 500 mg/kg of body weight/24 hr has been given in divided doses.

Hypocalcemia: 0.5 to 0.7 mEq/kg (1.1 to 1.5 ml/kg) 3 or 4 times daily.

Neonatal dose: *Elevate serum calcium in an emergency:* Up to 1 mEq (2.2 ml).

Hypocalcemia tetany: 2.4 mEq/kg of body weight/24 hr (5.2 ml/kg/24 hr) in divided doses.

Exchange transfusion: 0.45 mEq (1 ml) with each 100 ml of citrated blood.

Dilution: May be given undiluted or may be further diluted in up to 1,000 ml of normal saline solution for infusion.

Rate of administration: Undiluted, each 0.5 ml or fraction thereof over 1 minute. Diluted in 1,000 ml of normal saline, it may be given over 12 to 24 hours. Stop or slow infusion rate if patient complains of discomfort.

Actions: Calcium is a basic element prevalent in the human body. It affects bones, nerves, glands, cardiac and vascular tone, and normal coagulation of the blood. Crosses placental barrier and is secreted in breast milk. It is excreted in the urine and feces.

Indications and uses: (1) Calcium deficiency caused by hypoparathyroidism, osteomalacia, vitamin D deficiency, preeclampsia, uremia; (2) adjunctive therapy in sensitivity reactions, insect bites or stings, or acute symptoms of lead colic; (3) cardiac resuscitation only to treat hypocalcemia or hyperkalemia; (4) uterine inertia; (5) antidote for magnesium sulfate; (6) may be given after blood transfusions to maintain calcium/potassium ratio; (7) alkalosis.

Precautions: (1) Has only one-third the potency of calcium chloride. (2) IV use preferred in adults, mandatory for infants and young children. Necrosis and sloughing can occur with IM or SC injection or extravasation. Confirm patency of vein. (3) Solution should be warmed to body temperature. (4) Will increase digitalis toxicity. Use with extreme care in patients receiving digitalis. (5) Vitamin D aids absorption. (6) Inhibits tetracycline absorption. (7) Vasodilation may cause mild hypotension.

Contraindications: IM use in infants and small children, potential for existing digitalis toxicity.

Incompatible with: Amphotericin B (Fungizone), cefamandole (Mandol), cefazolin (Ancef), cephalothin (Keflin), chlortetracycline (Aureomycin), digitalis (e.g., digitoxin), dobutamine (Dobutrex), epinephrine (Adrenalin), hydrocortisone phosphate, kanamycin (Kantrex), magnesium sulfate, methylprednisolone (Solu Cortef), metoclopramide (Reglan), oxytetracycline (Terramycin), potassium phosphate, prochlorperazine (Compazine), promethazine (Phenergan), sodium bicarbonate, streptomycin, tetracycline. Calcium salts are not generally mixed with carbonates, phosphates, sulfates, or tartrates.

Side effects: Rare when given as recommended; bradycardia, calcium taste, cardiac arrest, depression of neuromuscular function, flushing, heat waves, prolonged state of cardiac contraction, tingling sensation.

Overdose: Coma, intractable nausea and vomiting, lethargy, markedly elevated plasma calcium level, weakness, and sudden death.

Antidote: If side effects occur, discontinue the drug and notify the physician. Further dilution or decrease in the rate of administration may be necessary. Resuscitate as necessary. Disodium edetate may be used with extreme caution as a calcium chelating agent if overdosage is critical. For extravasation inject affected area with 1% procaine hydrochloride and hyaluronidase to reduce venospasm and dilute calcium. Use a 27- or 25-gauge needle. Warm moist compresses may be helpful.

CARBENICILLIN DISODIUM pH 6.5 to 8.0

(Geopen)

Usual dose: 1 to 10 Gm every 4 to 6 hours (200 to 500 mg/kg of body weight/24 hr) depending on the severity of the infection. Not to exceed 40 Gm/24 hr; normal renal function is necessary for this dosage.

Pediatric dose: 50 to 500 mg/kg of body weight/24 hr in divided doses every 4 to 6 hours, depending on the severity of the infection. Not to exceed 500 mg/kg/24 hr or 40 Gm/24 hr, whichever is less.

Neonatal dose: *Under 2,000 Gm; age up to 7 days:* An initial dose of 100 mg/kg of body weight; then 75 mg/kg every 8 hours (225 mg/kg/24 hr). *Over 7 days:* 100 mg/kg every 6 hours (400 mg/kg/24 hr).

Over 2,000 Gm; age up to 3 days: An initial dose of 100 mg/kg of body weight; then 75 mg/kg every 6 hours (300 mg/kg/ 24 hr). *Over 3 days:* 100 mg/kg every 6 hours (400 mg/kg/24 hr).

Dilution: Each 1 Gm or fraction thereof is diluted with 2 to 2.6 ml of sterile water for injection. Further dilution of each gram with an additional 10 to 20 ml of sterile water for injection is required for direct IV administration. May be added to large volumes of standard IV fluids for infusion including 50 or 100 ml additive bottles.

Rate of administration: 1 Gm or fraction thereof over 5 minutes when given directly IV. Large doses may be given over 4 to 24 hours in an IV infusion.

Newborn dose: Administer over 15 minutes.

Too rapid injection may cause seizures.

Actions: An extended-spectrum penicillin. Bactericidal for many gram-positive, gram-negative, and anaerobic organisms including *Pseudomonas*, indole-positive *Proteus* strains, *Haemophilus influenzae*, and *Escherichia coli*. Not active against penicillinase-producing organisms. Appears in all body fluids. Appears in cerebrospinal fluid only if inflammation is present. Crosses the placental barrier. Excreted in the urine. Secreted in breast milk.

Indications and uses: (1) Urinary tract infections; (2) severe systemic infections and septicemia; (3) acute and chronic respiratory infections; (4) soft tissue infections.

Precautions: (1) Administer within 24 hours of preparation. (2) Sensitivity studies indicated to determine susceptibility of the causative organism to carbenicillin. (3) Oral probenecid is advised to achieve higher and more prolonged blood levels. (4) Reduce daily dose commensurate with amount of renal impairment. Intervals between injections should also be increased. (5) Watch for early symptoms of allergic reaction. (6) Avoid prolonged use of drug; superinfection caused by overgrowth of nonsusceptible organisms may result. (7) Periodic evaluation of renal, hepatic, and hematopoietic systems is recommended in prolonged therapy. (8) Electrolyte imbalance and cardiac irregularities resulting from high sodium content are very possible. (9) Confirm patency of vein, avoid extravasation or intraarterial injection. Slow infusion rate for pain along venipuncture site. (10) Frequently used concurrently with aminoglycosides (e.g., gentamicin [Garamycin]) but must be administered in separate infusions; inactivates aminoglycosides. (11) Inactivated by chloramphenicol, erythromycin, and tetracyclines. Bactericidal action is actually negated by these drugs. (12) Concomitant use with beta-adrenergic blockers (e.g., propranolol [Inderal]) may increase risk of anaphylaxis and inhibit treatment. (13) Risk of bleeding with anticoagulants (e.g., heparin) is increased. (14) Neuromuscular excitability or convulsions may be caused by higher than normal doses. (15) Elimination rate markedly reduced in neonates. (16) Decreases effectiveness of oral contraceptives; breakthrough bleeding or pregnancy could occur.

Contraindications: History of sensitivity to multiple allergens, known penicillin sensitivity, pregnancy.

Incompatible with: Aminoglycosides (e.g., amikacin, colistimethate, gentamicin, kanamycin, streptomycin, tobramycin), amphotericin B (Fungizone), bleomycin (Blenoxane), chloramphenicol, lincomycin, polymyxin B, promethazine (Phenergan), tetracycline (Achromycin), vitamin B with C.

Side effects: Abnormal clotting time or PT, anaphylaxis, anemia, convulsions, elevated temperature, elevated SGOT and SGPT, eosinophilia, hematuria, itching, nausea, neuromuscular irritability, thrombophlebitis, unpleasant taste in the mouth, urticaria.

Antidote: Notify the physician immediately of any adverse symptoms. For severe symptoms, discontinue the drug, treat allergic reaction (antihistamines, epinephrine, corticosteroids), and resuscitate as necessary. Hemodialysis is effective in overdose.

CARBOPLATIN pH 5.0 to 7.0

(Paraplatin)

Usual dose: *As a single agent:* With normal renal function (Crcl >60 ml/min), give 360 mg/M^2 on day 1 every 4 weeks. Platelets must be above 100,000/mm^3 and neutrophils above 2,000/mm^3. If the lowest weekly posttreatment neutrophil and platelet counts exceed 2,000/mm^3 and 100,000/mm^3, respectively, the dose may be increased to 125% of the starting dose (450 mg/M^2). No further dose increases are indicated regardless of circumstances. Maintain starting dose if the lowest weekly posttreatment neutrophil and platelet counts range from 500 to 2,000/mm^3 and 50,000 to 100,000/mm^3, respectively. Reduce dose to 75% of the starting dose (270 mg/M^2) if the lowest weekly posttreatment neutrophil and platelet counts are less than 500/mm^3 and 50,000/mm^3, respectively. With impaired renal function (Crcl 16 to 40 ml/min), give 200 mg/M^2. Adjust dose by percentages and criteria as indicated above under dose for normal renal function.

Dilution: *Specific techniques required, see Precautions.* Immediately before use dilute each 10 mg of carboplatin with 1 ml of sterile water for injection, 5% dextrose in water, or normal saline (50 mg with 5 ml, 150 mg with 15 ml, 450 mg with 45 ml). All yield 10 mg/ml. Should be further diluted with the same solutions to 1 to 4 mg/ml (add 10 ml additional diluent to each 10 mg to obtain 1 mg/ml and 2.5 ml to each 10 mg to obtain 4 mg/ml). Do not use needles or IV tubing with aluminum parts to mix or administer; a precipitate will form and potency is decreased.

Rate of administration: A single dose as an infusion over a minimum of 15 minutes. Extend administration time based on amount of diluent and patient condition.

Actions: An alkylating agent. An improved platinum-based compound similar to cisplatin but with improved therapeutic effects. Better tolerated by patients, carboplatin causes less nausea and vomiting, less neurotoxicity, and less nephrotoxicity than cisplatin. Myelosuppression is generally reversible and manageable with antibiotics and transfusions. Produces interstrand DNA cross-links and is cell cycle nonspecific. Not as heavily protein bound as cisplatin. Majority of carboplatin is excreted in the urine within 24 hours.

Indications and uses: Palliative treatment of recurrent ovarian cancer after prior chemotherapy including patients treated with cisplatin.

Investigational uses: To replace cisplatin in treatment of ovarian, cervical, endometrial, lung, and testicular cancer. Used as a single agent or in protocols instead of cisplatin.

Precautions: (1) Follow guidelines for handling cytotoxic agents recommended. See Appendix p. 677. (2) Usually administered by or under the direction of the physician specialist. (3) BUN and serum creatinine should be done before each dose. Creatinine clearance, differential white blood cell count, platelet count, and hemoglobin are recommended before each dose and weekly thereafter. Platelet count must be 100,000/mm^3 and neutrophils 2,000/mm^3 before a dose can be repeated. Anemia is frequent and cumulative. Transfusion is often indicated. (4) Excessive hydration or forced diuresis not required, but maintain adequate hydration and urinary output. (5) Nausea and vomiting are frequently severe but less than with cisplatin; generally last 24 hours. Prophylactic administration of antiemetics is indicated. Various protocols including metoclopramide (Reglan), dexamethasone (Decadron), and lorazepam (Ativan); droperidol (Inapsine) or haloperidol (Haldol) and dexamethasone; or prochlorperazine (Compazine) are used. (6) Bone marrow suppression is more severe in patients who have had prior therapy, especially with cisplatin, and when carboplatin is used with other bone marrow–suppressing therapies or radiation. Reduced dose may be indicated. Monitor carefully and manage dose and timing to reduce additive effects. (7) Peripheral neurotoxicity is infrequent, but may increase in patients over 65 years of age and in patients previously treated with cisplatin. (8) Observe for symptoms of allergic reaction during administration; epinephrine, corticosteroids, and antihistamines should be available. (9) Nephrotoxicity and ototoxicity potentiated by aminoglycosides (e.g., gentamicin [Garamycin]). Use caution if patient receiving both drugs. (10) Discontinue breast feeding. Safety for use in pregnancy and in men and women capable of conception not established. Embryotoxic and teratogenic to the fetus. (11) Store unopened vials at 15° to 30° C (59° to 86° F). Protect from light. Mix immediately before use and discard solution 8 hours after dilution.

Contraindications: Hypersensitivity to cisplatin or other platinum-containing compounds or mannitol; severe bone marrow depression; significant bleeding.

Incompatible with: Limited information available. Should be considered incompatible in syringe or solution with any other drug because of toxicity and specific use.

Side effects: Allergic reactions including anaphylaxis can occur during administration. Alopecia (rare), anemia, anorexia, bleeding, bone marrow suppression (usually reversible), bronchospasm, bruising, changes in taste, constipation, death, decreased urine output, decreased serum electrolytes, dehydration, diarrhea, elevated liver function tests, erythema, fatique, fever, hypotension, infection, laboratory test abnormalities (alkaline phosphatase, aspartate aminotransferase, BUN, serum creatinine, total bilirubin), neutropenia, nausea and vomiting (severe), ototoxicity, peripheral neuropathies, pruritus, rash, thrombocytopenia, urticaria, visual disturbances, weakness.

Antidote: Notify physician of all side effects. Symptomatic and supportive treatment is indicated. Withhold carboplatin until myelosuppression is reversed. Transfusions are indicated for anemia. Treat anaphylaxis with epinephrine, corticosteroids, oxygen, and antihistamines. No specific antidote exists.

CARMUSTINE (BCNU) (BiCNU)

pH 5.6 to 6.0

Usual dose: Initial dose is 200 mg/M^2. May be given as a single dose or one half of the calculated dose may be given initially and repeated the next day. Repeat every 6 weeks if bone marrow sufficiently recovered. Repeat doses adjusted according to hematological response of previous dose.

Dilution: *Specific techniques required, see Precautions.* Initially dilute 100 mg vial with supplied sterile diluent (3 ml of absolute ethanol). Further dilute with 27 ml of sterile water for injection. Each ml will contain 3.3 mg carmustine. Withdraw desired dose and further dilute in 100 to 500 ml 5% dextrose or sodium chloride for injection and give as an infusion.

Rate of administration: Each single dose must be given as an infusion over a minimum of 1 hour. Reduce rate for pain or burning at injection site, flushing of the skin, or suffusion of the conjunctiva. Usually given over 1 to 2 hours.

Actions: An alkylating agent of the nitrogen mustard group with antitumor activity, cell cycle phase nonspecific. Degraded to metabolites within 15 minutes of administration. Concurrent concentration higher in cerebrospinal fluid than in plasma. Excreted in changed form in urine. Small amounts excreted as respiratory CO_2.

Indications and uses: Suppress or retard neoplastic growth of brain tumors; multiple myeloma; GI, breast, bronchogenic, and renal carcinomas; meningeal leukemia; Hodgkin's disease; and some non-Hodgkin's lymphomas.

Precautions: (1) Follow guidelines for handling cytotoxic agents recommended. See Appendix, p. 677. (2) Administered by or under the direction of the physician specialist. (3) Adjust dose downward for platelet count below 75,000, leukocytes below 3,000, and when used with other myelosuppressive drugs. (4) Determine absolute patency and quality of vein and adequate circulation of extremity. Severe cellulitis may result from extravasation. (5) Delayed toxicity probable in 4 to 6 weeks; wait at least 6 weeks between doses; frequent leukocyte and platelet counts indicated. (6) Protect from light. Store in refrigerator (2° to 8° C [35° to 46° F]) in all forms. Stable up to 48 hours after dilution. Temperatures above 27° C (80° F) will cause liquefaction of the drug powder; discard immediately. (7) Often used with other antineoplastic drugs in reduced doses to achieve tumor remission. (8) Will produce teratogenic effects on the fetus. Has a mutagenic potential. (9) Nausea and vomiting can be severe. Prophylactic administration of antiemetics recommended. (10) Do not administer vaccine or chloroquine to patients receiving antineoplastic drugs. (11) Avoid contact of carmustine solution with the skin. (12) Potentiates or is potentiated by hepatotoxic or nephrotoxic medications and radiation therapy. (13) Potentiated by cimetidine (Tagamet), may cause toxicity. (14) Inhibits digoxin and phenytoin (Dilantin), may reduce serum levels. (15) Observe for any signs of infection. (16) Maintain hydration.

Contraindications: Hypersensitivity to carmustine, previous chemotherapy, or other causes that result in insufficient circulating platelets, leukocytes, or erythrocytes.

Incompatible with: Consider incompatible with any other drug in syringe or solution because of toxicity and specific use.

Side effects: Most are dose related and can be reversed. Bone marrow toxicity most pronounced at 4 to 6 weeks, can be severe and cumulative with repeated dosage. Anemia, elevated liver function test results, flushing of skin and suffusion of conjunctiva from too rapid infusion rate, hyperpigmentation and burning of skin (from actual contact with solution), nausea and vomiting, pulmonary infiltrates or fibrosis with long-term therapy, renal abnormalities, retinal hemorrage.

Antidote: Notify physician of all side effects. Most will decrease in severity with reduced dosage, increased time span between doses, or symptomatic treatment. May reduce therapeutic effectiveness. Hematopoietic depression may require withholding carmustine until recovery occurs. There is no specific antidote. Supportive therapy as indicated will help sustain the patient in toxicity. For extravasation, elevate extremity, consider injection of long-acting dexamethasone (Decadron LA) or hyaluronidase (Wydase) throughout extravasated tissue. Use a 27- or 25-gauge needle. Apply warm moist compresses.

CEFAMANDOLE NAFATE (Mandol)

pH 6.0 to 8.5

Usual dose: 500 mg to 2 Gm every 4 to 8 hours depending on severity of infection. Do not exceed 12 Gm/24 hr.

Perioperative prophylaxis: 1 or 2 Gm 30 minutes to 1 hour before incision. Follow with 1 to 2 Gm every 6 hours for 24 to 48 hours.

Pediatric dose: 50 to 150 mg/kg of body weight/24 hr in equally divided doses every 4 to 8 hours. Do not exceed maximum adult dose.

Perioperative prophylaxis; infants over 3 months of age: 50 to 100 mg/kg/24 hr in equally divided doses. Give first dose 30 minutes to 1 hour before incision and then every 6 hours for up to 72 hours.

Dilution: *Direct IV:* Each 1 Gm or fraction thereof must be diluted with at least 10 ml sterile water for injection, 5% dextrose in water, or normal saline.

Intermittent infusion: Further dilute in 100 ml dextrose in water or normal saline for infusion and give through Y-tube, three-way stopcock, or additive infusion set.

Continuous infusion: May be further diluted in up to 1,000 ml compatible infusion solutions (see literature).

Rate of administration: Each 1 Gm or fraction thereof over 3 to 5 minutes or longer as indicated by amount of solution and condition of the patient. Discontinue IV infusion solution during administration of cefamandole by intermittent infusion. Rate of continuous infusion should be by physician order.

Actions: A semisynthetic second-generation cephalosporin antibiotic that is bactericidal to specific gram-positive, gram-negative, and anaerobic organisms. Absorbed by most body fluids. Crosses the placental barrier. Excreted rapidly in the urine. Secreted in breast milk.

Indications and uses: (1) Treatment of serious respiratory tract, GU tract, bone, joint, soft tissue, and skin infections; septicemia; and peritonitis. Effective only if the causative organism is susceptible. (2) Perioperative prophylaxis.

Precautions: (1) Sensitivity studies indicated to determine susceptibility of the causative organism to cefamandole. (2) Watch for early symptoms of allergic reaction. (3) Reduce total daily dose if renal function impaired. Calculated according to degree of impairment. (4) Continue at least 2 to 3 days after all symptoms of infection subside. Avoid prolonged use of drug; superinfection caused by overgrowth of nonsusceptible organisms may result. (5) Administer within 24 hours of preparation if unrefrigerated or within 96 hours if refrigerated. (6) Use extreme caution in the penicillin-sensitive patient; cross-sensitivity may occur. (7) Adverse interaction may occur with promethazine (Phenergan), procainamide (Pronestyl), quinidine, muscle relaxants, potent diuretics, and aminoglycosides. Will produce symptoms of acute alcohol intolerance with alcohol. Abstain until at least 72 hours after discontinued. (8) Frequently used concomitantly with aminoglycosides in severe infections, but these drugs must never be mixed in the same infusion or given concurrently. Nephrotoxicity markedly increased when both drugs utilized. (9) Use only if absolutely necessary in pregnancy. (10) Probenecid inhibits excretion and may require reduction in dosage. (11) Forms carbon dioxide after initial dilution; use caution when drawing from vial; do not store in syringe. (12) Avoid concurrent administration of bacteriostatic agents; will inhibit bactericidal action. (13) Safety for use in infants under 1 month of age not established; immature renal function will increase blood levels. (14) Electrolyte imbalance and cardiac irregularities resulting from high sodium content are very possible. Each gram contains 3.3 mEq of sodium. (15) Will cause hypoprothrombinemia. 10 mg/week of prophylactic vitamin K is recommended.

Bleeding tendency increased with heparin and oral anticoagulants (warfarin [Coumadin]).

Contraindications: Known sensitivity to cephalosporins or related antibiotics (penicillins).

Incompatible with: All aminoglycosides (e.g., amikacin [Amikin], gentamicin [Garamycin], kanamycin [Kantrex]), calcium, carbenicillin (Geopen), cimetidine (Tagamet), lidocaine (Xylocaine), magnesium.

Side effects: Allergic reactions including anaphylaxis; anorexia; bleeding episodes; diarrhea; false positive reaction for urine glucose except with Tes-Tape or Keto-Diastix; jaundice; leukopenia; local site pain; nausea and vomiting; neutropenia; oral thrush; phlebitis; positive direct Coombs' test; pseudomembranous colitis; transient elevation of SGOT, SGPT, BUN, and alkaline phosphatase; proteinuria; seizures (large doses); and thrombophlebitis.

Antidote: Notify physician of any side effects. Discontinue the drug if indicated. Treat allergic reaction as indicated and resuscitate as necessary. Hemodialysis may be useful in overdose. Vitamin K, fresh frozen plasma, packed red cells, or platelet concentrates may be indicated in abnormal bleeding tendencies confirmed by laboratory evaluations. If bleeding due to platelet dysfunction, discontinue and use cefoperazone or moxalactam with extreme caution.

CEFAZOLIN SODIUM — pH 4.5 to 6.0

(Ancef, Kefzol, Zolicef)

Usual dose: 250 mg to 1.5 Gm every 6 to 8 hours. Up to 12 Gm in 24 hours has been used, depending on severity of infection. Normal renal function required.

Perioperative prophylaxis: 1 Gm 30 minutes to 1 hour before incision. 0.5 to 1 Gm may be repeated in 2 hours in the OR and every 6 to 8 hours for 24 hours or for up to 5 days in specific situations.

Pediatric dose: 25 to 50 mg/kg of body weight/24 hr in 3 or 4 equally divided doses. May be increased to 100 mg/kg/24 hr in severe infections. Do not exceed adult dose. Normal renal function required.

Dilution: Each 1 Gm or fraction thereof must be diluted with at least 10 ml of sterile water for injection. To reduce the incidence of thrombophlebitis, may be further diluted in 50 to 100 ml of 5% dextrose in water, normal saline for injection, or other compatible infusion solutions (see literature). Available premixed. May be administered through Y-tube, three-way stopcock, or additive infusion set.

Rate of administration: Each 1 Gm or fraction thereof over 5 minutes or longer as indicated by amount of solution and condition of patient.

Actions: A semisynthetic first-generation cephalosporin antibiotic that is bactericidal through inhibition of cell wall synthesis to some gram-positive and gram-negative organisms, including staphylococci and streptococci. A number of organisms are resistant to this cephalosporin. Absorbed by most body fluids. Crosses the placental barrier. Excreted rapidly in the urine. Secreted in breast milk.

Indications and uses: (1) Treatment of serious infections of the bone, joints, skin, soft tissue, bloodstream, cardiovascular system, respiratory tract, and GU tract. Effective only if the causative organism is susceptible. (2) Perioperative prophylaxis.

Precautions: (1) Sensitivity studies indicated to determine susceptibility of the causative organisms to cefazolin. (2) Watch for early symptoms of allergic reaction. (3) Reduce total daily dose if renal function impaired. Calculated according to degree of impairment. (4) Continue for at least 2 to 3 days after all symptoms of infection subside. Avoid prolonged use of drug; superinfection caused by overgrowth of nonsusceptible organisms may result. (5) Administer within 24 hours of preparation, or within 96 hours if under refrigeration (5° C [41° F]). (6) Continuous IV infusion not recommended; markedly increases incidence of phlebitis. (7) Use extreme caution in the penicillin-sensitive patient; cross-sensitivity may occur. (8) Adverse interaction may occur with promethazine (Phenergan), procainamide (Pronestyl), quinidine, muscle relaxants, aminoglycosides (e.g., gentamicin), and potent diuretics. (9)

Use only if absolutely necessary in pregnancy. (10) Higher blood levels obtained with probenecid. (11) Avoid concurrent administration of bacteriostatic agents; will inhibit bactericidal action. (12) Safety for use in infants under 1 month of age not established; immature renal function will increase blood levels. (13) Electrolyte imbalance and cardiac irregularities resulting from sodium content are very possible. Contains 2.1 mEq sodium/Gm.

Contraindications: Known sensitivity to cephalosporins or related antibiotics (penicillins).

Incompatible with: Amikacin (Amikin), amobarbital (Amytal), ascorbic acid, bleomycin (Blenoxane), calcium gluceptate, calcium gluconate, cimetidine (Tagamet), colistimethate (Coly-Mycin M), erythromycin, kanamycin (Kantrex), lidocaine (Xylocaine), pentobarbital (Nembutal), polymyxin B, tetracycline, vitamin B with C.

Side effects: Allergic reactions including anaphylaxis; anorexia; diarrhea; false positive reaction for urine glucose except with Tes-Tape or Keto-Diastix; leukopenia; local site pain; nausea and vomiting; neutropenia; oral thrush; phlebitis; positive direct and indirect Coombs' test; pseudomembranous colitis; transient elevation of SGOT, SGPT, BUN, and alkaline phosphatase; and seizures (large doses).

Antidote: Notify the physician of any side effects. Discontinue the drug if indicated, treat allergic reaction as indicated, and resuscitate as necessary.

CEFMETAZOLE SODIUM

pH 4.2 to 6.2

Usual dose: 2 Gm every 6, 8, or 12 hours. Dose based on severity of disease and patient's condition. Continue for 5 to 14 days (at least 2 to 3 days after all symptoms of infection subside). Reduce total daily dose if renal function impaired. Calculated according to degree of impairment (see literature).

Perioperative prophylaxis: Dose requirements and time

frames vary with specific surgery. In all situations repeat the preoperative dose if the surgery lasts more than 4 hours. Preoperative bowel preparation recommended.

Vaginal hysterectomy: 2 Gm 30 to 90 minutes before surgery as a single dose or 1 Gm 30 to 90 minutes before surgery, repeated in 8 hours and again in 16 hours.

Abdominal hysterectomy or high-risk cholecystectomy: 1 Gm 30 to 90 minutes before surgery. Repeat in 8 hours and again in 16 hours.

Colorectal surgery: 2 Gm 30 to 90 minutes before surgery. May be given as a single dose or repeated in 8 hours and again in 16 hours.

Cesarean section: 2 Gm after clamping the cord as a single dose or 1 Gm after clamping the cord, repeated in 8 hours and again in 16 hours.

Dilution: Initially dilute with sterile water for injection, bacteriostatic water for injection, or 0.9% sodium chloride. For 1 Gm use 3.7 ml (250 mg/ml) or 10 ml (100 mg/ml). For 2 Gm use 7 ml (250 mg/ml) or 15 ml (125 mg/ml). Shake to dissolve and let stand until clear. May be further diluted with normal saline, 5% dextrose in water, or lactated Ringer's injection to solutions containing 1 to 20 mg/ml. Usually given as an intermittent infusion, but may be given direct IV in otherwise healthy patients for surgical prophylaxis.

Rate of Administration: *Direct IV for surgical prophylaxis:* A single dose equally distributed over 3 to 5 minutes. *Intermittent IV:* A single dose over 10 to 60 minutes. Either route may be given through a Y-tube or three-way stopcock of infusion set. Temporarily discontinue other solutions infusing at the same site.

Actions: A semisynthetic, broad-spectrum second-generation cephalosporin antibiotic. Bactericidal through inhibition of cell wall synthesis to a wide range of selected aerobic and anaerobic gram-negative and gram-positive organisms. Onset of action is prompt, and serum levels are dose related. Half-life averages 1.2 hours. Effective concentrations are found in bile; the gallbladder wall; and vaginal, uterine, and adnexal tissue. 85% excreted unchanged in urine in 12 hours. Crosses placental barrier. Secreted in breast milk.

Indications and uses: (1) Treatment of serious urinary tract, lower respiratory tract, skin and skin structure, and intraabdominal infections. Most effective against specific organisms (see literature). (2) Perioperative prophylaxis. Not indicated for infections caused be methicillin-resistant staphylococci.

Precautions: (1) Specific sensitivity studies utilizing a 30 mcg cefmetazole disk are indicated to determine susceptibility of the causative organism to cefmetazole. (2) Watch for early symptoms of allergic reaction. Use caution in patients with histories of asthma or other allergies. (3) Use extreme caution in the penicillin-sensitive patient; cross-sensitivity with β-lactam antibiotics has occurred. (4) Avoid prolonged use of drug; superinfection caused by overgrowth of nonsusceptible organisms may result. (5) Use caution in patients with a history of GI disease, especially colitis. (6) Adverse interactions may occur with other highly protein-bound drugs (e.g., promethazine [Phenergan], procainamide [Pronestyl], quinidine, muscle relaxants, potent diuretics). (7) May be used concomitantly with aminoglycosides (e.g., gentamicin [Garamycin]) in severe infection, but these drugs must never be mixed in the same infusion or given concurrently. Nephrotoxicity may be increased when both drugs utilized. (8) Avoid concurrent administration of bacteriostatic agents. (9) May increase PT in patients with impaired hepatic or renal function, malnutrition, or receiving an extended course of antimicrobial therapy. Monitor PT; vitamin K may be indicated. (10) Produces a disulfiramlike reaction with alcohol (flushing, sweating, headache, tachycardia). Patient must abstain from alcohol during treatment and until at least 24 hours after completion. (11) Use only if absolutely necessary in pregnancy. Discontinue breast feeding until course of therapy complete. (12) Safety for use in children not established. Some testicular atrophy occurred in young rats given high doses. (13) May cause thrombophlebitis. Use small needles and large veins, and rotate infusion sites. (14) Electrolyte imbalance and cardiac irregularities resulting from sodium content are possible. Contains 2 mEq of sodium/Gm. (15) May cause a false positive reaction for glucose with Benedict's or Fehling's solution. (16)

Stable after dilution for 24 hours at room temperature, 7 days if refrigerated. May be frozen for up to 6 weeks after initial dilution; thaw at room temperature (see literature); do not refreeze.

Contraindications: Known hypersensitivity to cefmetazole, cephalosporins, or related antibiotics.

Incompatible with: Limited information available. Should be considered incompatible in syringe or solution with any other bacteriostatic agent; all aminoglycosides (e.g., kanamycin [Kantrex]).

Side effects: Generally well tolerated. Full scope of allergic reactions including anaphylaxis. Bleeding; burning, discomfort, and pain at injection site; candidiasis; changes in color perception; decreased serum albumin and total serum protein; diarrhea; dyspnea; elevated alkaline phosphatase, SGOT, SGPT, bilirubin, and LDH; elevated PT, PTT, and other differential blood cell abnormalities (e.g., lymphocytopenia); elevated serum glucose; epigastric pain; headache; hot flashes; hypotension; nausea and vomiting, pleural effusion; pseudomembranous colitis; seizures; shock. Many additional side effects are possible.

Antidote: Notify physician of any side effects. Discontinue the drug if indicated. Treat allergic reaction as indicated and resuscitate as necessary. Mild cases of colitis may respond to discontinuation of cefmetazole. Oral vancomycin (Vancocin) or metronidazole (Flagyl) is the treatment of choice for antibiotic-related pseudomembranous colitis. Overdose may precipitate seizures, especially in patients with renal impairment; may require anticonvulsants (e.g., diazepam [Valium]). Hemodialysis or peritoneal dialysis may be useful.

CEFONICID SODIUM pH 3.5 to 6.5

(Monocid)

Usual dose: 1 Gm/24 hr. Range is 0.5 to 2 Gm/ 24 hr.

Perioperative prophylaxis: 1 Gm IV 1 hour before incision except during cesarean birth. Given only after clamping the umbilical cord in cesarean birth. Daily dose may be repeated for 2 days in prosthetic arthroplasty or open heart surgery.

Dilution: *Direct IV:* Dilute 0.5 Gm with 2 ml of sterile water for injection and each 1 Gm with 2.5 ml.

Intermittent IV: A single dose may be further diluted or initially diluted with 50 to 100 ml of 5% dextrose in water, 0.9% sodium chloride, or other compatible infusion solution for injection (see literature). Shake well.

Rate of administration: *Direct IV:* A single dose equally distributed over 3 to 5 minutes. May be given through Y-tube or three-way stopcock of infusion set.

Intermittent IV: A single dose over 30 minutes.

Actions: A broad-spectrum second-generation cephalosporin antibiotic. Bactericidal to selected gram-negative, gram-positive, and anaerobic organisms. Effective against many otherwise resistant organisms. Absorbed by most body fluids. 99% excreted in the urine. Crosses placental barrier. Secreted in breast milk.

Indications and uses: (1) Treatment of serious lower respiratory tract, urinary tract, and skin and skin structure infections; and septicemia. Most effective against specific organisms (see literature). (2) Perioperative prophylaxis.

Precautions: (1) Sensitivity studies using the "Monocid" disk are indicated to determine susceptibility of the causative organism to cefonicid. (2) Watch for early symptoms of allergic reaction. (3) Reduce total daily dose if renal function impaired. Calculated according to degree of impairment. (4) Continue for at least 2 to 3 days after all symptoms of infection subside. Avoid prolonged use of drug; superinfection caused by overgrowth of nonsusceptible organisms may result. (5) Administer within 24 hours of preparation, or within

72 hours if refrigerated. Slight yellowing does not affect potency. (6) Use extreme caution in the penicillin-sensitive patient; cross-sensitivity may occur. (7) Adverse interaction may occur with promethazine (Phenergan), procainamide (Pronestyl), quinidine, muscle relaxants, potent diuretics, and aminoglycosides. (8) May be used concomitantly with aminoglycosides in severe infections, but these drugs must never be mixed in the same infusion or given concurrently. Nephrotoxicity markedly increased when both drugs utilized. (9) Use only if absolutely necessary in pregnancy and lactation. (10) Higher blood levels obtained with probenecid. (11) Avoid concurrent administration of bacteriostatic agents; will inhibit bactericidal action. (12) Single daily dose reduces incidence of thrombophlebitis. Use of small needles and large veins and rotation of infusion sites is still preferred. (13) Electrolyte imbalance and cardiac irregularities resulting from sodium con tent are possible. Contains 3.7 mEq sodium/Gm. (14) Safety for use in children not established. Immature renal function of infants and small children will increase blood levels of all cephalosporins.

Contraindications: Known sensitivity to cefonicid, cephalosporins, or related antibiotics (penicillins).

Incompatible with: Aminoglycosides (e.g., kanamycin [Kantrex]). Should be considered incompatible in syringe or solution with any other bacteriostatic agent.

Side effects: Full scope of allergic reactions including anaphylaxis. Burning, discomfort, and pain at injection site; diarrhea; increase in platelets and eosinophils; elevated alkaline phosphatase, SGOT, SGPT, GGTP, and LDH; positive direct Coombs' test; pseudomembranous colitis; and seizures (large doses).

Antidote: Notify physician of any side effects. Discontinue the drug if indicated. Treat allergic reaction as indicated and resuscitate as necessary. Mild cases of colitis may respond to discontinuation of cefonicid. Vancomycin (Vancocin) or metronidazole (Flagyl) is the treatment of choice for antibiotic-related pseudomembranous colitis. Hemodialysis may be useful in overdose.

CEFOPERAZONE SODIUM pH 4.5 to 6.5

(Cefobid)

Usual dose: 2 to 4 Gm/24 hr in equally divided doses every 12 hours. Total daily dose and frequency may be increased in severe infections. 12 to 16 Gm have been given in 24 hours.

Dilution: Each 1 Gm must be diluted with 5 ml sterile water. Difficult to put into solution. Shake vigorously to ensure solution, then allow to sit, and examine for clarity. Each 1 Gm may be further diluted with 20 to 40 ml 5% dextrose in water, normal saline, or other compatible solutions (see literature) to a maximum dilution of 50 mg/ml for intermittent infusion, or diluted to 2 to 25 mg/ml and given as a continuous infusion.

Rate of administration: *Direct IV:* A single dose equally distributed over 3 to 5 minutes. May be given through Y-tube or three-way stopcock of infusion set.

Intermittent IV: A single dose over 15 to 30 minutes. Discontinue primary infusion during administration.

Continuous infusion: 500 to 1,000 ml over 6 to 24 hours, depending on total dose and concentration.

Actions: A broad-spectrum third-generation cephalosporin antibiotic similar to cefamandole. Bactericidal to many gram-negative, gram-positive, and anaerobic organisms. Effective against organisms resistant to other second- and third-generation cephalosporins. Absorbed by most body fluids including inflamed meninges and bone tissue. Excreted in bile. Crosses placental barrier. Secreted in breast milk.

Indications and uses: Treatment of serious respiratory tract, intraabdominal, skin and skin structure, and gynecological infections; and bacterial septicemia. Most effective against specific organisms (see literature).

Precautions: (1) Sensitivity studies indicated to determine susceptibility of the causative organism to cefoperazone. (2) Watch for early symptoms of allergic reaction. (3) Reduce total daily dose if renal function impaired. Calculated according to degree of impairment. Immature renal function will increase blood levels in neonates. (4) Continue for at least 2 to 3 days after all symptoms of infection subside. Avoid prolonged use of drug; superinfection caused by overgrowth of nonsusceptible organisms may result. (5) Administer within 24 hours of preparation. Selected solutions may be preserved 5 days with refrigeration. (6) Use extreme caution in the penicillin-sensitive patient; cross-sensitivity may occur. (7) Adverse interaction may occur with promethazine (Phenergan), procainamide (Pronestyl), quinidine, muscle relaxants, potent diuretics, and aminoglycosides. Will produce symptoms of acute alcohol intolerance with alcohol. Abstain until at least 72 hours after discontinued. (8) Frequently used concomitantly with aminoglycosides in severe infections, but these drugs must never be mixed in the same infusion or given concurrently. Use individual secondary tubings and irrigate primary tubing between doses. Nephrotoxicity markedly increased when both drugs utilized. (9) Use only if absolutely necessary in pregnancy. (10) Use caution in patients with liver impairment. (11) Probenecid inhibits excretion and may require reduction in dosage. (12) Avoid concurrent administration of bacteriostatic agents; will inhibit bactericidal action. (13) May cause thrombophlebitis. Use small needles and large veins, and rotate infusion sites. (14) Electrolyte imbalance and cardiac irregularities resulting from sodium content are very possible. Contains 1.5 mEq sodium/Gm. (15) Will cause hypoprothrombinemia; 10 mg/week of prophylactic vitamin K is recommended. Platelet dysfunction can be avoided by limiting dose to 4 Gm/24 hr and using vitamin K. Bleeding tendency increased with heparin and oral anticoagulants (warfarin [Coumadin]).

Contraindications: Known sensitivity to cephalosporins or related antibiotics (penicillins). Not recommended for use in children.

Incompatible with: Labetalol (Trandate), perphenazine (Trilafon). Should be considered incompatible in syringe or solution with all aminoglycosides (e.g., kanamycin [Kantrex]) and any other bacteriostatic agent.

Side effects: Full scope of allergic reactions including anaphylaxis. Abnormal bleeding; decreased hemoglobin or decreased hematocrit; decreased PT; decreased platelet functions; diarrhea; dyspnea; eosinophilia; elevation of SGOT, SGPT, total bilirubin, alkaline phosphatase,

LDH, and BUN (transient); false positive reaction for urine glucose except with Tes-Tape or Keto-Diastix; fever; leukopenia; local site pain; pseudomembranous colitis; seizures (large doses); thrombocytopenia; thrombophlebitis; transient neutropenia; vaginitis; vomiting.

Antidote: Notify the physician of any side effects. Discontinue the drug if indicated. Treat allergic reaction as indicated and resuscitate as necessary. Hemodialysis may be useful in overdose. Vitamin K, fresh frozen plasma, packed red cells, or platelet concentrates may be indicated in abnormal bleeding tendencies confirmed by laboratory evaluations. If bleeding due to platelet dysfunction, discontinue and use cefamandole or moxalactam with caution.

CEFORANIDE — pH 5.5 to 8.5

(Precef)

Usual dose: 0.5 to 1 Gm/12 hr.

Perioperative prophylaxis: 0.5 to 1 Gm IV 1 hour before incision. Daily dose may be repeated for 2 days in prosthetic arthroplasty or open heart surgery.

Pediatric dose: 20 to 40 mg/kg of body weight/24 hr in equally divided doses every 12 hours.

Dilution: *Direct IV:* Dilute each 0.5 Gm with 5 ml of sterile water or normal saline for injection.

Intermittent IV: A single dose may be further diluted in 50 to 100 ml of 5% dextrose in water, 0.9% sodium chloride, or other compatible infusion solution for injection (see literature). Shake well.

Rate of administration: *Direct IV:* A single dose equally distributed over 3 to 5 minutes. May be given through Y-tube or three-way stopcock of infusion set.

Intermittent IV: A single dose over 30 minutes.

Actions: A broad-spectrum second-generation cephalosporin antibiotic. Bactericidal to selected gram-negative, gram-positive, and anaerobic organisms. Effective against many otherwise resistant organisms. Therapeutic levels absorbed into the gallbladder, myocardium, bone, skeletal muscle, vaginal tissue, pericardial fluid, synovial fluid, and bile. Excreted unchanged in the urine. Crosses placental barrier. May be secreted in breast milk.

Indications and uses: (1) Treatment of serious lower respiratory tract, urinary tract, skin and skin structure, and bone and joint infections; and endocarditis. Most effective against specific organisms (see literature). (2) Perioperative prophylaxis.

Precautions: (1) Specific sensitivity studies are indicated to determine susceptibility of the causative organism to ceforanide. (2) Watch for early symptoms of allergic reaction. (3) Reduce total daily dose if renal function impaired. Calculated according to degree of impairment. (4) Continue for 2 to 3 days after all symptoms of infection subside. Avoid prolonged use of drug; superinfection caused by overgrowth of nonsusceptible organisms may result. (5) Administer within 24 hours of preparation. Will be light yellow to amber in color depending on concentration and diluent. (6) Use extreme caution in the penicillin-sensitive patient; cross-sensitivity may occur. (7) Adverse interaction may occur with promethazine (Phenergan), procainamide (Pronestyl), quinidine, muscle relaxants, potent diuretics, and aminoglycosides. (8) May be used concomitantly with aminoglycosides in severe infections, but these drugs must never be mixed in the same infusion or given concurrently. Nephrotoxicity markedly increased when both drugs utilized. (9) Use only if absolutely necessary in pregnancy and lactation. (10) Probenecid does not increase blood levels as it does with other cephalosporins. (11) Avoid concurrent administration of bacteriostatic agents; will inhibit bactericidal action. (12) May cause thrombophlebitis. Use small needles and large veins, and rotate infusion sites. (13) Ceforanide is sodium free. (14) Safety for use in infants under 1 year of age not established. Immature renal function of infants and small children will increase blood levels of all cephalosporins.

Contraindications: Known sensitivity to ceforanide, cephalosporins, or related antibiotics (penicillins).

Incompatible with: Should be considered incompatible in syringe or solution with any other bacteriostatic agent and all aminoglycosides (e.g., kanamycin [Kantrex]).

Side effects: Full scope of allergic reactions including anaphylaxis. Burning, discomfort, and pain at injection site; diarrhea; elevated alkaline phosphatase, SGOT, SGPT, and BUN; nausea and vomiting; positive direct Coombs' test; pseudomembranous colitis; seizures (large doses); transient thrombocytosis.

Antidote: Notify physician of any side effects. Discontinue the drug if indicated. Treat allergic reaction as indicated and resuscitate as necessary. Mild cases of colitis may respond to discontinuation of ceforanide. Vancomycin (Vancocin) or metronidazole (Flagyl) is the treatment of choice for antibiotic-related pseudomembranous colitis. Hemodialysis may be useful in overdose.

CEFOTAXIME SODIUM pH 4.5 to 7.0

(Claforan)

Usual dose: Depends on seriousness of infection. 1 to 2 Gm every 4 to 6 or 8 hours. Usually 1 Gm every 6 to 8 hours. Maximum daily dose is 12 Gm. Higher doses often reduced with positive clinical response.

Perioperative prophylaxis: 1 Gm 30 to 90 minutes before incision. Then 1 Gm 30 to 120 minutes later. May be repeated in a lengthy procedure. In cesarean birth give initial dose after cord is clamped, then 1 Gm at 6 and 12 hours postoperatively.

Pediatric dose: *Newborn to 1 week:* 50 mg/kg of body weight every 12 hours.

1 to 4 weeks: 50 mg/kg every 8 hours.

1 month to 12 years: Weight less than 50 kg, 50 to 180 mg/kg/day in 4 to 6 divided doses.

Dilution: Each single dose must be diluted with 10 ml sterile water, 5% dextrose in water, 0.9% sodium chloride, or other compatible infusion solution for injection (see literature). Available premixed. May be further diluted with compatible solutions and given as an intermittent infusion or added to larger volumes and given as a continuous infusion.

Rate of administration: *Direct IV:* A single dose equally distributed over 3 to 5 minutes. May be given through Y-tube or three-way stopcock of infusion set.

Intermittent IV: A single dose over 30 minutes. Discontinue primary infusion during administration.

Continuous infusion: 500 to 1,000 ml over 6 to 24 hours, depending on total dose and concentration.

Actions: A broad-spectrum third-generation cephalosporin antibiotic. Bactericidal to many gram-negative, gram-positive, and anaerobic organisms. Effective against many otherwise resistant organisms. Absorbed by most body fluids including inflamed meninges. Some metabolites formed. Excreted in the urine. Crosses placental barrier. Secreted in breast milk.

Indications and uses: (1) Treatment of serious lower respiratory tract, urinary tract, skin and skin structure, intraabdominal, bone and joint, CNS, and gynecological infections; bacteremia/septicemia; disseminated gonococcal infection; and gonococcal ophthalmia. Most effective against specific organisms (see literature). (2) Perioperative prophylaxis.

Precautions: (1) Sensitivity studies indicated to determine susceptibility of the causative organism to cefotaxime. (2) Watch for early symptoms of allergic reaction. (3) Reduce total daily dose if renal function impaired. Calculated according to degree of impairment. (4) Continue for 2 to 3 days after all symptoms of infection subside. Avoid prolonged use of drug; superinfection caused by overgrowth of nonsusceptible organisms may result. (5) Administer within 24 hours of preparation, or within 5 days if refrigerated. (6) Use extreme caution in the penicillin-sensitive patient; cross-sensitivity may occur. (7) Adverse interaction may occur with promethazine (Phenergan), procainamide (Pronestyl), quinidine, muscle relaxants, potent diuretics, and aminoglycosides. (8) Frequently used concomitantly with aminoglycosides in severe infections, but these drugs must never be mixed in the same infusion or given concurrently. (9) Use only if absolutely necessary in pregnancy. (10) Probenecid inhibits excretion and may require reduction in dosage. (11) Avoid concurrent administration of bacteriostatic agents; will inhibit bactericidal actions. (12) May cause thrombophlebitis. Use small needles and large veins, and rotate infusion sites. (13) Electrolyte imbalance and cardiac irregularities resulting from high sodium content are very possible. Contains 2.2 mEq sodium/Gm.

Contraindications: Known sensitivity to cephalosporins or related antibiotics (penicillins).

Incompatible with: Should be considered incompatible in syringe or solution with any other bacteriostatic agent; all aminoglycosides (e.g., kanamycin [Kantrex]); all diluents with a pH of 7.5 or more (e.g., aminophylline and sodium bicarbonate).

Side effects: Full scope of allergic reactions including anaphylaxis. Decreased hemoglobin or decreased hematocrit; decreased PT; decreased platelet functions; diarrhea; dyspnea; elevation of SGOT, SGPT, total bilirubin, alkaline phosphatase, LDH, and BUN (transient); eosinophilia; false positive reaction for urine glucose except with Tes-Tape or Keto-Diastix; fever; leukopenia; local site pain; nausea; oral thrush; positive direct Coombs' test; pseudomembranous colitis; seizures (large doses) thrombocytopenia; thrombophlebitis; transient neutropenia; vaginitis; vomiting.

Antidote: Notify the physician of any side effects. Discontinue the drug if indicated. Oral vancomycin (Vancocin) or metronidazole (Flagyl) is the treatment of choice for antibiotic-related pseudomembranous colitis. Treat allergic reaction as indicated and resuscitate as necessary. Hemodialysis may be useful in overdose.

CEFOTETAN DISODIUM pH 4.5 to 6.5

(Cefotan)

Usual dose: 1 or 2 Gm every 12 hours for 5 to 10 days. Do not exceed 6 Gm/24 hr.

Perioperative prophylaxis: 1 to 2 Gm IV 30 to 60 minutes before incision except during cesarean birth. Given only after clamping the umbilical cord in cesarean birth.

Dilution: *Direct IV:* Dilute each 1 Gm with 10 ml of sterile water for injection (2 Gm with 20 ml).

Intermittent IV: A single dose may be further diluted or initially diluted with 50 to 100 ml of 5% dextrose in water or 0.9% sodium chloride. Shake well and let stand until clear.

Rate of administration: *Direct IV:* A single dose equally distributed over 3 to 5 minutes.

Intermittent IV: A single dose over 30 minutes. May be given through Y-tube or three-way stopcock of infusion set. Discontinue primary infusion during administration.

Actions: A broad-spectrum third-generation cephalosporin antibiotic. Bactericidal to selected gram-negative, gram-positive, and anaerobic organisms. Effective against many otherwise resistant organisms. Absorbed by many body fluids and tissues. Primarily excreted in the urine. Crosses placental barrier. Secreted in breast milk.

Indications and uses: (1) Treatment of serious lower respiratory tract, urinary tract, skin and skin structure, gynecological, intraabdominal, and bone and joint infections. Most effective against specific organisms (see literature). (2) Perioperative prophylaxis.

Precautions: (1) Sensitivity studies using the Cefotan 30 mcg disk are indicated to determine susceptibility of the causative organism to cefotetan. (2) Watch for early symptoms of allergic reaction. (3) Reduce total daily dose if renal function impaired. Calculated according to degree of impairment. (4) Continue for at least 2 or 3 days after all symptoms of infection subside. Avoid prolonged use of drug; superinfection caused by overgrowth of nonsusceptible organisms may result. (5) Administer within 24 hours of preparation, or within 96 hours if refrigerated. Stable after dilution for 1 week if frozen; thaw at room temperature before use, discard remaining solution, do not refreeze. Slight yellowing does not affect potency. (6) Use extreme caution in the penicillin-sensitive patient; cross-sensitivity may occur. (7) Adverse interaction may occur with promethazine (Phenergan), procainamide (Pronestyl), quinidine, muscle relaxants, potent diuretics, and aminoglycosides. (8) May be used concomitantly with aminoglycosides in severe infections, but these drugs must never be mixed in the same infusion or given concurrently. Nephrotoxicity markedly increased when both drugs utilized. (9) Bleeding tendency increased with heparin or oral anticoagulants (warfarin [Coumadin]). (10) Will produce symptoms of acute alcohol intolerance with alcohol. Abstain until at least 72 hours after discontinued. (11) May cause hypoprothrombinemia. Monitor PT in cases of renal or hepatic impairment and in patients with poor nutritional status. (12) Use caution in patients with a history of GI disease, especially colitis. (13) Use only if absolutely necessary in pregnancy and lactation. (14) Higher blood levels possible with probenecid. (15) Avoid concurrent administration of bacteriostatic agents; will inhibit bactericidal action. (16) May cause thrombophlebitis. Use small needles and large veins, and rotate infusion sites. (17) Electrolyte imbalance and cardiac irregularities resulting from sodium content are possible. Contains 3.5 mEq sodium/Gm. (18) Safety for use in children not established. Immature renal function of infants and small children will increase blood levels of all cephalosporins.

Contraindications: Known sensitivity to cefotetan, cephalosporins, or related antibiotics.

Incompatible with: Should be considered incompatible in syringe or solution with any other bacteriostatic agent; all aminoglycosides (e.g., kanamycin [Kantrex]), doxapram (Dopram), heparin, tetracyclines.

Side effects: Full scope of allergic reactions including anaphylaxis. Bleeding episodes; burning, discomfort, and pain at injection site; diarrhea; eosinophilia; elevated alkaline phosphatase, SGOT, SGPT, and LDH; false increases in creatinine levels with Jaffe method; false positive for urine glucose with Benedict's or Fehling's solution; positive direct Coombs' test; nausea; pseudomembranous colitis; seizures (large doses); thrombocytosis.

Antidote: Notify physician of any side effects. Discontinue the drug if indicated. Treat allergic reaction as indicated and resuscitate as necessary. Mild cases of colitis may respond to discontinuation of cefotetan. Oral vancomycin (Vancocin) or metronidazole (Flagyl) is the treatment of choice for antibiotic-related pseudomembranous colitis. Bleeding episodes may respond to Vitamin K or require discontinuation of drug. Hemodialysis may be useful in overdose.

CEFOXITIN SODIUM — pH 4.2 to 7.0

(Mefoxin)

Usual dose: 1 to 2 Gm every 6 to 8 hours depending on severity of the infection.

Perioperative prophylaxis: 2 Gm 30 minutes to 1 hour before incision. Follow with 2 Gm every 6 hours for 24 to 72 hours. During cesarean birth, give after clamping the umbilical cord. Repeat in 4 hours times two then every 6 hours for 24 hours.

Pediatric dose: *Infants and children over 3 months of age:* 80 to 160 mg/kg of body weight/24 hours in equally divided doses every 4 to 6 hours. Do not exceed adult dose.

Perioperative prophylaxis in infants and children over 3 months of age: 30 to 40 mg/kg every 6 hours.

Dilution: Each 1 Gm or fraction thereof must be diluted with at least 10 ml of sterile water, 5% dextrose in water, or normal saline for injection. A single dose may be further diluted in 50 to 1,000 ml of most common infusion solutions (see literature) and given through a Y-tube, three-way stopcock, additive infusion set, or as a continuous infusion.

Rate of administration: Each 1 Gm or fraction thereof over 3 to 5 minutes or longer as indicated by amount of solution and condition of the patient. Discontinue IV infusion solution during administration of cefoxitin by intermittent infusion. Rate of continuous infusion should be by physician order.

Actions: A semisynthetic second-generation cephalosporin antibiotic that is bactericidal to many gram-positive, gram-negative, and anaerobic organisms. Absorbed by most body fluids including inflamed meninges and bone tissue. Crosses the placental barrier. Excreted rapidly in the urine. Secreted in breast milk.

Indications and uses: (1) Treatment of serious respiratory, GU, intraabdominal, gynecological, bone and joint, and skin and skin structure infections; and septicemia. Effective only if the causative organism is susceptible. (2) Perioperative prophylaxis.

Precautions: (1) Sensitivity studies indicated to determine susceptibility of the causative organism to cefoxitin. (2) Watch for early symptoms of allergic reaction. (3) Reduce total daily dose if renal function impaired; calculated according to degree of impairment. (4) Continue for at least 2 to 3 days after all symptoms of infection subside. Avoid prolonged use of drug; superinfection caused by overgrowth of nonsusceptible organisms may result. (5) Administer within 24 hours of preparation, or up to 1 week if refrigerated. (6) Use extreme caution in the penicillin-sensitive patient; cross-sensitivity may occur. (7) Adverse interaction may occur with promethazine (Phenergan), procainamide (Pronestyl), quinidine, muscle relaxants, potent diuretics, and aminoglycosides. (8) Frequently used concomitantly with aminoglycosides in severe infections, but these drugs must never be mixed in the same infusion or given concurrently. Nephrotoxicity markedly increased when both drugs utilized. (9) Use only if absolutely necessary in pregnancy. (10) Probenecid inhibits excretion and may require reduction in dosage. (11) Use of scalp-vein needles may reduce incidence of phlebitis. (12) Safety for infants and children under 3 months not established; immature renal function will increase blood levels. (13) Electrolyte imbalance and cardiac irregularities resulting from high sodium content are very possible. Contains 2.3 mEq sodium/Gm. (14) Avoid concurrent use of bacteriostatic agents; will inhibit bactericidal action.

Contraindications: Known sensitivity to cephalosporins or related antibiotics (penicillins).

Incompatible with: All aminoglycosides (e.g., gentamicin [Garamycin], tobramycin [Nebcin]), amikacin (Ami kin), carbenicillin (Geopen).

Side effects: Allergic reactions including anaphylaxis; anorexia; false positive reaction for urine glucose except with Tes-Tape or Keto-Diastix; leukopenia; local site pain; nausea and vomiting; neutropenia; oral thrush; phlebitis; positive direct Coombs' test; transient elevation of SGOT, SGPT, BUN, and alkaline phosphatase; proteinuria; pseudomembranous colitis; seizures (large doses); and thrombophlebitis.

Antidote: Notify physician of any side effects. Discontinue the drug if indicated. Oral vancomycin (Vancocin) or metronidazole (Flagyl) is the treatment of choice for antibiotic-related pseudomembranous colitis. Treat allergic reaction as indicated and resuscitate as necessary.

CEFPIRAMIDE SODIUM — pH 6.0 to 8.0

Usual dose: 1 to 2 Gm every 12 hours or 2 to 3 Gm once a day. Dosage based on severity of disease and patient's condition. Continue for at least 2 to 3 days after all symptoms of infection subside. Treat infections caused by *Streptococcus pyogenes* for at least 10 days.

Dilution: *Direct IV:* Dilute each 1 Gm with 9.4 ml of sterile water for injection; 5% dextrose in water, lactated Ringer's injection, Normosol-M, 0.2% or 0.9% sodium chloride; normal saline; or lactated Ringer's injection (100 mg/ml). Add an additional 10 ml to each 1 Gm for a 50 mg/ml dilution. Shake well.

Infusion: A single 1 Gm dose may be diluted in 49 to 99 ml of the above solutions and given as an infusion; 49 ml results in 20 mg/ml and 99 ml in 10 mg/

ml. A 2 Gm dose diluted in the same amounts will result in 40 mg/ml and 20 mg/ml.

Rate of administration: *Direct IV:* A single dose equally distributed over 3 to 5 minutes.

Intermittent IV: A single dose over 30 minutes. May be given through Y-tube or three-way stopcock of infusion set.

Actions: A semisynthetic, broad-spectrum third-generation cephalosporin antibiotic. Bactericidal through inhibition of cell wall synthesis to selected gram-negative and gram-positive organisms. Prolonged serum levels maintained after a single dose. Half-life averages 5.7 hours. Serum concentrations increase with larger doses. Elimination pathways are not clear, but high concentrations are found in bile and small amounts in the urine. Crosses placental barrier. Secreted in breast milk.

Indications and uses: Treatment of serious respiratory tract, and skin and skin structure infections (including pneumonia). Most effective against specific organisms (see literature).

Precautions: (1) Specific sensitivity studies utilizing a 30 mcg cefpiramide disk are indicated to determine susceptibility of the causative organism to cefpiramide. (2) Watch for early symptoms of allergic reaction. Use caution in patients with history of asthma or other allergies. (3) Use extreme caution in the penicillin-sensitive patient; cross-sensitivity has occurred. (4) Impaired renal function usually does not require dose adjustment; however, in some patients serum half-life doubles. Monitor and adjust dose if indicated. (5) Avoid prolonged use of drug; superinfection caused by overgrowth of nonsusceptible organisms may result. (6) Not recommended for patients with known or suspected hepatic dysfunction; use caution in patients with a history of GI disease, especially colitis. (7) Adverse interactions may occur with other highly protein-bound drugs (e.g., phenytoin [Dilantin], warfarin [Coumadin], quinidine). (8) Nephrotoxicity may increase with aminoglycoside antibiotics (e.g., gentamicin [Garamycin]) and furosemide (Lasix). (9) Avoid concurrent administration of bacteriostatic agents. (10) May increase PT in patients with impaired vitamin K synthesis, malnutrition, or taking warfarin (Coumadin). Monitor PT; vitamin K may be indicated. (11) Produces a disulfiramlike reaction with alcohol (flushing, sweating, headache, tachycardia). Patient must abstain from alcohol during treatment and until at least 1 week after completion. (12) Use only if absolutely necessary in pregnancy. Discontinue breast feeding until course of therapy complete. (13) Safety for use in children not established. Testicular atrophy occurred in young rats given high doses. (14) May cause thrombophlebitis. Use small needles and large veins, and rotate infusion sites. (15) Consider 2.5 mEq sodium content/Gm in patients with cardiac or electrolyte problems. (16) Stable before and after dilution for 3 days at room temperature, 6 days if refrigerated. May congeal under refrigeration, warm to room temperature before administration; will liquify with no adverse changes. May be frozen for up to 2 months after initial dilution; thaw at room temperature (see literature); do not refreeze.

Contraindications: Known hypersensitivity to cefpiramide, cephalosporins, or related antibiotics.

Incompatible with: Limited information available. Should be considered incompatible in syringe or solution with any other bacteriostatic agent; all aminoglycosides (e.g., kanamycin [Kantrex]).

Side effects: Generally well tolerated. Full scope of allergic reactions including anaphylaxis. Burning, discomfort, and pain at injection site; diarrhea; elevated alkaline phosphatase, SGOT, SGPT, and GGT; elevated PT, PTT, and other differential blood cell abnormalities (e.g., eosinophilia); elevated serum amylase, BUN, and creatinine; headache; nausea and vomiting; pseudomembranous colitis.

Antidote: Notify physician of any side effects. Discontinue the drug if indicated. Treat allergic reaction as indicated and resuscitate as necessary. Mild cases of colitis may respond to discontinuation of cefpiramide. Oral vancomycin (Vancocin) or metronidazole (Flagyl) is the treatment of choice for antibiotic-related pseudomembranous colitis. Overdose may precipitate seizures, especially in patients with renal impairment; may require anticonvulsants (e.g., diazepam [Valium]).

CEFTAZIDIME pH 5.0 to 8.0

(Ceptaz, Fortaz, Tazicef, Tazidime)

Usual dose: 1 Gm every 8 to 12 hours. Range is from 250 mg to 2 Gm every 8 to 12 hours. Dosage based on severity of disease and condition of the patient. Normal renal function required. Continue for at least 2 days after all symptoms of infection subside.

Pediatric dose: *1 month to 12 years:* 30 to 50 mg/kg of body weight every 8 hours. Do not exceed 6 Gm/24 hr.

Neonatal dose: *Up to 4 weeks:* 30 mg/kg every 12 hours.

Dilution: *Direct IV:* Dilute 0.5 Gm with 5 ml of sterile water; 1 Gm or more with 10 ml of sterile water for injection. Shake well. Dilution generates CO_2. Invert vial and completely depress plunger of syringe. Insert needle through stopper and keep it within the solution. Expel bubbles from solution in syringe before injection.

Intermittent IV: A single dose may be further diluted in 50 to 100 ml of 5% dextrose in water, 0.9% sodium chloride, or other compatible infusion solutions for injection (see literature).

Rate of administration: *Direct IV:* A single dose equally distributed over 3 to 5 minutes.

Intermittent IV: A single dose over 30 minutes. May be given through Y-tube or three-way stopcock of infusion set. Discontinue primary IV during administration.

Actions: A broad-spectrum third-generation cephalosporin antibiotic. Bactericidal to selected gram-negative, gram-positive, and anaerobic organisms. Effective against many otherwise resistant organisms. Therapeutic levels absorbed into many body fluids and tissues. Excreted unchanged in the urine. Crosses placental barrier. May be secreted in breast milk.

Indications and uses: Treatment of serious lower respiratory tract, urinary tract, skin and skin structure, bone and joint, gynecological, intraabdominal, and CNS infections (including meningitis); and bacterial septicemia. Most effective against specific organisms (see literature).

Precautions: (1) Specific sensitivity studies utilizing a 30 mcg ceftazidime disk are indicated to determine susceptibility of the causative organism to ceftazidime. (2) Watch for early symptoms of allergic reaction. (3) Reduce total daily dose if renal function impaired. Calculated according to degree of impairment. (4) Avoid prolonged use of drug; superinfection caused by overgrowth of nonsusceptible organisms may result. (5) Administer within 18 hours of preparation, or refrigerate for up to 7 days. May be frozen for up to 3 months after initial dilution; thaw at room temperature (see instructions); do not refreeze. Will be light yellow to amber in color depending on concentration and diluent. (6) Use extreme caution in the penicillin-sensitive patient; cross-sensitivity may occur. (7) Adverse interaction may occur with promethazine (Phenergan), procainamide (Pronestyl), quinidine, muscle relaxants, potent diuretics, and aminoglycosides. (8) May be used concomitantly with aminoglycosides, vancomycin, and clindamycin in severe infections, but these drugs must never be mixed in the same infusion or given concurrently. (9) Use only if absolutely necessary in pregnancy and lactation. (10) Probenecid does not increase blood levels as it does with other cephalosporins. (11) Avoid concurrent administration of bacteriostatic agents; will inhibit bactericidal action. (12) May cause thrombophlebitis. Use small needles and large veins, and rotate infusion sites. (13) Electrolyte imbalance and cardiac irregularities resulting from sodium content are possible. Contains 2.3 mEq of sodium/Gm. (14) Immature renal function of infants and small children will increase blood levels of all cephalosporins.

Contraindications: Known sensitivity to ceftazidime, cephalosporins, or related antibiotics.

Incompatible with: Should be considered incompatible in syringe or solution with any other bacteriostatic agent; all aminoglycosides (e.g., kanamycin [Kantrex]).

Side effects: Full scope of allergic reactions including anaphylaxis. Burning, discomfort, and pain at injection site; diarrhea; elevated alkaline phosphatase, SGOT, SGPT, GGT, and BUN; nausea and vomiting; positive direct Coombs' test; pseudomembranous colitis; seizures (large doses).

Antidote: Notify physician of any side effects. Discontinue the drug if indicated. Treat allergic reaction as indicated and resuscitate as necessary. Mild cases of colitis may respond to discontinuation of ceftazidime. Oral vancomycin (Vancocin) or metronidazole (Flagyl) is the treatment of choice for antibiotic-related pseudomembranous colitis. Hemodialysis may be useful in overdose.

CEFTIZOXIME SODIUM pH 6.0 to 8.0

(Cefizox)

Usual dose: Dependent on seriousness of infection. Range is 500 mg to 4 Gm every 8 to 12 hours. Higher doses often reduced with positive clinical response.

Pediatric dose: *Children over 6 months of age:* 50 mg/kg of body weight every 6 to 8 hours. Up to 200 mg/kg has been used, but do not exceed adult dose.

Dilution: Each 1 Gm must be diluted with 10 ml sterile water. Shake well. May be further diluted with 50 to 100 ml of sodium chloride or other compatible solutions and given as an intermittent infusion. Available premixed. Not given as a continuous infusion.

Rate of administration: *Direct IV:* A single dose equally distributed over 3 to 5 minutes. May be given through Y-tube or three-way stopcock of infusion set.
Intermittent IV: A single dose over 30 minutes.

Actions: A broad-spectrum third-generation cephalosporin antibiotic similar to cefamandole. Bactericidal to many gram-negative, gram-positive, and anaerobic organisms. Effective against many otherwise resistant organisms. Absorbed by most body fluids including inflamed meninges and bone tissue. Excreted in the urine. Crosses placental barrier. Secreted in breast milk.

Indications and uses: Treatment of serious infections of the lower respiratory tract, urinary tract; intraabdominal, skin and skin structure, and bone and joint infections; septicemia; and gonorrhea. Most effective against specific organisms (see literature).

Precautions: (1) Sensitivity studies indicated to determine susceptibility of the causative organism to ceftizoxime.

(2) Watch for early symptoms of allergic reaction. (3) Reduce total daily dose if renal function impaired. Calculated according to degree of impairment. (4) Continue for at least 2 to 3 days after all symptoms of infection subside. Avoid prolonged use of drug; superinfection caused by overgrowth of nonsusceptible organisms may result. (5) Administer within 8 hours of preparation, or within 48 hours if refrigerated. (6) Use extreme caution in the penicillin-sensitive patient; cross-sensitivity may occur. (7) Adverse interaction may occur with promethazine (Phenergan), procainamide (Pronestyl), quinidine, muscle relaxants, potent diuretics, and aminoglycosides. (8) Frequently used concomitantly with aminoglycosides in severe infections; but these drugs must never be mixed in the same infusion or given concurrently. Nephrotoxicity markedly increased when both drugs utilized. (9) Use only if absolutely necessary in pregnancy. (10) Probenecid inhibits excretion and may require reduction in dosage. (11) Avoid concurrent administration of bacteriostatic agents; will inhibit bactericidal action. (12) May cause thrombophlebitis. Use small needles and large veins, and rotate infusion sites. (13) Electrolyte imbalance and cardiac irregularities resulting from sodium content are very possible. Contains 2.6 mEq sodium/Gm.

Contraindications: Known sensitivity to cephalosporins or related antibiotics (penicillins). Not recommended for use in children under 6 months of age.

Incompatible with: Should be considered incompatible in syringe or solution with any other bacteriostatic agent; all aminoglycosides (e.g., kanamycin [Kantrex]).

Side effects: Full scope of allergic reactions including anaphylaxis. Decreased hemoglobin or decreased hematocrit; decreased PT; decreased platelet functions; diarrhea; dyspnea; elevation of SGOT, SGPT, total bilirubin, alkaline phosphatase, LDH, and BUN (transient); eosinophilia; false positive reaction for urine glucose except with Tes-Tape or Keto-Diastix; fever; leukopenia; local site pain; nausea; oral thrush; positive direct Coombs' test; pseudomembranous colitis; seizures (large doses); thrombocytopenia; thrombophlebitis; vaginitis; vomiting.

Antidote: Notify the physician of any side effects. Discontinue the drug if indicated. Oral vancomycin (Vancocin) or metronidazole (Flagyl) is the treatment of choice for antibiotic-related pseudomembranous colitis. Treat allergic reaction as indicated and resuscitate as necessary. Hemodialysis may be useful in overdose.

CEFTRIAXONE SODIUM pH 6.7

(Rocephin)

Usual dose: 1 to 2 Gm/24 hr. May be given as a single dose every 24 hours or equally divided into 2 doses and given every 12 hours. Do not exceed a total dose of 4 Gm/24 hr.

Lyme disease: 4 Gm/24 hr equally divided into 2 doses every 12 hours. Treat for 14 days.

Perioperative prophylaxis: 1 Gm IV 30 minutes to 2 hours before incision. Used primarily in patients undergoing coronary artery bypass surgery.

Pediatric dose: 50 to 75 mg/kg of body weight/24 hr in equally divided doses every 12 hours. Do not exceed a total dose of 2 Gm/24 hr. In meningitis increase the dosage to 100 mg/kg/24 hr. Do not exceed a total dose of 4 Gm/24 hr.

Dilution: Initially dilute each 250 mg with 2.4 ml (500 mg with 4.8 ml, etc.) of sterile water, normal saline, or 5% or 10% dextrose in water or saline for injection. Each ml will contain 100 mg. A single dose must be further diluted with 50 to 100 ml normal saline or 5% or 10% dextrose in water or saline and be given as an intermittent infusion. Shake well. Concentrations of 10 mg/ml to 40 mg/ml are recommended for intermittent infusion.

Rate of administration: *Intermittent IV:* A single dose over 30 minutes.

Actions: A broad-spectrum third-generation cephalosporin antibiotic. Bactericidal to selected gram-negative, gram-positive, and anaerobic organisms. Effective against many otherwise resistant organisms. Absorbed by most body fluids. Excreted through bile and urine. Crosses placental barrier. Secreted in breast milk.

Indications and uses: (1) Treatment of serious lower respiratory tract, urinary tract, skin and skin structure, bone and joint, and intraabdominal infections; pelvic inflammatory disease; bacterial septicemia; and meningitis. Most effective against specific organisms (see literature). (2) Perioperative prophylaxis.

Unlabeled use: Treatment of Lyme disease.

Precautions: (1) Sensitivity studies are indicated to determine susceptibility of the causative organism to ceftriaxone. (2) Watch for early symptoms of allergic reaction. (3) Reduction of total daily dose in impaired renal function is not necessary if dose does not exceed 2 Gm/24 hr. Monitor serum levels in patients with severe renal impairment or both renal and hepatic function impairment. (4) Alterations in PT have occurred. Monitor PT; vitamin K may be required. May cause bleeding episodes with anticoagulants. (5) Continue for at least 2 to 3 days after all symptoms of infection subside. Usual course of therapy 4 to 14 days. Avoid prolonged use of drug; superinfection caused by overgrowth of nonsusceptible organisms may result. (6) Stable at room temperature for at least 24 hours in stated solutions or up to 10 days if refrigerated. Stability and color (clear to yellow) depend on concentration and diluent. Thaw frozen solutions at room temperature before use. Discard unused portions; do not re freeze. (7) Use extreme caution in the penicillin-sensitive patient; cross-sensitivity may occur. (8) Adverse interaction may occur with promethazine (Phenergan), procainamide (Pronestyl), quinidine, muscle relaxants, potent diuretics, and aminoglycosides. (9) May be used concomitantly with aminoglycosides in severe infections, but these drugs must never be mixed in the same infusion or given concurrently. Nephrotoxicity markedly increased when both drugs utilized. (10) Use only if absolutely necessary in pregnancy and lactation. (11) Higher blood levels possible with probenecid. (12) Avoid concurrent administration of bacteriostatic agents; will inhibit bactericidal action. (13) Single daily dose reduces incidence of thrombophlebitis. Use of small needles, large veins, and rotation of infusion sites is still preferred. (14) Electrolyte imbalance and cardiac irregularities resulting from sodium content are possible but not likely with single daily dose. Contains 3.6 mEq sodium/Gm. (15) Immature renal function of infants and small children will increase blood levels of all cephalosporins. (16) Use caution in GI diseases or patients with a history of colitis.

Contraindications: Known sensitivity to ceftriaxone or other cephalosporins.

Incompatible with: Should be considered incompatible in syringe, solution, or IV tubing with any other bacteriostatic agent; clindamycin and all aminoglycosides (e.g., kanamycin [Kantrex]).

Side effects: Full scope of allergic reactions including anaphylaxis are possible. Bleeding episodes; burning, discomfort, and pain at injection site; casts in urine; diarrhea; dizziness; eosinophilia; elevated alkaline phosphatase, bilirubin, BUN, creatinine, SGOT, and SGPT; headache; leukopenia; prolonged PT; pseudomembranous colitis; seizures (large doses); thrombocytosis.

Antidote: Notify physician of any side effects. Discontinue the drug if indicated. Treat allergic reaction as indicated and resuscitate as necessary. Mild cases of colitis may respond to discontinuation of ceftriaxone. Oral vancomycin (Vancocin) or metronidazole (Flagyl) is the treatment of choice for antibiotic-related pseudomembranous colitis. Vitamin K may be useful in bleeding episodes, or drug may have to be discontinued. Hemodialysis not useful in overdose.

CEFUROXIME SODIUM — pH 6.0 to 8.5

(Kefurox, Zinacef)

Usual dose: Dependent on seriousness of infection. Range is from 750 mg to 3 Gm every 8 hours for 5 to 10 days. 1.5 Gm every 6 hours is used for life-threatening infections.

Acute pelvic inflammatory disease: 150 mg/kg of body weight/day equally divided into 4 doses. May be given in combination with erythromycin, sulfisoxazole, or tetracycline. Continue IV until 2 days after symptoms subside. Continue other agents orally for 14 days.

Perioperative prophylaxis: 1.5 Gm IV 30 minutes to 1 hour before incision; then 750 mg every 8 hours for 24 hours or 1.5 Gm every 12 hours to total dose of 6 Gm in open heart surgery.

Pediatric dose: *Infants and children over 3 months of age:* 50 to 100 mg/kg of body weight/24 hr in equally divided doses every 6 to 8 hours. Increase to 200 to 240 mg/kg/day in bacterial meningitis.

Acute pelvic inflammatory disease in children over 7 years of age: 30 mg/kg/day equally divided into 3 doses. See adult regimen for rest of protocol.

Dilution: Each 750 mg must be diluted with 9 ml sterile water, 5% dextrose in water, 0.9% sodium chloride, or other compatible infusion solution for injection (see literature). Shake well. May be further diluted with compatible solutions to 50 or 100 ml and given as an intermittent infusion, or added to 500 to 1,000 ml and given as a continuous infusion.

Rate of administration: *Direct IV:* A single dose equally distributed over 3 to 5 minutes. May be given through Y-tube or three-way stopcock of infusion set.

Intermittent IV: A single dose over 30 minutes. Discontinue primary infusion during administration.

Continuous infusion: 500 to 1,000 ml over 6 to 24 hours, depending on total dose and concentration.

Actions: A broad-spectrum second-generation cephalosporin antibiotic. Bactericidal to selected gram-negative, gram-positive, and anaerobic organisms. Effective against many otherwise resistant organisms. Absorbed by most body fluids including inflamed meninges and bone tissue. Excreted in the urine. Crosses placental barrier. Secreted in breast milk.

Indications and uses: (1) Treatment of serious lower respiratory tract, urinary tract, and skin and skin structure infections; septicemia; meningitis; and gonorrhea. Most effective against specific organisms and when mixed organisms are present (see literature). (2) Perioperative prophylaxis.

Precautions: (1) Sensitivity studies indicated to determine susceptibility of the causative organism to cefuroxime. (2) Watch for early symptoms of allergic reaction. (3) Reduce total daily dose if renal function impaired. Calculated according to degree of impairment. (4) Continue for at least 2 to 3 days after all symptoms of infection subside. Avoid prolonged use of drug; superinfection caused by overgrowth of nonsusceptible organisms may result. (5) Administer within 24 hours of preparation, or within 48 hours if refrigerated. (6) Use extreme caution in the penicillin-sensitive patient; cross-sensitivity may occur. (7) Adverse interaction may occur with promethazine (Phenergan), procainamide (Pronestyl), quinidine, muscle relaxants, potent diuretics, and aminoglycosides. (8) Frequently used concomitantly with aminoglycosides in severe infections, but these drugs must never be mixed in the same infusion or given concurrently. Nephrotoxicity markedly increased when both drugs utilized. (9) Use only if absolutely necessary in pregnancy. (10) Probenecid inhibits excretion and may require reduction in dosage. (11) Avoid concurrent administration of bacteriostatic agents; will inhibit bactericidal action. (12) May cause thrombophlebitis. Use small needles and large veins, and rotate infusion sites. (13) Electrolyte imbalance and cardiac irregularities resulting from high sodium content are very possible. Contains 2.4 mEq sodium/Gm. (14) Safety for infants under 3 months of age not established; immature renal function will increase blood levels. (15) May cause a false negative reaction in specific blood glucose tests (ferricyanide).

Contraindications: Known sensitivity to cephalosporins or related antibiotics (penicillins).

Incompatible with: Should be considered incompatible in syringe or solution with any other bacteriostatic agent; all aminoglycosides (e.g., kanamycin [Kantrex]).

Side effects: Full scope of allergic reactions including anaphylaxis. Decreased hemoglobin, hematocrit, PT, or platelet functions; diarrhea; dyspnea; elevation of SGOT, SGPT, total bilirubin, alkaline phosphatase, LDH, and BUN (transient); eosinophilia; false positive reaction for urine glucose except with Tes-Tape or Keto-Diastix; fever; leukopenia; local site pain; nausea; oral thrush; positive direct Coombs' test; pseudomembranous colitis; transient neutropenia; seizures (large doses); thrombocytopenia; thrombophlebitis; vaginitis; vomiting.

Antidote: Notify physician of any side effects. Discontinue the drug if indicated. Treat antibiotic-related pseudomembranous colitis with oral vancomycin (Vancocin) or metronidazole (Flagyl). Treat allergic reaction and resuscitate as necessary. Hemodialysis may be useful in overdose.

CEPHALOTHIN SODIUM pH 6.0 to 8.5

(✱ Ceporacin, Keflin)

Usual dose: 1 to 2 Gm every 4 to 6 hours. Not to exceed 12 Gm/24 hr, depending on severity of infection.

Perioperative prophylaxis: 1 to 2 Gm 30 minutes to 1 hour before incision. May be repeated in OR and every 6 hours for 24 hours.

Pediatric dose: 80 to 160 mg/kg of body weight/24 hr in equally divided doses. *Do not exceed adult dose.*

Perioperative prophylaxis: 20 to 30 mg/kg. Give first dose 30 minutes to 1 hour before incision. May be repeated in OR and every 6 hours for 24 hours.

Dilution: Each 1 Gm or fraction thereof must be diluted with at least 10 ml of sterile water for injection. To reduce incidence of thrombophlebitis, may be further diluted in 50 ml or more of 5% dextrose in water, normal saline, or other compatible infusion solutions (see literature). Available premixed. May be administered through Y-tube, three-way stopcock, or additive infusion set.

Rate of administration: 1 Gm over 3 to 5 minutes or longer as indicated by amount of solution and condition of patient. Discontinue IV infusion solution during administration of cephalothin. May be given as a continuous infusion.

Actions: A broad-spectrum first-generation cephalosporin antibiotic. Bactericidal against some gram-positive and gram-negative organisms. Absorbed by all body fluids except bile and spinal fluid. Excreted rapidly in the urine. Crosses the placental barrier. Secreted in breast milk.

Indications and uses: (1) Treatment of severe infections of bone, joints, skin, soft tissue, bloodstream, cardiovascular system, respiratory tract, GU tract, and GI tract; peritonitis; septic abortion; and staphylococcal and pneumococcal meningitis (if more effective antibiotics are contraindicated); (2) perioperative prophylaxis.

Precautions: (1) Sensitivity studies necessary to determine susceptibility of the causative organism to cephalothin. (2) Watch for early symptoms of allergic reaction. (3) Reduce total daily dose if renal function impaired. Calculated according to degree of impairment. (4) Continue use for at least 2 to 3 days after all symptoms of infection subside. Avoid prolonged use of drug; superinfection caused by overgrowth of nonsusceptible organisms may result. (5) *Pseudomonas* is almost always resistant to cephalothin. (6) Administer within 24 hours of preparation. Warm to body temperature if precipitate forms on refrigeration. Agitate to dissolve. (7) Sometimes given to the penicillin-sensitive patient. Use extreme caution; cross-sensitivity is common (see Contraindications). (8) Rotation of vein sites is recommended at least every 3 days. Use larger veins when possible. Addition of hydrocortisone may reduce inci dence of thrombophlebitis. (9) Adverse interaction may occur with promethazine (Phenergan), procainamide (Pronestyl), quinidine, muscle relaxants, aminoglycosides (e.g., gentamicin), and potent diuretics. Potentiates nephrotoxic effects of polypeptide antibiotics (e.g., colistimethate). (10) Use only if absolutely necessary in pregnancy. (11) Higher blood levels obtained with probenecid. (12) Electrolyte imbalance and cardiac irregularities resulting from sodium content are very possible. Contains 2.4 mEq sodium/Gm. (13) Immature renal function will increase blood levels in neonates. (14) IM route will cause severe discomfort. (15) Avoid concurrent administration of bacteriostatic agents; will inhibit bactericidal action.

Contraindications: Known penicillin or cephalothin sensitivity.

Incompatible with: Alkaline earth metals, amikacin (Amikin), aminophylline, amobarbital (Amytal), bleomycin (Blenoxane), calcium chloride, calcium gluceptate, calcium gluconate, chlorpromazine (Thorazine), chlortetracycline (Aureomycin), cimetidine (Tagamet), colistimethate (Coly-Mycin M), diphenhydramine (Benadryl), dopamine (Intropin), doxorubicin (Adriamycin), epinephrine (Adrenalin), ergonovine (Ergotrate), erythromycin (Iloytcin, Erythrocin), gentamicin (Garamycin), heparin, kanamycin (Kantrex), levarterenol (Levophed), metaraminol (Aramine), methylprednisolone (Solu-Medrol), metoclopramide (Reglan), penicillin G, potassium or sodium salt, pentobarbital (Nembutal), phenobarbital (Luminal), phenytoin (Dilantin), phytonadione (Aquamephyton), polymyxin B sulfate (Aerosporin), prochlorperazine (Compazine), succinylcholine (Anectine), tetracycline, thiopental (Pentothal), warfarin (Coumadin).

Side effects: Allergic reactions including anaphylaxis; diarrhea; false positive reaction for urine glucose except with Tes-Tape and Keto-Diastix; local site pain; neutropenia and hemolytic anemia; positive direct Coombs' test; pseudomembranous colitis; redness; seizures (large doses); and thrombophlebitis.

Antidote: Notify the physician immediately of any adverse symptoms. Discontinue the drug if indicated. Treat antibiotic-related pseudomembranous colitis with oral vancomycin (Vancocin) or metronidazole (Flagyl). Treat allergic reaction as indicated and resuscitate as necessary.

CEPHAPIRIN SODIUM pH 6.5 to 8.5

(Cefadyl)

Usual dose: 500 mg to 1 Gm every 4 to 6 hours. 8 to 12 Gm/24 hr has been given in severe infections.

Perioperative prophylaxis: 1 to 2 Gm 30 minutes to 1 hour before incision. May be repeated in OR and every 6 hours for 24 hours, or up to 5 days in specific situations.

Pediatric dose: 40 to 80 mg/kg of body weight/24 hr in 4 equally divided doses. *Do not exceed adult dose.*

Dilution: Each 1 Gm or fraction thereof must be diluted with at least 10 ml of sterile water for injection. To reduce incidence of thrombophlebitis, may be further diluted in 50 to 100 ml of 5% dextrose in water, normal saline for injection, or other compatible infusion solutions (see literature). Available premixed. May be administered through Y-tube, three-way stopcock, or additive infusion set.

Rate of administration: Each 1 Gm or fraction thereof over 5 minutes or longer as indicated by amount of solution and condition of patient. Discontinue IV infusion solution during administration of cephapirin.

Actions: A semisynthetic first-generation cephalosporin antibiotic that is bactericidal through inhibition of cell wall synthesis to some gram-positive and gram-negative organisms, including staphylococci and streptococci. A number of organisms are resistant to this cephalosporin. Absorbed by most body fluids and excreted in the urine. Crosses the placental barrier. Secreted in breast milk.

Indications and uses: (1) Treatment of moderate to severe infections of the skin, soft tissue, respiratory tract, and GU tract. Effective only if the causative organism is susceptible. (2) Perioperative prophylaxis.

Precautions: (1) Sensitivity studies necessary to determine susceptibility of the causative organism to cephapirin. (2) Watch for early symptoms of allergic reaction. (3) Reduce total daily dose if renal function impaired. Calculated according to degree of impairment. (4) Continue for at least 2 to 3 days after all symptoms of infection subside. Avoid prolonged use of drug; superinfection caused by overgrowth of nonsusceptible organisms may result. (5) Administer within 24 hours of preparation. (6) Use extreme caution in the penicillin-sensitive patient; cross-sensitivity can occur. (7) Use only if absolutely necessary in pregnancy. (8) Adverse interaction may occur with promethazine (Phenergan), procainamide (Pronestyl), quinidine, muscle relaxants, aminoglycosides (e.g., gentamicin), and potent diuretics. (9) Higher blood levels obtained with probenecid. (10) Avoid concurrent administration of bacteriostatic agents; will inhibit bactericidal action. (11) Safety for use in infants under 3 months of age not established. Immature renal function will increase blood levels. (12) Electrolyte imbalance and cardiac irregularities resulting from sodium content are very possible. Contains 2.36 mEq sodium/Gm.

Contraindications: Known sensitivity to cephalosporins or related antibiotics (penicillins).

Incompatible with: Amikacin (Amikin), aminophylline, chlortetracycline (Aureomycin), epinephrine (Adrenalin), gentamicin (Garamycin), kanamycin (Kantrex), levarterenol (Levophed), mannitol, phenytoin (Dilantin), tetracycline (Achromycin), thiopental (Pentothal).

Side effects: Allergic reactions including anaphylaxis; anemia; diarrhea; false positive reaction for urine glucose except with Tes-Tape or Keto-Diastix; jaundice; leukopenia; local site pain; neutropenia; phlebitis; positive direct and indirect Coombs' test; pseudomembranous colitis; seizures (large doses); and transient elevation of SGOT, SGPT, BUN, and alkaline phosphatase.

Antidote: Notify the physician of any side effects. Discontinue the drug if indicated, treat allergic reaction as indicated, and resuscitate as necessary. Treat antibiotic-related pseudomembranous colitis with oral vancomycin (Vancocin) or metronidazole (Flagyl).

CEPHRADINE SODIUM pH 8.5 to 9.5

(Velosef)

Usual dose: 500 mg to 1 Gm every 4 to 6 hours. Not to exceed 8 Gm/24 hr, depending on severity of infection. *Perioperative prophylaxis:* 1 Gm 30 to 90 minutes before incision. Repeat in 4 to 6 hours and every 6 hours for 24 hours if indicated.

Pediatric dose: 50 to 100 mg/kg of body weight/24 hr in equally divided doses every 6 hours. *Do not exceed adult dose.*

Dilution: Each 500 mg or fraction thereof must be diluted with at least 5 ml of sterile water for injection. To reduce incidence of thrombophlebitis or for doses of 2 Gm or over, further dilute each 500 mg in at least 10 to 20 ml of 5% dextrose in water, normal saline for injection, or other compatible infusion solutions. Available premixed. May be administered through Y-tube, three-way stopcock, or additive infusion set.

Rate of administration: Each 1 Gm or fraction thereof over 3 to 5 minutes or longer as indicated by amount of solution and condition of patient.

Actions: A semisynthetic first-generation cephalosporin antibiotic that is bactericidal through inhibition of cell wall synthesis to some gram-positive and gram-negative organisms, including staphylococci and streptococci. A number of organisms including *Pseudomonas* are resistant to this cephalosporin. Readily absorbed by most body fluids and rapidly excreted in the urine. Crosses the placental barrier. Secreted in breast milk.

Indications and uses: (1) Treatment of serious infections of the bone, joints, skin, soft tissue, GI tract, respiratory tract, GU tract, and bloodstream; peritonitis; and meningococcal meningitis. Effective only if the causative organism is susceptible. (2) Perioperative prophylaxis.

Precautions: (1) Sensitivity studies necessary to determine susceptibility of the causative organism to cephradine. (2) Watch for early symptoms of allergic reaction. (3) Reduce total daily dose if renal function impaired. Calculated according to the degree of impairment. (4) Continue for at least 2 to 3 days after all signs of infection subside. Avoid prolonged use of drug; superinfection caused by overgrowth of nonsusceptible organisms may result. (5) Administer within 2 hours of preparation. Stable for 10 hours in compatible infusion fluids; 24 hours if refrigerated. Protect solution from direct sunlight. (6) Continuous IV infusion may increase incidence of phlebitis. Rotation of vein sites is recommended at least every 3 days. Use larger veins when possible. (7) Use extreme caution in the penicillin-sensitive patient; cross-sensitivity may occur. (8) Use only if absolutely necessary in pregnancy. (9) Probenecid inhibits excretion; may require reduction of dosage. (10) Adverse interaction may occur with promethazine (Phenergan), procainamide (Pronestyl), quinidine, muscle relaxants, aminoglycosides (e.g., gentamicin), and potent diuretics. (11) Avoid concurrent administration of bacteriostatic agents; will inhibit bactericidal action. (12) Electrolyte imbalance and cardiac irregularities resulting from high sodium content are very possible. Contains 6 mEq of sodium/Gm. (13) Safety for use in infants under 1 month of age not established. Immature renal function will increase blood levels. (14) May cause false positive urinary protein reactions.

Contraindications: Known sensitivity to cephalosporins or related antibiotics (penicillins).

Incompatible with: Do not mix in syringe or solution with any other antibiotic; calcium salts; epinephrine (Adrenalin); lidocaine (Xylocaine); Ringer's injection; or tetracyclines.

Side effects: Allergic reactions including anaphylaxis; diarrhea; dizziness; dyspnea; edema; false positive reaction for urine glucose except with Tes-Tape, Clinistix, and Keto-Diastix; headache; joint pains; candidal overgrowth; nausea; paresthesia; pseudomembranous colitis; seizures (large doses); thrombophlebitis; transient leukopenia and neutropenia; transient elevated SGOT, SGPT, total bilirubin, alkaline phosphatase, LDH, BUN, and serum creatinine; vaginitis; and vomiting.

Antidote: Notify the physician of any side effects. Discontinue the drug if indicated, treat allergic reaction as indicated, and resuscitate as necessary. Treat antibiotic-related pseudomembranous colitis with oral vancomycin (Vancocin) or metronidazole (Flagyl).

CHLORAMPHENICOL SODIUM SUCCINATE

pH 6.4 to 7.0

(Chloromycetin)

Usual dose: *Adults and children:* 50 mg/kg of body weight/24 hr in equally divided doses every 6 hours. Exceptional cases may require up to 100 mg/kg/24 hr, but this dose must be reduced as soon as possible.

Infant dose: *Under 2,000 Gm:* 25 mg/kg of body weight once daily.

Over 2,000 Gm; age up to 7 days: 50 mg/kg once daily.

Over 7 days: 50 mg/kg/24 hr in equally divided doses every 12 hours.

Dilution: Each 1 Gm should be diluted with 10 ml of sterile water or 5% dextrose in water for injection to prepare a 10% solution. May be further diluted in 50 to 100 ml of 5% dextrose in water for infusion. Give through Y-tube, three-way stopcock, or additive infusion set.

Rate of administration: 1 Gm or fraction thereof over at least 1 minute. Diluted in 50 to 100 ml, give as an infusion over 30 to 60 minutes.

Actions: Effective against many life-threatening organisms, both bacteriostatic and bactericidal. Acts by inhibiting protein synthesis. Quickly absorbed, well distributed in therapeutic doses throughout the body, especially in the liver and kidneys. Lowest concentrations are found in the brain and spinal fluid. Excreted in urine, bile, and feces. Crosses the placental barrier. Secreted in breast milk.

Indications and uses: (1) Only in serious infections in which potentially less dangerous drugs are ineffective or contraindicated; acute *Salmonella typhi* infections, meningeal infections, bacteremia, Rocky Mountain spotted fever, lymphogranuloma psittacosis, and others; (2) cystic fibrosis regimens.

Precautions: (1) *This is a lethal drug.* (2) Observe baseline blood studies at least every 2 to 3 days during therapy and discontinue drug if indicated. Desired blood level range is 5 to 20 mcg/ml. (3) Potentiates chlorpropamide, cyclophosphamide, hydantoins (e.g., phenytoin

[Dilantin]), oral anticoagulants, oral antidiabetics, and phenobarbital. Concurrently with penicillin it extends its own half-life while inhibiting the action of penicillin. (4) This drug causes irreversible bone marrow depression. Avoid concurrent therapy with other similarly acting drugs. (5) Has a cumulative potency effect in impaired or immature liver and kidney metabolic functions. (6) Superinfection caused by overgrowth of nonsusceptible organisms, including fungi, is possible. (7) Avoid repeated courses of the drug. (8) For IV use only; not effective IM. Reduce dose and/or initiate oral therapy as soon as feasible. (9) Sensitivity studies mandatory to determine susceptibility of the causative organism not only to chloramphenicol but to other less dangerous drugs. (10) Use caution in infants and children; causes gray syndrome. (11) Inhibits iron dextran. Inhibited by rifampin. (12) Use caution in patients with acute intermittent porphyria or glucose 6-phosphate dehydrogenase deficiency.

Contraindications: Known chloramphenicol sensitivity; pregnancy, labor, delivery, and lactation.

Incompatible with: Ampicillin (Polycillin), amobarbital (Amytal), ascorbic acid, carbenicillin (Geopen), chlorpromazine (Thorazine), digitoxin (Crystodigin), erythromycins (Ilotycin, Erythrocin), glycopyrrolate (Robinul), hydrocortisone phosphate, hydroxyzine (Vistaril), metoclopramide (Reglan), oxacillin (Prostaphlin), pentobarbital (Nembutal), phenytoin (Dilantin), polymyxin B (Aerosporin), procaine (Novocain), prochlorperazine (Compazine), promazine (Sparine), promethazine (Phenergan), solutions with a pH below 5.5 or above 7.0, tetracyclines (Aureomycin, Achromycin, Terramycin), thiopental (Pentothal), tripelennamine hydrochloride (Pyribenzamine), vancomycin (Vancocin), warfarin (Coumadin).

Side effects: Anaphylaxis, aplastic anemia, bone marrow depression, confusion, depression, diarrhea, fever, granulocytopenia, gray syndrome of newborns and infants, headache, hypoplastic anemia, leukemia, nausea, optic and peripheral neuritis, paroxysmal nocturnal hemoglobinuria, rashes, stomatitis, thrombocytopenia, vomiting, and many others. *May be fatal.*

Antidote: Notify the physician immediately of any adverse symptoms. Discontinue the drug if indicated, treat allergic reaction as indicated, and resuscitate as necessary.

CHLORDIAZEPOXIDE HYDROCHLORIDE

pH 2.5 to 3.5

(Librium)

Usual dose: 50 to 100 mg initially. Repeat 25 to 100 mg in 2 to 4 hours if indicated, or 25 to 50 mg 3 or 4 times in 24 hours. Maximum dose is 300 mg in a 6- to 24-hour period.

Dilution: Each 100 mg ampoule of sterile powder should be diluted with 5 ml of normal saline or sterile water for injection. Agitate gently to dissolve completely. *(Do not use diluent provided; for IM use only)*. May not be mixed with infusion fluids. Give through Y-tube or three-way stopcock of infusion set. Observe closely for occurrence of fine white precipitate.

Rate of administration: 100 mg or fraction thereof over a minimum of 1 minute.

Actions: A CNS depressant that produces a calming effect. Also relaxes skeletal muscles. Wide margin of safety between therapeutic and toxic doses. Response is extremely rapid by IV route. Slowly metabolized and excreted very slowly in the urine.

Indications and uses: (1) Acute or severe agitation; (2) tremor; (3) anxiety; (4) acute alcoholism withdrawal.

Precautions: (1) Use only freshly prepared solutions; discard unused portion. (2) Bed rest required for a minimum of 3 hours after IV injection. (3) Withdrawal symptoms possible after long-term use. (4) Potentiates or is potentiated by narcotics, phenothiazines (e.g., prochlorperazine [Compazine]), antihistamines, barbiturates, MAO inhibitors (e.g., pargyline [Eutonyl]), alcohol, other CNS depressants, cimetidine (Tagamet), digoxins, phenytoin (Dilantin), and tricyclic antidepressants (e.g., imipramine [Tofranil-PM]). Concomitant use is not recommended, or reduce dose by one third. (5) Reduce dose for the elderly, debilitated, children over 12 years of age, and in impaired renal or hepatic function. (6) Inhibited by oral anticoagulants. (7) Use caution in depressed patients; may develop suicidal tendencies. (8) Keep resuscitation equipment available.

Contraindications: Known hypersensitivity to chlordiazepoxide; children under 12 years; known psychoses; pregnancy, childbirth, or lactation; shock or comatose states; untreated narrow-angle glaucoma.

Incompatible with: Ascorbic acid, benzquinamide (Emete-Con), heparin, pentobarbital (Nembutal), phenytoin (Dilantin), promethazine (Phenergan), Ringer's injection, secobarbital (Seconal), sodium chloride 0.9%.

Side effects: *Average dose:* Blood dyscrasias, constipation, EEG changes, hiccups, hypotension, menstrual irregularities, nausea, skin eruptions, syncope, tachycardia, urinary retention, urticaria.

Overdose: May be caused by too rapid injection. Apnea, ataxia, bradycardia, cardiovascular collapse, confusion, coma, diminished reflexes, drowsiness, edema, hypotension (severe), paradoxical reactions, somnolence.

Antidote: Notify the physician of all side effects. Reduction of dosage may be required. Discontinue the drug for paradoxical reactions including hyperexcitability, hallucinations, and acute rage. Do not treat with barbiturates or CNS stimulants. Treat hypotension with dopamine (Intropin). For overdose, symptomatic and supportive treatment is indicated. Promote excretion with fluid and electrolyte administration and osmotic diuretics (e.g., mannitol). Consider hemodialysis. Physostigmine 0.5 to 4 mg at 1 mg/min may reverse symptoms of anticholinergic overdose (e.g., confusion), but may also cause seizures. Resuscitate as necessary.

CHLOROTHIAZIDE SODIUM pH 9.2 to 10.0

(Diuril)

Usual dose: 0.5 to 2.0 Gm once or twice every 24 hours as indicated. Sometimes given every second or third day.

Dilution: Each 0.5 Gm must be diluted with at least 18 ml of sterile water for injection. May be further diluted in dextrose or sodium chloride IV solutions.

Rate of administration: 0.5 Gm or fraction thereof over 5 minutes.

Actions: A nonmercurial diuretic and antihypertensive drug with carbonic anhydrase inhibitor and thiazide effects. Related to the sulfonamides. Effectiveness is noted within 15 to 30 minutes. Apparently acts in the renal tubules to excrete sodium, chlorides, potassium, water, and, in high doses, some bicarbonate. Potassium excretion is usually not excessive, and rigid low salt intake is never indicated. Rapidly absorbed and excreted unchanged in the urine.

Indications and uses: (1) Edema of any etiology; (2) toxemia of pregnancy when edema results from pathological causes; (3) antidiuretic in diabetes insipidus.

Precautions: (1) Use of oral form preferred. (2) Discard reconstituted solution after 24 hours. (3) Do not give simultaneously with whole blood or its derivatives. (4) Determine absolute patency of vein. Avoid extravasation. For IV use only. (5) May precipitate excessive diuresis with water and electrolyte depletion. Routine checks on electrolyte panel, CO_2, and BUN are necessary during therapy. Potassium chloride replacement may be required. (6) Has antihypertensive actions. Reduced dosage of both agents is required when used concurrently with other antihypertensive drugs. (7) Monitor blood pressure frequently. (8) Hypotensive effect increased by alcohol, barbiturates, and narcotics; decreased by indomethacin (Indocin). (9) Discontinue 48 hours before elective surgery. (10) Use caution in impaired liver or renal function and bronchial asthma. (11) May cause excessive potassium depletion with corticosteroids; cardiac dysrhythmias with digitalis; changes in insulin and oral antidiabetic agent requirements in diabetes; and exacerbation of symptoms of gout or lupus erythematosus. (12) Potentiates amantadine, calcium salts, lithium, quinidine, salicylates, muscle relaxants (e.g., tubocurarine), hypotensive effect of other diuretics, and MAO inhibitors (e.g., pargyline [Eutonyl]). (13) Inhibits oral anticoagulants, antineoplastics (e.g., methotrexate), and pressor amines (e.g., norepinephrine). (14) Potentiated by anticholinergics (e.g., atropine) and tetracyclines. (15) May alter laboratory test results, especially potassium, BUN, uric acid, glucose, and protein-bound iodine.

Contraindications: Anuria, increasing azotemia and oliguria; known sulfonamide sensitivity; not recommended for children; pregnancy and lactation except in preeclampsia.

Incompatible with: Amikacin (Amikin), ascorbic acid, chlorpromazine (Thorazine), codeine, hydralazine (Apresoline), insulin (aqueous), ionosol solutions, levarterenol (Levophed), levorphanol (Levo-Dromoran), methadone, morphine, Normosol solutions, polymyxin B (Aerosporin), procaine (Novocain), prochlorperazine (Compazine), promazine (Sparine), promethazine (Phenergan), protein hydrolysate, streptomycin, tetracycline, triflupromazine (Vesprin), vancomycin (Vancocin), vitamin B with C, warfarin (Coumadin).

Side effects: *Minor:* Diarrhea, dizziness, fatigue, hyperglycemia, hyperuricemia, muscle cramps, nausea, orthostatic hypotension, paresthesias, photosensitivity, purpura, rash, urticaria, vertigo, vomiting, weakness.

Major: Anaphylaxis, blood volume reduction, circulatory collapse, dehydration, excessive diuresis, hematuria, hypokalemia, metabolic acidosis, vascular thrombosis or embolism.

Antidote: If minor side effects are noted, discontinue the drug and notify the physician, who may treat the side effects and continue the drug. If side effects are progressive or any major side effect occurs, discontinue the drug immediately and notify the physician. Treatment of major side effects is symptomatic and aggressive. Resuscitate as necessary.

CHLORPHENIRAMINE MALEATE

pH 4.0 to 5.2

(Chlor-Pro-10, Chlor-Trimeton, ♦ Chlor-Tripolon)

Usual dose: 5 to 20 mg; usually 10 mg initially. 10 mg may be repeated as necessary (before administration of each unit of blood), but do not exceed 40 mg/24 hr. In anaphylactic reactions 10 to 20 mg may be given initially.

Pediatric dose: 0.35 mg/kg of body weight/24 hr (10 mg/M^2/24 hr) in divided doses every 6 hours.

Dilution: May be given undiluted.

Rate of administration: 10 mg or fraction thereof over 1 minute. Extend injection time when possible.

Actions: An antihistamine, acts by blocking the effects of histamine at various receptor sites. Either eliminates an allergic reaction or greatly modifies it. Readily absorbed, widely distributed, and excreted in changed form in the urine.

Indications and uses: (1) Prophylaxis of allergic (not pyrogenic) transfusion reactions; (2) treatment of anaphylactic reactions; (3) treatment of other allergic reactions if IV route is indicated.

Precautions: (1) IM or SC use is indicated in all situations except the above specific indications. (2) Note label; only the 10 mg/ml chlorpheniramine may be used IV. (3) Do not add to unit of blood. Give direct IV only. (4) Protect from light to prevent discoloration. (5) Use with caution for severe asthmatic patients. (6) Increases effectiveness of epinephrine and is often used in conjunction with it. (7) Antagonizes heparin. (8) Reduce dosage for the elderly and debilitated.

Contraindications: Hypersensitivity to antihistamines, pregnancy, lactation, newborn or premature infants, patients taking MAO inhibitors (e.g., pargyline [Eutonyl]), narrow-angle glaucoma, stenosing peptic ulcer, symptomatic prostatic hypertrophy, asthmatic attack, bladder neck obstruction, pyloroduodenal obstruction.

Incompatible with: Calcium chloride, iodipamide meglumine (Cholografin), kanamycin (Kantrex), levarterenol (Levophed), pentobarbital (Nembutal).

Side effects: Occur infrequently.

Minor: Drowsiness, headache, nervousness, polyuria, transitory stinging at injection site.

Major: Acute CNS excitement, convulsions, death, diaphoresis, pallor, transitory hypotension, weak pulse.

Antidote: For major side effects, discontinue the drug and notify the physician. The side effects will usually subside within an hour or may be treated symptomatically. Treat hypotension promptly, may lead to cardiovascular collapse. Use dopamine (Intropin), norepinephrine, or phenylephrine. Epinephrine is contraindicated for hypotension; further hypotension will occur. Propranolol (Inderal) is the drug of choice for ventricular dysrhythmias. Treat convulsions with phenytoin (Dilantin). Anticonvulsant barbiturates, diazepam (Valium), or analeptics (e.g., doxapram [Dopram]) will increase toxicity. Epinephrine must be available to treat anaphylaxis. Resuscitate as necessary.

CHLORPROMAZINE HYDROCHLORIDE pH 3.0 to 5.0

(♣ Ormazine, Thorazine)

Usual dose: *Nausea and vomiting and perioperative:* 1 mg. May repeat at 2-minute intervals as indicated. Do not exceed 0.5 mg/kg.

Intractable hiccups: 25 to 50 mg in 500 to 1,000 ml of normal saline.

Tetanus: 0.5 mg/kg of body weight every 6 to 8 hours.

Pediatric dose: *Children over 6 months of age: Nausea and vomiting:* 1 mg. May repeat at 2-minute intervals as indicated. Maximum is usually 12 mg. IV route rarely used for children.

Tetanus: 0.5 mg/kg of body weight every 6 to 8 hours. Do not exceed 40 mg/24 hours for up to 23 kg and 75 mg/24 hours for up to 50 kg.

Dilution: Each 25 mg (1 ml) must be diluted with 24 ml of normal saline for injection. 1 ml will equal 1 mg. May be further diluted in 500 to 1,000 ml of normal saline and given as an infusion.

Rate of administration: Direct IV administration; each 1 mg or fraction thereof over 2 minutes. Given by very slow IV infusion. Titrate to symptoms and vital signs. Never exceed direct IV rate. *See Precautions.*

Actions: A phenothiazine derivative with effects on the central, autonomic, and peripheral nervous systems. Decreases anxiety and tension, relaxes muscles, produces sedation, and tranquilizes. Has an antiemetic effect, some antihistamine action, and potentiates CNS depressants. Onset of action is prompt and of short duration in small IV doses. Excretion is slow through the kidneys.

Indications and uses: (1) Treatment of acute nausea, vomiting, hiccups, restlessness, or retching; primarily used during operative procedures; (2) tetanus; (3) treatment of drug-induced hypertension (e.g., methylergonovine [Methergine]), lysergic acid (LSD) intoxication, and amphetamine overdose (IM injection preferred); (4) preoperative sedation of the psychotic patient.

Precautions: (1) IV use is limited to above specific indications. IM injection preferred. (2) Sensitive to light. Slightly yellow color does not alter potency. Discard if markedly discolored. (3) Handle carefully; may cause contact dermatitis. (4) Keep patient in supine position. Monitor blood pressure and pulse before administration and between doses. (5) Use caution in cardiovascular, liver, and chronic respiratory diseases, and acute respiratory diseases of children. (6) Cough reflex is often depressed. (7) May discolor urine pink to reddish brown. (8) Photosensitivity of skin is possible. (9) May mask diagnosis of brain tumor, drug intoxication, and intestinal obstruction. (10) Potentiates CNS depressants such as narcotics, alcohol, anesthetics, barbiturates, MAO inhibitors (e.g., pargyline [Eutonyl]), anticholinergics, antihistamines, antihypertensives, hypnotics, muscle relaxants, and Rauwolfia alkaloids. Reduce dosage of any medication potentiated by phenothiazines by one fourth to one half. (11) May reduce anticonvulsant activity of barbiturates and other anticonvulsants. (12) Contraindicated with quinidine, dipyrone, epinephrine, thiazide diuretics, and orphenadrine. (13) Capable of innumerable other interactions. (14) May cause paradoxical excitation in children and the elderly. (15) Use phenothiazines with extreme caution in children with a history of sleep apnea, a family history of SIDS, or in the presence of Reye's syndrome.

Contraindications: Bone marrow depression, cerebral arteriosclerosis, children under 6 months, circulatory collapse, coronary disease, comatose or severely depressed states, hypersensitivity to phenothiazines, lactation, Parkinson's disease, pregnancy, severe hypotension or hypertension, subcortical brain damage (even if only suspected).

Incompatible with: Aminophylline, amphotericin B (Fungizone), ampicillin, atropine, caffeine and sodium benzoate, cephalothin (Keflin), chloramphenicol (Chloromycetin), chlorothiazide (Diuril), dimenhydrinate (Dramamine), epinephrine (Adrenalin), folic acid, hydrocortisone (Solu-Cortef), kanamycin (Kantrex), magnesium sulfate, methicillin (Staphcillin), methohexital (Brevital), methylprednisolone (Solu-Medrol), paraldehyde, penicillin G potassium, pentobarbital (Nembutal), phenobarbital (Luminal), ranitidine (Zantac), secobarbital (Seconal), sodium bicarbonate, tetracycline (Achromycin), thiopental (Pentothal).

Side effects: Usually transient if drug discontinued, but may require treatment if severe. Anaphylaxis, cardiac arrest, distorted Q and T waves, excitement, extrapyramidal symptoms (e.g., abnormal positioning, extreme restlessness, pseudoparkinsonism, weakness of extremities), fever, hypersensitivity reactions, hypertension, hypotension, tachycardia, and many others. Overdose can cause convulsions, hallucinations, and death.

Antidote: Discontinue the drug at onset of any side effect and notify the physician. Counteract hypotension with dopamine (Intropin) or phenylephrine (Neo-Synephrine) and IV fluids. Counteract extrapyramidal symptoms with benztropine (Cogentin) or diphenhydramine (Benadryl). Use diazepam (Valium) or phenobarbital for convulsions or hyperactivity. Epinephrine is contraindicated for hypotension; further hypotension will occur. Phenytoin may be helpful in ventricular dysrhythmias. Avoid analeptics such as caffeine and sodium benzoate in treating respiratory depression and unconsciousness; they may cause convulsions. Resuscitate as necessary.

CIMETIDINE pH 3.8 to 6.0

(Tagamet)

Usual dose: *Direct or intermittent IV:* 300 mg every 6 hours. Increase frequency of dose, not amount, if necessary for pain relief. Do not exceed 2,400 mg/day. Increase intervals between injections to achieve pain relief with least frequent dosage in impaired renal function.

Continuous IV: 900 mg evenly distributed over 24 hours (37.5 mg/hr). May be preceded by a loading dose of 150 mg if indicated to rapidly increase pH (total dose up to 1,050 mg/24 hr). To maintain intragastric acid secretory rates at 10 mEq/hr or less, dose range may be higher in patients with pathological hypersecretory states. Product insert mentions a study that used a range of 40 to 600 mg/hr averaging 160 mg/hr; well beyond usual doses. Any dose beyond the normal should be administered with extreme caution.

Prevention of aspiration pneumonitis: 300 mg 60 to 90 minutes before anesthesia.

Dilution: *Direct IV:* Each 300 mg must be diluted with 20 ml of normal saline for injection.

Intermittent infusion: Each 300 mg may be diluted in 50 to 100 ml of 5% dextrose in water or other compatible infusion solution and given piggyback. Available premixed. Do not use premixed plastic containers in series connections; may cause air embolism.

Continuous infusion: Total daily dose may be diluted in 100 to 1,000 ml of 5% dextrose in water or other compatible infusion solution.

Rate of administration: *Direct IV:* Each 300 mg or fraction thereof over a minimum of 2 minutes.

Intermittent infusion: Each 300 mg dose over 15 to 20 minutes.

Continuous infusion:: Give loading dose at intermittent infusion rate and distribute balance of daily dose equally over 24 hours. Use of infusion pump preferred, especially with volumes of 250 ml or less, to avoid complications of overdose or too rapid administration (note side effects).

Actions: A histamine H_2 antagonist, it inhibits both daytime and nocturnal basal gastric acid secretion. It also inhibits gastric acid secretion stimulated by food, histamine, pentagastrin, caffeine, and insulin. Onset of action is prompt and effective for 4 to 5 hours. Excreted in the urine. Crosses placental barrier. Secreted in breast milk.

Indications and uses: Short-term treatment of active duodenal ulcers, active benign gastric ulcers, and pathological hypersecretory conditions.

Unlabeled use: Preoperatively to prevent aspiration pneumonia; treatment of itching and flushing of anaphylaxis, pruritus, urticaria, and contact dermatitis; treatment of acetaminophen overdose (helps to reduce hepatotoxicity).

Precautions: (1) IV bolus administration has precipitated rare instances of cardiac dysrhythmias, hypotension, and death. (2) Use antacids concomitantly to relieve pain. (3) May potentiate warfarin-type anticoagulants; monitor prothrombin times. (4) Gastric malignancy may be present even though patient is asymptomatic. (5) Stable at room temperature for 48 hours after dilution. (6) Gastric pain and ulceration may recur after medication stopped. (7) Usually discontinued after 4 to 8 weeks; effects maintained with oral dosage. (8) Potentiates effects of antimalarials (e.g., chloroquine), some benzodiazepines (e.g., diazepam [Valium]), beta blockers (e.g., propranolol [Inderal]), caffeine, calcium channel blockers (e.g., verapamil), carbamazepine, ethanol, hydantoins (e.g., phenytoin [Dilantin]), lidocaine, metronidazole (e.g., Flagyl), pentoxifylline (Trental), procainamide (Pronestyl), quinidine, sulfonylureas, tricyclic antidepressants (e.g., imipramine [Tofranil]), theophyllines (e.g., aminophylline), triamterene (Dyrenium), and warfarin. (9) May inhibit digoxin absorption. (10) Clinical effect (inhibition of nocturnal gastric secretion) reversed by cigarette smoking. (11) May precipitate apnea, confusion, and muscle twitching with morphine. (12) May cause increased myelosuppression with alkylating agents (e.g., carmustine). (13) Many unconfirmed reports of inhibiting pharmacologic action of other drugs. (14) Discontinue breast feeding.

Contraindications: Known hypersensitivity to cimetidine. Pregnant and lactating women and children under 16 years of age should be considered.

Incompatible with: Aminophylline, amphotericin B (Fungizone), barbiturates, cefamandole (Mandol), cefazolin (Ancef), cephalothin (Keflin). Do not add any other drugs to premixed cimetidine in plastic containers.

Side effects: *Average dose:* Bradycardia, confusion, diarrhea, delirium, dizziness, elevated SGOT, fever, galactorrhea, hallucinations, impotence, interstitial nephritis, muscular pain, rash.

Overdose: Cardiac dysrhythmias, death, hypotension, respiratory failure, tachycardia.

Antidote: Notify physician of all side effects. May be treated symptomatically or may respond to decrease in frequency of dosage. Resuscitate as necessary for overdosage. Physostigmine may be useful to reverse CNS toxicity.

CIPROFLOXACIN pH 3.3 to 4.6

(Cipro I.V.)

Usual dose: 400 mg every 12 hours except dose is reduced to 200 mg every 12 hours in mild to moderate urinary infections. Dose based on severity and nature of the infection, susceptibility of the causative organism, integrity of host-defense mechanisms, and renal and hepatic status. Continue for 7 to 14 days (at least 2 days after all symptoms of infection subside). Bone and joint infections may require treatment for 4 to 6 weeks or more. May be transferred to oral dosing when appropriate. Reduce time between doses (200 to 400 mg every 18 to 24 hours) if creatinine clearance is less than 30 ml/min (see literature for additional information).

Dilution: Available as a 0.2% solution in plastic infusion containers ready for use (200 mg in 100 ml 5% dextrose, 400 mg in 200 ml 5% dextrose). Do not hang plastic containers in a series, may cause air embolism. Also available in 20 and 40 ml vials containing 10 mg/ml (1% solution), which must be diluted with normal saline or 5% dextrose in water to a final concentration of 0.5 to 2 mg/ml. Stable for up to 14 days refrigerated or at room temperature in the final diluted concentration.

Rate of administration: A single dose must be equally distributed over 60 minutes as an infusion. Too rapid administration and/or the use of a small vein may increase incidence of anaphylaxis, local site inflammation, and other side effects. May be given through a Y-tube or three-way stopcock of infusion set. Temporarily discontinue other solutions infusing at the same site.

Actions: A synthetic broad-spectrum antimicrobial agent, a fluoroquinolone. Bactericidal to a wide range of aerobic gram-negative and gram-positive organisms through interference with the enzyme needed for synthesis of bacterial DNA. Onset of action is prompt, and serum levels are dose related. Half-life averages 5 to 6 hours. Readily distributed to body fluids (saliva, nasal and bronchial secretions, sputum, skin blister fluid, lymph, peritoneal fluid, bile and prostatic secretions). Found in lung, skin, fat, muscle, cartilage, and bone. Distribution to cerebrospinal fluid and eye fluids is lower than plasma levels. Excreted as unchanged drug in the urine, usually within 24 hours. Crosses placental barrier. Secreted in breast milk.

Indications and uses: Treatment of mild, moderate, severe, and complicated urinary tract infections and mild to moderate lower respiratory, skin and skin structure, and bone and joint infections. (Most effective against specific organisms (see literature). Additional appropriate therapy required if anaerobic organisms are suspected of contributing to the infection.

Precautions: (1) Culture and sensitivity studies utilizing a 5 mcg ciprofloxacin disk indicated to determine susceptibility of the causative organism to ciprofloxacin. (2) *Pseudomonas aeruginosa* may develop resistance during treatment. Ongoing culture and sensitivity studies indicated. (3) Use of large veins recommended to dilute toxicity, reduce incidence of allergic reactions, and reduce incidence of local irritation. Symptoms of local irritation do not preclude further administration of ciprofloxacin unless they recur or worsen. Generally resolve when infusion complete. (4) May cause serious or fatal reactions with theophylline (e.g., cardiac arrest, respiratory failure, seizures, status epilepticus). If must be used concomitantly, monitor serum levels of theophylline and decrease dose as appropriate. Observe closely with caffeine intake, may cause similar problems. (5) May cause anaphylaxis with the first or succeeding doses, even in patients without known hypersensitivity. Emergency equipment must always be available. (6) Maintain adequate hydration and acidity of urine throughout treatment. Will form crystals in alkaline urine. (7) Monitor hematopoietic, hepatic, and renal systems during prolonged treatment. (8) Use with cyclosporine may cause an increase in serum creatinine. (9) May potentiate oral anticoagulants (e.g., warfarin [Coumadin]), monitor prothrombin times. (10) Potentiated by probenicid; may require dose adjustment. (11) Prolonged use may cause superinfection because of overgrowth of nonsusceptible organisms. Monitor carefully. (12) Avoid excessive sunlight, phototoxicity has been reported and may cause severe sunburn. (13)

Use caution in patients with impaired hepatic function and known CNS disorders (e.g., epilepsy, severe cerebral arteriosclerosis, or any other factors that predispose to seizures). (14) Safety for use in pregnancy not established, use only if benefit justifies risk to fetus. (15) Discontinue breast feeding. Safety for use in children under 18 years of age not established. May erode cartilage of weight-bearing joints or other signs of arthropathy in infants and children. (16) A clear, colorless to slightly yellow solution. Store at room temperature before dilution; protect from light, excessive heat, and freezing.

Contraindications: Known hypersensitivity to ciprofloxacin or any other quinolone antimicrobial agent (e.g., norfloxacin [Noroxin].

Incompatible with: Manufacturer recommends ciprofloxacin be administered separately.

Side effects: Allergic reactions (anaphylaxis, cardiovascular collapse, death, dyspnea, edema [facial or pharyngeal], eosinophilia, fever, hepatic necrosis, itching, jaundice, loss of consciousness, rash, urticaria); cardiac arrest; CNS stimulation (confusion, hallucinations, lightheadedness, restlessness, seizures, tingling, toxic psychosis, tremors); decreased hemoglobin, hematocrit, and platelet count; diarrhea; elevation of eosinophil and platelet counts, blood glucose, BUN, serum creatine, serum creatinine phosphokinase, uric acid, and triglycerides; headache; hepatic enzyme abnormalities (elevation of alkaline phosphatase, AST [SGOT], ALT [SGPT], LDH, serum bilirubin); increased intracranial pressure; local site reactions; nausea; pseudomembranous colitis; respiratory failure; status epilepticus. Capable of numerous other reactions in less than 1% of patients.

Antidote: Death may result from some of these side effects. Discontinue ciprofloxacin at the first appearance of a skin rash or any other sign of hypersensitivity, at the onset of any CNS symptom, or the onset of pseudomembranous colitis. Treat allergic reaction with epinephrine (Adrenalin), airway management, oxygen, IV fluids, antihistamines (diphenhydramine [Benadryl], corticosteroids (Solu-cortef), and pressor amines (dopamine [Intropin] as indicated. Treat CNS symptoms as indicated. May require diazepam (Valium) for seizures. Mild cases of colitis may respond to discontinuation of ciprofloxacin. Oral vancomycin (Vancocin) or metronidazole (Flagyl) is the treatment of choice for antibiotic-related pseudomembranous colitis. Keep physician informed of all side effects. Many will require symptomatic treatment, monitor closely. Maintain hydration in overdose. No specific antidote, up to 10% may be excreted by hemodialysis or peritoneal dialysis. Maintain patient until drug excreted.

CISPLATIN pH 3.5 to 5.5

(CDDP, Platinol, Platinol-AQ)

Usual dose: *Metastatic testicular tumors:* 20 mg/M^2 daily for 5 days every 3 weeks for 3 courses. Bleomycin and vinblastine also indicated.

Metastatic ovarian tumors: 50 mg/M^2 once every 3 weeks, with doxorubicin.

As a single agent: 50 to 70 mg/M^2 once every 3 to 4 weeks. All doses adjusted based on prior radiation therapy or chemotherapy.

Dilution: *Specific techniques required, see Precautions.* Initially dilute each 10 (50) mg vial with 10 (50) ml of sterile water for injection. Platinol-AQ is prediluted to 1 mg/ml. Withdraw desired dose. Immediately before use, each one half of a single dose should be diluted in 1 liter of 5% dextrose in 0.2% or 0.45% saline containing 37.5 Gm of mannitol. Will decompose if adequate chloride ion not available.

Rate of administration: Each 1 liter of infusion solution over 3 to 4 hours. Give total dose (2 liters) over 6 to 8 hours.

Actions: A heavy metal complex (platinum and chloride atoms). Has properties similar to alkylating agents and is cell cycle nonspecific. Concentrates in liver, kidneys, large and small intestines. Little is absorbed into normal cerebrospinal fluid but is absorbed into intracerebral tumors. Heavily protein bound. Only one fourth to one half of the drug is excreted in the urine by the end of 5 days. Secreted in breast milk.

Indications and uses: Suppress or retard neoplastic growth of metastatic tumors of the testes, ovaries, and bladder. Most commonly used in specific combinations with other chemotherapeutic drugs.

Precautions: (1) Follow guidelines for handling cytotoxic agents recommended. See Appendix p. 677. (2) Administered by or under the direction of the physician specialist. (3) Hydrate patient with 1 to 2 liters of infusion fluid for 8 to 12 hours before injection. (4) Maintain adequate hydration and urinary output for 24 hours after each dose. (5) Frequent kidney function tests, blood counts, and electrolytes are indicated. Repeat doses may not be given unless serum creatinine is below 1.5 mg/100 ml and/or the BUN is below 25 mg/100 ml; platelets should be 100,000/mm^3 and leukocytes 4,000/mm^3; verify auditory acuity as within normal limits. (6) Refrigerate dry powder only. Reconstituted solutions must be kept at room temperature. Discard after 20 hours. Use immediately if contains mannitol. (7) Do not use needles or IV tubing with aluminum parts to administer; a precipitate will form and potency is decreased. (8) Will produce teratogenic effects on the fetus. Has a mutagenic potential. (9) Nausea and vomiting are frequently severe and prolonged (up to a week). Prophylactic administration of antiemetics recommended. Metoclopramide (Reglan), dexamethasone, or droperidol are effective in most patients. (10) Ototoxicity is cumulative, test hearing before administration and regularly during treatment. Ototoxicity increased in children. (11) Ototoxicity and nephrotoxicity are potentiated with aminoglycosides (e.g., gentamicin) and ethacrynic acid (Edecrin). (12) Neuropathies may occur with higher doses, greater frequency of average doses or prolonged therapy. (13) Allopurinol may be indicated to reduce uric acid levels. (14) May inhibit phenytoin (Dilantin).

Contraindications: Hypersensitivity to cisplatin or other platinum-containing compounds, myelosuppressed patients, preexisting impaired renal function or hearing deficit.

Incompatible with: Metoclopramide (Reglan). Should be considered incompatible in syringe or solution with any other drug (except for mannitol) because of toxicity and specific use. Inactivated by alkaline solutions (e.g., sodium bicarbonate), sodium bisulfite, sodium thiosulfate.

Side effects: Are frequent, can occur with the initial dose, and will become more severe with succeeding doses. Anaphylaxis (facial edema, hypotension, tachycardia, and wheezing within minutes of administration), hyperuricemia, myelosuppression, nausea and vomiting, nephrotoxicity (often noted in the second week after a dose), ototoxicity including tinnitus and hearing loss in the high-frequency range, and peripheral neuropathy (may be irreversible).

Antidote: Notify physician of all side effects. Cisplatin may have to be discontinued permanently or until recovery. Symptomatic and supportive treatment is indicated. Treat anaphylaxis with epinephrine, corticosteroids, oxygen, and antihistamines. There is no specific antidote.

CLINDAMYCIN PHOSPHATE pH 6.0 to 6.3

(Cleocin Phosphate)

Usual dose: 600 to 2,700 mg/24 hr in 2, 3, or 4 equally divided doses. Up to 4.8 Gm has been given in life-threatening infections.

Acute pelvic inflammatory disease: 600 mg every 6 hours for 4 days. Concurrent administration of 2 mg/kg of body weight of gentamicin as an initial dose and 1.5 mg/kg every 8 hours thereafter is recommended. Complete 10- to 14-day treatment program with oral clindamycin.

Pediatric dose: *Children over 1 month of age:* 15 to 25 mg/kg of body weight/24 hr (350 mg/M^2/24 hr) in 3 or 4 equally divided doses for serious infections. Up to 40 mg/kg/24 hr (450 mg/M^2/24 hr) may be used for more serious infections if necessary.

Dilution: Each 300 mg or fraction thereof must be diluted with a minimum of 50 ml of 5% dextrose in water, normal saline for injection, or other compatible infusion solution.

Acute pelvic inflammatory disease: May be further diluted in larger amounts of compatible infusion solutions and given as a continuous infusion after the initial dose.

Rate of administration: Each 300 mg or fraction thereof over a minimum of 10 minutes. Do not give more than 1,200 mg in single 1-hour infusion.

Acute pelvic inflammatory disease: To maintain serum levels at 4 (5 or 6) mcg/ml give initial dose at 10 (15 or 20) mg/min over 30 minutes. Follow with maintenance infusion at 0.75 (1.00 or 1.25) mg/min.

Severe hypotension and cardiac arrest can occur with too rapid injection.

Actions: A semisynthetic antibiotic that quickly converts to active clindamycin. It inhibits protein synthesis in the bacterial cell, producing irreversible changes in the protein-synthesizing ribosomes. Widely distributed in most body fluids, tissues, and bones. There is no clinically effective distribution to cerebrospinal fluid. Excreted in urine and feces in small amounts. Most excreted in inactive form in the urine. Crosses placental barrier. Secreted in breast milk.

Indications and uses: (1) Treatment of serious infections caused by susceptible anaerobic bacteria; or susceptible aerobic bacterial infections in penicillin-sensitive patients; or infections that do not respond or are resistant to other less toxic antibiotics, such as penicillins or cephalosporins; (2) treatment of acute pelvic inflammatory disease.

Precautions: (1) A highly toxic drug, to be used only when absolutely necessary and an alternate drug (e.g., erythromycin) is not acceptable. (2) Sensitivity studies indicated to determine susceptibility of the causative organism to clindamycin. (3) Avoid prolonged use; superinfection caused by overgrowth of nonsusceptible organisms may result. (4) Capable of causing severe, even fatal, colitis; observe for symptoms of diarrhea. (5) Periodic blood cell counts and liver and kidney studies are indicated in prolonged therapy. (6) May potentiate other neuromuscular blocking agents (e.g., kanamycin, streptomycin). (7) Antagonized by erythromycin. (8) Use caution with a history of GI, severe renal, or liver disease. (9) Each ml contains 9.45 mg benzyl alcohol. Monitor organ system functions if used in infants.

Contraindications: Known hypersensitivity to clindamycin or lincomycin; lactation, pregnancy, and newborns.

Incompatible with: Aminophylline, ampicillin, barbiturates, calcium gluconate, magnesium sulfate, phenytoin (Dilantin), ranitidine (Zantac), Ringer's solution, tobramycin (Nebcin).

Side effects: Abdominal pain, allergic reactions, anaphylaxis, cardiac arrest, colitis, diarrhea, hypotension, jaundice, nausea, thrombophlebitis, vomiting.

Antidote: Notify the physician of any side effects. Discontinue the drug if indicated (colitis, diarrhea, allergic reactions, etc.), treat allergic reaction as indicated, and resuscitate as necessary. Do not treat diarrhea with opiates or diphenoxylate with atropine (Lomotil). Condition will worsen. Treat colitis with fluid, electrolyte, and protein supplements, systemic corticosteroids, and corticoid retention enemas. Hemodialysis or CAPD will not decrease blood levels in toxicity.

COLCHICINE pH 6.0 to 7.2

Usual dose: 2 mg (4 ml) as initial dose. Follow with 0.5 mg (1 ml) every 6 hours. Do not exceed 4 mg (8 ml) in 24 hours. Maintenance doses of 0.5 to 2 mg (1 to 4 ml)/24 hr may be given or divided into 2 doses every 24 hours.

Dilution: May be given undiluted or diluted with 0.9% sodium chloride without a bacteriostatic agent.

Rate of administration: Each single dose over 2 to 5 minutes.

Actions: An alkaloid. Its mode of action has not been determined, but it has a distinct antiinflammatory and analgesic effect. IV administration is preferred for rapid response and fewer GI side effects. Readily absorbed into the liver, spleen, kidneys, and intestinal tract. Excreted in urine and feces.

Indications and uses: Specific for the treatment of acute gout.

Precautions: (1) Must be given IV. Will cause severe local reaction IM or SC. Maintain absolute patency of vein; severe irritation will occur with leakage along vein pathway. (2) Use only clear solutions. (3) Use with caution for the elderly and debilitated. Safety for use in pregnancy, lactation, and children not established. (4) Reduce dosage if weakness, anorexia, nausea, vomiting, or diarrhea occurs. (5) Symptoms of overdosage do not occur immediately. The patient must be continuously observed while hospitalized and well informed of all side effects when treated outside the hospital. (6) Thrombophlebitis can occur at the injection site. (7) Inhibited by acidifying agents; potentiated by alkalinizing agents. (8) May alter absorption of vitamin B_{12}. (9) Potentiates CNS depressants and sympathomimetic agents (agents for glaucoma, bronchodilators, decongestants, mydriatics, vasopressors).

Contraindications: *Absolute:* IM and SC use.

Incompatible with: Specific information not available. Interaction with other drugs does occur. Should be considered incompatible with any other drug in a syringe.

Side effects: Rare when recommended dose is not exceeded but may be latent.

Average dose: Abdominal pain, aplastic anemia, bone marrow depression, diarrhea, nausea, thrombocytopenia, thrombophlebitis at injection site, vomiting.

Overdose: Usual side effects plus ascending CNS paralysis; burning sensations in the throat, stomach, and skin; convulsions; delirium; electrolyte imbalance; hematuria; hemorrhagic gastroenteritis; muscular weakness; oliguria; respiratory depression; severe bloody diarrhea; shock; death.

Antidote: Discontinue the drug at initial onset of symptoms and notify the physician. For acute overdosage, treatment is symptomatic and includes treatment of shock and electrolyte imbalance and respiratory assistance as necessary. Morphine and atropine may be used to relieve pain. Hemodialysis or peritoneal dialysis may promote elimination of the drug.

COLISTIMETHATE SODIUM pH 7.0 to 8.0

(Coly-Mycin M)

Usual dose: *adults, children, and infants:* 2.5 to 5.0 mg/kg of body weight/24 hr (150 mg/M^2/24 hr) equally divided into 2 doses and given every 12 hours. Normal renal function is necessary for this dosage.

Dilution: 150 mg vial is diluted with 2 ml of sterile water for injection. 1 ml equals 75 mg. Further dilute each single dose with 20 ml of sterile water for injection for direct IV administration. May be further diluted with 50 ml or more of 5% dextrose in water, isotonic saline, lactated Ringer's solution, or 10% invert sugar solution and given as an infusion through the Y-tube, three-way stopcock, or additive infusion tubing.

Rate of administration: Direct IV administration. Each 75 mg or fraction thereof over 5 minutes. Initial dose should be direct IV. Second dose often given in 1 to 2 hours as a continuous infusion at 5 to 6 mg/hr.

Actions: A polypeptide antibiotic with neuromuscular blocking action. Bactericidal against specific gram-negative bacilli. Serum and urine levels remain adequate for up to 6 to 8 hours. Crosses the placental barrier. Excreted through the kidneys.

Indications and uses: Acute and chronic infections, especially of the urinary tract, caused by gram-negative bacilli, such as *Pseudomonas aeruginosa, Aerobacter aerogenes, Escherichia coli,* and *Klebsiella pneumoniae.*

Precautions: (1) Read the label carefully. Only a specific powder can be diluted for IV use. (2) Sensitivity studies indicated to determine susceptibility of the causative organism to colistimethate. (3) Reduce daily dose if renal function is impaired. Calculated according to degree of impairment. (4) Watch for decrease in urine output and for rising BUN and serum creatinine. Dosage may require decreasing. (5) Be especially observant in infants, children, and the elderly. (6) Potentiated by anesthetics, other neuromuscular blocking antibiotics (e.g., kanamycin, streptomycin), anticholinesterases (e.g., edrophonium [Tensilon]), cephalosporins (e.g., cefoperazone), and muscle relaxants (e.g., tubocurarine). *Apnea can occur.* (7) Avoid prolonged use of drug; superinfection caused by overgrowth of nonsusceptible organisms may result. (8) Motor coordination impaired; supervise ambulation. (9) Store reconstituted drug in refrigerator for up to 7 days. Discard solutions diluted for infusion after 24 hours. (10) Use during pregnancy only when absolutely necessary.

Contraindications: History of sensitivity to multiple allergens, known colistimethate sensitivity. Not effective against *Proteus* or *Neisseria.*

Incompatible with: Administer separately as recommended by manufacturer. Cefazolin (Kefzol), cephalothin (Keflin), chlortetracycline (Aureomycin), erythromycin (Erythrocin), hydrocortisone (Solu-Cortef), hydroxyzine (Vistaril), kanamycin (Kantrex).

Side effects: *Average dose:* Circumoral paresthesia, dizziness, formication of extremities, numbness of extremities, pruritus, slurring of speech, tingling of extremities, vertigo.

Overdose: Anaphylaxis, apnea, decreased urine output, elevated BUN, elevated serum creatinine, muscle weakness, renal insufficiency.

Antidote: Side effects are expected with an average dose; notify the physician. Reduction of dose will usually alleviate symptoms. If any symptom of overdose occurs, discontinue the drug immediately and notify the physician. Nephrotoxicity is reversible. Maintain an adequate airway and artificial ventilation as indicated. Treat allergic reactions symptomatically with antihistamines, pressor amines, and corticosteroids.

CONJUGATED ESTROGENS pH 7.2 to 7.4

(Premarin Intravenous)

Usual dose: 25 mg in 1 injection. May be repeated in 6 to 12 hours if indicated.

Dilution: Withdraw all air from the vial of powder. Carefully withdraw contents from ampoule of sterile diluent provided. Direct flow of diluent gently against the side of the vial of powder. Mix solution by rotating the vial between the palms of the hands. Do not shake.

Rate of administration: 5 mg or fraction thereof over 1 minute. Must be given direct IV or through IV tubing close to needle site. Infusion solution must be compatible (normal saline, dextrose, and invert sugar solutions).

Actions: Produces a prompt increase in circulating prothrombin and accelerator globulin and decrease in antithrombin activities of the blood. The coagulability of the blood, especially in capillary beds, is enhanced. Promptly corrects bleeding due to estrogen deficiency. It is probably excreted in the urine. Secreted in breast milk.

Indications and uses: Dysfunctional uterine bleeding caused by hormonal imbalance in the absence of organic pathology.

Unlabeled use: Postcoital contraception.

Precautions: (1) Dilution in an IV infusion is not recommended. (2) Must be refrigerated before and after reconstitution. Most frequently used promptly, but it is stable for up to 60 days if protected from light. (3) Do not use if discolored or precipitate present. (4) Even though bleeding is controlled, the etiology of the bleeding must be determined and definitive therapy instituted. (5) Follow immediately with oral estrogens as recommended for dysfunctional uterine bleeding. (6) Potentiates oral antidiabetics and oxytocin injections. (7) May increase blood glucose levels. (8) Use with caution in epilepsy, hypercalcemia, migraine, asthma, or cardiac or renal disease; induces salt and water retention. (9) Estrogens are carcinogenic; use only for specific indications. (10) May increase neuromuscular blocking effects of succinylcholine (Anectine). (11)

Safety for use in children not established. Has adverse effects on epiphyseal closure of bone.

Contraindications: Breast cancer except selected metastatic disease, estrogen-dependent neoplasia, pregnancy, thrombophlebitis or thromboembolic disorders, undiagnosed abnormal genital bleeding. Other specific contraindications for estrogens must be considered.

Incompatible with: Ascorbic acid, lactated Ringer's injection, protein hydrolysate, Ringer's injection, sodium lactate injection (1/6 molar lactate), any solution with an acid pH.

Side effects: Rare when used as directed; flushing, nausea, vomiting.

Antidote: No toxicity has been reported throughout years of clinical use.

CORTICOTROPIN INJECTION pH 2.5 to 6.0

(ACTH, Acthar)

Usual dose: 10 to 25 units/24 hr as an initial dose. Up to 80 units as a single injection has been used after the initial dose for diagnostic testing.

Dilution: Dilute lyophilized powder initially with 2 ml water or sodium chloride for injection. Withdraw desired dose of corticotropin and further dilute in 500 ml of 5% glucose in water. An isotonic saline solution may be used unless salt is restricted.

Rate of administration: Given as a continuous IV infusion over an 8-hour period.

Actions: Synthesized anterior pituitary hormone, a polypeptide, not absorbed through the GI tract. Given IV, it rapidly disappears from the bloodstream and little effect remains 6 hours after termination of the infusion. Effective only when the adrenal glands are normal and can respond to its stimulation. A normal increase in plasma cortisol rules out primary adrenocortical failure. Excreted in the urine.

Indications and uses: (1) Diagnosis of adrenocortical function; (2) treatment of idiopathic thrombocytopenic purpura.

Precautions: (1) Skin test for allergy if a known sensitivity exists to polypeptides or to hogs. (2) Vial must state "for IV use." (3) Continuous observation for at least the first 30 minutes is mandatory. Observe frequently throughout administration. (4) Check blood pressure frequently; may cause elevated blood pressure and salt and water retention. (5) May increase insulin needs in diabetes. (6) Use with caution in hypothyroidism and cirrhosis. (7) Refrigerate remainder of medication after initial dilution. (8) Prolonged therapy may be initiated as an adjunctive measure if no acute response (increase in plasma cortisol) to this diagnostic test. (9) Do not vaccinate for smallpox during therapy. (10) May require increased doses of anticoagulants; hemorrhagic episodes may occur. (11) May block effects of nondepolarizing neuromuscular blockers (e.g., pancuronium, tubocurarine). (12) Potassium depleting diuretics (e.g., acetazolamide [Diamox]) and amphotericin B may cause hypokalemia and enhance wasting effect. Monitor serum potassium. (13) Amphotericin B may decrease adrenocortical responsiveness.

Contraindications: Do not use in ocular herpes simplex, acute psychoses, scleroderma, osteoporosis, systemic fungal infections, or recent surgery.

Relative contraindications: Active or latent peptic ulcer, congestive heart failure, diabetes mellitus, diverticulitis, hypertension, lactation, pregnancy (especially during the first trimester), protein sensitivity, psychotic tendencies, renal insufficiency, thromboembolic tendencies, active or healed tuberculosis.

Incompatible with: Aminophylline, sodium bicarbonate. Many drug interactions are possible with corticosteroids. Some drugs markedly potentiate their effects and others necessitate increased doses.

Side effects: Do occur, but are usually reversible; alteration of glucose metabolism including hyperglycemia, Cushing's syndrome (moon face, fat pads), electrolyte imbalance, increased blood pressure, increased intracranial pressure with papilledema, masking of infection, pancreatitis, perforation and hemorrhage from aggravation of peptic ulcer, protein catabolism with negative nitrogen balance, psychic disturbances (especially euphoria), suppression of growth, thromboembolism, and many others including anaphylaxis.

Antidote: Notify the physician of any side effect so that it can be treated as necessary. Dosage may be reduced. Resuscitate as necessary for anaphylaxis and notify the physician. Keep epinephrine immediately available.

COSYNTROPIN

pH 5.5 to 7.5

(Cortrosyn)

Usual dose: 250 mcg (0.25 mg). Up to 750 mcg (0.75 mg) has been used.

Pediatric dose: May use adult dose for children over 2 years of age, but 125 mcg (0.125 mg) is usually adequate.

Dilution: Diluent provided (1.1 ml vial of 0.9% sodium chloride for injection). May be given direct IV after this initial dilution or further diluted in 5% dextrose or 0.9% saline solution and given as an infusion. (250 mcg in 250 ml equals 1 mcg/ml.)

Rate of administration: *Direct IV:* A single dose over 2 minutes.

Infusion: A single dose evenly distributed over 4 to 8 hours.

Actions: A synthetic form of adrenocorticotropic hormone (ACTH). Stimulates the adrenal cortex to secrete cortisol, corticosterone, androgenic substances, and aldosterone. Does not increase cortisol secretion in patients with primary adrenocortical insufficiency. Peak serum concentrations occur 45 to 60 minutes after direct IV injection.

Indications and uses: Diagnostic aid for adrenocortical insufficiency.

Precautions: (1) Preferable to ACTH because it is less likely to cause allergic reactions. May be used in patients who have had an allergic reaction to ACTH. (2) Plasma cortisol may be falsely elevated for patients taking spironolactone when fluorometric procedure used, patients receiving corticosteroids, and individuals with increased plasma bilirubin levels or free hemoglobin in the plasma. (3) Infusion method used if greater stimulus needed to effect results. (4) Use caution in pregnancy and lactation. (5) Stable after reconstitution for 24 hours at room temperature and 21 days if refrigerated. Infusion stable 12 hours at room temperature.

Contraindications: Hypersensitivity to cosyntropin.

Incompatible with: Blood and blood products. Should be considered incompatible with any other drug because of specific use.

Side effects: Bradycardia, dizziness, dyspnea, fainting, fever, flushing, irritability, rash, seizures, urticaria.

Antidote: Notify the physician of any side effect. Keep epinephrine and diphenhydramine available to treat anaphylaxis. Resuscitate as necessary.

CYCLOPHOSPHAMIDE pH 3.0 to 7.5

(Cytoxan, Cytoxan Lyophilized, Neosar, ✤ Procytox)

Usual dose: Initial dose may be up to a maximum of 40 to 50 mg/kg of body weight, usually given in divided doses (10 to 20 mg/kg/24 hr) over 2 to 5 days. This dose is reduced by one third to one half if hematological disease is present or there has been extensive radiation therapy. Maintenance doses vary from 3 to 5 mg/kg twice weekly to 10 to 15 mg/kg every 7 to 10 days. Dose based on average weight in presence of edema or ascites.

Reduced dose may be required in the adrenalectomized patient and in impaired renal or hepatic function.

Polymyositis: (investigational): 500 mg every 1 to 3 weeks as an IV infusion over 1 hour.

Dilution: *Specific techniques required, see Precautions.* Each 100 mg must be diluted with 5 ml of sterile water or bacteriostatic water for injection (paraben-preserved only). Shake solution gently and allow to stand until clear. Additional diluent (up to 250 ml 5% glucose or normal saline) recommended by some researchers to reduce side effects. Do not use heat to facilitate dilution.

Rate of administration: Each 100 mg or fraction thereof may be given over 1 minute. Cyclophosphamide may be given IV through the lumen of the rubber tubing or the three-way stopcock if the IV solution is glucose or saline.

Actions: An alkylating agent of the nitrogen mustard group with antitumor activity, cell cycle phase nonspecific, and most effective in S phase. It is an inert compound but is activated in the body (probably in the liver) by an unknown action to produce regression in the size of malignant tumors, to relieve pain and fever, and to increase appetite, strength, and a sense of well-being. Well absorbed, this drug or its metabolites are excreted in the urine. Secreted in breast milk.

Indications and uses: (1) To suppress or retard neoplastic growth. Good response has been experienced in hematopoietic malignancies such as Hodgkin's disease and leukemia, multiple myeloma, and in solid malignancies of the breast and ovary. (2) Treatment of biopsy-proven nephrotic syndrome in children when disease fails to respond to primary therapy or primary therapy causes intolerable side effects.

Investigational uses:: severe rheumatological conditions, polyarteritis nodosa, and alone or in combination with corticosteroids to treat polymyositis.

Precautions: (1) Follow guidelines for handling cytotoxic agents recommended. See Appendix, p. 677. (2) Administered by or under the direction of the physician specialist. (3) Marked leukopenia will occur after the initial dose. Recovery should begin in 7 to 10 days. Maintenance doses are regulated by an acceptable leukocyte count (2,500 to 4,000 cells/mm^3) and the absence of serious side effects. The maximum effective maintenance dose should be used. Monitor neutrophils and platelets and examine urine for red blood cells on a regular basis. (4) Do not store cyclophosphamide in temperatures over 37° C (90° F). (5) Diluted solution is not stable and must be used within 24 hours. Stable up to 6 days if refrigerated. (6) Use antiemetics for patient comfort. (7) Use caution in cases of leukopenia, thrombocytopenia, bone marrow infiltrated with malignant cells, recent radiation therapy, and severe hepatic or renal disease. Observe continuously for infection. (8) Wait 5 to 7 days after a major surgical procedure before beginning treatment. May interfere with normal wound healing. (9) Cyclophosphamide interacts with numerous drugs, including allopurinol, antidiabetics, barbiturates, chloramphenicol, corticosteroids, succinylcholine (Anectine), thiazide diuretics, and other alkylating agents to produce potentially serious reactions. (10) Often used with other antineoplastic drugs in reduced doses to achieve tumor remission. (11) Discontinue breast feeding. May produce teratogenic effects on the fetus. Has a mutagenic potential. (12) Potentiates anticoagulants. (13) Administer before 4 PM to decrease amount of drug remaining in bladder overnight. Encourage fluid intake and frequent voiding to prevent cystitis. (14) Do not administer any vaccine or chloroquine to patients receiving antineoplastic drugs. (15) May inhibit digoxin. (16) May cause syndrome of inappropriate antidiuretic hormone (SIADH) with normal doses because of fluid loading. (17) May result in reversible hemorrhagic ureteritis or renal tubular necrosis.

Contraindications: Previous hypersensitivity, severely depressed bone marrow function.

Incompatible with: Limited information available. Note Precautions. Give separately.

Side effects: *Minor:* Alopecia (regrowth may be slightly darker), amenorrhea, gonadal suppression, leukopenia (see Precautions), mucosal ulcerations, nausea and vomiting, skin and fingernails become darker, susceptibility to infection.

Major: Bone marrow depression; hemorrhagic ureteritis (reversible), pulmonary fibrosis, renal tubular necrosis (reversible), secondary neoplasia, SIADH, sterile hemorrhagic cystitis; which can be fatal.

Antidote: Minor side effects will be treated symptomatically if necessary. Discontinue the drug and notify the physician of hematuria immediately. There is no specific antidote. Supportive therapy as indicated will help sustain the patient in toxicity. Will respond to hemodialysis.

CYCLOSPORINE

(Sandimmune)

Usual dose: 5 to 6 mg/kg of body weight as a single dose 4 to 12 hours before transplantation. Repeat once each day until oral solution can be tolerated. Individualized adjustment is imperative and may be required on a daily basis.

Dilution: Each 50 mg should be diluted immediately before use with 20 to 100 ml of normal saline or 5% dextrose in water and given as an infusion. May leach phthalate from polyvinylchloride containers; use diluents in glass infusion bottles.

Rate of administration: A single dose properly diluted over 2 to 6 hours.

Actions: A potent immunosuppressive agent. Prolongs survival of kidney, liver, and heart allogeneic transplants in the human. 24-hour trough values of 250 to 800 ng/ml of whole blood or 50 to 300 ng/ml of plasma minimize side effects and rejection events. Extensively metabolized to metabolites and excreted in bile and urine. Crosses the placental barrier. Secreted in breast milk.

Indications and uses: (1) Prophylaxis of organ rejection in kidney, liver, and heart allogeneic transplants in conjunction with adrenocortical steroids; (2) treatment of chronic rejection in patients previously treated with other immunosuppressive agents.

Investigational uses: Prophylaxis of organ rejection in pancreas, bone marrow, and heart/lung transplantation.

Precautions: (1) Oral dosage preferred; begin as soon as feasible. (2) Dilute immediately before use and discard unused portion. Protect diluted solution from light. (3) Usually administered in the hospital by or under the direction of a physician experienced in immunosuppressive therapy and management of organ transplant patients. Adequate laboratory and supportive medical resources must be available. (4) Monitor bone marrow function, red and white blood cell counts, and platelet count. Monitor BUN, creatinine, serum bilirubin, and liver enzymes frequently. Timing and amount of rise in

BUN and creatinine and degree of nephrotoxicity or hepatotoxicity distinguish between need for dosage reduction or symptoms of organ rejection. (5) Given concomitantly with adrenocortical steroids only. Do not administer any other immunosuppressive agent. (6) Monitoring of cyclosporine blood levels may be helpful. (7) In impaired renal function, if rejection is severe, try other immunosuppressive therapy or allow rejection and removal of the kidney rather than increase dose of cyclosporine. (8) Observe constantly for signs of infection (fever, sore throat, tiredness) or unusual bleeding or bruising. (9) Safety for use in pregnancy and in men and women capable of conception not established. Embryotoxic and fetotoxic in rats. Discontinue breast feeding. (10) May cause lymphomas. (11) Potentiated by other nephrotoxic drugs (e.g., amphotericin B, ketoconazole, ethacrynic acid [Edecrin], aminoglycosides [e.g., gentamicin]); use extreme caution. Increased blood levels hazardous.

Contraindications: Hypersensitivity to cyclosporine or polyoxyethylated castor oil.

Incompatible with: Sufficient information not available. Administer separately.

Side effects: Acne, convulsions, cramps, diarrhea, gum hyperplasia, headache, hepatotoxicity, hirsutism, hypertension, infection, leukopenia, lymphoma, nausea and vomiting, paresthesia, renal dysfunction, and tremor. Mild allergic reactions have occurred.

Antidote: Notify the physician of all side effects. Most can be treated symptomatically. Drug may be decreased or discontinued or other immunosuppressive agents utilized. Nephrotoxicity, hepatotoxicity, or hematopoietic depression may require temporary reduction of dosage or permanent withholding of treatment. Dialysis is not effective in overdose.

CYSTEINE HYDROCHLORIDE pH 1.0 to 2.5

(L-Cysteine hydrochloride)

Usual dose: Individually ordered by neonatologist.

Dilution: Each 0.5 Gm dose must be initially diluted with 12.5 Gm of Aminosyn 5%, then must be further diluted with 250 ml or less of 50% dextrose. Equal volumes of Aminosyn and dextrose equal a final solution of 2.5% Aminosyn and 25% dextrose/ml.

Rate of administration: Should be specifically ordered by the neonatologist. Usually begin with 1 ml/kg of body weight/hr of properly diluted solution. May be gradually increased to 2 ml/kg/hr. A protein (amino acid) product. *Total daily dose should be evenly distributed over the 24-hour period. Maintain a constant drip rate.* Use of infusion pump and microfilter is recommended.

Actions: A sulfur-containing amino acid naturally synthesized in the adult. The enzyme necessary to accomplish this conversion is missing in newborn infants. An essential amino acid in infants. Provided as an additive to Aminosyn 5% to be mixed immediately before administration.

Indications and uses: Meet the IV amino acid nutritional requirements of infants receiving total parenteral nutrition via central venous infusion.

Precautions: (1) For use only after dilution with Aminosyn 5% and dextrose 50%. (2) Suitable for administration by central venous infusion only. (3) Cysteine is unstable over time and will precipitate. Begin administration within 1 hour of mixing, or may be refrigerated and must be used within 24 hours. (4) See all precautions listed under protein (amino acid) products.

Contraindications: Known hypersensitivity to any component.

After mixing with Aminosyn and dextrose: Acidosis, anuria, azotemia, severe liver disease, metabolic disorders with impaired nitrogen utilization.

Incompatible with: Any other drug in syringe. Note incompatibilities under protein (amino acid) products.

Side effects: All side effects under protein (amino acid) products are possible; i.e., abdominal pains, anaphylaxis, convulsions, edema at the site of injection, electrolyte imbalances, glycosuria, hyperammonemia, hyperglycemia, hyperpyrexia, hyperchloremia, metabolic acidosis and/or alkalosis, neuromuscular paresthesias, osmotic dehydration, phlebitis and thrombosis, rebound hypoglycemia, septicemia, vasodilation, vomiting, and weakness.

Antidote: Notify the physician of all side effects. Amounts of cysteine, glucose, or other additives may be adjusted to correct the problem. Many of the side effects possible will respond to a reduced rate. Some will require catheter insertion at a new site. Treat symptomatically and resuscitate as necessary.

CYTARABINE pH 5.0

(ARA-C, ♣ Cytosar, Cytosar-U, Cytosine Arabinoside)

Usual dose: *Acute lymphocytic leukemia in adults and children:* In combination chemotherapy, variable depending on specific regime or protocol. 2 to 6 mg/kg daily or 100 to 200 mg/M^2/24 hr as a continuous infusion or direct IV in divided doses every 12 hours. Repeat daily for 5 to 10 days depending on regimenn. Maintain treatment until therapeutic effect or toxicity occurs. Modify on a day-to-day basis for maximum individualized effectiveness.

Acute myelocytic leukemia remission induction in adults and children: As a single agent, 200 mg/M^2/24 hr for 5 days as a continuous infusion. Total dose is 1,000 mg/M^2. Repeat every 2 weeks.

Refractory acute leukemia remission induction: As a single agent, 3 Gm/M^3 as an IV infusion over 2 to 3 hours every 12 hours for 4 to 12 doses. Repeat at 2 to 3 week intervals.

Dilution: *Specific techniques required, see Precautions.* Each 100 mg must be initially diluted with 5 ml (500 mg with 10 ml) of sterile water for injection with benzyl alcohol 0.9%. Solution pH about 5.0. May be given by direct IV administration as is or further diluted in 50 to 100 ml or more of normal saline or 5% dextrose in water and given as an infusion. Direct IV administration should be through a free-flowing IV tubing.

Rate of administration: *IV injection:* Each 100 mg or fraction thereof over 1 to 3 minutes.

IV infusion: Single daily dose properly diluted over 30 minutes to 24 hours, depending on amount of infusion solution and dosage regimen.

Actions: An antimetabolite and pyrimidine antagonist that interferes with the synthesis of DNA and RNA. Cell cycle specific for S phase. Through various chemical processes this deprivation acts more quickly on rapidly growing cells and causes their death. Cytotoxic and cytostatic. A potent bone marrow depressant. Crosses the blood-brain barrier. Metabolized in the liver and excreted in the urine.

Indications and uses: Induction of remission in acute myelocytic leukemia of adults and children and other acute leukemias in adults and children.

Precautions: (1) Follow guidelines for handling cytotoxic agents. See Appendix, p. 677. (2) Administered by or under the direction of the physician specialist. (3) Remissions induced by cytarabine are brief unless followed by maintenance therapy. (4) Refrigerate until after dilution, then stable at room temperature for 48 hours. Use only clear solutions. (5) Leukocyte and platelet counts should be monitored daily. Discontinue therapy for platelet count under 50,000 or polymorphonuclear granulocytes under 1,000 cells/mm^3. (6) Use caution with impaired liver function. (7) Monitor bone marrow, liver, and renal function at intervals during therapy. (8) Higher doses tolerated by IV injection compared with IV infusion, but the incidence and intensity of nausea and vomiting are increased. Prophylactic administration of antiemetics recommended. (9) May produce teratogenic effects on the fetus, especially during the first trimester. (10) Usually used with other antineoplastic drugs in specific doses to achieve tumor remission. (11) Dosage based on average weight in presence of edema or ascites. (12) Potentiates anticoagulants, may inhibit digoxin absorption. (13) Be alert for signs of bone marrow depression, bleeding, or infection. These side effects are dose- and schedule-dependent. (14) Do not administer any vaccines or chloroquine to patients receiving antineoplastic drugs. (15) Monitor uric acid levels; maintain hydration; allopurinol may be indicated. (16) May cause acute pancreatitis in patients who previously received L-asparaginase. (17) Benzyl alcohol may cause a fatal "gasping syndrome" in premature infants.

Contraindications: Hypersensitivity to cytarabine, preexisting drug-induced bone marrow depression.

Incompatible with: Fluorouracil, methylprednisolone sodium succinate (Solu-Medrol). Consider toxicity and specific use.

Side effects: Anemia, abdominal pain, bone marrow depression, bone pain, chest pain, conjunctivitis, diarrhea, esophagitis, fever, hepatic dysfunction, hyperuricemia, leukopenia, malaise, megaloblastosis, mucosal bleeding, myalgia, nausea, oral ulceration, rash, stomatitis, thrombocytopenia, thrombophlebitis, vomiting. Higher than usual dose regimens may cause severe coma, GI ulcerations and peritonitis, personality changes, pulmonary toxicity, somnolence, or death.

Antidote: Notify the physician of all side effects. Most will be treated symptomatically. Some toxicity is necessary to produce remission. Discontinue the drug for serious hematological depression. Drug must be restarted as soon as signs of bone marrow recovery occur or its effectiveness will be lost. Use corticosteroids for cytarabine syndrome (fever, myalgia, bone pain, occasional chest pain, maculopapular rash, conjunctivitis, malaise). Usually occurs in 6 to 12 hours after administration. Continue cytarabine if patient responds to corticosteroids. There is no specific antidote; supportive therapy as indicated will help to sustain the patient in toxicity.

CYTOMEGALOVIRUS IMMUNE GLOBULIN INTRAVENOUS (HUMAN)

(CMV-IGIV)

Usual dose: 150 mg/kg of body weight as a single dose IV infusion. This initial dose must be given within 72 hours of transplant. Do not exceed this dose. Follow with an infusion containing 100 mg/kg at 2, 4, 6, and 8 weeks post transplant. Reduce dose to 50 mg/kg per infusion at weeks 12 and 16 post transplant.

Dilution: Absolute sterile technique required at all steps of reconstitution; contains no preservatives. Each 2,500 mg vial must be diluted with 50 ml of sterile water for injection (provided) to provide a final concentration of 50 mg/ml. Supplied in an evacuated vial so diluent will transfer by suction. A syringe and needle or a double-ended transfer needle may be used. Prepare or puncture diluent first, then insert into CMV-IGIV vial. Release any residual vacuum before withdrawing needle. Rotate gently to moisten all powder, do not shake, avoid foaming. Will take up to 30 minutes to dissolve completely. Reenter vial only 1 time to withdraw desired dose. Use only if clear and colorless. Initiate infusion within 6 hours and must be completely infused within 12 hours of dilution. Filters are not required.

Rate of administration: Use of a constant infusion pump (e.g., IVAC) is required. Begin with a rate of 15 mg/kg/hr. May be increased to 30 mg/kg/hr in 30 minutes if no discomfort or adverse effects. May be increased in another 30 minutes to 60 mg/kg/hr if no discomfort or adverse effects. Do not exceed the 60 mg/kg/hr rate or allow the volume infused to exceed 75 ml/hr regardless of mg/kg/hr dose. Slow rate of infusion at onset of patient discomfort or any adverse reactions. Infusion must be complete within 12 hours of dilution. Subsequent doses may be increased at 15 minute intervals using the same mg/kg/hr rates and adhering to the volume maximum of 75 ml/hr.

Actions: A sterile lyophilized powder of immunoglobulin G (IgG). Derived from pooled adult human plasma selected for high titers of antibody for cytomegalovirus (CMV). Purified by a specific process. Can raise the relevant antibody levels sufficiently to attenuate or reduce the incidence of serious CMV disease. Antibody levels will last 2 to 3 weeks.

Indications and uses: Attenuation of primary (1°) CMV disease associated with kidney transplantation. Intended for use in all kidney transplant recipients who are seronegative for CMV and who receive a kidney from a CMV seropositive donor.

Precautions: (1) Continuous monitoring of vital signs is preferred. Must be monitored before infusion, at every rate change, the midpoint, at the conclusion, and several times after completion. (2) All supplies for emergency treatment of acute anaphylatic reaction must be available (see Antidote). (3) 75% of untreated recipients would be expected to develop CMV disease. Use of CMV-IGIV has effected a 50% reduction in this disease rate. Effective results have been obtained with a variety of immunosupressive regimens (e.g., combinations of azathioprine, cyclosporine, prednisone). (4) A fatal CMV infection occurred even with ganciclovir treatment in one patient, who inadvertently missed a single injection. Adherence to the prescribed regimen is imperative. (5) Defer vaccination with any live virus vaccine (e.g., measles, mumps, rubella) until 3 months after CMV-IGIV administration. (6) Safety for use during pregnancy not established. Use only if clearly needed. (7) Distributed by the American Red Cross. Store dry powder in refrigerator between 2° to 8° C (35° to 46° F).

Contraindications: History of a prior severe reaction associated with any human immunoglobulin preparations. Individuals with selective immunoglobulin A deficiency may develop antibodies to IgA and are at risk for anaphylaxis.

Incompatible with: Administration through a separate infusion line recommended. If absolutely necessary, may be piggy-backed into a preexisting line containing normal saline, 0.45% saline, dextrose 2.5%, 5%, 10%, or 20% in water or saline. Do not dilute CMV-IGIV more than one part to two parts of any of these solutions.

Side effects: Incidence related to rate of administration; back pain, chills, fever, flushing, hypotension, muscle cramps, nausea, vomiting, wheezing. Allergic reactions including anaphylaxis are possible.

Antidote: With onset of any minor side effect reduce rate of infusion immediately or discontinue temporarily. Discontinue CMV-IGIV if symptoms persist and notify the physicain. May be treated symptomatically, and infusion resumed at a slower rate if symptoms subside. Discontinue CMV-IGIV if hypotension or anaphylaxis occur and treat immediately. Epinephrine (Adrenalin), diphenhydramine (Benadryl), oxygen, vasopressors (e.g., dopamine [Intropin]), corticosteroids, and ventilation equipment must always be available. Resuscitate as necessary.

DACARBAZINE

pH 3.0 to 4.0

(DTIC, DTIC-Dome, Imidazole carboxamide)

Usual dose: *Malignant melanoma:* 2 to 4.5 mg/kg of body weight/24 hr for 10 days. May be repeated at 4-week intervals. May administer 250 mg/M^2 for 5 days. Repeat in 3 weeks. Has proved as effective in lesser doses as in larger doses. Individualized response determines dosage of succeeding treatments.

Hodgkin's disease: 150 mg/M^2/day for 5 days. Repeat every 4 weeks. Used in combination with other drugs in a specific regimen.

Dilution: *Specific techniques required, see Precautions.* Each 100 mg vial is diluted with 9.9 ml (200 mg with 19.7 ml) of sterile water for injection (10 mg/ml). Additional diluent may be used. May be given through Y-tube or three-way stopcock of infusion set. Administration through a free-flowing IV tubing is preferred. May be further diluted in 50 to 250 ml of 5% dextrose in water or normal saline for infusion.

Rate of administration: Total dose over 1 minute. If diluted with 50 to 250 ml, administer over 30 minutes.

Actions: An antineoplastic agent. Exact mechanism of action is not known; may inhibit DNA and RNA synthesis. It is an alkylating agent, cell cycle phase nonspecific. Probably localizes in the liver and is excreted in the urine.

Indications and uses: Induction of remission of (1) malignant melanoma with metastasis after surgical excision of the tumor; (2) Hodgkin's disease; (3) soft tissue sarcomas.

Precautions: (1) Follow guidelines for handling cytotoxic agents. See Appendix, p. 677. (2) Administered by or under the direction of the physician specialist. (3) Determine absolute patency of vein; a stinging or burning sensation indicates extravasation; severe cellulitis and tissue necrosis will result. Discontinue injection; use another vein. (4) Diluted solution stable for 72 hours only if refrigerated at 4° C (39° F); discard in 6 to 8 hours if kept at room temperature. (5) Used with other antineoplastic drugs and radiation therapy in reduced doses to achieve tumor remission. (6) Monitor bone marrow function, white and red blood cell and platelet count frequently. (7) Nausea and vomiting may be reduced by restricting oral intake of fluid and foods for 4 to 6 hours before administration. Use antiemetics. (8) Dosage based on average weight in presence of edema or ascites. (9) Safety for use in pregnancy or lactation and in men and women capable of conception not established. (10) Do not administer any vaccines or chloroquine to patients receiving antineoplastic drugs. (11) Use caution in impaired liver and renal function. (12) Inhibited by phenobarbital and phenytoin (Dilantin). Potentiates allopurinol. (13) Be alert for signs of bone marrow depression, bleeding, or infection. (14) Alert patient to photosensitivity skin reaction.

Contraindications: Known hypersensitivity to dacarbazine.

Incompatible with: Limited information available; heparin, hydrocortisone sodium succinate, hydrocortisone sodium phosphate, lidocaine. Should be considered incompatible in syringe or solution with any other drug because of toxicity and specific use.

Side effects: Leukopenia and thrombocytopenia may be serious enough to cause death. Alopecia, anaphylaxis, anorexia, facial flushing, facial paresthesias, fever, hepatotoxicity, malaise, myalgia, nausea, skin necrosis, vomiting.

Antidote: Notify physician of all side effects. Most will be treated symptomatically. Hematopoietic depression may require temporary or permanent withholding of treatment. There is no specific antidote. Supportive therapy as indicated will help sustain the patient in toxicity. For extravasation elevate extremity, consider injection of long-acting dexamethasone (Decadron LA) or hyaluronidase (Wydase) throughout extravasated tissue. Use a 27- or 25-gauge needle. Apply moist warm compresses.

DACTINOMYCIN pH 5.5 to 7.0

(ACT, Actinomycin D, Cosmegen)

Usual dose: 0.5 mg/24 hr for up to 5 days. May be repeated after 3 weeks if all signs of toxicity have disappeared. Do not exceed 15 mcg/kg of body weight/ day in adults or children.

Pediatric dose: 0.015 mg (15 mcg)/kg of body weight/24 hr for 5 days. May be repeated after 3 weeks if all signs of toxicity have disappeared.

Dilution: *Specific techniques required, see Precautions.* Dilute each 0.5 mg vial with 1.1 ml of sterile water for injection without preservative (0.5 mg/ml). Sterile water with preservative (benzyl alcohol or paraben) will cause precipitation. Use 2.2 ml to yield 0.25 mg/ml (vent vial to relieve pressure). May be given direct IV (see Precautions), through the Y-tube or three-way stopcock of a free-flowing infusion of compatible solutions, or further diluted in 50 ml 5% dextrose in water or normal saline for infusion. Do not use a filter smaller than 5 microns. Loss of potency will occur.

Rate of administration: *Direct IV:* Each 0.5 mg or fraction thereof over 1 minute.

IV infusion: A single dose over 10 to 15 minutes.

Actions: A highly toxic antibiotic antineoplastic agent, cell cycle phase nonspecific. Cytotoxic, it interferes with cell division by binding DNA to slow production of RNA. Found in high concentrations in the kidney, liver, and spleen.

Indications and uses: To suppress or retard neoplastic growth in (1) Wilms' tumor; (2) rhabdomyosarcoma; (3) carcinoma of the testis and uterus; (4) choriocarcinoma; (5) Ewing's sarcoma; (6) botryoid sarcoma.

Precautions: (1) Follow guidelines for handling cytotoxic agents. See Appendix, p. 677. (2) Administered by or under the direction of the physician specialist. (3) Determine absolute patency of vein; a stinging or burning sensation indicates extravasation; severe cellulitis and tissue necrosis will result. Discontinue injection; use another vein. (4) Use sterile two-needle technique for direct IV administration: one needle to dilute and withdraw and one needle to inject into the vein (rinse with blood before removing). (5) Dosage based on average weight in presence of edema or ascites. (6) Light sensitive in dry form. (7) Discard any unused portion. (8) Used with other antineoplastic drugs in reduced doses to achieve tumor remission. (9) Reduce dose of dactinomycin and radiation therapy when used concurrently, if either has been used previously, or if previous chemotherapy has been employed. (10) Radiation therapy potentiates dactinomycin. (11) Dactinomycin alone may reactivate erythema from previous radiation therapy. (12) May produce teratogenic effects on the fetus; use caution in men and women capable of conception. (13) Monitor renal, hepatic, and bone marrow function frequently. (14) Except for immediate nausea and vomiting, side effects may not appear for 2 to 4 days. Always observe closely. Use prophylactic antiemetics. (15) Do not administer any vaccines or chloroquine to patients receiving antineoplastic drugs. (16) Inhibits action of penicillin. (17) Allopurinol, increased fluid intake, and alkalinization of the urine may be required to reduce uric acid levels. (18) May interfere with bioassay procedures used in determining antibacterial drug levels.

Contraindications: Exposure to chickenpox, known sensitivity to dactinomycin, infants under 6 months of age.

Incompatible with: Specific information not available. Should be considered incompatible in syringe or solution with any other drug.

Side effects: Abdominal pain, acne, alopecia, anaphylaxis, anemia, anorexia, ascites; cheilitis, diarrhea, dysphagia, erythema flare-up, esophagitis, fatigue, fever, GI ulceration, hepatitis, hepatomegaly, hypocalcemia, lethargy, leukopenia, liver function test abnormalities, malaise, myalgia, nausea, pharyngitis, proctitis, skin eruptions, thrombocytopenia, ulcerative stomatitis, vomiting.

Antidote: Any side effect can result in death. Notify the physician of all side effects. Most will be treated symptomatically. Hematopoietic depression may require withholding dactinomycin until recovery occurs. There is no specific antidote. Supportive therapy as indicated will help sustain the patient in toxicity. For extravasation elevate extremity, apply cold compresses, flush area with normal saline, and inject long-acting dexamethasone (Decadron LA) or hyaluronidase (Wydase) throughout extravasated tissue. Use a 27- or 25-gauge needle.

DANTROLENE SODIUM — pH 9.5

(Dantrium Intravenous)

Usual dose: 1 mg/kg of body weight as an initial dose. Repeat as necessary until symptoms subside or a cumulative dose of 10 mg/kg is reached. Entire regimen may be repeated if symptoms reappear. Dosage required depends on degree of susceptibility to malignant hyperthermia, length of time of exposure to triggering agent, and time lapse between onset of crisis and beginning of treatment.

Dilution: Each 20 mg must be diluted with 60 ml sterile water for injection without a bacteriostatic agent. Shake until solution is clear. May be administered through a Y-tube or three-way stopcock of infusion tubing.

Rate of administration: Each single dose should be given by rapid continuous IV push. Follow immediately with subsequent doses as indicated.

Actions: A direct-acting skeletal muscle relaxant. Inhibits excitation-contraction coupling by interfering with the release of the calcium ion from the sarcoplasmic reticulum to reverse the physiological cause of malignant hyperthermia. Has no appreciable effect on cardiovascular or respiratory function. Onset of action is prompt and lasts about 5 hours. Metabolized in the liver and excreted in urine.

Indications and uses: To manage the fulminant hypermetabolism of skeletal muscle characteristic of malignant hyperthermia crisis (tachycardia, tachypnea, central venous desaturation, hypercapnia, metabolic acidosis, skeletal muscle rigidity, cyanosis, mottling of skin, fever, increased use of anesthesia circuit CO_2 absorber).

Precautions: (1) Discontinue all anesthetic agents immediately when onset of malignant hyperthermia is recognized. (2) Monitor ECG, vital signs, electrolytes, and urine output continuously. Oxygen needs are increased; manage metabolic acidosis; institute cooling measures. (3) Confirm absolute patency of vein; avoid extravasation. (4) Protect diluted solution from direct light and discard after 6 hours. Store between 15° and 30° C (59° and 86° F). (5) Oral dantrolene indicated preoperatively in known susceptible patients and postoperatively for 1 to 3 days to follow emergency IV treatment. (6) Ability to bind to plasma proteins inhibited by warfarin and clofibrate; increased by tolbutamide. (7) Use caution in pregnancy, lactation, and children under 5 years.

Contraindications: None when used as indicated.

Incompatible with: Specific information not available.

Side effects: None when used as short-term therapy for this specific indication.

Antidote: No specific antidote is available or needed when used correctly. Notify physician and initiate supportive measures (adequate airway and ventilation, monitor ECG) in overdosage. Large amounts of IV fluids may be needed to prevent crystalluria. Treat anaphylaxis and resuscitate as necessary.

DAUNOROBICIN HYDROCHLORIDE

pH 4.5 to 6.5

(Cerubidine, DNR)

Usual dose: *Single agent:* Up to 60 mg/M^2/day for 3 days. Repeat every 3 to 4 weeks.

Adult acute nonlymphocytic leukemia: 45 mg/M^2/day in adults under age 60 (adults over age 60 may require reduction to 30 mg/M^2/day) for 3 days in combination with cytarabine 100 mg/M^2/day for 7 days. Repeat daunorubicin, 30 to 45 mg/M^2/day depending on age for only 2 days in subsequent courses every 3 to 4 weeks. Cytarabine 100 mg/M^2/day given daily for 5 days in subsequent courses.

Adult acute lymphocytic leukemia: 45 mg/M^2/day IV on days 1, 2, and 3 in combination with vincristine 2 mg IV on days 1, 8, and 15; prednisone 40 mg/M^2/day orally on days 1 through 22 (taper prednisone dose from day 22 to 29); L-asparaginase 500 IU/kg/day IV for 10 days from days 22 through 32.

Normal liver and kidney function required. When remission is complete, an individual maintenance program should be established.

Pediatric dose: *Pediatric acute lymphocytic leukemia:* 25 mg/M^2/day on day 1 each week, vincristine 1.5 mg/M^2 on day 1 each week, and prednisone 40 mg/M^2 orally daily. Remission should be obtained in 4 to 6 weeks.

Dilution: *Specific techniques required, see Precautions.* Each 20 mg must be diluted with 4 ml of sterile water for injection (5 mg/ml). Agitate gently to dissolve completely. Further dilute each dose with 10 to 15 ml of normal saline. Do not add to IV solutions. Must be given through Y-tube or three-way stopcock of a free-flowing infusion of 5% dextrose or normal saline.

Rate of administration: A single dose of properly diluted medication over 3 to 5 minutes.

Actions: A highly toxic antibiotic antineoplastic agent. Rapidly cleared from plasma, it inhibits synthesis of DNA. Cell cycle specific for S phase; exact method of action is unknown; antimitotic, cytotoxic, and immunosuppressive. Does not cross blood-brain barrier. Slowly excreted in bile and urine.

Indications and uses: (1) To induce remission of acute nonlymphocytic leukemia in adults; (2) combination therapy for acute lymphocytic leukemia in adults and children.

Precautions: (1) Follow guidelines for handling cytotoxic agents. See Appendix, p. 677. (2) Administered by or under the direction of the physician specialist. (3) Determine absolute patency of vein; a stinging or burning sensation indicates extravasation; severe cellulitis; tissue necrosis will result. Discontinue injection; use another vein. (4) Diluted solution stable 24 hours at room temperature, 48 hours if refrigerated; then discard. (5) Protect from sunlight. (6) Urine may be reddish color (from dye not hematuria). (7) Monitoring of white blood cells, red blood cells, platelet count, liver function, kidney function, ECG, chest x-ray, echocardiography, and systolic ejection fraction indicated before and during therapy. (8) May produce teratogenic effects on the fetus. (9) Observe closely for all signs of infection. (10) Use extreme caution in preexisting drug-induced bone marrow suppression, existing heart disease, previous treatment with doxorubicin (Adriamycin), or radiation therapy encompassing the heart. (11) May cause acute congestive heart failure with total cumulative doses over 550 mg/M^2 (400 mg/M^2 if previous treatment with doxorubicin or radiation therapy in area of heart). (12) Reduce dose up to one half if liver or renal function impaired. (13) Prophylactic antiemetics may reduce nausea and vomiting and increase patient comfort. (14) Monitor uric acid levels; maintain hydration; allopurinol may be indicated. (15) Dosage based on average weight if edema or ascites present. (16) Do not administer any vaccines or chloroquine to patients receiving antineoplastic drugs.

Contraindications: Not absolute; preexisting bone marrow suppression, impaired cardiac function, preexisting infection (see Precautions).

Incompatible with: Dexamethasone (Decadron), heparin. Should be considered incompatible with any other drug because of toxicity and specific use.

Side effects: Acute congestive heart failure, alopecia (reversible), bone marrow suppression (marked with average doses), chills, decrease in systolic ejection fraction, depressed QRS voltage, diarrhea, fever, gonadal suppression, mucositis, myocarditis, nausea, pericarditis, skin rash, vomiting.

Antidote: Most side effects will be tolerated or treated symptomatically. Keep physician informed. Close monitoring of accumulated dosage, bone marrow, ECG, chest x-ray, echocardiography, and systolic ejection fraction may prevent most serious and potentially fatal side effects. There is no specific antidote. Supportive therapy as indicated will help sustain the patient in toxicity. For extravasation aspirate as much infiltrated drug as possible, flood site with normal saline and inject hydrocortisone sodium succinate (Solu-Cortef) or hyaluronidase (Wydase) throughout extravasated tissue. Use a 27- or 25-gauge needle. Cold moist compresses may be helpful, elevate extremity. Site should be observed promptly by a reconstructive surgeon.

DEFEROXAMINE MESYLATE — pH 4.0 to 6.0

(Desferal)

Usual dose: *Acute iron intoxication:* An initial dose of 1 Gm may be followed by doses of 500 mg every 4 hours as indicated by clinical response. *Do not exceed 6 Gm in 24 hours by way of any or all routes—IV, IM, clysis, or oral.*

Chronic iron overload: 2 Gm with each unit of blood. Use a separate vein.

Pediatric dose: 50 mg/kg of body weight up to 2 Gm every 6 hours. *Do not exceed 6 Gm in 24 hours.*

Dilution: Each 500 mg must be diluted in 2 ml of sterile water for injection. When completely dissolved, deferoxamine must be further diluted in an IV solution; normal saline, glucose in water, and Ringer's lactate solution are compatible.

Rate of administration: The fully diluted solution must not exceed a rate of 15 mg/kg of body weight/hr. Deferoxamine, 2 Gm in 1,000 ml of infusion fluid, equally distributed over 24 hours, constitutes a reasonably safe dose for anyone weighing over 25 kg.

Actions: An iron-chelating agent, deferoxamine complexes with iron to form ferrioxamine, a stable chelate that prevents the iron from entering into further chemical reactions. Readily soluble in water, it passes easily through the kidney, giving the urine a characteristic reddish color. It will remove iron from free serum iron, ferritin, and transferrin, but not from hemoglobin or cytochromes. Metabolized by plasma enzymes.

Indications and uses: To facilitate the removal of iron in the treatment of acute iron intoxication or chronic iron overload from multiple transfusions.

Investigational use: Manage accumulation of aluminum in bone of renal failure patients and in aluminum-induced dialysis encephalopathy.

Precautions: (1) Deferoxamine is adjunctive therapy. Standard measures for treating acute iron intoxication are also indicated: induction of emesis and/or gastric lavage; suction and maintenance of a clear airway; control of shock with IV fluids, blood, oxygen, and vasopressors; and correction of acidosis. (2) IM administration is preferred. May be given SC by hypodermoclysis. IV administration should be used only in a state of cardiovascular shock or chronic iron overload. (3) For long-term therapy, check for cataract development. (4) Use only if clearly needed during early pregnancy or during childbearing years. (5) Use in children under 3 years only if there is iron mobilization greater than 1 mg/24 hours. (6) Under sterile conditions, deferoxamine diluted with sterile water may be stored at room temperature for 1 week. (7) Protect from light.

Contraindications: Severe renal disease or anuria.

Incompatible with: Must be diluted in specific IV solutions. *Do not mix with any other IV medication.*

Side effects: Occur more frequently with too rapid administration; abdominal discomfort, allergic type of reactions including anaphylaxis, blurring of vision, diarrhea, flushing of the skin, fever, hypotension, leg cramps, shock, tachycardia, urticaria.

Antidote: At first sign of side effects, decrease rate of administration. If side effects persist, discontinue drug and notify physician. Further dilution and decrease in rate of administration may be necessary. Resuscitate as indicated.

DESLANOSIDE INJECTION pH 5.9 to 6.5

(✱ Cedilanid, Cedilanid-D)

Usual dose: 1.2 to 1.6 mg (6 to 8 ml) for digitalization. May be given as a single dose or equally divided over approximately 12 hours. Maintenance dose is usually about one fourth of the digitalizing dose. Give one half of the maintenance dose every 12 hours.

Pediatric dose: Total digitalizing dose for newborns is 0.022 mg/kg of body weight; for children 2 weeks to 3 years of age it is 0.025 mg/kg; 3 years and over, 0.022 mg/kg. Give in divided doses every 3 to 4 hours or in a single dose if necessary.

Dilution: May be given undiluted or further diluted with 10 ml sodium chloride injection (preferred). Do not mix with infusion fluids. Give through Y-tube or three-way stopcock of IV infusion tubing.

Rate of administration: 0.2 mg (1 ml) or fraction thereof over 1 minute.

Actions: This is a rapid-acting derivative of lanatoside C. Effective within 5 to 15 minutes and lasts 2 to 3 days. It increases the strength of myocardial contraction. It alters myocardial automaticity, conduction velocity, and refractory period. Results are a slower, stronger beat with increased cardiac output. Venous pressure falls, coronary circulation is increased, and heart size may become more normal. It is widely distributed throughout the body and excreted in the urine.

Indications and uses: (1) Congestive heart failure; (2) atrial fibrillation; (3) atrial flutter; (4) paroxysmal tachycardia; (5) cardiogenic shock; (6) ventricular dysrhythmias with congestive heart failure; (7) preoperative, intraoperative, and postoperative need for digitalis because of stress on the heart.

Precautions: (1) IV administration is the preferred route until oral therapy is feasible. (2) Do not give digitalized patients calcium; death has occurred. (3) Potassium depletion makes the heart sensitive to digitalis intoxication. Check electrolytes during therapy. (4) Use with caution in patients with hypercalcemia or liver or kidney disease. (5) Reduce dose in impaired renal function and partially digitalized patients. (6) Potentiated by phenytoin sodium (Dilantin); thyroid preparations; *Veratrum* alkaloids (Unitensen); reserpine; quinidine; propranolol (Inderal); verapamil; mercurial, thiazide, and loop diuretics; pressor agents (epinephrine); and others. (7) Inhibited by potassium salts, spironolactone (Aldactone), triamterene (Dyrenium), and others. (8) ECG monitoring suggested.

Contraindications: Digitalis toxicity, ventricular tachycardia, or known sensitivity to deslanoside.

Relative contraindications: Myocardial infarction or angina pectoris without congestive heart failure.

Incompatible with: Acids, alkalies, calcium chloride, calcium disodium edetate, calcium gluceptate, calcium gluconate.

Side effects: Seldom last more than 3 days after drug is discontinued. Any form of digitalis may cause partial or AV block and almost any dysrhythmia, including paroxysmal tachycardia, atrial tachycardia, fibrillation, or standstill. *First ECG signs of toxicity* are ST segment sagging, PR prolongation, and possible bigeminal rhythm. *Clinical signs of toxicity* are mostly GI and visual: abdominal discomfort or pain, anorexia, blurred vision, confusion, diarrhea, disturbed color (yellow) vision, headache, nausea, salivation, vomiting.

Antidote: Discontinue the drug at first sign of toxicity and notify the physician. Dosage may be decreased or discontinued. For severe toxicity, digoxin immune Fab is a specific antidote. Depending on symptoms, use one or more of the following for supportive treatment: atropine, phenytoin (Dilantin), potassium salts (potassium chloride), procainamide (Pronestyl), or disodium edetate (EDTA disodium). Resuscitate as necessary.

DESMOPRESSIN ACETATE pH 3.5 to 4.0

(DDAVP, 1-Deamino-8-D-Arginine Vasopressin, Stimate)

Usual dose: *Diabetes insipidus:* 0.5 to 1.0 ml (2 to 4 mcg) daily in 2 divided doses. Adjust each dose individually for an adequate diurnal rhythm of water turnover. Ten times more potent than intranasal desmopressin. Reduce dose accordingly when transferring from intranasal to IV administration.

Hemophilia A and von Willebrand's disease (Type 1): 0.3 mcg/kg of body weight. Administer 30 minutes preoperatively.

Dilution: *Diabetes insipidus:* May be given undiluted.

Hemophilia A and von Willebrand's disease (Type 1): Dilute a single dose in 10 ml of normal saline for children under 10 kg; and 50 ml for adults and children over 10 kg. Must be given as an IV infusion.

Rate of administration: *Diabetes insipidus:* A single dose direct IV over 1 minute.

Hemophilia A and von Willebrand's disease (Type 1): A single dose as an IV infusion over 15 to 30 minutes.

Actions: A synthetic analog of the natural hormone arginine vasopressin (human antidiuretic hormone—ADH). It is more potent than arginine vasopressin in increasing plasma levels of factor VIII activity in patients with hemophilia A and von Willebrand's disease (Type 1). Onset of action as an antidiuretic is prompt and lasts from 8 to 20 hours. Clinically effective antidiuretic doses are usually below the levels needed to affect vascular or visceral smooth muscle. Produces dose-related increase in factor VIII levels within 30 minutes and peaks in 90 to 120 minutes.

Indications and uses: (1) Antidiuretic replacement therapy in the management of central (cranial) diabetes insipidus; (2) management of the temporary polyuria and polydipsia following head trauma or surgery in the pituitary region; (3) maintain hemostasis in patients with hemophilia A or von Willebrand's disease during surgical procedures and postoperatively; (4) stop bleeding in patients with hemophilia A or von Willebrand's disease with episodes of spontaneous or trauma-induced injuries.

Precautions: (1) When antidiuretic effect is not needed, caution patients (especially the young and the elderly) to limit fluid intake to satisfy thirst needs only; this decreases potential occurrence of water intoxication and hyponatremia. (2) Use caution in patients with coronary artery insufficiency or hypertension. (3) May produce hypertension with other vasopressors (e.g., dopamine [Intropin]). (4) Use only when clearly indicated in pregnancy and lactation. (5) May be potentiated by chlorpropamide, clofibrate, or carbamazepine.

Diabetes insipidus: (1) Not effective for the treatment of nephrogenic diabetes insipidus. (2) Confirm diagnosis of diabetes insipidus by the water deprivation test, the hypertonic saline infusion test, and the response to ADH. Monitor continued response by measuring urine volume and osmolality. Plasma osmolality may be needed. Accuracy and effectiveness of dose measured by duration of sleep and adequate, not excessive, water turnover.

Hemophilia A: (1) May be considered for use in patients with factor VIII activity levels from 2% to 5% with careful monitoring. Generally used only when the factor VIII activity level is above 5%. (2) Not indicated in patients with hemophilia B or those with factor VIII antibodies. (3) Monitor factor VIII coagulant, factor VIII antigen, factor VIII ristocetin cofactor, and activated PTT.

Von Willebrand's disease (Type 1): (1) Most effective when factor VIII activity level above 5%. (2) Monitor bleeding time, factor VIII activity levels, ristocetin cofactor activity, and von Willebrand factor antigen during therapy to ensure adequate levels. (3) Not indicated for treatment of severe classic von Willebrand's disease (Type 1), Type 2B von Willebrand's disease (will induce platelet aggregation), or if there is evidence of an abnormal molecular form of factor VIII antigen.

Hemophilia and von Willebrand's: (1) Sometimes used with aminocaproic acid. (2) Monitor blood pressure and pulse during infusion.

Contraindications: Children under 12 years with diabetes insipidus, infants under 3 months with hemophilia A or von Willebrand's disease, known hypersensitivity to desmopressin.

Incompatible with: Specific information not available.

Side effects: Are infrequent. High doses may produce facial flushing, headache, hypertension (slight), mild abdominal cramps, nausea, and vulval pain. May cause burning, local erythema, and swelling at site of injection; hyponatremia; and water intoxication.

Antidote: Notify physician of all side effects. Most will respond to reduction of dose or rate of administration, or symptomatic treatment. May need to discontinue drug. Resuscitate as necessary.

DEXAMETHASONE SODIUM PHOSPHATE

pH 7.0 to 8.5

(Ak-Dek, Dalalone, Decadrol, Decadron, Decadron Phosphate, Decaject, Dexacen-4, Dexasone, Dexone, Hexadrol Phosphate, Solurex)

BETAMETHASONE SODIUM PHOSPHATE

pH 8.5

(Celestone Phosphate, Cel-U-Jec, Selestoject)

Usual dose: ***Dexamethasone:*** 0.5 to 9 mg daily. May be divided into 2 to 4 doses. Larger doses may be justified by patient's condition. Repeat until adequate response; then decrease dose as indicated. Total dose usually does not exceed 80 mg/24 hr. Dosage must be individualized.

Unresponsive shock: 1 to 6 mg/kg of body weight (maximum 40 mg) as a single injection. Repeat every 2 to 6 hours while shock persists.

Antiemetic in management of emetic-inducing chemotherapy: One protocol calls for 20 mg 40 minutes before administration of chemotherapeutic agent. Given concurrently with metoclopramide and lorazepam or diphenhydramine. Another protocol calls for 10 mg 30 minutes before administration of chemotherapeutic agent. Given concurrently with oral dexamethasone 8 mg beginning prior evening, 4 mg every 4 to 6 hours continuing through treatment day, and droperidol or haloperidol.

Betamethasone: *Respiratory distress syndrome of premature infants:* Up to 12 mg daily.

Dilution: May be given undiluted or added to IV glucose or saline solutions and given as an infusion.

Rate of administration: A single dose over 1 minute or less if necessary. As an IV infusion, give at prescribed rate.

Actions: An antiinflammatory glucocorticoid. A synthetic adrenocortical steroid with little sodium retention. Very soluble in water. Seven times as potent as prednisolone and 20 to 30 times as potent as hydrocortisone. May be used in conjunction with other forms of therapy, such as epinephrine for acute allergic reactions or antibiotics for acute infections. Crosses the placental barrier. Excreted in urine and secreted in breast milk.

Indications and uses: (1) Supplementary therapy for severe allergic reactions; (2) reduction of acute edematous states (cerebral edema); (3) acute life-threatening infections with massive antibiotic therapy; (4) acute exacerbations of disease for patients receiving steroid therapy; (5) viral hepatitis; (6) thyroid crisis; (7) diagnostic aid to distinguish adrenocortical hyperplasia or tumor; (8) adrenocortical insufficiency: total, relative, and operative; (9) chemotherapy; (10) antiemetic for cisplatin-induced vomiting; (11) prevention and treatment of acute mountain sickness; (12) shock unresponsive to conventional therapy (controversial); (13) betamethasone is used in the prevention of respiratory distress syndrome of premature infants.

Precautions: (1) Use diluted solutions within 24 hours. (2) Sensitive to heat. (3) Protect from freezing. (4) May cause hypertension, but often effects diuresis rather than salt and water retention. (5) May mask signs of infection. (6) Inhibited by hydantoins (e.g., phenytoin [Dilantin]), barbiturates (e.g., phenobarbital), ephedrine, oral contraceptives, rifampin, and troleandomycin. (7) Inhibits anticoagulants, isoniazid, and salicylates. (8) Potentiates theophyllines and cyclosporine. (9) May cause hypokalemia with digitalis products, amphotericin B, or potassium-depleting diuretics. (10) Dose adjustments may be required with cyclophosphamide. (11) Withdrawal from therapy should be gradual to avoid precipitation of symptoms of adrenal insufficiency. The patient is observed, especially under stress, for up to 2 years. (12) Maintain on ulcer regimen and antacids prophylactically. (13) If used in cerebral edema, results of brain scan may be altered because of poor uptake of radioactive material. (14) May increase insulin needs in diabetes. (15) Salt and potassium replacement may be necessary. (16) Do not vaccinate with attenuated-virus vaccines (e.g., smallpox) during therapy. (17) Use with caution in hypothyroidism and cirrhosis. (18) Altered protein-binding capacity will impact effectiveness of this drug. (19) Administer a single dose before 9 AM to reduce suppression of individual's own adrenocortical activity.

Contraindications: Hypersensitivity to any product component including sulfites, systemic fungal infections.

Relative contraindications: Active or latent peptic ulcer, acute or healed tuberculosis, acute or chronic infections (especially chickenpox and vaccinia), acute psychoses, diabetes mellitus, diverticulitis, fresh intestinal anastomoses, myasthenia gravis, ocular herpes simplex, osteoporosis, pregnancy, psychotic tendencies, renal insufficiency, septic shock, thromboembolic tendencies.

Incompatible with: Amikacin (Amikin), daunorubicin (Cerubidine), doxorubicin (Adriamycin), metaraminol (Aramine), prochlorperazine (Compazine), vancomycin (Vancocin). Limited information available. Give other drugs concurrently through a three-way stopcock.

Side effects: Do occur but are usually reversible: burning, Cushing's syndrome, electrolyte imbalance, embolism, euphoria, glycosuria, headache, hyperglycemia, hypersensitivity reactions including anaphylaxis, hypertension, menstrual irregularities, peptic ulcer, perforation and hemorrhage, perineal burning, protein catabolism, sweating, thromboembolism, tingling, weakness, and many others.

Antidote: Notify the physician of any side effect. Will probably treat the side effect. Resuscitate as necessary for anaphylaxis and notify physician. Keep epinephrine immediately available.

DEXPANTHENOL pH 5.0 to 7.0

(Ilopan)

Usual dose: 2 ml (500 mg) every 6 hours until effective peristalsis returns. Treatment may be required for 72 hours or more.

Dilution: Each 2 ml (500 mg) or fraction thereof must be diluted in 500 ml or more of 5% dextrose in water or lactated Ringer's solution and given as an infusion.

Rate of administration: Each single dose properly diluted should be slowly and consistently infused over 3 to 6 hours.

Actions: A coenzyme precursor that helps to promote acetylcholine synthesis. Smooth muscle contraction is increased, promoting improved intestinal motility.

Indications and uses: (1) Paralytic ileus; (2) intestinal atony; (3) postoperative or postpartum retention of flatus or delay in resumption of intestinal motility; (4) prophylactic use immediately after major abdominal surgery.

Precautions: (1) IM administration preferred; rarely given IV. (2) Allergic reactions of unknown cause have occurred when dexpanthenol is used concomitantly with antibiotics, narcotics, and barbiturates. (3) Must not be given within 12 hours of neostigmine (Prostigmin), other parasympathomimetics, or anticholinesterases, or within 1 hour of succinylcholine (Anectine). (4) Hypokalemia will impede effect of dexpanthenol. (5) Safety for use in children and during pregnancy and lactation not established.

Contraindications: Hemophilia, ileus caused by mechanical obstruction.

Incompatible with: Specific information not available. Note Precautions.

Side effects: Rarely occur, but respiratory depression and allergic reactions are possible.

Antidote: Discontinue the drug and notify the physician of any symptoms of respiratory depression or allergic reaction. Treat anaphylaxis with epinephrine, antihistamines (e.g., diphenhydramine [Benadryl]), vasopressors (e.g., dopamine [Intropin]), aminophylline, and corticosteroids as indicated. Maintain a patent airway and resuscitate as necessary.

DEXTRAN, HIGH MOLECULAR WEIGHT

pH 3.0 to 7.0

(Dextran 70, Dextran 75, Gentran 75, Macrodex)

Usual dose: Variable, depending on amount of fluid loss and resultant hemoconcentration. Initially 500 ml. Total dose should not exceed 20 ml/kg of body weight/24 hr for adults and children.

Dilution: Available as a 6% solution in 500 ml bottles properly diluted in normal saline or 5% dextrose in water and ready for use. Dextran 70 is available in a 250 ml bottle.

Rate of administration: Variable, depending on indication, present blood volume, and patient response. Initial 500 ml may be given at 20 to 40 ml/min. If additional high molecular weight dextran is required, reduce flow to lowest rate possible to maintain hemodynamic status desired.

Actions: Approximates colloidal properties of human albumin. Provides hemodynamically significant plasma volume expansion in excess of the amount infused for about 24 hours. Dilutes total serum proteins and hematocrit values. A glucose polymer, it is degraded to glucose and excreted in the urine.

Indications and uses: Treatment of shock or impending shock caused by burns, hemorrhage, surgery, or trauma.

Precautions: (1) For IV use only. (2) Used when whole blood or blood products are not available. Not a substitute for whole blood or plasma proteins. (3) Monitor pulse, blood pressure, central venous pressure, and urine output every 5 to 15 minutes for the first hour and hourly thereafter while indicated. (4) Maintain hydration of patient with additional IV fluids; dextran promotes tissue dehydration. Avoid overhydration with dilution of electrolyte balance. (5) Change IV tubing or flush well with normal saline before infusing blood. Dextran will promote coagulation of blood in the tubing (glucose content). (6) Use caution in heart disease, renal shutdown, congestive heart failure, pulmonary edema, in patients with edema and sodium retention, and in patients taking corticosteroids. (7) May reduce coagulability of the circulating blood. Observe patient for increased bleeding; maintain hematocrit above 30%. (8) Draw blood for laboratory tests and type and cross-match before giving dextran, or notify laboratory of its use. May alter blood sugar and total bilirubin evaluation. (9) May produce elevated urine specific gravity (also symptom of dehydration) and increase SGOT and SGPT. (10) Crystallization of dextran can occur at low temperatures. Submerge in warm water and dissolve all crystals before administration. (11) Hemoglobin, hematocrit, electrolyte, and serum protein evaluations are necessary during therapy. (12) Use only clear solution. Store at constant temperature not above 25° C (76° F). Discard partially used solution; no preservative added.

Contraindications: Severe bleeding disorders, marked hemostatic defects (e.g., thrombocytopenia, hypofibrinogenemia) even if drug induced (e.g., heparin, warfarin), known hypersensitivity to dextran, lactation and pregnancy unless a lifesaving measure, severe congestive cardiac failure, renal failure.

Incompatible with: Ascorbic acid, chlortetracycline (Aureomycin), phytonadione (Aquamephyton), promethazine (Phenergan). Do not add any drug to a bottle of dextran solution.

Side effects: Bleeding, dehydration, fever, hypotension, joint pain, nausea, overhydration, tightness of the chest, urticaria, vomiting, wheezing. Severe anaphylaxis and death have occurred. Excessive doses have caused wound hematoma, seroma, and bleeding; distant bleeding (hematuria, melena); and pulmonary edema.

Antidote: Notify the physician of any side effect. Discontinue the drug immediately at the first sign of an allergic reaction, provided other means of sustaining the circulation are available. Use epinephrine (Adrenalin) and/or antihistamines (diphenhydramine [Benadryl]) as indicated. Factor VIII infusion may reverse excessive bleeding. Resuscitate as necessary.

DEXTRAN, LOW MOLECULAR WEIGHT

pH 3.0 to 7.0

(Dextran 40, Gentran 40, L.M.D. 10%, Rheomacrodex)

Usual dose: 20 ml/kg of body weight total over first 24 hours. 10 ml/kg total over each succeeding 24 hours. Discontinue infusion after 5 days of therapy.

Prophylaxis: 10 mg/kg of body weight on day of surgery. 500 ml daily for 2 to 3 days, then 500 ml every 2 to 3 days up to 2 weeks.

As priming fluid: 10 to 20 ml/kg of body weight. Do not exceed this dose.

Dilution: Available as a 10 solution in 500 ml bottles properly diluted in normal saline or 5% dextrose in water and ready for use.

Rate of administration: Initial 500 ml may be given over 15 to 30 minutes. Remainder of any desired daily dose should be evenly distributed over 8 to 24 hours depending on use.

Actions: A low molecular weight, rapid, but short-acting plasma volume expander. A colloid hypertonic solution, it increases plasma volume by once or twice its own volume. Helps to restore normal circulatory dynamics, increasing arterial and pulse pressure, central venous pressure, and cardiac output. Improves microcirculatory flow and prevents sludging in venous channels. Mobilizes water from body tissues and increases urine output. Each 1 Gm of dextran will hold 25 ml of water in the vascular space.

Indications and uses: (1) Adjunctive therapy in the treatment of shock caused by hemorrhage, burns, trauma, or surgery; (2) prophylaxis during surgical procedures with a high incidence of venous thrombosis and pulmonary embolism; (3) pump priming during extracorporeal circulation.

Precautions: (1) For IV use only. (2) Monitor pulse, blood pressure, central venous pressure, and urine output every 5 to 15 minutes for the first hour and hourly thereafter while indicated. Slow rate or discontinue dextran for rapid increase of central venous pressure (normal 7 to 14 mm H_2O pressure). If anuric or oliguric after 500 ml of dextran, discontinue the dextran. Mannitol may help increase urine flow. (3) Maintain hydration of patient with additional IV fluids; dextran promotes tissue dehydration. Avoid overhydration with dilution of electrolyte balance. (4) Change IV tubing or flush well with normal saline before superimposing blood. Dextran will promote coagulation of blood in the tubing (glucose content). (5) Use caution in heart disease, renal shutdown, congestive heart failure, pulmonary edema, patients with edema and sodium retention, and patients taking corticosteroids. (6) May reduce coagulability of the circulating blood slightly. Combined with increased volume, additional blood loss is possible. Maintain hematocrit above 30%. (7) Draw blood for laboratory tests and type and cross-match before giving dextran, or notify laboratory of its use. May alter blood sugar and total bilirubin evaluation. (8) May produce elevated urine specific gravity (also a symptom of dehydration) and increase SGOT and SGPT. (9) Crystallization can occur at low temperatures. Submerge in warm water and dissolve all crystals before administration. (10) Use only clear solution. Store at constant temperature not above 25° C (76° F). Discard partially used solution; no preservative added.

Contraindications: Severe bleeding disorders, marked hemostatic defects (e.g., thrombocytopenia, hypofibrinogenemia) even if drug induced (e.g., heparin, warfarin), known hypersensitivity to dextran, lactation and pregnancy unless a lifesaving measure, severe congestive cardiac failure, renal failure.

Incompatible with: Ascorbic acid, chlortetracycline (Aureomycin), phytonadione (Aquamephyton), promethazine (Phenergan). Do not add any drug to a bottle of dextran solution.

Side effects: Bleeding, dehydration, fever, hypotension, joint pain, nausea, overhydration, tightness of chest, urticaria, vomiting, wheezing. Severe anaphylaxis and death can occur. Excessive doses have caused wound hematoma, wound seroma, wound bleeding, distant bleeding (hematuria, melena), and pulmonary edema.

Antidote: Notify the physician of any side effect. Discontinue the drug immediately at the first sign of an allergic reaction, provided other means of sustaining the circulation are available. Use epinephrine (Adrenalin) and/or antihistamines (diphenhydramine [Benadryl]) as indicated. Factor VIII infusion may reverse excessive bleeding. Resuscitate as necessary.

DEXTRAN 1

(Promit)

Usual dose: 20 ml (150 mg/ml) 1 to 2 minutes before every IV clinical dextran infusion. If 15 minutes or more elapses before the clinical dextran infusion is started, a full dose of dextran 1 must be repeated before the infusion.

Pediatric dose: 0.3 ml/kg of body weight. To be given in same manner as adult dose.

Dilution: May be given undiluted. May be given through Y-tube or three-way stopcock of an infusion set if there is minimum dilution with the primary IV. May not be diluted with or administered through an IV tubing containing clinical dextran infusion.

Rate of administration: A single dose over 1 minute.

Actions: A monovalent hapten, it binds to one of two available sites on dextran-reacting antibodies. An adequate dose (molar excess) given just before the IV administration of clinical dextran solution prevents the formation of immune complexes with the polyvalent clinical dextrans and helps to prevent anaphylaxis. Incidence of anaphylaxis is 15 to 20 times less. Rapidly excreted in urine.

Indications and uses: Prophylaxis of serious anaphylactic reactions associated with IV infusion of clinical dextran solutions.

Precautions: (1) For IV use only. (2) Will not prevent mild allergic reactions induced by clinical dextran solutions. (3) If any reaction occurs to dextran 1, *do not administer clinical dextran infusion.* (4) May cause severe hypotension and bradycardia.

Contraindications: Do not give if clinical dextran is contraindicated (severe bleeding disorders, marked hemostatic defects [e.g., thrombocytopenia, hypofibrinogenemia], even if drug induced [e.g., heparin, warfarin], lactation and pregnancy unless a lifesaving measure, severe congestive cardiac failure, renal failure).

Incompatible with: Dextran, low molecular weight; dextran, high molecular weight.

Side effects: Bradycardia, cutaneous reactions, hypotension (moderate to severe), nausea, pallor, shivering.

Antidote: Discontinue the drug immediately and notify the physician at the first sign of an allergic reaction or side effect. Do not administer clinical dextran solution. Use epinephrine (Adrenalin) and/or antihistamines (diphenhydramine [Benadryl]) as indicated. Resuscitate as necessary.

DEXTROSE

pH 3.5 to 6.5

(Glucose)

Usual dose: Depends on use and age, weight, and clinical condition of the patient.

50 to 1,000 ml 2½% (25 Gm/L) and 5% (50 Gm/L) dextrose. May be repeated as indicated. Consider total amount of fluid.

5 ml of 10% dextrose. May repeat as necessary.

500 to 1,000 ml of 10% dextrose (100 Gm/L) once or twice every 24 hours as indicated.

500 ml of 20% dextrose (200 Gm/L) once or twice every 24 hours as indicated.

50 ml of 50% dextrose (25 Gm). 10 to 25 Gm for insulin-induced hypoglycemia. May repeat if indicated.

500 to 1,500 ml/24 hr of 30% (300 Gm/L), 38.5% (385 Gm/L), 40% (400 Gm/L), 50% (500 Gm/L), 60% (600 Gm/L), 70% (700 Gm/L) as dextrose for nutrition.

Neonatal dose: *Acute symptomatic hypoglycemia:* 250 to 500 mg/kg of body weight of 25% dextrose.

Dilution: May be given undiluted in prepared solutions.

Rate of administration: 2½ and 5% solution, rate dependent on amount.

10% solution, 5 ml over 10 to 15 seconds.

10% solution, 1,000 ml over at least 3 hours.

20% solution, 500 ml over 30 to 60 minutes.

50% solution, 10 ml over 1 minute.

500 ml of 30% to 70% solution over 4 to 12 hours, depending on body weight. A rate of 0.5 Gm/kg/hr will not cause glycosuria. At 0.8 Gm/kg/hr 95% is retained and will cause glycosuria.

Actions: A monosaccharide, it provides glucose calories for metabolic needs. Its oxidation provides water to sustain volume. It lowers excess ketone production, protects body proteins, and prevents loss of electrolytes. Hypertonic solutions (20% to 50%) act as a diuretic and reduce CNS edema. Readily excreted by the kidneys, producing diuresis.

Indications and uses: (1) To provide calories by peripheral infusion when calories and fluid are required (2½%,

5%, 10%); (2) to provide calories by central IV infusion in conditions requiring a minimum volume of fluid (20%); (3) to provide calories by central IV infusion in combination with other amino acid solutions as total parenteral nutrition (10% to 70%); (4) treatment of insulin hypoglycemia (50%); (5) treatment of acute symptomatic episodes of hypoglycemia in the neonate and infant (25%); (6) cerebral and meningeal edema (e.g., eclampsia, acute glomerulonephritis) (50% solution); (7) shock (sustain blood volume) (10% to 70% solution); (8) diuresis (20% to 50% solution); (9) hyperkalemia (20% solution); (10) as a diluent for IV administration of medications (2½% to 10% solutions usually); (11) a sclerosing solution (50% solution, 3 to 20 ml).

Precautions: (1) Use caution in severe kidney damage. (2) Do not use as a diluent for blood or administer simultaneously through the same infusion set; dextrose in any dilution causes clumping of red blood cells unless sodium chloride is added. (3) Dextrose solutions are excellent media for bacterial growth. Do not use unless the solution is entirely clear and the vial is sterile. Do not store after adding additives. (4) For concentrations over 12.5% (hypertonic) very large (central) veins and slow administration are absolutely necessary. (5) Confirm patency of vein; avoid extravasation. (6) 50% dextrose can be used as a sclerosing agent and will cause thrombosis. (7) Insulin requirements may be increased. Monitor blood glucose. (8) Potassium and vitamins are readily depleted. Watch for any signs of beginning deficiency and replace as needed. Add other electrolytes and minerals as required by fluid and electrolyte status. (9) Can cause fluid or solute overload. May result in dilution of serum electrolyte concentrations, overhydration, congested states, or pulmonary edema. (10) Use caution in infants of diabetic mothers, in patients with carbohydrate intolerance or subclinical or overt diabetes, and in patients receiving corticosteroids. (11) Rapid administration of hypertonic solutions will cause hyperglycemia (over 0.5 Gm/kg/hr) and may cause hyperosmolar syndrome. (12) Concentrated dextrose solutions must not be withdrawn abruptly. Will cause reactive hypoglycemia. Reduce rate of administration gradually and then follow with administration of 5% or 10% dextrose solution.

Contraindications: Delirium tremens with dehydration, diabetic coma while blood sugar is excessive, intracranial or intraspinal hemorrhage, glucose-galactose malabsorption syndrome.

Incompatible with: Cyanocobalamin (vitamin B_{12}), kanamycin (Kantrex), sodium bicarbonate, warfarin (Coumadin), whole blood.

Side effects: Rare in small doses administered slowly: acidosis, alkalosis, fluid overload (congested states, pulmonary edema, overhydration, dilution of serum electrolyte concentrations), hyperglycemia (during infusion), hyperosmolar syndrome (mental confusion, loss of consciousness), hypokalemia, hypovitaminosis, reactive hypoglycemia (after infusion), thrombosis.

Antidote: Discontinue the drug and notify the physician of the side effect. Symptomatic treatment is probable.

DEZOCINE pH 4.0

(Dalgan)

Usual dose: 5 mg initially. Range is 2.5 to 10 mg. Repeat every 2 to 4 hours as necessary. Larger doses have been given IM.

Reduce dosages for the elderly and debilitated; in impaired liver or renal function; in patients with limited pulmonary reserve; and in the presence of other CNS depressants.

Dilution: May be given undiluted.

Rate of administration: Each 5 mg or fraction thereof evenly distributed over 2 to 3 minutes.

Actions: A synthetic narcotic agonist-antagonist with a potent analgesic action. Analgesia similar to morphine or butorphanol is produced. Does produce respiratory depression, but this does not increase markedly with larger doses. Pain relief is effected within 15 minutes. Length of pain relief is related to the initial dose (i.e., 2 hours with a 5 mg dose and 3 to 4 hours with a 10 mg dose). Relief in some patients may last up to 6 hours. Metabolized in the liver. Primarily excreted in urine.

Indications and uses: (1) Relief of moderate to severe postoperative pain (e.g., abdominal, gynecologic, orthopedic).

Precautions: (1) Naloxone (Narcan), oxygen, and controlled ventilation equipment must be available. (2) Observe patient frequently and monitor vital signs. (3) Use caution in respiratory depression or difficulty from any source, head injury, increased intracranial pressure, biliary surgery, history of drug abuse, the elderly or debilitated, and in impaired liver or kidney function. Reduced doses may be indicated. (4) Use caution with CNS depressants such as narcotic analgesics (e.g., morphine), general anesthetics, alcohol, anticholinergics (e.g., atropine), antihistamines (e.g., diphenhydramine [Benadryl]) barbiturates (e.g., phenobarbital), cimetidine (Tagamet), hypnotics, sedatives, psychotropic agents, MAO inhibitors (e.g., pargyline [Eutonyl]), and neuromuscular blocking agents (e.g., tubocurarine). Reduced doses of both drugs may be indicated. (5) Do not drive or operate hazardous machinery until all effects have subsided. (6) Mild narcotic antagonist. May precipitate withdrawal symptoms in patients accustomed to narcotics. (7) Low addictive element but can produce dependency. (8) Use during pregnancy only if benefit justifies risk to the fetus and in labor and delivery only if the physician considers it essential. Safety for these uses, nursing mothers, and in children under 18 years of age not yet established. (9) Store at room temperature, protect from light, inspect visually for particulate matter, discard if contains a precipitate.

Contraindications: Hypersensitivity to dezocine or its components; contains sodium metabisulfite (can cause anaphylaxis from a sulfite sensitivity reaction). Not recommended for nursing mothers or children under 18 years of age.

Incompatible with: Specific information not available.

Side effects: Dizziness, injection site reactions, nausea and vomiting are most common. Abdominal pain, allergic reactions including anaphylaxis or severe asthmatic episodes (especially in the sulfite sensitive patient), atelectasis, blurred vision, chest pain, chills, confusion, constipation, crying, deliriums, delusions, depression, diarrhea, diplopia, edema, erythema, flushing, headache, hiccups, hypertension, hypotension, irregular pulse, low hemoglobin, muscle pain, pallor, pruritis, rash, respiratory depression, sleep disturbances, slurred speech, sweating, tinnitus, thrombophlebitis, and urinary frequency, hesitancy, and retention have been reported.

Antidote: With increasing severity of any side effect or onset of symptoms of overdose (e.g., respiratory depression) or allergic reaction, discontinue the drug and notify the physician. Treat side effects symptomatically. Naloxone hydrochloride (Narcan) will reverse respiratory depression. A patent airway, artificial ventilation, oxygen therapy, and other symptomatic treatment must be instituted promptly. Treat anaphylaxis with epinephrine (Adrenalin), diphenhydramine (Benadryl), and corticosteroids as indicated.

DIAZEPAM pH 6.2 to 6.9

(Valium, Zetran)

Usual dose: 2 to 10 mg (0.4 to 2 ml) every 3 to 4 hours. May be repeated in 1 hour. Maximum dose is 30 mg in 8 hours.

Status epilepticus: 5 to 10 mg. May be repeated at intervals of 5 to 10 minutes up to a total dose of 30 mg. Some specialists start with 20 mg and titrate the total dose over 10 minutes or until seizures stop. Maximum dose in 24 hours is 100 mg.

Cardioversion: 5 to 15 mg (1 to 3 ml) before procedure begins.

Endoscopy: Up to 20 mg before procedure begins if a narcotic is not used. Titrate to desired sedation.

Pediatric dose: *Tetanus in infants over 30 days:* 1 to 2 mg every 3 to 4 hours.

Tetanus in children 5 years or older: 5 to 10 mg every 3 to 4 hours.

Status epilepticus in infants over 30 days: 0.2 to 0.5 mg every 2 to 5 minutes to maximum 5 mg dose.

Status epilepticus in children 5 years or older: 0.5 to 1 mg every 2 to 5 minutes to maximum 10 mg dose.

Dilution: Do not dilute or mix with any other drug. Do not add to any IV solution.

Rate of administration: 5 mg (1 ml) or fraction thereof over 1 minute. Give total dose over a minimum of 3 minutes in infants and children.

Actions: Depresses the central, autonomic, and peripheral nervous systems in an undetermined manner. Exerts antianxiety, sedative/hypnotic, amnesic, anticonvulsant, skeletal muscle relaxant, and antitremor effects. Diminishes patient recall. Stays in the body in appreciable amounts for several days and is excreted very slowly in the urine. Crosses the placental barrier. Secreted in breast milk.

Indications and uses: (1) Moderate to severe psychoneurotic reactions; (2) acute alcohol withdrawal; (3) acute stress reactions; (4) muscle spasm; (5) status epilepticus and severe recurrent convulsive seizures, including tetany; (6) preoperative medication, including endoscopic procedures; (7) cardioversion.

Precautions: (1) Should be given directly into the vein. Not soluble in any solution. Inject into IV tubing close to vein site only when direct IV injection is not feasible. Some precipitation or absorption into plastic tubing may take place. Consider heparin lock for frequent injection. Change site every 2 to 3 days. If dilution imperative add diluent solution to diazepam not diazepam to diluent. Consult pharmacist. (2) To reduce incidence of thrombophlebitis, avoid smaller veins. Extravasation or arterial administration hazardous. (3) Respiratory assistance must be available. (4) Bed rest required for a minimum of 3 hours after IV injection. (5) Drug of choice for initial treatment of status epilepticus. Some specialists administer phenytoin simultaneously to facilitate long-term control (onset of action is not as immediate as diazepam). Oral phenytoin or phenobarbital may be used for maintenance. (6) May not be effective if seizures are due to acute brain lesions. (7) Potentiates narcotics, phenothiazines (e.g., prochlorperazine [Compazine]), antihistamines, barbiturates, MAO inhibitors (e.g., pargyline [Eutonyl]), and tricyclic antidepressants (e.g., imipramine [Tofranil-PM]) for up to 48 hours. Potentiated by cimetidine (Tagamet), alcohol, and other CNS depressants. (8) Inhibits antiparkinson effects of levodopa. (9) Inhibited by oral contraceptives and valproic acid. (10) Reduce dosages for the elderly and debilitated and in those with impaired liver or renal function or limited pulmonary reserve. (11) Withdrawal symptoms will occur for several weeks after extended or large doses. (12) Intended for short-term use only.

Contraindications: Acute narrow-angle glaucoma; infants and children under 12 years, except in tetany and status epilepticus; manifestation of allergic reaction; known psychoses; pregnancy, childbirth, and lactation; shock; coma; acute alcoholic intoxication with depression of vital signs. Safety for use in neonates not established.

Incompatible with: Any other drug or solution in syringe or solution. Precipitation will occur.

Side effects: Apnea, ataxia, blurred vision, bradycardia, cardiac arrest, cardiovascular collapse, coma, confusion, coughing, depressed respiration, depression, diminished reflexes, drowsiness, dyspnea, headache, hiccups, hyperexcited states, hyperventilation, laryngospasm, neutropenia, nystagmus, somnolence, syncope, venous thrombosis and phlebitis at injection site, vertigo.

Antidote: Notify the physician of all side effects. Reduction of dosage may be required. Discontinue the drug for major side effects or paradoxical reactions including hyperexcitability, hallucinations, and acute rage. Treat allergic reaction, or resuscitate as necessary and notify the physician. In overdose maintain an adequate airway and ventilation, and promote excretion through fluid and electrolyte administration and osmotic diuretics (e.g., mannitol). Effectiveness of hemodialysis is not confirmed but should be considered. Caffeine and sodium benzoate effectively combat CNS depression of diazepam overdose. Use dopamine (Intropin), levarterenol (Levophed), or metaraminol (Aramine) for hypotension. Physostigmine 0.5 to 4 mg at 1 mg/min may reverse symptoms of anticholinergic overdose (e.g., confusion), but may also cause seizures.

DIAZOXIDE pH 11.6

(Hyperstat IV)

Usual dose: 150 mg (10 ml) initially. 1 to 3 mg/kg of body weight may be used to calculate exact dose (preferred). May be repeated in 5 to 15 minutes if an adequate response is not obtained. This second injection may effect a greater response. Repeat as indicated at intervals of 4 to 24 hours to maintain desired blood pressure. For short-term use until a regimen of oral antihypertensive medication is effective.

Pediatric dose: 1 to 3 mg/kg of body weight.

Dilution: Should be given undiluted.

Rate of administration: Rapidly as a single dose over 10 to 30 seconds. Not as effective when administered at a slower rate.

Actions: A potent, rapid-acting antihypertensive agent. Produces vasodilation by relaxing the smooth muscle of peripheral arterioles. Increases cardiac output while maintaining coronary and cerebral blood flow. Effects on renal blood flow not significant. Effective in patients not responsive to other antihypertensive agents. Acts within 1 to 5 minutes. Usually no further decrease in blood pressure after 30 minutes, but a gradual increase over 2 to 12 hours. Crosses placental barrier; probably secreted in breast milk.

Indications and uses: Malignant and nonmalignant hypertensive emergencies.

Precautions: (1) Give only into a peripheral vein; avoid extravasation. (2) Maintain patient in recumbent position during injection and for at least 30 minutes after injection. (3) Check blood pressure every 5 minutes until stabilized and hourly thereafter. (4) Take blood pressure with patient in standing position before ambulation. (5) Use caution in diabetes; monitor blood glucose levels. May cause hyperglycemia. (6) Diuresis may be required to reverse sodium and water retention before diazoxide can be effective. (7) Use caution in impaired cerebral or cardiac circulation. (8) Potentiates coumarin and its derivatives; a reduced dose of anticoagulant may be required. (9) Potentiated by thiazides and other diuretics; side effects increased. (10) Inhibits phenytoin (Dilantin). (11) Profound hypotension will result if used with peripheral vasodilators (e.g., hydralazine [Apresoline], nitroprusside sodium [Nipride]). (12) Do not use for more than 10 days. (13) Protect from light and freezing. Best to store in refrigerator 2° to 30° C (36° to 86° F). (14) Safety for use in children not established. May produce fetal or neonatal hyperbilirubinemia, thrombocytopenia, altered carbohydrate metabolism, and other adverse reactions if given before delivery. Discontinue breast feeding.

Contraindications: Compensatory hypertension (e.g., arteriovenous shunt or coarctation of the aorta), known sensitivity to thiazides, labor and delivery, not effective in pheochromocytoma.

Incompatible with: Do not mix in syringe or solution with any other drug.

Side effects: Abdominal discomfort, cerebral ischemia, confusion, congestive heart failure, convulsions, edema, flushing, headache, hyperglycemia, hypotension (severe), ileus, lightheadedness, myocardial ischemia, nausea, orthostatic hypotension, palpitations, paralysis, sensations of warmth, sensitivity reactions, sodium and water retention, supraventricular tachycardia, sweating, vomiting, weakness.

Antidote: Notify the physician of all side effects. Some will subside spontaneously; others will require symptomatic treatment. Treat sensitivity reaction as indicated and resuscitate as necessary. Treat undesirable hypotension with dopamine (Intropin); if no response, diazoxide is probably not the cause of the hypotension. Excessive hyperglycemia may be treated with insulin. Hemodialysis or peritoneal dialysis may be required in overdose.

DIETHYLSTILBESTROL DIPHOSPHATE

pH 9.0 to 10.5

(♣ Honvol, Stilphostrol)

Usual dose: 0.5 Gm/24 hr initially. Increase to 1 Gm/24 hr beginning with second day, and give 1 Gm/24 hr for 5 days or as indicated by patient response. 0.25 to 0.5 Gm once or twice weekly as maintenance dose.

Dilution: A single daily dose must be diluted in 300 ml of saline or dextrose solutions for infusion.

Rate of administration: 20 gtt/min for the first 15 minutes; then increase rate to complete infusion within 1 hour of starting time.

Actions: An estrogen hormone. In the diphosphate form there are fewer side effects, and large doses can be given. May be directly cytotoxic to malignant cells or may simply slow the growth. Does decrease the percentage of cells actively proliferating in a tumor mass. Metabolized in the liver. Excreted in the urine.

Indications and uses: Palliative treatment of prostatic carcinoma. Particularly useful in advanced stages.

Precautions: (1) IV route used when oral route ineffective or not practical. (2) Will cause salt and water retention. Monitor weight and encourage a low salt diet. (3) Used with other antineoplastic drugs to achieve tumor remission. (4) Feminization in the male and uterine bleeding in postmenopausal women are expected. (5) Use caution in cardiac, liver, or renal disease and diabetes.

Contraindications: Markedly impaired liver function, a past history of or active thrombophlebitis, thromboembolic disorders or cerebral apoplexy, estrogen-dependent neoplasia.

Incompatible with: Sufficient information not available. Calcium gluconate.

Side effects: Burning and local pain in the perineal region and metastatic sites are expected and last only a few moments. Other side effects are abdominal cramps, anemia, decreased libido, dizziness, elevated prothrombin time, headache, hypercalcemia, myocardial infarction, nausea, painful swelling of breasts, pulmonary embolism, thrombophlebitis, and vomiting. All side effects associated with estrogens are possible.

Antidote: Notify the physician of all side effects. Most will be treated symptomatically. Hypercalcemia is reversible when detected early (limit oral calcium, push fluids, record output, ambulate to keep calcium in the bones). There is no specific antidote. Supportive therapy as indicated will help sustain the patient in toxicity.

DIGOXIN IMMUNE FAB (OVINE) pH 6.0 to 8.0

(Digibind)

Usual dose: Testing for sensitivity to sheep serum may be indicated before use (see Precautions). Dose in number of vials based on ingested dose is calculated by dividing the body load of digoxin or deslanoside in milligrams by 0.6 (mg/vial). Each vial contains 40 mg and will bind 0.6 mg digoxin or deslanoside. Dose may also be based on serum digoxin levels (see literature). If ingested dose or serum digoxin is not available, give 20 vials (800 mg). This dose should provide adequate treatment of most life-threatening ingestions in adults and children (will bind approximately 60 [0.25 mg] tablets of Lanoxin). Usually given as an infusion through a 0.22 micron filter. May be given as an IV bolus if cardiac arrest is imminent. A single dose may be repeated in several hours if toxicity has not reversed or appears to recur.

Dilution: Each vial (40 mg) must be diluted with 4 ml of sterile water for injection (10 mg/ml). Mix gently. May be given in this initial dilution or may be further diluted with any desired amount of normal saline (36 ml normal saline/vial yields 1 mg/ml). Consider volume overload in children when further diluting in normal saline. Administer to infants after initial dilution using a tuberculin syringe to deliver an accurate dose with less volume or for extremely small doses dilute to 1 mg/ml before administration.

Rate of administration: Must be given through a 0.22 micron membrane filter. A single dose as an IV infusion equally distributed over 30 minutes. May be given as an IV bolus injection if cardiac arrest is imminent. Be prepared to treat anaphylaxis.

Actions: Antigen binding fragments (Fab) prepared from specific antidigoxin antibodies produced in sheep are isolated and purified. Fab fragments bind molecules of digoxin and make them unavailable for binding at their site of action. Freely distributed in extracellular space. Onset of action is prompt with improvement in symptoms of toxicity within 30 minutes. Excreted in urine.

Indications and uses: (1) Treatment of patients with life-threatening digoxin intoxication or overdose; (2) also indicated when potassium concentrations are above 5 mEq/L with digitalis intoxication.

Precautions: (1) Cardiac arrest can result from ingestion of more than 10 mg digoxin by healthy adults, 4 mg digoxin by healthy children, or serum digoxin levels above 10 ng/ml. (2) Although allergy testing is not required before treating life-threatening digitalis toxicity, patients allergic to ovine proteins or those who have previously received antibodies or Fab fragments produced from sheep are at risk. Determine patient response to any previous injections of serum of any type and history of any allergic-type reactions. (3) Test for sensitivity if indicated. Make a 1:100 solution by diluting 0.1 ml of initially diluted solution (10 mg/ml) with 10 ml sterile normal saline (100 mcg/ml).

Scratch test: Make a ¼ inch skin scratch through a drop of 1:100 dilution in normal saline. Inspect the site in 20 minutes. An urticarial wheal surrounded by a zone of erythema is a positive reaction.

Skin test: Inject 0.1 ml (10 mcg) of 1:100 dilution intradermally. Inspect the site in 20 minutes. An urticarial wheal surrounded by a zone of erythema is a positive reaction. Concomitant use of antihistamines may interfere with sensitivity tests. If skin testing causes a systemic reaction, place a tourniquet above the testing site and treat anaphylaxis.

(4) Consider that multiple drugs may have been used and are producing toxicity in suicide attempts. (5) Use reconstituted solution promptly or store in refrigerator

for up to 4 hours. (6) Larger doses act more quickly but increase the possibility of febrile or allergic reaction. (7) Obtain serum concentrations if possible. High margin of error will occur if drawn soon after ingestion. Six to eight hours is required after the last digitalis dose to obtain an accurate serum concentration. (8) Monitor temperature, blood pressure, ECG, and potassium concentration frequently during and after drug administration. (9) Will cause a precipitous rise in total serum digoxin, but most will be bound to the Fab fragment. Will interfere with digitalis immunoassay measurements until Fab fragment is completely eliminated. (10) Potassium may be shifted from inside to outside the cell causing increased renal excretion. May appear to have hyperkalemia while there is a total body deficit of potassium. When the digitalis effect is reversed hypokalemia may develop rapidly. (11) Do not redigitalize until all Fab fragments have been eliminated from the body. May take several days. May take longer in severe renal impairment, and reintoxication may occur by release of newly unbound digoxin into the blood. (12) Use caution in impaired cardiac function. Inability to use cardiac glycosides may endanger patient. Support with dopamine (Intropin) or vasodilators. (13) Catecholamines may aggravate digitalis dysrhythmias. (14) Use only when clearly indicated and benefits outweigh hazards in pregnancy, lactation, and infants.

Contraindications: None known when used for specific indications. If hypersensitivity exists and treatment is necessary, preload with corticosteroids and diphenhydramine, and prepare to treat anaphylaxis.

Incompatible with: Specific information not available. Do not mix with any other drug in syringe or solution because of specific use.

Side effects: Acute anaphylaxis with urticaria, respiratory distress, and vascular collapse is possible. Exacerbation of congestive heart failure and low cardiac output states and increased ventricular response in atrial fibrillation may occur because of withdrawal of digitalis effects. Hypokalemia may be life threatening.

Antidote: Notify the physician of all side effects. Discontinue the drug and treat anaphylaxis immediately. Corticosteroids, epinephrine (Adrenalin) and diphenhydramine (Benadryl), oxygen, vasopressors (dopamine), and ventilation equipment must always be available. Resuscitate as necessary. Treat hypokalemia cautiously when necessary. Support exacerbated cardiac conditions as necessary.

DIGOXIN INJECTION

pH 6.8 to 7.2

(Lanoxin)

Usual dose: 0.5 to 1 mg (2 to 4 ml) for digitalization. 0.25 to 0.5 mg (1 to 2 ml) as the initial dose, followed by 0.25 to 0.5 mg (1 to 2 ml) at 4- to 6-hour intervals until digitalized (approximately 4 to 6 hours). Maintenance dose is usually 0.125 to 0.5 mg daily.

Pediatric dose: *Use 0.1 mg/ml pediatric injection.*

Premature infants: 15 to 25 mcg/kg of body weight.

Maintenance dose: 25% to 35% of total loading dose divided and given every 12 hours. Individualized doses.

Full-term infants: 20 to 30 mcg/kg.

Ages 1 to 24 months: 30 to 50 mcg/kg.

2 to 5 years: 25 to 35 mcg/kg.

5 to 10 years: 15 to 30 mcg/kg.

Over 10 years: 8 to 12 mcg/kg.

Give one half of total daily dose initially, then 2 doses of one fourth of total dose at 8-hour intervals.

Maintenance dose: 20% to 30% of total loading dose divided and given every 12 hours. Individual adjustments required.

Dilution: May be given undiluted or each 1 ml may be diluted in 4 ml sterile water, normal saline, or 5% dextrose for injection. Less diluent will cause precipitation. Use diluted solution immediately. Give through Y-tube or three-way stopcock of IV infusion set.

Rate of administration: Each single dose over a minimum of 5 minutes.

Actions: A crystalline cardiac glycoside obtained from *Digitalis lanata,* this is a fast-acting hydrolytic product of lanatoside C. Onset of action is within 5 to 30 minutes and lasts 2 to 3 days. It has positive inotropic action, increasing the strength of myocardial contraction. It also alters the electric behavior of heart muscle through actions on myocardial automaticity, conduction velocity, and refraction. Results are a slower, stronger beat with increased cardiac output. Venous pressure falls, coronary circulation is increased, and heart size may become more normal. Widely distributed throughout the body and rapidly excreted in the urine. Excretion reduces toxicity period in overdigitalization.

Indications and uses: (1) Congestive heart failure; (2) atrial fibrillation; (3) atrial flutter; (4) paroxysmal tachycardia; (5) cardiogenic shock; (6) ventricular dysrhythmias with congestive heart failure; (7) preoperative, intraoperative, and postoperative need for digitalis because of stress on the heart.

Precautions: (1) IV administration is preferred. (2) Do not give digitalized patients calcium. Death has occurred. (3) Potassium depletion makes the heart sensitive to digitalis intoxication. Check electrolytes during therapy. (4) Use with caution in patients with hypercalcemia or liver or kidney disease. (5) Reduce dose in partially digitalized patients and patients with impaired kidney function. (6) Potentiated by aminoglycosides (e.g., gentamicin), phenytoin (Dilantin), tetracyclines, thyroid preparations, *Veratrum* alkaloids (Unitensen), reserpine, quinidine, propranolol (Inderal), verapamil, diuretics, pressor agents (epinephrine), and others. (7) Inhibited by antineoplastics (e.g., bleomycin), potassium salts, spironolactone (Aldactone), triamterene (Dyrenium), and others. (8) ECG monitoring suggested.

Contraindications: Digitalis intoxication. Not absolute. Used in ventricular paroxysmal tachycardia or ventricular fibrillation only if heart failure is present and the etiology is not digitalis intoxication.

Incompatible with: Acids, alkalies, calcium chloride, calcium disodium edetate, calcium gluceptate, calcium gluconate.

Side effects: Seldom last more than 3 days after drug is discontinued. Any form of digitalis may cause partial or AV block and almost any dysrhythmia, including paroxysmal tachycardia, atrial tachycardia, fibrillation, or standstill. *First ECG signs of toxicity* are ST segment sagging, PR prolongation, and possible bigeminal rhythm. *Clinical signs of toxicity* are mostly abdominal discomfort or pain, anorexia, blurred vision, confusion, diarrhea, disturbed color (yellow) vision, headache, nausea, vomiting, and weakness.

Antidote: Discontinue the drug at the first sign of toxicity and notify the physician. Dosage may be decreased or discontinued. For severe toxicity digoxin immune Fab is a specific antidote. Depending on symptoms, use one or more of the following if necessary: atropine, phenytoin (Dilantin), potassium salts (potassium chloride), procainamide (Pronestyl), or disodium edetate (EDTA disodium).

DIHYDROERGOTAMINE MESYLATE (D.H.E. 45)

pH 3.2 to 4.0

Usual dose: 1 mg (1 ml). May be repeated in 1 hour. No more than 2 doses (2 mg total) may be given IV in 24 hours. Do not exceed 6 mg in 1 week.

Dilution: May be given undiluted.

Rate of administration: 1 mg or fraction thereof over 1 minute.

Actions: A vasoconstrictor, it probably acts on distended cerebral arteries. It also paralyzes the effector cells connected with adrenergic nerves. Probably detoxified in the liver and excreted in the urine. Secreted in breast milk.

Indications and uses: Vascular headaches (migraine, histamine cephalalgia).

Experimental use: Enhance heparin effects in preventing postoperative deep vein thrombosis after total hip replacement.

Precautions: (1) IM use is preferred but may be given IV to obtain a more rapid effect. (2) Protect the ampoules from light and heat. (3) Discontinue breast feeding. (4) Safety for use in children not established. (5) Potentiated by oral nitroglycerin. (6) May cause hypertensive crisis in combination with other vasoconstrictors (e.g., epinephrine).

Contraindications: Coronary artery disease, hepatic or renal disease, hypersensitivity, hypertension, lactation, malnutrition, peripheral vascular disease, pregnancy or women who may become pregnant, pruritus, sepsis.

Incompatible with: Any other drug in syringe or solution.

Side effects: Rare in therapeutic doses, but may include angina pectoris, blindness, gangrene, muscle pains, muscle weakness, nausea, numbness and tingling of the fingers and toes, thirst, uterine bleeding, and vomiting.

Antidote: Discontinue the drug and notify the physician of any side effects. Another drug will probably be chosen if further treatment is indicated. Vasodilators (nitroprusside) and CNS stimulants (e.g., caffeine and sodium benzoate) are indicated as an antidote. Heparin and low molecular weight dextran may be used to reduce thrombosis due to excessive vasoconstriction. Hemodialysis may be indicated. Resuscitate as necessary.

DIMENHYDRINATE

pH 6.4 to 7.2

(Dinate, Dommanate, Dramanate, Dramamine, Dramocen, Dramoject, Dymenate, ✤ Gravol, Hydrate, Marmine, ✤ Nauseatol, Reidamine)

Usual dose: 50 to 100 mg every 4 hours.

Pediatric dose: 5 mg/kg of body weight divided into 4 equal doses over 24 hours. Do not exceed 300 mg. Note Precautions.

Dilution: Each 50 mg (1 ml) must be diluted in 10 ml of sodium chloride injection.

Rate of administration: Each 50 mg or fraction thereof, properly diluted, is injected over 2 minutes.

Actions: An antihistamine and CNS depressant. Specific mode of action is not exactly known, but depression of hyperstimulated labyrinthine functions and associated neural pathways does occur. Threshold of susceptibility, especially to motion sickness, is raised. Excreted in changed form in the urine. Secreted in breast milk.

Indications and uses: Treatment of motion sickness, nausea and vomiting, vertigo, and diseases affecting the vestibular system (labyrinthitis and Ménière's disease).

Precautions: (1) Will induce drowsiness; this is often a desirable reaction. (2) Will cause irreversible ototoxicity because of masking of infection or toxicity symptoms when given in conjunction with some antibiotics such as dihydrostreptomycin, gentamicin (Garamycin), kanamycin (Kantrex), neomycin, streptomycin, and vancomycin (Vancocin). (3) Reduce dosage for the elderly and debilitated. (4) Alcohol and CNS depressants will produce an additive effect. (5) Use caution in children under 7 years of age, pregnancy, prostatic hypertrophy, peptic ulcer, pyloroduodenal obstruction, bladder neck obstruction, narrow-angle glaucoma, cardiac dysrhythmias, and asthma. (6) Antimuscarinic effect may inhibit lactation. Discontinue breast feeding.

Contraindications: Hypersensitivity to dimenhydrinate, neonates.

Incompatible with: Alkaline solutions, aminophylline, ammonium chloride, amobarbital (Amytal), butorphanol (Stadol), chlordiazepoxide (Librium), chlorpromazine (Thorazine), diphenhydramine (Benadryl), glycopyrrolate (Robinul), heparin, hydrocortisone (Solu-Cortef), hydroxyzine (Vistaril), iodipamide meglumine 52% (Cholografin), midazolam (Versed), pentobarbital (Nembutal), phenobarbital (Luminal), phenytoin (Dilantin), prednisolone (Hydeltrasol), prochlorperazine (Compazine), promazine (Sparine), promethazine (Phenergan), tetracyclines, trifluoperazine (Stelzine), thiopental (Pentothal).

Side effects: Rare when used as indicated. The primary side effect is drowsiness. Overdose produces CNS excitation in children, convulsions, hallucinations, hyperpyrexia, marked irritability, and death.

Antidote: For exaggerated drowsiness or other major side effects, discontinue the drug and notify the physician.

Side effects will usually subside within a few hours or may be treated symptomatically. Treat convulsions with diazepam (Valium) initially; they may then be controlled with phenobarbital. Resuscitate as necessary.

DIPHENHYDRAMINE HYDROCHLORIDE

pH 5.0 to 6.0

(Bena-D 10/50, Benadryl, Benahist 10/50, Ben-Allergin-50, Bendylate, Benoject 10/50, Diphenacen-50, Hyrexin-50, Nordryl, Wehdryl)

Usual dose: 10 to 50 mg. Up to 100 mg may be given. Total dosage should not exceed 400 mg/24 hr.

Pediatric dose: *Children after neonatal period:* 5 mg/kg of body weight/24 hr. Divide this into 4 equal doses. Never exceed a total dosage of 300 mg/24 hr.

Dilution: May be given undiluted.

Rate of administration: 25 mg or fraction thereof over 1 minute. Extend injection time in nonemergency situations.

Actions: A potent antihistamine, it is capable of blocking the effects of histamines at various receptor sites, either eliminating allergic reaction or greatly modifying it. It is also an anticholinergic (antispasmodic), an antiemetic, and has sedative effects. Readily absorbed, widely distributed, and easily metabolized, it is excreted in changed form in the urine. Some secretion may occur in breast milk.

Indications and uses: (1) Allergic reactions to blood or plasma; (2) supplemental therapy to epinephrine in anaphylaxis and angioneurotic edema; (3) preoperative or generalized sedation; (4) antidote for parkinsonism-like syndrome caused by some phenothiazines (e.g., prochlorperazine [Compazine]); (5) severe nausea and vomiting; (6) motion sickness.

Precautions: (1) IV administration is used only in emergency situations. (2) Avoid SC or perivascular injection. (3) Will induce drowsiness. (4) Use with extreme caution in infants, children, elderly, or debilitated individuals, lactation and pregnancy, asthmatic attack, bladder neck obstruction, narrow-angle glaucoma, lower respiratory tract infections, prostatic hypertrophy, pyloroduodenal obstruction, and stenosing peptic ulcer. (5) Increases effectiveness of epinephrine and is often used in conjunction with it. (6) Potentiates anticholinergics (e.g., Atropine); alcohol, hypnotics, sedatives, tranquilizers, and other CNS depressants (e.g., reserpine, antipyretics); thioridazine (Mellaril); procarbazine (Matulane); and others. Reduced dose of potentiated drug may be indicated. (7) Inhibits anticoagulants, corticosteroids, and others. (8) Effectiveness of many drugs is reduced in combination with diphenhydramine because of increased metabolism. (9) May cause paradoxical excitation, especially in children and the elderly. (10) May inhibit lactation.

Contraindications: Hypersensitivity to antihistamines, pregnancy, lactation, newborn or premature infants, patients taking MAO inhibitors (e.g., pargyline [Eutonyl]), narrow-angle glaucoma, stenosing peptic ulcer, symptomatic prostatic hypertrophy, asthmatic attack, bladder neck obstruction, pyloroduodenal obstruction.

Incompatible with: Amobarbital (Amytal), amphotericin B (Fungizone), cephalothin (Keflin), dexamethasone (Decadron), diatrizoate meglumine (Renografin-60), furosemide (Lasix), iodipamide meglumine (Cholografin), methylprednisolone (SoluMedrol), pentobarbital (Nembutal), phenobarbital (Luminal), phenytoin (Dilantin), secobarbital (Seconal), thiopental (Pentothal).

Side effects: Rare when used as indicated: anaphylaxis; blurring of vision; confusion; constipation; diarrhea; difficulty in urination; diplopia; drowsiness; drug rash; dryness of mouth, nose, and throat; epigastric distress; headache; hemolytic anemia; hypotension; insomnia; nasal stuffiness; nausea; nervousness; palpitations; photosensitivity; rapid pulse; restlessness; thickening of bronchial secretions; tightness of the chest and wheezing; tingling, heaviness, weakness of hands; urticaria; vertigo; vomiting. Overdose may cause convulsions, hallucinations, and death in children.

Antidote: For exaggerated drowsiness or other disturbing side effects, discontinue the drug and notify the physician. Side effects will usually subside within a few hours or may be treated symptomatically. Treat hypotension promptly; may lead to cardiovascular collapse. Use dopamine (Intropin), norepinephrine, or phenylephrine. Epinephrine is contraindicated for hypotension; further hypotension will occur. Propranolol (Inderal) is the drug of choice for ventricular dysrhythmias. Treat convulsions with diazepam (Valium). Some convulsions may require physostigmine. Avoid analeptics (e.g., caffeine); will cause convulsions. Epinephrine must be available to treat anaphylaxis. Resuscitate as necessary.

DIPHTHERIA ANTITOXIN

Usual dose: Testing for sensitivity to horse serum required before use (see Precautions). Suggested ranges for adults and children to be given as a single dose.

Pharyngeal or laryngeal disease of 48 hours duration: 20,000 to 40,000 units.

Nasopharyngeal lesions: 40,000 to 60,000 units.

Extensive disease (3 or more days duration or anyone with brawny swelling of the neck): 80,000 to 120,000 units.

Dilution: May be given undiluted as an IV infusion. Warm to 32° to 35° C (90° to 95° F).

Rate of administration: To be given as a slow IV infusion. Titrate carefully to patient reaction.

Actions: A sterile solution of purified antitoxic substances prepared from the blood serum of horses immunized against diphtheria toxin. Neutralizes the toxins produced by *Corynebacterium diphtheriae.*

Indications and uses: Treatment of patients with clinical symptoms of diphtheria.

Precautions: (1) Read drug literature supplied with antitoxin completely before use. Essential to evaluate symptoms and individual status of each patient. (2) Determine patient response to any previous injections of serum of any type and history of any allergic-type reactions. (3) Hospitalize patient if possible. (4) Test every patient without exception for sensitivity to horse serum (1 ml vial of 1:10 dilution horse serum supplied). Conjunctival test and skin test recommended for maximum safety. Always begin with the conjunctival test.

Conjunctival test: Instill 1 drop 1:10 horse serum into conjunctival sac for adults (1 drop 1:100 dilution for children). Itching, redness, burning, and/or lacrimation within 30 minutes is a positive reaction. A drop of normal saline in the opposite eye is used as a control and should be asymptomatic. Reverse adverse effects of positive reaction with 1 drop epinephrine ophthalmic solution.

Scratch test: Make a ¼ inch skin scratch through a drop of 1:100 dilution in normal saline. Make a similar scratch through a drop of normal saline on a comparable skin site as a control. Compare sites in 20 minutes. An urticarial wheal surrounded by a zone of erythema is a positive reaction.

Skin test: Inject 0.02 to 0.1 ml of 1:100 horse serum intradermally. In patients with a history of allergies use a 1:1,000 solution. A like injection of normal saline can be used as a control. An urticarial wheal surrounded by a zone of erythema is a positive reaction. Compare in 20 minutes.

Other testing methods may be used. Use at least two. Concomitant use of antihistamines may interfere with sensitivity tests. (5) Bacteriological confirmation of the disease is not necessary to initiate treatment. Begin treatment as soon as possible. Each hour delay increases dosage requirements and decreases effectiveness. (6) Continue treatment until all symptoms controlled or bacteriological confirmation of another disease entity confirmed. (7) Use of full therapeutic doses of antimicrobial agents recommended in conjunction with diphtheria antitoxin. (8) All contacts must be evaluated and immunized if necessary.

Contraindications: Hypersensitivity to horse serum unless only treatment available for a life-threatening situation. Several techniques including preload of antihistamines and/or desensitization may be considered (see literature).

Incompatible with: Specific information not available. Do not mix with any other drug in syringe or solution because of specific use.

Side effects: Acute anaphylaxis with urticaria, respiratory distress, and vascular collapse. Serum sickness may occur. Usually appears in 7 to 12 days. Local pain, local erythema, and urticaria without systemic reaction can occur.

Antidote: Discontinue the drug and notify the physician of all side effects. Treat anaphylaxis immediately. Epinephrine (Adrenalin) and diphenhydramine (Benadryl), oxygen, vasopressors (dopamine), corticosteroids, and ventilation equipment must always be available. Resuscitate as necessary.

DIPYRIDAMOLE pH 2.2 to 3.2

(Persantine IV)

Usual dose: 0.57 mg/kg of body weight equally distributed over 4 minutes (0.142 mg/kg/min). A 70 kg adult would receive a total dose of 39.9 mg (10 mg/min). Never exceed 0.57 mg/kg dose. Thallium should be injected within 5 minutes following the 4-minute infusion of dipyridamole.

Dilution: Each 1 ml (5 mg) must be diluted with a minimum of 2 ml 5% dextrose in water, 0.45% normal saline, or normal saline. Total volume should range from a minimum of 20 ml to 50 ml (39.9 mg [8 ml] would be diluted in a minimum of 16 ml for a total infusion of 24 ml; additional diluent can be used to facilitate titration). May not be given undiluted, will cause local irritation.

Rate of administration: A single dose must be equally distributed over 4 minutes (0.142 mg/kg/min).

Actions: A coronary vasodilator that will cause an increase in coronary blood flow velocity of from 3.8 to 7 times greater than resting velocity. Action may result from the inhibition of adenosine uptake. Peak velocity is reached in 2.5 to 8.7 minutes. Will cause a 20% increase in heart rate and a mild but significant decrease in systolic and diastolic blood pressure in the supine position. Vital signs may take up to 30 minutes to return to baseline measurements. Used in combination with thallium, visualization shows dilation with sustained enhanced flow of intact vessels, leaving reduced pressure and flow across areas of hemodynamically important coronary vascular constriction. Results achieved are comparable to exercise-induced thalium imaging. Metabolized in the liver. Excreted in bile. Secreted in breast milk.

Indications and uses: An alternative to exericse in thallium myocardial perfusion imaging for the evaluation of coronary artery disease in patients who cannot exercise adequately.

Precautions: (1) Administered by or under the direction of the cardiologist. (2) Full facilities for treatment of any airway, allergic, or cardiac emergency, including laboratory analysis, must be available. (3) Theophylline (aminophylline) and other emergency drugs must be immediately available. (4) An IV line with a Y-tube or three-way stop-cock must be in place. Monitor vital signs continuously during infusion and for at least 15 minutes after or until return to baseline. ECG monitoring using at least 1 chest lead should be continuous. (5) Patient is usually in a supine position, but tests have been conducted in a sitting position. Lower to supine with head tilted down (Trendelenburg) if hypotension occurs. (6) This drug has caused two fatal myocardial infarctions as well as other serious side effects in a small percentage of patients; clinical information to be gained must be weighed against risk to the patient. (7) Patients with a history of unstable angina or a history of asthma may be at greater risk; use extreme caution. (8) May experience a false negative thallium imaging result if the patient takes maintenance doses of theophylline. (9) May inhibit adenosine. (10) Safety for use during pregnancy not established. Use only if clearly needed. (11) Temporarily discontinue nursing. (12) Safety for use in children not established. (13) Undiluted drug should be stored at controlled room temperature and protected from direct light; avoid freezing.

Contraindications: Hypersensitivity to dipyridamole.

Incompatible with: Specific information not available. Consider specific use.

Side effects: *Average:* Blood pressure lability, chest pain/angina pectoris, dizziness, dyspnea, ECG abnormalities (e.g., extrasystoles, ST-T changes, tachycardia), fatigue, flushing, headache, hypertension, hypotension, nausea, pain (unspecified), paresthesia. Numerous other side effects occur in less than 1% of patients.

Major: Bronchospasm, cerebral ischemia (transient), fatal and nonfatal myocardial infarction, ventricular fibrillation, ventricular tachycardia (symptomatic) occurred in 0.3% of patients.

Antidote: Physician will be present throughout test administration. Theophylline (aminophylline) is an adenosine receptor antagonist and will reverse the vasodilatory effect of dipyridamole. If bronchospasm or chest pain occur, administer 50 to 250 mg of theophylline (aminophylline) at a rate not to exceed 50 mg over 30 seconds. If symptoms are not relieved by 250 mg of theophylline (aminophylline), sublingual nitroglycerin may be helpful. Persistent chest pain may indicate impending potentially fatal myocardial infarction. If patient condition permits, thallium may be injected and allowed to circulate for 1 minute before injection of theophylline (aminophylline); this will permit initial thallium perfusion imaging before reversal of vasodilatory effects of dipyridamole on coronary circulation. Use head-down supine position for hypotension before administering theophylline (aminophylline). After reversal of vasodilatory action, treat dysrhythmias as indicated. Resuscitate as necessary.

DOBUTAMINE HYDROCHLORIDE

pH 2.5 to 5.5

(Dobutrex)

Usual dose: 2.5 to 10 mcg/kg of body weight/min initially. Adjust rate to effect desired response. Up to 40 mcg/kg/min has been used in some instances.

Dilution: Each 250 mg ampoule should be initially diluted with 10 ml of sterile water or 5% dextrose for injection. An additional 10 ml may be used if necessary to completely dissolve. Must be further diluted to at least 50 ml. Any amount of infusion solution desired above 50 ml may be used. (250 mg in 1 liter equals 250 mcg/ml; 250 mg in 500 ml equals 500 mcg/ml; 250 mg in 250 ml equals 1 mg/ml). Adjust to fluid requirements of the patient. Use of 5% dextrose, 0.9% sodium chloride, or sodium lactate is recommended.

Rate of administration: Begin with recommended dose for body weight and seriousness of condition. Gradually increase to effect desired response. May take up to 10 minutes to achieve peak effect of a specific dose. Maintain at correct therapeutic level with microdrip (60 gtt/ml) or infusion pump. Half-life of dobutamine is only about 2 minutes.

Actions: A synthetic catecholamine chemically related to dopamine, it is a direct-acting inotropic agent possessing beta-stimulator activity. Induces short-term increases in cardiac output by improving stroke volume with minimum increases in rate and blood pressure, minimum rhythm disturbances, and decreased peripheral vascular resistance. Usually most effective for only a few hours. May improve atrioventricular conduction. Peak effect obtained in 2 to 10 minutes. Has a very short duration of action and is excreted in the urine.

Indications and uses: Short-term inotropic support in cardiac decompensation resulting from depressed contractility (organic heart disease or cardiac surgical procedures).

Investigational use: Increase cardiac output in children with congenital heart disease undergoing cardiac catheterization.

Precautions: (1) Observe patient's response continuously; monitor heart rate, ectopic activity, blood pressure, urine flow, and central venous pressure. Measure pulmonary wedge pressure and cardiac output if possible. (2) Use digitalis preparation before starting dobutamine in patients with atrial fibrillation with rapid ventricular response. (3) Compatible through common tubing with dopamine, lidocaine, tobramycin, nitroprusside, potassium chloride, and protamine sulfate. (4) Correct hypovolemia and acidosis as indicated before initiating treatment. (5) May be ineffective if beta-blocking drugs (e.g., propranolol [Inderal]) have been given. (6) Use extreme caution in myocardial infarction; may increase size of infarction. (7) Produces higher cardiac output and lower pulmonary wedge pressure when given concomitantly with nitroprusside. (8) May cause serious dysrhythmias in presence of cyclopropane or halogen anesthetics, severe hypertension with oxytocic drugs. Use extreme caution and reduced dose, one tenth of calculated amount, in patients taking MAO inhibitors (e.g., isocarboxazid [Marplan]). (9) Will produce severe hypotension and seizures with phenytoin (Dilantin). (10) May increase insulin requirements in diabetics. (11) Refrigerate reconstituted solution up to 48 hours, or keep at room temperature 6 hours. When mixed in infusion solution, use within 24 hours. (12) Pink coloring of solution does not affect potency; will crystallize if frozen.

Contraindications: Idiopathic hypertrophic subaortic stenosis; shock without adequate fluid replacement. Safety in pregnant women and in children not established.

Incompatible with: Acyclovir (Zovirax), alkaline solutions (e.g., aminophylline, sodium bicarbonate), bretylium (Bretylol), bumetamide, calcium chloride, calcium gluconate, cefamandole (Mandol), cefazolin (Kefzol), cephalothin (Keflin), diazepam (Valium), digoxin, furosemide (Lasix), heparin, hydrocortisone, insulin, magnesium sulfate, penicillin, phenytoin (Dilantin), potassium phosphate, sodium ethacrynate (Edecrin).

Side effects: Anginal pain, chest pain, headache, hypertension, increased ventricular ectopic activity, nausea, palpitations, shortness of breath, tachycardia.

Antidote: Notify physician of all side effects. Decrease infusion rate and notify physician immediately if number of PVCs increases or there is a marked increase in pulse rate (30 or more beats) or blood pressure (50 or more mm Hg systolic). For accidental overdose reduce rate or temporarily discontinue until condition stabilizes.

DOPAMINE HYDROCHLORIDE pH 2.5 to 4.5

(Dopastat, Intropin, ✦ Revimine)

Usual dose: 2 to 5 mcg/kg of body weight/min initially in patients likely to respond to minimum treatment. 5 to 10 mcg/kg/min may be required initially to correct hypotension in the seriously ill patient. Gradually increase by 5 to 10 mcg/kg/min at 10- to 30-minute increments until optimum response occurs. Average dose is 20 mcg/kg/min; over 50 mcg/kg/min has been required in some instances.

Dilution: Each 5 ml (200 mg) ampoule must be diluted in 250 to 500 ml of the following IV solutions and given as an infusion: normal saline, 5% dextrose in water, 5% dextrose in 0.9% or 0.45% sodium chloride, 5% dextrose in lactated Ringer's injection, ⅙ molar sodium lactate, or lactated Ringer's injection. Diluted in 250 ml of solution, each ml contains 800 mcg dopamine. Diluted in 500 ml of solution, each ml contains 400 mcg dopamine. More concentrated solutions may be used if absolutely necessary to reduce fluid volume. Available prediluted in 250 ml or 500 ml of 5% dextrose in water. Dopamine content varies: choose 0.8 mg/ml, 1.6 mg/ml, or 3.2 mg/ml.

Rate of administration: Begin with recommended dose for body weight and seriousness of condition. Gradually increase by 5 to 10 mcg/kg of body weight/min to effect desired response. Use slowest possible rate to maintain adequate or preset systolic blood pressure. Use a microdrip (60 gtt/ml) or an infusion pump for accuracy. Optimum urine flow determines correct evaluation of dosage.

Actions: Dopamine is a chemical precursor of epinephrine, possessing alpha- and beta-receptor-stimulating actions. Increases cardiac output with minimum increase in myocardial oxygen consumption. Dilates renal and mesenteric blood vessels at doses lower than those required to elevate systolic blood pressure. Therapeutic doses effect little change on diastolic blood pressure. Has short duration of action and is promptly excreted in changed form in the urine.

Indications and uses: To correct hemodynamic imbalances including hypotension resulting from shock syndrome of myocardial infarction, trauma, endotoxic septicemia, open heart surgery, renal failure, and chronic cardiac decompensation.

Precautions: (1) Recognition of signs and symptoms and prompt treatment with dopamine will improve prognosis. (2) Alkaline solutions, including sodium bicarbonate, inactivate dopamine. (3) Check blood pressure every 2 minutes until stabilized at the desired level. Check every 5 minutes thereafter during therapy. Avoid hypertension. Check central venous pressure or pulmonary wedge pressure before administration and as ordered thereafter. (4) Use larger veins (antecubital fossa) and avoid extravasation; may cause necrosis and sloughing of tissue. (5) If possible, correct hypovolemia with whole blood or plasma as indicated; correct acidosis if present. (6) Discard diluted solution after 24 hours. (7) Use caution in pregnant women, children, and the presence of cyclopropane or other similar anesthetics. (8) Monitor urine flow continuously. (9) Reduce dose to one tenth of the calculated amount for individuals being treated with MAO inhibitors (e.g., isocarboxazid [Marplan]) and other sympathomimetics. (10) May cause severe hypertension with ergonovine or oxytocin. (11) Antagonizes effects of morphine, reducing analgesic effect. (12) Potentiated by tricyclic antidepressants and diuretics. (13) Therapy may be continued until the patient can maintain his own hemodynamic and renal functions. (14) β-receptor effects blocked by propranolol (Inderal), and dopamine antagonizes β-blocking effects of propranolol (Inderal). (15) Will cause severe bradycardia and hypotension with phenytoin (Dilantin).

Contraindications: Pheochromocytoma, uncorrected tachyarrhythmias, ventricular fibrillation.

Incompatible with: Acyclovir (Zovirax), alkaline solutions, amphotericin B, cephalothin (Keflin), gentamicin (Garamycin), sodium bicarbonate.

Side effects: Aberrant conduction, anginal pain, azotemia, bradycardia, dyspnea, ectopic beats, headache, hypertension, hypotension, nausea, palpitation, piloerection, tachycardia, vasoconstriction, vomiting, widened QRS complex.

Antidote: Notify the physician of all side effects. Decrease infusion rate and notify the physician immediately for decrease in established urine flow rate, disproportionate rise in diastolic blood pressure, increasing tachycardia, or new dysrhythmias. For accidental overdosage with hypertension, reduce rate or temporarily discontinue until condition stabilizes. Phentolamine may be required. To prevent sloughing and necrosis in areas where extravasation has occurred, with a fine hypodermic needle inject 5 to 10 mg of phentolamine (Regitine) diluted in 10 to 15 ml normal saline liberally throughout the tissue in the extravasated area. Begin as soon as extravasation recognized.

DOXAPRAM HYDROCHLORIDE

pH 3.5 to 5.0

(Dopram)

Usual dose: 0.5 to 1.0 mg/kg of body weight. Up to 1.5 mg/kg may be given as a single injection, or up to 2 mg/kg may be divided and given as several injections at 5-minute intervals. Maximum dosage equals 2 mg/kg. Repeat every 1 to 2 hours as necessary to maintain respiration, or follow with an infusion. *Do not exceed 3 Gm/24 hr. Minimum effective dosage is recommended. Repetitive doses are to be used only if the initial dose elicits a positive response.*

Chronic obstructive pulmonary disease: 400 mg in specific amount of diluent over no more than 2 hours.

Dilution: May be given undiluted or diluted with equal parts of sterile water for injection; or dilute 250 mg (12.5 ml) in 250 ml 5% or 10% dextrose in water or normal saline solution and give as an infusion.

Chronic obstructive pulmonary disease: Dilute 400 mg in 180 ml infusion fluid (2 mg/ml).

Rate of administration: Total desired dose of undiluted medication over 5 minutes. Infusion rate may start at 5 mg/min, decrease to 1 to 3 mg/min with observance of respiratory response. If an infusion is used after the initial priming dose, rate may start at 1 to 3 mg/min depending on patient response. Discontinue use after 2 hours, wait 1 to 2 hours, and repeat entire process. Use an infusion pump or microdrip (60 gtt/ml) for accuracy.

Chronic obstructive pulmonary disease: Specific dose over a 2-hour period. Begin at 1 mg/min. *Do not exceed 3 mg/min.*

Actions: An analeptic CNS stimulant. Affects medullary respiratory center to increase the depth of respiration and to slightly increase the rate. Achieves maximum effect in 2 minutes and lasts about 10 to 12 minutes with a single dose. Elevates blood pressure and heart rate. Rapidly metabolized.

Indications and uses: (1) Respiratory stimulation and return of protective reflexes (laryngopharyngeal) postanesthesia; (2) CNS depressant drug overdose (except muscle relaxant and narcotic overdose); (3) chronic obstructive pulmonary disease with acute hypercapnia (to prevent CO_2 retention).

Precautions: (1) Maintain an adequate airway at all times. Oxygen and facilities for controlled ventilation must be available. (2) Observe patient continuously and monitor blood pressure, pulse, and deep tendon reflexes during therapy until 1 hour after doxapram is discontinued. Adjust rate if indicated. (3) Arterial blood gas measurements are desirable to determine effective ventilation. (4) Failure to respond to treatment may indicate CNS source for sustained coma; requires neurological evaluation; repeat doses are not indicated. (5) Not effective for muscle relaxant– or narcotic-induced respiratory depression. (6) Adjunctive therapy only. Does not inhibit depressant drug metabolism. (7) Stimulates systemic epinephrine increase. (8) Use care in agitation, asthma, cardiac dysrhythmias or disease, cerebral edema, gastric surgery, hyperthyroidism, increased intracranial pressure, pheochromocytoma, tachycardia, and ulcers. (9) Potentiated by MAO inhibitors (e.g., pargyline [Eutonyl]) and inhalant anesthetics (e.g., halothane, cyclopropane). (10) Confirm patency of vein; vascular extravasation and thrombophlebitis can result from extended usage. (11) In chronic obstructive pulmonary disease, arterial blood gases before administration and every 30 minutes thereafter are mandatory; do not use in conjunction with mechanical ventilation. Adjust rate of infusion and oxygen concentration as indicated by arterial blood gases and patient response. Consider increased work of breathing. Observe for CO_2 retention and acidosis. Repeat infusions not recommended.

Contraindications: Cerebrovascular accidents, children under 12 years, convulsive states of any etiology, coronary artery disease, head injury, hypertension, inadequate ventilation capacity, known hypersensitivity to doxapram, pregnancy, severe pulmonary dysfunction.

Incompatible with: Alkaline drugs, aminophylline, ascorbic acid, carbenicillin (Geopen), cefoperazone (Cefobid), cefotaxime (Claforan), cefotetan (Cefotan), cefuroxime (Zinacef), dexamethasone (Decadron), diazepam (Valium), digoxin, dobutamine (Dobutrex), folic acid (Folvite), furosemide (Lasix), hydrocortisone sodium phosphate (Hydrocortone), hydrocortisone sodium succinate (Solu-Cortef), ketamine (Ketalar), methylprednisolone (Solu-Medrol), minocycline (Minocin), pentobarbital (Nembutal), phenobarbital (Luminal), secobarbital (Seconal), sodium bicarbonate, thiopental (Pentothal), ticarcillin (Ticar).

Side effects: *Minor:* Confusion, cough, diaphoresis, dizziness, dyspnea, fever, hiccups, hyperactivity, nausea, salivation, urinary retention or urgency, vomiting, warmth.

Major: Aggravated deep tendon reflexes, bilateral Babinski sign, bronchospasm, convulsions, hypertension, hypotension, laryngospasm, PVCs, respiratory alkalosis, skeletal muscle spasm, tachycardia.

Chronic obstructive pulmonary disease: Acidosis and CO_2 retention.

Antidote: Notify the physician of any side effect; depending on severity, physician may elect to continue the drug at a reduced rate of administration or discontinue it. Discontinue doxapram with onset of sudden hypotension or dyspnea. IV diazepam (Valium) or pentobarbital sodium (Nembutal) may be useful in overdose. Discontinue doxapram if blood gases deteriorate. Resuscitate as necessary.

DOXORUBICIN HYDROCHLORIDE

pH 3.8 to 6.5

(ADR, Adriamycin PFS, Adriamycin RDF, Rubrex)

Usual dose: 60 to 75 mg/M^2 of body surface as a single injection every 21 days.

Alternate dose schedule: 30 mg/M^2 of body surface as a single injection each day for 3 days. Repeat every 4 weeks. Normal liver and kidney function required.

Elevated serum bilirubin: Give 50% of above doses for serum bilirubin from 1.2 to 3.0 mg/ml and 25% for serum bilirubin above 3.0 mg/ml.

Pediatric dose: 30 mg/M^2 of body surface as a single injection each day for 3 days. Repeat every 4 weeks.

Dilution: *Specific techniques required, see Precautions.* Each 10 mg must be diluted with 5 ml of sodium chloride for injection. An additional 5 ml of diluent for each 10 mg is recommended. Shake to dissolve completely. Do not use bacteriostatic diluent. Available in preservative-free solutions.

Rate of administration: A single dose of properly diluted medication over a minimum of 3 to 5 minutes. Do not add to IV solutions. Should be given through Y-tube or three-way stopcock of a free-flowing infusion of normal saline or 5% dextrose. Slow injection rate further for erythematous streaking along the vein or facial flushing.

Actions: A highly toxic antibiotic antineoplastic agent that is cell cycle specific for the S phase. Rapidly cleared from plasma, it interferes with cell division by binding with DNA to slow production of RNA. Tissue levels remain constant for 7 to 10 days. Does not cross blood-brain barrier. Slowly excreted in bile and urine.

Indications and uses: To suppress or retard neoplastic growth. Regression has been produced in soft tissue, osteogenic, and other sarcomas; Hodgkin's disease; non-Hodgkin's lymphomas; acute leukemias; breast, GU, thyroid, lung, and stomach carcinoma; neuroblastoma; and many other carcinomas.

Precautions: (1) Follow guidelines for handling cytotoxic agents recommended. See Appendix, p. 677. (2) Usually administered in hospital by or under the direction of the physician specialist. (3) Use only large veins. Avoid veins over joints or in extremities with compromised venous or lymphatic drainage. Determine absolute patency of vein. A stinging or burning sensation indicates extravasation; severe cellulitis and tissue necrosis will result. Discontinue injection; use another vein. (4) Recent studies suggest that cardiotoxicity may be reduced and doses may be increased by administration on a weekly basis or as a prolonged infusion (48 to 96 hours). A central venous catheter or infuse-a-port would be necessary. (5) Diluted solution stable 24 hours at room temperature, 48 hours if refrigerated; then discard. (6) Protect from sunlight. (7) Urine will be reddish color for several days (from dye, not hematuria). (8) Monitoring of white blood cells, red blood cells, platelet count, uric acid levels, liver function, kidney function, ECG, chest x-ray, and echocardiogram is necessary before and during therapy. (9) Wash thoroughly if powder or solution contacts skin or mucosa. (10) Used cautiously with other antineoplastic drugs to achieve tumor remission. (11) Will produce teratogenic effects on the fetus. Toxic to embryo with mutagenic potential. Give with caution in men and women capable of conception. (12) May exacerbate cyclophosphamide-induced hemorrhagic cystitis or increase hepatotoxicity of 6-mercaptopurine. Many drug interactions possible; observe patient closely. (13) Do not administer any vaccines or chloroquine to patients receiving antineoplastic drugs. (14) Increased toxicity including skin redness and exfoliative changes possible when given concurrent with or after radiation. (15) Maintain adequate hydration. (16) Allopurinol may prevent formation of uric acid crystals. (17) Be alert for signs of bone marrow depression, bleeding, or infection. (18) Prophylactic antiemetics are indicated.

Contraindications: Myelosuppression resulting from treatment with other antineoplastic agents, impaired cardiac function, or previous treatment with complete cumulative doses of doxorubicin and/or daunorubicin.

Incompatible with: Aminophylline, cephalothin (Keflin), dexamethasone, diazepam (Valium), fluorouracil, heparin, hydrocortisone sodium succinate, and methotrexate. Should be considered incompatible with any other drug because of toxicity and specific use.

Side effects: Acute cardiac failure, alopecia (complete), bone marrow depression, depressed QRS voltage, diarrhea, esophagitis, gonadal suppression, hyperpigmentation of nail beds and dermal creases, hyperuricemia, nausea, stomatitis, vomiting.

Antidote: Most side effects will either be tolerated or treated symptomatically. Keep the physician informed. Hematopoietic toxicity may require cessation of therapy. Acute cardiac failure occurs suddenly (most common when total cumulative dosage approaches 550 mg/M^2) and frequently does not respond to currently available treatment. Close monitoring of accumulated dosage, bone marrow, ECG, chest x-ray, echocardiography, and systolic ejection fraction may prevent most serious and potentially fatal cardiac side effects. There is no specific antidote. Supportive therapy as indicated will help sustain the patient in toxicity. For extravasation flood the area with normal saline and inject long-acting dexamethasone (Decadron LA) or other injectable corticosteroid throughout extravasated tissue. Use a 27- or 25-gauge needle. Apply cold compresses, elevate extremity. Site should be observed promptly by a reconstructive surgeon.

DOXYCYCLINE HYCLATE pH 1.8 to 3.3

(Doxy 100, Doxy 200, ✤ Vibramycin, Vibramycin IV)

Usual dose: *Adults and children over 45 kg:* 200 mg the first day in 1 or 2 infusions followed by 100 to 200 mg/24 hr on subsequent days, depending on severity of the infection.

Pediatric dose: *Children under 45 kg (but over 8 years):* 4.4 mg/kg of body weight/24 hr in 2 equally divided doses. Follow with 2.2 mg/kg/24 hr given once daily or in 2 equally divided doses on subsequent days.

Dilution: Each 100 mg or fraction thereof is diluted with 10 ml of sterile water or normal saline for injection. Further dilute each 10 ml with 100 to 1,000 ml of a compatible infusion solution such as sodium chloride, 5% dextrose injection, Ringer's injection, 10% invert sugar in water, lactated Ringer's injection with or without 5% dextrose, Normosol-M or -R in 5% dextrose in water, or other compatible solutions (see literature). Recommended concentrations 0.1 to 1 mg/ml. 1,000 ml diluent equals 0.1 mg/ml, 100 ml equals 1 mg/ml.

Rate of administration: Each 100 mg or fraction thereof, properly diluted, over a minimum of 1 to 4 hours. 100 mg diluted in 100 ml equals 1 mg/ml and must be given over a minimum of 2 hours. 100 mg diluted in 200 ml equals 500 mcg/ml and can be given in 1 hour if absolutely necessary. Infusion must be completed in 6 hours when diluted in Ringer's lactate injection with or without dextrose 5% and in 12 hours when diluted in other compatible solutions.

Actions: A broad-spectrum antibiotic that is bacteriostatic against many gram-positive and gram-negative organisms. Thought to interfere with the protein synthesis of microorganisms. Tetracyclines are well distributed in most body tissues and often bound to plasma protein. Doxycycline may penetrate normal meninges, the eye, and the prostate more easily than most tetracyclines. Concentrated in the liver and excreted through the bile to urine and feces in a biologically active state. Crosses the placental barrier. Secreted in breast milk.

Indications and uses: (1) Infections caused by susceptible strains or organisms such as rickettsiae, spirochetal agents, viruses, and many other gram-negative and gram-positive bacteria; (2) to substitute for contraindicated penicillin or sulfonamide therapy; (3) drug of choice when a tetracycline is indicated for treatment of an extrarenal infection in patients with renal impairment; (4) adjunct to amebicides in acute intestinal amebiasis.

Precautions: (1) Initiate oral therapy as soon as possible. (2) Check expiration date. Outdated ampoules may cause nephrotoxicity. (3) Must be stored away from heat and light; protect from direct sunlight during infusion. (4) Buffered with ascorbic acid. (5) After reconstitution, must be stored at 2° to 8° C (36° to 46° F) and used within 72 hours. (6) Sensitivity studies indicated to determine susceptibility of the causative organism to doxycycline. (7) Avoid prolonged use of drug; superinfection caused by overgrowth of nonsusceptible organisms may result. (8) Use caution in impaired liver function. Doxycycline serum concentrations and liver function tests are indicated. (9) May cause skeletal retardation in the fetus and infants and permanent tooth discoloration in children under 8 years, including in utero or through mother's milk. Do not use during pregnancy; discontinue nursing. (10) Inhibits oral contraceptives; may result in pregnancy or breakthrough bleeding. (11) Monitor blood glucose; may reduce insulin requirements. (12) May alter lithium levels. (13) Inhibits bactericidal action of all penicillins (e.g., ampicillin, oxacillin, methicillin). May be toxic with sulfonamides. (14) May potentiate digoxin and anticoagulants; reduced dosage of these drugs may be necessary. (15) Potentiated by alcohol and hepatotoxic drugs (e.g., methoxyflurane [Penthrane]); severe liver damage may result. (16) Inhibited by alkalinizing agents; barbiturates; calcium, iron, and magnesium salts; carbamazepine (Tegretol); cimetidine (Tagamet); hydantoins (e.g., phenytoin); riboflavin; sodium bicarbonate; and others. (17) Alert patient to photosensitive skin reaction. (18) Determine absolute patency of vein and avoid extravasation; thrombophlebitis may occur. (19) Organisms resistant to one tetracycline are usually resistant to others. (20) If syphilis is suspected, perform a dark-field examination before initiating tetracyclines.

Contraindications: Known hypersensitivity to tetracyclines, pregnancy, lactation. Not recommended in children under 8 years.

Incompatible with: Cephalothin. 5% dextrose in lactated Ringer's and lactated Ringer's injection may present compatibility problems with some drugs. Administer separately.

Side effects: Relatively nontoxic in average doses. More toxic in large doses or if given too rapidly.

Minor: Anogenital lesions, anorexia, blood dyscrasias, diarrhea, dysphagia, enterocolitis, nausea, skin rashes, vomiting.

Major: Hypersensitivity reactions including anaphylaxis; blurred vision and headache (benign intracranial hypertension); bulging fontanels in infants; liver damage; photosensitivity; systemic candidiasis; thrombophlebitis.

Antidote: Notify the physician of all side effects. If minor side effects are progressive or any major side effect occurs, discontinue the drug, treat allergic reaction, or resuscitate as necessary.

DROPERIDOL pH 3.0 to 3.8

(Inapsine)

Usual dose: *Antiemetic:* 0.5 mg every 4 hours. May increase dose if required. Often used in an antiemetic regimen with dexamethasone in chemotherapy (unlabeled use).

Premedication: 2.5 to 10 mg 30 to 60 minutes preoperatively or before procedure. Repeat 1.25 to 2.5 mg as indicated.

Induction of anesthesia: 2.5 mg/10 to 12 kg of body weight.

Maintenance of anesthesia: 1.25 to 2.5 mg as indicated.

Reduce dose of narcotics and all CNS depressants to one fourth or one third of usual dose before, during, and for 24 hours after injection of droperidol. If other CNS depressants (e.g., narcotics) have been given previously, reduce dose of droperidol. Reduce dose for elderly, debilitated, and poor-risk patients, and impaired kidney or liver function.

Pediatric dose: Children 2 to 12 years: 1 to 1.5 mg/10 to 12 kg of body weight. Decrease dose as indicated in Usual dose.

Dilution: Given undiluted. Give through Y-tube or three-way stopcock of the infusion set. May be added to selected infusion solutions (5% dextrose in water, normal saline, or lactated Ringer's). 20 mg in 1,000 ml equals 20 mcg/ml or 1 mg/50 ml.

Rate of administration: 10 mg or fraction thereof over 1 minute. Titrate by desired patient response. Infusion must be titrated by desired dose and patient response.

Actions: An antianxiety agent that produces marked tranquilization and sedation. Has an antiemetic action also. It is an alpha adrenergic blocker and produces peripheral vascular dilation. May decrease an abnormally high pulmonary arterial pressure. Effective in 3 to 10 minutes with maximum results in 30 minutes. Lasts 2 to 4 hours. Some effects persist for 12 hours. Metabolized in the liver. Excreted in urine and feces. Crosses placental barrier very slowly.

Indications and uses: (1) Preoperative sedation; (2) induction and maintenance of anesthesia, regional or general. Frequently given concurrently with narcotic analgesics such as fentanyl (Sublimaze) to produce neuroleptanalgesia. (3) Antiemetic, used in surgical and diagnostic procedures.

Unlabeled use: Antiemetic in cancer chemotherapy.

Precautions: (1) Primarily used by or under direct observation of the anesthesiologist. (2) A potent drug. Monitor the patient closely. Resuscitation equipment, a narcotic antagonist (if a narcotic has been used concurrently), IV infusion line, and drugs to manage hypotension must be readily available. (3) Use caution with known Parkinson's disease. (4) Orthostatic hypotension is common; move and position patients with care. (5) EEG pattern may be slow in returning to normal postoperatively. (6) Physically compatible for at least 15 minutes in a syringe with atropine, butorphanol (Stadol), chlorpromazine (Thorazine), diphenhydramine (Benadryl), fentanyl, glycopyrrolate (Robinul), hydroxyzine (Atarax [IM use only]), meperidine, morphine, perphenazine (Trilafon), promazine (Sparine), promethazine (Phenergan), and scopolamine. See each individual drug for requirements of administration. (7) Rarely used during pregnancy (see Contraindications). Exceptions are selected use during cesarean section and as a continuous infusion to treat hyperemesis gravidarum in the 2nd and 3rd trimester. Secretion in breast milk is unconfirmed, use caution in the nursing mother.

Contradictions: Known hypersensitivity to droperidol, children under 2 years, pregnancy.

Incompatible with: Barbiturates, epinephrine.

Side effects: *Minor:* Abnormal EEG, chills, dizziness, hallucinations, hypotension, restlessness, shivering, tachycardia.

Major: Apnea, extrapyramidal symptoms, hypotension (severe), respiratory depression.

Antidote: Notify the physician of any side effect. Minor side effects will probably be transient; for major side effects discontinue the drug, treat symptomatically, and notify the physician. Treat hypotension with fluid therapy (rule out hypovolemia) and vasopressors such as dopamine hydrochloride (Intropin) or levarterenol (Levophed).

Epinephrine is contraindicated for hypotension. Further hypotension will occur. Treat extrapyramidal symptoms with benztropine mesylate (Cogentin) or diphenhydramine hydrochloride (Benadryl). Resuscitate as necessary.

EDETATE DISODIUM pH 6.5 to 7.5

(Chealamide, Disotate, EDTA disodium, Endrate)

Usual dose: 50 mg/kg of body weight/24 hr as indicated. Total dose should not exceed 3 Gm/24 hr. Usually given for 5 days, held for 2 days. Regimen may be repeated to a total of 15 doses.

Pediatric dose: 40 mg/kg of body weight/24 hr as indicated. Do not exceed 70 mg/kg/24 hr or adult dose, whichever is less.

Dilution: Recommended dose must be diluted in 500 ml dextrose or isotonic saline solution and given as IV infusion. A 0.5% solution will reduce the risk of thrombophlebitis. Do not exceed cardiac reserve in any patient. Use less diluent if necessary in children. Must be diluted to at least a 3% solution.

Rate of administration: Must not exceed more than 15 mg of actual medication over 1 minute. Total dose usually given over 3 to 4 hours. Reduce rate and further dilute solution for pain at injection site.

Actions: A calcium-chelating agent. Attracts calcium ions immediately on injection and becomes calcium disodium edetate. Capable of severely depleting the body of calcium stores. Exerts a negative inotropic effect on the heart. It is well distributed in extracellular fluids and rapidly excreted in the urine.

Indications and uses: (1) Cardiac dysrhythmias (atrial and ventricular, especially when caused by digitalis toxicity); (2) hypercalcemia.

Precautions: (1) Used only when the severity of disease indicates necessity. (2) May produce hypocalcemia quickly, especially if used for purposes other than chelating calcium. (3) Use repeatedly only with caution because of potential for nephrotoxicity and mobilization of extracirculatory calcium stores. (4) Monitor vital signs and ECG before and during therapy. (5) Confirm patency of vein. Avoid extravasation; can cause tissue necrosis. (6) Routine electrolyte panel (potassium deficiency) and urine specimens for casts and cells necessary during therapy. Magnesium deficiency can occur in prolonged therapy. (7) Inhibits coagulation of blood (transient). (8) Use caution in cardiac disease (may adversely affect myocardial contractility), diabetes (lower blood sugar may require less insulin), severe renal disease, liver disease, congestive heart failure (1 Gm of sodium in each 5 Gm), and limited cardiac reserve. (9) Inhibits mannitol. (10) Potentiates neuromuscular blocking antibiotics (e.g., gentamicin [Garamycin]). (11) Obtain blood for serum calcium levels just before beginning a new infusion. Specific laboratory methods must be used for accurate evaluation. (12) Keep patient in supine position during and after administration (15 to 30 minutes) to avoid postural hypotension. (13) Safety for use in pregnancy or lactation not established. Use with extreme caution and only if clearly needed. (14) Store at room temperature.

Contraindications: Anuria, known sensitivity to edetate disodium, patients with seizures or intracranial lesions, renal disease.

Incompatible with: 5% dextrose in 5% alcohol. Will chelate any metal. Not recommended to mix in syringe or solution with any other drug.

Side effects: *Minor:* Anorexia, arthralgia, circumoral paresthesias, fatigue, fever, glycosuria, headache, hypotension, malaise, nasal congestion, nausea, sneezing, tearing, thirst, thrombophlebitis, urinary urgency, vomiting.

Major: Anaphylaxis, anemia, dermatitis, hemorrhage, hypocalcemic tetany, prolonged QT interval, renal tubular destruction (reversible), death.

Antidote: Notify the physician of any side effect. For progression of minor side effects or any major side effect, discontinue drug immediately and notify the physician. Calcium gluconate is the antidote of choice and should be available for infusion at all times (use extreme caution if patient digitalized). Treat anaphylaxis and resuscitate as necessary.

EDROPHONIUM CHLORIDE pH 5.4

(Enlon, Reversol, Tensilon)

Usual dose: 1 to 10 mg (0.1 to 1 ml) at specified intervals depending on usage. Maximum dose should never exceed 40 mg (4 doses of 10 mg each).

Myasthenia gravis diagnosis: 10 mg (1 ml) in tuberculin syringe. Give 2 mg (0.2 ml). If no reaction occurs in 45 seconds, give remaining 8 mg (0.8 ml). Test may be repeated after 30 minutes.

Myasthenia treatment evaluation: 1 to 2 mg (0.1 to 0.2 ml) 1 hour after oral intake of drug being used for treatment.

Myasthenia crisis evaluation: 2 mg (0.2 ml) in tuberculin syringe. Give 1 mg (0.1 ml). If the patient's condition does not deteriorate, give 1 mg (0.1 ml) after 60 seconds. Improvement in cardiac status and respiration should occur.

Curare antagonist: 10 mg (1 ml). May be repeated as necessary up to 4 doses.

Antiarrhythmic: 5 to 10 mg. Repeat once in 10 minutes if necessary.

Pediatric dose: *Myasthenia gravis diagnosis:* 0.5 for infants. 1 mg for children under 34 kg; if no response in 30 to 45 seconds, give 1 mg every 30 to 45 seconds up to 5 mg. Over 34 kg, give 2 mg; if no response in 30 to 45 seconds, give 1 mg every 30 to 45 seconds up to 10 mg.

Antiarrhythmic: 2 mg (0.2 ml) administered slowly.

Dilution: May be given undiluted. In the treatment of myasthenia crisis, this drug may be given as a continuous IV drip. Use an infusion pump or microdrip (60 gtt/ml).

Rate of administration: 2 mg (0.2 ml) or fraction thereof over 15 to 30 seconds. As a curare antagonist give a single dose over 30 to 45 seconds.

Actions: An anticholinesterase and antagonist of skeletal muscle relaxants. Inhibits the enzyme cholinesterase, allowing acetylcholine to accumulate at the myoneural junction. Restores normal transmission of nerve impulses. Acts within 30 to 60 seconds and has an extremely short duration of action, seldom exceeding 10 minutes. Produces vagal stimulation, shortens refractory period of atrial muscle, and slows conduction through the AV node.

Indications and uses: (1) Diagnosis of myasthenia gravis; (2) evaluation of adequate treatment of myasthenia gravis; (3) treatment of myasthenia crisis; (4) an antagonist to curare, tubocurarine; gallamine triethiodide (Flaxedil), and dimethyl tubocurarine.

Investigational use: Termination of supraventricular tachycardia.

Precautions: (1) Atropine 1 mg must be available and ready for injection at all times. (2) A physician should be present when this drug is used. (3) Anticholinesterase insensitivity may develop; withhold drugs and support respiration as necessary. (4) Use caution in patients with bronchial asthma, cardiac dysrhythmias, or myasthenia gravis treated with anticholinesterase drugs. (5) May be inhibited by corticosteroids and magnesium. (6) Antagonizes anesthetics (e.g., ether), ganglionic blocking agents (e.g., trimethaphan [Arfonad]), and aminoglycoside antibiotics (e.g., gentamycin [Garamycin]); neuromuscular block may be accentuated. Prolongs muscle relaxant effect of succinylcholine chloride (Anectine). (7) May cause bradycardia with digitalis glycosides. (8) Continuously observe patient reactions.

Contraindications: Apnea, known hypersensitivity to anticholinesterase agents, mechanical intestinal and urinary obstructions, patients taking mecamylamine, pregnancy.

Incompatible with: An extremely specific drug. Should be considered incompatible in syringe or solution with any other drug.

Side effects: Abdominal cramps, anorexia, anxiety, bradycardia, bronchiolar spasm, cardiac dysrhythmias and arrest, cold moist skin, contraction of the pupils, convulsions, diarrhea, dysphagia, fainting, increased lacrimation, increased pulmonary secretion, increased salivation, insomnia, irritability, laryngospasm, muscle weakness, nausea, perspiration, ptosis, respiratory arrest (either muscular or central), urinary frequency and incontinence, vomiting.

Antidote: If side effects occur, discontinue the drug and notify the physician. Atropine sulfate in doses of 0.4 to 0.5 mg IV will counteract most side effects and may be repeated every 3 to 10 minutes. Pralidoxime chloride 50 to 100 mg/min to 1 Gm may be used with extreme caution as a cholinesterase reactivator. Endotracheal intubation or tracheostomy is considered prophylactic in anesthesia or crises. Artificial ventilation, oxygen therapy, cardiac monitoring, adequate suctioning, and treatment of shock or convulsions must be instituted and maintained as necessary. Treat allergic reactions with epinephrine.

ENALAPRIL MALEATE pH 4.5 to 6.5

(Vasotec IV)

Usual dose: 1.25 mg every 6 hours. Dosage is the same when converting from oral to IV therapy. Doses up to 5 mg every 6 hours have been tolerated for up to 36 hours, but clinical studies have not shown a need for dosage over 1.25 mg. Reduce initial dose to 0.625 mg in patients taking diuretics, patients with a creatinine clearance less than 30 ml/min (serum creatinine greater than 3 mg/dl), and dialysis patients. If the 0.625 dose is not clinically effective after 1 hour, it may be repeated. Additional doses of 1.25 mg may be given every 6 hours, reduce by one half for dialysis patients.

Dilution: May be given undiluted through the port of a free-flowing infusion of normal saline; 5% dextrose in water, normal saline, or lactated Ringer's injection; or Isolyte E. May also be diluted in up to 50 ml of any of the same solutions and given in infusion.

Rate of administration: A single dose must be evenly distributed over 5 minutes.

Actions: An antihypertensive agent. An angiotensin-converting enzyme inhibitor that prevents conversion of angiotensin I to angiotensin II. Peripheral arterial resistance is reduced in hypertensive patients. In patients with heart failure, significant reduction in peripheral vascular resistance, blood pressure (afterload), pulmonary capillary wedge pressure (preload), and heart size occurs, as well as an increase in cardiac output (stroke index) and exercise tolerance time. Initial response may take 15 minutes to 1 hour. Peak blood pressure reduction occurs in 4 to 6 hours, and effects last up to 24 hours. Peak effects of subsequent doses may be greater than the initial dose. Excreted in bile and urine.

Indications and uses: (1) Treatment of hypertension; (2) treatment of patients in heart failure not adequately responsive to diuretics and digitalis. Enalapril is used in addition to digitalis and diuretics.

Precautions: (1) Stable for up to 24 hours after dilution. (2) Has been used IV for up to 7 days. (3) Monitor vital signs very frequently. May cause precipitous drop in blood pressure following the first dose. Use extreme caution in fluid-depleted patients. Patients with congestive heart failure may become hypotensive at any time. Dysrhythmias or conduction defects may occur. (4) Monitor BUN and serum creatinine. An increase in either may require a decrease in dose of enalapril or discontinuation of a diuretic. (5) Diuretics given concomitantly may cause a precipitous drop in blood pressure within the first hour of the initial dose; observe the patient closely. Severe dietary salt restriction or dialysis will aggravate this effect. (6) May cause oliguria or progressive azotemia in patients with severe congestive heart failure whose renal function is dependent on the activity of the renin-angiotensin-aldosterone system. Acute renal failure and death are possible. (7) Use caution in patients with aortic stenosis; afterload reduction may not be adequate. (8) May cause hyperkalemia. May cause a significant increase in serum potassium with potassium-sparing diuretics (e.g., spironolactone) or potassium supplements. Use with caution and only in documented hypokalemia. Use salt substitutes with caution. Monitor serum potassium levels. (9) Use caution in surgery, with anesthesia, or with any agents that produce hypotension. (10) May be used concomitantly with other antihypertensive agents, e.g., thiazide diuretics (chlorothiazide [Diuril]). Effects are additive. (11) Hypersensitivity reactions may increase in combination with allopurinol. (12) Use caution and consider lower doses when administering nitroglycerin, nitroprusside sodium, other nitrates, or other vasodilators (e.g., hydralazine). (13) May decrease hemoglobin and hematocrit slightly. (14) Potentiated by probenicid. (15) Safety for use during pregnancy and lactation not established. Has caused reversible acute renal failure in a premature infant whose mother received enalapril. Use with extreme caution, and only when clearly indicated. (16) Safety for use in children not established. (17) Blood levels markedly increased in the elderly. (18) Average dose for conversion to oral therapy is 5 mg/day as a single dose. May be adjusted by patient response. When a reduced dose of enalapril IV has been indicated (e.g., diuretics, impaired renal function, dialysis), reduce initial oral dose to 2.5 mg/day as a single dose. Adjust by patient response.

Contraindications: Hypersensitivity to enalapril or its components.

Incompatible with: Must be diluted or infused with specific solutions; see Dilution.

Side effects: Abdominal pain, angioedema, chest pain, cough, diarrhea, dizziness, dyspnea, fatigue, headache, hyperkalemia, hypotension (severe), impotence, insomnia, muscle cramps, nausea, palpitations, paresthesias, pruritus, rash, somnolence, vomiting.

Antidote: For minor side effects, notify the physician. Most will be tolerated or treated symptomatically. If symptoms progress or any major side effect occurs (angioedema, precipitous hypotension, hyperkalemia), discontinue drug and notify the physician immediately. Hypotension should respond to IV fluids if the patient's condition allows their use. Other drugs in the regimen may need to be discontinued or the dosage reduced. Use epinephrine immediately for angioedema. Maintain the patient as indicated. If cardiac dysrhythmias occur, treat appropriately.

EPHEDRINE SULFATE pH 4.5 to 7.0

Usual dose: 12.5 to 25 mg, may be repeated every 3 to 4 hours. 150 mg/24 hr is the maximum total dose. Smaller doses, 5 to 25 mg, encouraged for IV use.

Pediatric dose: Rarely used IV in children, but the dose is 3 mg/kg of body weight/24 hr divided into 4- to 6-hour doses.

Dilution: May be given undiluted. Not usually added to IV solutions. May be injected through Y-tube or three-way stopcock of infusion set.

Rate of administration: Each 10 mg or fraction thereof over 1 minute.

Actions: An alkaloid sympathomimetic drug and a CNS stimulant, it is less potent but longer acting than epinephrine. It has positive inotropic action, increasing the strength of myocardial contraction. It increases the heart rate and elevates the blood pressure. Some arteriolar vasoconstriction occurs. Relaxes the smooth muscle of the bronchi and dilates the pupils. Metabolic rate and respiratory rate are increased. Widely distributed in body fluids, ephedrine crosses the blood-brain barrier. It is excreted in urine. Secreted in breast milk.

Indications and uses: (1) Bronchospasm; (2) hypotension; (3) bradycardia and atrioventricular block; (4) pressor agent during spinal anesthesia; (5) Stokes-Adams syndrome; (6) allergic disorders (epinephrine preferred); (7) narcotic, barbiturate, and alcohol poisoning.

Precautions: (1) Check blood pressure every 5 minutes. (2) Note label; only specific solutions can be given IV. (3) Vasoconstriction-induced tissue sloughing can occur. Avoid administering in areas of limited blood supply (e.g., fingers, toes) or if peripheral vascular disease is present. (4) Use caution in heart disease, angina, diabetes, hyperthyroidism, and prostatic hypertrophy. (5) Has a cumulative effect. (6) Hypertensive crisis may occur in conjunction with MAO inhibitors (e.g., pargyline [Eutonyl]) or furazolidone (Furoxone). (7) May cause cardiac dysrhythmias with digitalis or mercurial diuretics. (8) May cause severe hypertension with ergonovine or oxytocin; hypotension and bradycardia with hydantoins (e.g., phenytoin [Dilantin]). (9) Inhibits guanethidine. (10) Tolerance may develop, but effectiveness is usually restored if the drug is discontinued temporarily. (11) Potentiated by anesthetics (e.g., halothane, cyclopropane), tricyclic antidepressants, antihistamines, sodium levothyroxine, and urinary alkalizers. (12) Antagonized by β-adrenergic blockers (e.g., propranolol [Inderal]) and α-adrenergic blockers (e.g., phentolamine [Regitine]). (13) Inhibited by ergot alkaloids and phenothiazines (e.g., prochlorperazine [Compazine]). (14) Inhibits insulin and oral hypoglycemic agents; increased dose may be required. (15) Interacts with many other drugs.

Contraindications: Known hypersensitivity to ephedrine, labor and delivery if maternal blood pressure exceeds 130/80 mm Hg, narrow-angle glacoma. Do not use to treat overdosage of phenothiazines (e.g., chlorpromazine [Thorazine]). A further drop in blood pressure and irreversible shock may result.

Incompatible with: Alkaline solutions, hydrocortisone (Solu-Cortef), pentobarbital (Nembutal), phenobarbital (Luminal), secobarbital (Seconal), thiopental (Pentothal).

Side effects: Rare in therapeutic doses; anorexia, cardiac dysrhythmias, headache, insomnia, nausea, nervousness, painful urination, palpitations, precordial pain, sweating, tachycardia, urinary retention, vertigo, vomiting. Confusion, delirium, euphoria, and hallucinations may occur with higher doses. Convulsions, pulmonary edema, and respiratory failure may occur with overdose.

Antidote: If side effects occur, discontinue the drug and notify the physician. Side effects may be treated symptomatically. Treat hypotension with IV fluids; vasopressors (e.g., dopamine [Intropin]) are contraindicated. Treat hypertension with phentolamine (Regitine) and convulsions with diazepam (Valium). Treat cardiac dysrhythmias with β blockers (e.g., propranolol [Inderal]). Resuscitate as necessary.

EPINEPHRINE HYDROCHLORIDE

pH 2.5 to 5.0

(Adrenalin chloride)

Usual dose: 0.2 to 0.5 mg of 1:10,000 solution. May be repeated as necessary.

Cardiac arrest: 0.5 to 1.0 mg of 1:10,000 solution IV; may repeat every 5 minutes. Larger initial doses are being used in some emergency rooms. 1.0 mg of 1:10,000 solution may be given through the endotracheal tube before an IV is established.

Maintenance dose: 1 to 8 mcg/min.

Pediatric dose: *Cardiac arrest:* 5 to 10 mcg/kg of body weight of 1:10,000 solution by IV administration. Give intracardiac only if no other route is available.

Dilution: Each 1 mg (1 ml) of 1:1,000 solution must be diluted in at least 10 ml of normal saline for injection to prepare a 1:10,000 solution. For maintenance, may be further diluted in 500 ml 5% dextrose in water. Give through Y-tube or three-way stopcock of infusion set.

Rate of administration: Each 1 mg or fraction thereof over 1 minute or longer. May be given more rapidly in cardiac resuscitation.

Actions: A naturally occurring hormone secreted by the adrenal glands. A sympathomimetic drug, it imitates almost all actions of the sympathetic nervous system. It is a vasoconstrictor and delays the absorption of many drugs; a potent cardiac stimulant, it strengthens the myocardial contraction (positive inotropic effect) and increases cardiac rate (positive chronotropic effect). A potent dilator or relaxant of smooth muscle, especially bronchial muscle. Decreases blood supply to the abdomen and increases blood supply to skeletal muscles. Elevates systolic blood pressure, lowers diastolic pressure, and increases pulse pressure. It is seldom used as a vasopressor because of its short duration of action. It is rapidly inactivated in the body by various enzymes and excreted in changed form in the urine.

Indications and uses: (1) Drug of choice for anaphylactic shock; (2) antidote of choice for histamine overdose and allergic reactions including bronchial asthma, urticaria, and angioneurotic edema; (3) cardiac resuscitation; (4) Stokes-Adams syndrome.

Precautions: (1) Usual route is SC or IM. (2) Effects are instantaneous IV. Start with a small dose, giving only as much of the drug as required to alleviate undesirable symptoms, and repeat as necessary, gradually increasing the dose depending on need. Check blood pressure every 5 minutes. (3) Vasoconstriction-induced tissue sloughing can occur. Avoid administering in areas of limited blood supply (e.g., fingers, toes) or if peripheral vascular disease is present. (4) Deteriorates rapidly. Protect from light. Do not use if brown in color or if a sediment is present. (5) Check the label. Not all epinephrine solutions can be given IV. (6) Intracardiac injection or IV injection in cardiac arrest must be accompanied by cardiac massage to perfuse drug into the myocardium and permit effective defibrillation. (7) Use caution in elderly people, diabetics, in hypotension (except in anaphylactic shock), patients receiving thyroid preparations, and those with long-term emphysema or bronchial asthma. (8) *May be used alternately with isoproterenol (Isuprel), but they may not be used together.* Both are direct cardiac stimulants and death will result. An adequate interval between doses must be maintained. (9) Simultaneous use with oxytocics (e.g., ergonovine), MAO inhibitors (e.g., pargyline [Eutonyl]), or furazolidone (Furoxone) may cause hypertensive crisis; with propranolol (Inderal) will cause hypertension. (10) Potentiated by anesthetics (e.g., halothane, cyclopropane), tricyclic antidepressants, antihistamines, sodium levothyroxine, and urinary alkalizers. (11) Antagonized by β-adrenergic blockers (e.g., propranolol [Inderal]) and α-adrenergic blockers (e.g., phentolamine [Regitine]). (12) Inhibited by ergot alkaloids and phenothiazines (e.g., prochlorperazine [Compazine]). (13) Inhibits insulin and oral hypoglycemic agents; increased dose may be required. (14) Interacts with many other drugs. (15) Often used with corticosteroids in treatment of anaphylactic shock.

Contraindications: Anesthesia with inhalant anesthetics (e.g., chloroform, trichloroethylene, cyclopropane), cerebral arteriosclerosis, hypertension, during labor, hyperthyroidism, narrow-angle glaucoma, nervous instability, organic brain damage, patients receiving digitalis, shock. Do not use to treat overdosage of adrenergic blocking agents (e.g., phenoxybenzamine [Dibenzyline]), phenothiazines (e.g., chlorpromazine [Thorazine]), methotrimeprazine (Levoprome); a further drop in blood pressure will occur and irreversible shock may result.

Incompatible with: Any other drug in a syringe. Readily destroyed by alkalis, alkaline solutions, and oxidizing agents. Unstable in any solution with a pH over 5.5, aminophylline, cephapirin (Cephadyl), mephentermine (Wyamine), sodium bicarbonate, warfarin (Coumadin).

Side effects: Often transitory and sometimes occur with average doses.

Average dose: Anxiety, dizziness, dyspnea, glycosuria, pallor, palpitations.

Overdose (frequently caused by too-rapid injection): Cerebrovascular hemorrhage, collapse (rapid), fibrillation, headache (severe), hypertension, hypotension (irreversible), pulmonary edema, pupillary dilation, restlessness, tachycardia, weakness, death.

Antidote: If side effects from the average dose become progressively worse, discontinue the drug and notify the physician. IM or SC route may be preferable. For a severe reaction caused by toxicity, treat the patient for shock and administer an antihypertensive agent such as phentolamine (Regitine) or nitroprusside (Nipride). Treat cardiac dysrhythmias with a β-adrenergic blocker (propranolol [Inderal]). Resuscitate as necessary.

EPOETIN ALFA pH 6.6 to 7.2

(Epogen, Erythropoietin, EPO, Procrit)

Usual dose: *Anemia of chronic renal failure:* 50 to 100 units/kg of body weight 3 times a week. Median dose is 75 units/kg. A 55 kg (120 lb) individual would receive 2,750 units at 50 units/kg, 4,125 units at 75 units/kg, and 5,500 units at 100 units/kg. Larger doses may be required especially in dialysis patients (see literature). Reduce dose by 25 units/kg when the hematocrit reaches the target range (30% to 33%) or rises more than 4 points in any 2-week period.

Increase dose by 25 μ/kg if the hematocrit does not increase by 5 to 6 points after 8 weeks of therapy and is below target range.

Maintenance dose: Individually titrated. After reaching target range, reduce by 25 units/kg. Adjust dose by 25 units/kg increments at 2- to 6-week intervals to keep hematocrit in target range.

Zidovudine-induced anemia in HIV infected patients: 100 units/kg 3 times a week for 8 weeks. Obtain endogenous serum erythropoietin level (prior to transfusion) before initiating therapy (see Precautions). After 8 weeks of therapy, the dose may be increased by 50 to 100 units/kg 3 times a week (total dose of 150 to 200 units/kg). Evaluate response every 4 to 8 weeks and adjust dose accordingly by 50 to 100 units/kg (total dose of 200 to 300 units/kg). Not likely to be effective if doses of 300 units/kg 3 times a week have not corrected the anemia.

Maintenance dose: When desired response is attained (i.e., reduced transfusion requirements or increased hematocrit) titrate dose to maintain the response. Consider variations in zidovudine (AZT) dose and presence of infectious or inflammatory episodes. If the hematocrit exceeds 40%, discontinue until the hematocrit drops to 36%. Reduce dose by 25% when treatment is resumed and titrate carefully to maintain desired hematocrit.

In all situations dosage based on average weight if edema is present. Rate of hematocrit increase is dose dependent and varies between patients. Availability of iron stores, baseline hematocrit, and concurrent medical problems affect the rate and extent of response.

Dilution: May be given undiluted as an IV bolus. Do not shake during preparation; will render it biologically inactive. Use only 1 dose per vial. Do not reenter vial. Discard unused portions.

Rate of administration: A single dose over at least 1 minute.

Actions: An amino acid glycoprotein manufactured by recombinant DNA technology. Has the same biological effects as erythropoietin produced naturally by the kidneys. Stimulates bone marrow to produce red blood cells; increasing the reticulocyte count within 10 days and the red cell count, hemoglobin, and hematocrit within 2 to 6 weeks. Normal iron stores are necessary because it steps up red blood cell production to a rate above what the body usually makes. New cells need iron, which is quickly depleted. Detectable levels remain in plasma for up to 24 hours. Continued therapy will maintain improved red blood cell levels and decrease need for transfusions. Within 2 months most patients are transfusion independent. Considered replacement therapy as insulin is to diabetics.

Indications and uses: (1) To treat anemia associated with chronic renal failure and decrease the need for transfusions in patients receiving dialysis (end-stage renal disease) and those not receiving dialysis; (2) treatment of zidovudine (AZT, Retrovir)-induced anemias in HIV-infected patients.

Investigational uses: Other drug-induced anemias; to increase potential for procurement in individuals who choose autologous blood transfusions before elective surgery; rheumatoid arthritis and other chronic inflammatory diseases; and sickle cell anemia.

Precautions: (1) May be given IV or SC in patients not receiving dialysis. May be given to dialysis patients into the venous line at the end of the dialysis procedure to eliminate additional venous access. (2) Hypertension must be controlled before initiation of therapy. Monitor blood pressure frequently and control aggressively; generally rises when hematocrit is increasing rapidly. 25% of renal patients require an increase in antihypertensive therapy and dietary restrictions. Exacerbation of hypertension has not been observed in zidovudine (AZT)-treated HIV-infected patients receiving epoetin alfa (Procrit); however, any indication may require a decrease in dose of epoetin if blood pressure difficult to control or withhold epoetin until blood pressure is controlled. (3) CBC with differential and platelet counts; BUN; uric acid; creatinine; phosphorus; and potassium are required before treatment is initiated and at regular intervals during therapy. Modest increases are expected. Changes in dialysis treatment may be required. (4) Can cause polycythemia. Baseline hematocrit required. Repeat twice weekly until stabilization in the target range (30% to 33%). Continue monitoring at regular intervals. After any dose adjustment, twice-weekly hematocrit is required for 2 to 6 weeks to evaluate outcome and make further dose adjustments. If hematocrit exceeds 36%, withhold doses and check hematocrit twice weekly until it reaches 33%. Reduce dose as indicated in Usual dose. (5) Normal iron stores required to support epoetin-stimulated erythropoiesis. Transferrin saturation should be at least 20% and ferritin at least 100 ng/ml. Monitor before and during therapy. Supplemental iron (ferrous sulfate 325 mg orally 3 times a day) is usually required to increase and maintain transferrin saturation. (6) Seizures rare, but more occur in the first 90 days. Observe blood pressure and neurological symptoms. Caution against driving or operating heavy machinery. (7) Dialysis patients may require additional anticoagulation with heparin to prevent clotting of artificial kidney or clotting of the vascular access (AV shunt) and to maintain efficiency of the dialysis procedure. (8) Monitor patients with preexisting vascular disease carefully; increase in hematocrit may precipitate a cerebrovascular accident, transient ischemic attack, or myocardial infarction. (9) Compliance with dialysis and/or dietary restrictions is mandatory. (10) Monitor fluid and electrolyte balance carefully in patients not receiving dialysis. Improved sense of well-being may mask need for dialysis. (11) Effectiveness in HIV-infected patients seems to be dependent on an endogenous serum erythropoietin level less than 500 mU/ml (normal levels are 4 to 26 mU/ml) and a dose of zidovudine (AZT, Retrovir) of less than 4,200 mg/wk. (12) In addition to low baseline hematocrit and inadequate iron stores, delayed or diminished response may result from concurrent medical problems (infections, inflammatory or malignant processes, occult blood loss, underlying hematological disease, folic acid or vitamin B_{12} deficiency, hemolysis, aluminum intoxication, osteitis fibrosa cystica). (13) Not intended for use in anemias caused by iron or folate deficiencies, hemolysis, or gastrointestinal bleeding. (14) As anemia is corrected, elevated bleeding time decreases toward normal with epoetin treatment as it does with transfusion. (15) Use with caution in patients with porphyria; may exacerbate disease. (16) Not a substitute for emergency transfusion in patients requiring immediate correction of severe anemia. (17) May present risk to fetus; use only if benefit justifies risk during pregnancy. (18) Menses may resume; possibility of pregnancy. Contraception may be indicated. (19) Use caution in nursing mothers. (20) Safety for use in children not established.

Contraindications: Known hypersensitivity to albumin (human) or to mammalian cell–derived products, uncontrolled hypertension.

Incompatible with: Any other drug in syringe or solution because of specific use and manufacturer's recommendation.

Side effects: Generally well tolerated. Increased hypertension is common, and hypertensive encephalopathy and seizures can occur. Clotted vascular access (AV shunt) and clotting of the artificial kidney may occur during dialysis. Too-rapid increase in hematocrit (over 4 points in 2 weeks) or a hematocrit over 36% (polycythemia) often occurs.

Reported side effects are those common to chronic renal failure, HIV infection, or zidovudine, and not necessarily attributable to epoetin and include: allergic reactions, arthralgias, asthenia, bone marrow fibrosis, cerebrovascular accident or transient ischemic attack, chest pain, cough, CVA/TIA, diarrhea, dizziness, edema, fatigue, fever, headache, hyperkalemia, myocardial infarction, nausea, rash, respiratory congestion, shortness of breath, tachycardia, and vomiting.

Antidote: Notify physician of all side effects; most will be treated symptomatically. Excessive hypertension may require discontinuation of epoetin until blood pressure is controlled or may respond to reduction in dose of epoetin or to an increase in antihypertensive therapy. Reduce dose of epeotin in patients with an increase in hematocrit over 4 points in 2 weeks or any patient with a hematocrit over 36% to 40% depending on reason for administration. May need to withhold epoetin until hematocrit falls to 33%. Additional heparin may be required during dialysis to prevent clotting. Treat minor allergic reactions symptomatically. Discontinue drug and treat anaphylaxis as indicated; resuscitate as necessary.

ERGONOVINE MALEATE pH 2.7 to 3.5

(Ergotrate Maleate)

Usual dose: 1 ml (0.2 mg or gr 1/300). Repeat in 2 to 4 hours if necessary.

Investigational use: 0.05 to 0.2 IV during coronary angiography (see Precautions).

Dilution: May be given undiluted. Do not add to IV solutions. Give through Y-tube or three-way stopcock of infusion set.

Rate of administration: 0.2 mg or fraction thereof over 1 minute.

Actions: An oxytocic, it exerts a direct stimulation on the smooth muscle of the uterus, causing contraction of the uterus itself and vasoconstriction of uterine vessels. In therapeutic doses the prolonged initial contraction is followed by periods of relaxation and contraction. Effective within 1 minute for up to 3 hours. The least toxic of the ergot derivatives, it is probably detoxified in the liver and excreted in bile and urine.

Indications and uses: Prevents or controls postpartum or postabortal hemorrhage.

Investigational use: Diagnosis of Prinzmetal's angina.

Precautions: (1) Not recommended for use before the delivery of the placenta. (2) IV administration is for emergency use only. IM or oral route is preferred and should be used after the initial IV dose. (3) Monitor blood pressure. (4) Uterine response may be poor in calcium-deficient patients and will require calcium replacement for effective response. (5) Should be refrigerated; may not be stored at room temperature more than 60 days. (6) Check expiration date on vial. Ergonovine deteriorates with age. (7) Severe hypertension and cerebrovascular accidents can result in the presence of regional anesthesia (caudal or spinal) and with ephedrine, epinephrine, methoxamine (Vasoxyl), and other vasopressors. Chlorpromazine (Thorazine) IV will reduce this hypertension. (8) Use caution in patients with cardiac, renal, or liver disease and in febrile or septic states. (9) Potentiated by nitrates. (10) Simulates spontaneous coronary arterial spasms responsible for Prinzmetal's angina when injected during coronary arteriography. These spasms are reversible with nitroglycerin. This use has precipitated dysrhythmias including ventricular tachycardia and myocardial infarction.

Contraindications: Known hypersensitivity to ergot alkaloids, pregnancy before the third stage of labor.

Incompatible with: Amobarbital (Amytal), ampicillin (Polycillin), cephalothin (Keflin), chloramphenicol (Chloromycetin), chlortetracycline (Aureomycin), epinephrine (Adrenalin), heparin, methicillin (Staphcillin), pentobarbital (Nembutal), thiopental (Pentothal), warfarin (Coumadin).

Side effects: Rare in therapeutic doses, but may include the following.

Average dose: Allergic phenomena, blindness, confusion, diarrhea, dilated pupils, dizziness, headache, hypertension, hypotension, nausea, numb and/or cold extremities, vomiting, weakness.

Overdose: Abortion, convulsions, excitement, gangrene, hypercoagulability, shock, tachycardia, thirst, tremor, uterine bleeding.

Antidote: Discontinue the drug immediately at the onset of any side effect and notify the physician. Most side effects are transient unless there is severe toxicity and will be treated symptomatically. Severe poisoning is treated with vasodilator drugs, sedatives, calcium gluconate to relieve muscular pain, and other supportive treatment. Heparin is used to control hypercoagulability.

ERYTHROMYCIN LACTOBIONATE

pH 6.5 to 7.7

(Erythrocin IV)

Usual dose: 15 to 20 mg/kg of body weight/24 hr in divided doses every 6 hours or preferably in a continuous infusion. Up to 4 Gm/24 hr has been given.

Pediatric dose: 10 to 20 mg/kg of body weight/24 hr in divided doses every 6 hours is recommended.

Dilution: Each 500 mg or fraction thereof must be diluted with 10 ml of sterile water for injection without preservatives to form a 5% solution and avoid precipitation. To administer direct IV, further dilute in 80 to 250 ml of a compatible IV fluid (normal saline, lactated Ringer's solution, or Normosol-R). Add sodium bicarbonate (Neut) 1 ml if final dilution is less than 250 ml. Administer with a volume control set. Most often further diluted to 1 mg/ml in above infusion solutions or dextrose in water or saline and given as a continuous infusion. Shake well to ensure dilution.

Rate of administration: 1 Gm or fraction thereof in at least 100 ml over 20 to 60 minutes. Slow infusion rate for pain along injection site. IV infusion of a 0.1% to 0.2% solution by continuous drip over 6 hours is preferable.

Actions: Macrolide antibiotic, bactericidal and bacteriostatic, used as a substitute for penicillin or tetracyclines. Effective against a number of gram-positive and some gram-negative organisms. Very effective against penicillin-resistant staphylococci. Well distributed in body fluids, except for spinal fluid. Excreted in urine and bile. Crosses placental barrier. Secreted in breast milk.

Indications and uses: (1) Staphylococci, pneumococci, and streptococci infections; (2) prophylaxis against endocarditis preoperatively in patients with a history of rheumatic fever or congenital heart disease; (3) gonorrhea; (4) syphilis in penicillin-sensitive patients; (5) active diphtheria in conjunction with antitoxin; (6) Legionnaires' disease.

Precautions: (1) Sensitivity studies indicated to determine susceptibility of the causative organism to erythromycin. (2) Begin oral therapy as soon as practical. (3) Superinfection caused by overgrowth of nonsusceptible organisms is rare unless this drug is given in combination with other antibacterial agents. (4) Not stable if final pH less than 5.5. Give within 4 hours or use 1 ml sodium bicarbonate (Neut) to 100 ml solution to stabilize. (5) Use caution in impaired liver function, pregnancy, and lactation. (6) Refrigerate after dilution. Maintains potency for up to 7 days. (7) Antagonized by clindamycin and lincomycin. (8) Inhibits penicillins. (9) Will increase serum levels of cyclosporine, digoxin, methylprednisolone, theophyllines, and warfarin.

Contraindication: Known erythromycin sensitivity.

Incompatible with: Do not add any drug to solution unless effects on chemical and physical stability are determined. Amikacin (Amikin), aminophylline, ascorbic acid, carbenicillin (Geopen), cephalothin (Keflin), cephapirin (Cefadyl), chloramphenicol (Chloromycetin), colistimethate (Coly-Mycin M), heparin, lincomycin (Lincocin), metaraminol (Aramine), metoclopramide (Reglan), pentobarbital (Nembutal), phenobarbital (Luminal), phenytoin (Dilantin), prochlorperazine (Compazine), secobarbital (Seconal), sodium chloride solutions until after initial dilution, sodium salts, tetracycline (Achromycin), thiopental (Pentothal), vancomycin (Vancocin), vitamin B complex with C, warfarin (Coumadin).

Side effects: Relatively free from side effects when given as directed. Urticaria and mild local venous discomfort. Increased incidence of reversible ototoxicity with larger doses. Anaphylaxis may occur.

Antidote: Notify the physician of early or mild symptoms. For severe symptoms, discontinue the drug, treat allergic reactions, or resuscitate as necessary and notify physician.

ESMOLOL HYDROCHLORIDE pH 3.5 to 5.5

(Brevibloc)

Usual dose: 100 mcg/kg of body weight/min is an average dose. Range is 50 to 200 mcg/kg/min. Dosage must be individualized by titration. Each step in the process consists of a loading dose followed by a maintenance dose. Begin with a loading dose of 500 mcg/kg/min for 1 minute only. Follow with a maintenance infusion of 50 mcg/kg/min for 4 minutes. If desired therapeutic effect does not occur in the next 5 minutes, repeat the loading dose and increase the maintenance infusion to 100 mcg/kg/min. Continue this two-step process by repeating the same loading dose while increasing the maintenance infusion by 50 mcg/kg/min. As the desired heart rate is approached or a safety end-point (falling blood pressure) occurs, omit the loading dose and reduce the maintenance dose from 50 mcg/kg/min to 25 mcg/kg/min or lower. Interval between titration steps may be increased from 5 to 10 minutes if desired. Hypotension is common and is dose related. Doses greater than 200 mcg/kg/min are not recommended.

Dilution: 5 Gm (two 10 ml ampoules) must be initially diluted with 20 ml of one of the following solutions (withdraw from the 500 ml bottle): 5% dextrose in water, 5% dextrose in Ringer's injection, 5% dextrose in 0.9% or 0.45% sodium chloride, lactated Ringer's injection, 0.9% or 0.45% sodium chloride. Must be further diluted in the remaining 480 ml of the same solution and given as an infusion. (Final dilution is 10 mg/ml.)

Rate of administration: Titrate infusion according to procedure outlined in Usual dose.

Actions: A β-adrenergic blocker with antiarrhythmic effects. Decreases heart rate and blood pressure in a dose-related titratable manner. Hemodynamically similar to propranolol, but vascular resistance is not increased. Onset of action occurs within 1 to 2 minutes and lasts about 20 to 30 minutes. Metabolized in the liver. Some excreted in the urine.

Indications and uses: (1) Management of supraventricular tachycardia (atrial fibrillation or atrial flutter) in situations requiring short-term control of ventricular rate with a short-acting agent (perioperative, postoperative, or other emergent circumstances); (2) management of noncompensatory tachycardia when heart rate requires specific intervention.

Precautions: (1) Continuous observation of the patient and ECG and blood pressure monitoring are mandatory during administration. Hypotension should reverse within 30 minutes after decreasing the infusion rate or discontinuing the drug. (2) Well tolerated if administered through a central vein. Incidence of inflammation or thrombophlebitis increases with dilutions greater than 10 mg/ml. (3) Intended for short-term use only. Transfer to an alternative antiarrhythmic agent (e.g., propranolol [Inderal], digoxin [Lanoxin], verapamil [Calan]) is required after stable clinical status and heart rate control are obtained. Thirty minutes after first dose of alternative agent reduce dose of esmolol by 50%. Monitor patient carefully. One hour after the second dose of alternative agent discontinue esmolol infusion if condition remains satisfactory. (4) Stable at room temperature for 24 hours. (5) Potentiates digoxin blood levels. (6) IV morphine increases esmolol steady-state levels by 46%. (7) While it has not been a problem with esmolol, it is recommended that the dose of β-adrenergic blockers be reduced gradually to avoid rebound angina, myocardial infarction, or ventricular dysrhythmias. Use caution. (8) β-Adrenergic blockers antagonize antihistamines, antiinflammatory agents, isoproterenol (Isuprel), ritodrine, and others. (9) β-Blockers are potentiated by general anesthetics, cimetidine (Tagamet), furosemide, phenothiazines (e.g., promethazine [Phenergan]), phenytoin (Dilantin), and urethane. Death can occur. (10) β-Blockers potentiate antidiabetics, barbiturates, catecholamine-depleting drugs (e.g., reserpine), insulin, lidocaine, narcotics, mus cle relaxants, theophyllines, and thyroid agents; dosage adjustment may be required. Increased CNS depression may cause death. (11) Use with extreme caution in asthmatics, diabetics, or patients with a history of hypoglycemia. May cause hypoglycemia and mask the symptoms. (12) Epinephrine concurrently is contraindicated. (13) Use with clonidine may precipitate acute hypertension. (14) Use with verapamil may potentiate both drugs and result in severe depression of myocardium and AV conduction. (15) May cause severe bradycardia in patients with Wolff-Parkinson-White syndrome. (16) May aggravate rebound hypertension if clonidine stopped abruptly. (17) Safety for use in pregnant and lactating women and in children not established. Use only when clearly indicated.

Contraindications: Not intended for use in chronic settings when transfer to another agent is anticipated. Bradycardia; cardiogenic shock; congestive heart failure not secondary to a tachycardia responsive to β-adrenergic blockers; overt cardiac failure; second- or third-degree heart block.

Incompatible with: Furosemide (Lasix), sodium bicarbonate. Manufacturer recommends not mixing with any other drug before full dilution in a compatible infusion solution.

Side effects: Hypotension and inflammation or induration of the infusion site are the major side effects. Asthenia, confusion, fever, flushing, lightheadedness, midscapular pain, pallor, paresthesia, rhonchi, somnolence, speech disorders, taste disorders, and urinary retention have occurred. One grand mal seizure has been reported.

Antidote: Notify the physician of all side effects. Decrease rate or discontinue drug if hypotension occurs. Notify physician immediately. Hypotension should reverse within 30 minutes. Trendelenburg position may be appropriate. May require treatment with IV fluids or vasopressors (e.g., dopamine [Intropin], norepinephrine [Levarterenol]) but protracted severe hypotension may result. Use atropine for bradycardia, digitalis and diuretics for cardiac failure. Treat other side effects symptomatically and resuscitate as necessary.

ETHACRYNIC ACID pH 6.3 to 7.7

(✱ Edecrin, Sodium Edecrin)

Usual dose: 0.5 to 1 mg/kg of body weight. 50 mg for average adult. Do not exceed 100 mg in a single dose.

Pediatric dose: 1 mg/kg of body weight. Do not exceed adult dose.

Dilution: Add 50 ml sodium chloride injection to reconstitute, 5% dextrose may be used if pH is adjusted upward; without adjustment of pH, solution will be hazy, do not use. Do not add to IV solutions. May be injected through Y-tube or three-way stopcock of infusion set.

Rate of administration: Each 10 mg or fraction thereof (approximately 10 ml) may be given over 1 minute. Infusion of total dose over 30 minutes is preferred.

Actions: A saluretic-diuretic agent. Extremely potent and has a rapid onset of action. Effectiveness is noted within 5 to 10 minutes; peak effect noted in 1 to 2 hours after administration and may last for 8 hours. Has a mild hypotensive effect. Apparently acts on the proximal and distal ends of the tubule and the ascending limb of the loop of Henle to excrete sodium, chlorides, and potassium. Will produce diuresis in alkalosis or acidosis. Rapidly absorbed and distributed, it is excreted in the urine.

Indications and uses: (1) Congestive heart failure; (2) acute pulmonary edema; (3) renal edema; (4) hepatic cirrhosis with ascites; (5) nephrotic syndrome in children; (6) edema unresponsive to other diuretic agents; (7) ascites due to malignancy; (8) short-term management of hospitalized pediatric patients with congenital heart disease.

Precautions: (1) For IV use only. (2) Use a new injection site for each dose to avoid thrombophlebitis. (3) May precipitate excessive diuresis with water and electrolyte depletion. (4) Routine checks on electrolyte panel, CO_2, and BUN are necessary during therapy. Potassium chloride replacement may be required. (5) Do not give simultaneously with whole blood or its derivatives. (6) Use only clear, colorless solutions. Discard reconstituted solution after 24 hours. (7) Use caution in patients with advanced cirrhosis of the liver, electrolyte imbalance, or hepatic encephalopathy. (8) May precipitate an acute attack of gout. (9) Has caused permanent deafness when given in conjunction with other ototoxic drugs (e.g., cisplatin, dihydrostreptomycin, gentamicin). (10) Potentiates antihypertensive drugs, oral antidiabetics, oral anticoagulants, some muscle relaxants (e.g., curare, tubocurarine), and tetracyclines. (11) Inhibited by indomethacin (Indocin). (12) May cause cardiac dysrhythmias with digitalis or furosemide (Lasix). (13) Not recommended for use in children except for specialized indications.

Contraindications: Anuria; infants; pregnancy and lactation; severe, progressive renal disease with increasing azotemia and oliguria; severe watery diarrhea; women during childbearing years.

Incompatible with: Any other drug in a syringe, whole blood and its derivatives, drugs and solutions with pH below 5.0, hydralazine (Apresoline), Normosol-M, procainamide (Pronestyl), reserpine, tolazine (Priscoline), triflupromazine (Vesprin).

Side effects: Usually occur with prolonged therapy or in seriously ill patients.

Minor: Anorexia, deafness (transient), dysphagia, hyperglycemia, hyperuricemia, hypokalemia, hypochloremic alkalosis, muscle cramps, nausea, thirst, vomiting, weakness.

Major: Acute necrotizing panacreatitis, blood volume reduction, circulatory collapse, deafness (permanent), dehydration, diarrhea (watery), embolism, hepatic coma, hypokalemia (severe), vascular thrombosis, death.

Antidote: If minor side effects are noted, discontinue the drug and notify the physician, who may treat the side effects symptomatically and continue the drug. If side effects are progressive or any major side effect occurs, discontinue the drug immediately and notify the physician. Treatment of major side effects is symptomatic and aggressive. Resuscitate as necessary.

ETIDRONATE DISODIUM pH 4.0 to 5.5

(Didronel IV)

Usual dose: 7.5 mg/kg of body weight/24 hr daily for 3 days. In selected situations, patients have been treated for 7 days during the first course of therapy. If hypercalcemia recurs, a second course of therapy limited to 3 days may be given. Begin at least 7 days after completion of first course. The day after the last infusion, begin follow-up treatment with oral etidronate 20 mg/kg/day. Usually continues for 30 days but may be extended up to 90 days if serum calcium levels remain normal or within clinically acceptable parameters. Normal renal function required.

Dilution: Must be diluted in 250 ml or more of normal saline and given as an infusion.

Rate of administration: 250 ml of diluted solution over a minimum of 2 hours. Extend infusion time if larger amounts of fluid are used.

Actions: Reduces normal and abnormal bone resorption and bone formation. Does not appear to alter renal tubular absorption of calcium. Not effective in hyperparathyroidism where increased calcium resorption may contribute to the cause of hypercalcemia. In hypercalcemia of malignancy the renal tubules become less able to concentrate urine, and this reduces the ability of the kidneys to eliminate excess calcium. By inhibiting excess bone resorption, etidronate interrupts this process. Not metabolized. Within 24 hours about one half of this drug is chemically absorbed to bone and the remainder is excreted in the urine. Half-life in bone is 3 to 6 months.

Indications and uses: (1) Hypercalcemia of malignancy inadequately managed by dietary modification or oral hydration or persisting after adequate hydration has been restored; (2) oral form has other uses.

Precautions: (1) Carefully assess renal status and reduce dose in renal impairment (see Contraindications). (2) Diluted solution stable at room temperature for 48 hours. (3) Increased risk of hypocalcemia in patients treated over 3 days IV. (4) Monitor total serum calcium and renal function with serum creatinine or BUN. (5) Must be adequately hydrated and have adequate urine output. Pretreatment and simultaneous treatment with IV saline and loop diuretics (furosemide [Lasix], ethacrynic acid [Edecrin], or bumetanide [Bumex]) is recommended and will increase calcium excretion. Rate of renal calcium excretion is directly related to renal sodium excretion. (6) Avoid overhydration in the elderly and in cardiac failure. (7) Safety for use in pregnancy or lactation not established. Use only when clearly indicated. (8) Safety for use in children not established. (9) Renal toxicity may be potentiated by nephrotoxic drugs (e.g., aminoglycosides [gentamicin]), ethacrynic acid (Edecrin). (10) Maintain adequate nutrition including calcium and vitamin D. (11) Use caution in patients with enterocolitis. (12) Delay treatment in patients with fractures until callus is evident (especially fractures of long bones). (13) Hypercalcemia of hyperparathyroidism may coexist in patients with malignancy. Etidronate will probably not be effective.

Contraindications: Known hypersensitivity, serum creatinine greater than 5 mg/dl.

Incompatible with: Specific information not available. Consider specific use and required dilution in normal saline.

Side effects: Diarrhea, elevated serum creatinine and BUN, hypersensitivity reactions (angioedema, pruritus, rash, urticaria), hypocalcemia, loss of taste or metallic taste (temporary), nausea, renal insufficiency. Bleeding and ECG changes have occurred in animals with too-rapid injection or excessive doses (27 mg/kg).

Antidote: Notify the physician of any side effect. May respond to symptomatic treatment or to decrease in rate of infusion, or dose may be divided and given every 12 hours. Hypocalcemia is rare but can be treated with IV calcium gluconate. Treatment is symptomatic and supportive. Resuscitate as necessary.

ETOPOSIDE pH 3.0 to 4.0

(VePesid, VP-16-213)

Usual dose: *Testicular cancer:* 50 to 100 mg/M^2 daily for 5 days or 100 mg/M^2/day on days 1, 3, and 5. Repeat at 3- to 4-week intervals.

Small cell lung cancer: 35 mg/M^2/day for 4 days to 50 mg/M^2/day for 5 days. Repeat at 3- to 4-week intervals.

Modify dose if indicated based on myelosuppressive effects of other drugs administered in combination, and any previous radiation therapy or chemotherapy (compromised bone marrow reserve). Frequently given in combination with cisplatin, bleomycin, and doxorubicin. Dosage based on average weight in presence of ascites or edema.

Dilution: *Specific techniques required, see Precautions.* Each 100 mg (5 ml) must be diluted in at least 250 ml of 5% dextrose in water or normal saline and given as an infusion (0.4 mg/ml). 500 ml of solution may be used to yield 0.2 mg/ml. Monitor closely for precipitation from dilution to completion of infusion.

Rate of administration: Total desired dose, properly diluted (0.2 to 0.4 mg/ml) and evenly distributed over at least 30 to 60 minutes. Rapid infusion may cause marked hypotension.

Actions: A semisynthetic derivative of podophyllotoxin. Cell cycle specific for the G_2 phase, it inhibits DNA synthesis. Half-life is from 3 to 12 hours. Primarily excreted through urine and feces.

Indications and uses: To suppress or retard neoplastic growth in (1) refractory testicular tumors (used in combination with other agents after previous surgery, chemotherapy, and radiotherapy); (2) small cell lung cancer (used in combination with other chemotherapeutic agents as first-line treatment).

Unlabeled uses: Treatment of acute nonlymphocytic leukemias, Hodgkin's disease, non-Hodgkin's lymphomas, carcinoma of the breast, Kaposi's sarcoma, and neuroblastoma. Additional tumors have shown up to 20% response. Used alone or in combination with other agents.

Precautions: (1) Follow guidelines for handling cytotoxic agents. See Appendix, p. 677. (2) Administered by or under the direction of the physician specialist. (3) Stable after dilution at room temperature for at least 48 hours. (4) Determine absolute patency and quality of vein and adequate circulation of extremity. Avoid extravasation. (5) Use caution to prevent bone marrow depression. Platelet count, hemoglobin, white blood cell count, and differential must be completed before start of therapy and before each dose. Withhold therapy if platelets less than 50,000/mm^3 or absolute neutrophil count less than 500/mm^3. Do not restart until adequate recovery. Monitor between courses also. (6) Bone marrow recovery from a course is usually complete within 20 days. No cumulative toxicity has been reported as yet. (7) Carcinogenic; wear gloves, wash skin or mucosa thoroughly and immediately with soap and water after accidental contact. (8) Teratogenic and embryocidal in rats, must be given with caution in men and women capable of conception. Discontinue breast feeding. (9) Do not administer any vaccine or chloroquine to patients receiving antineoplastic drugs. (10) May potentiate warfarin with concomitant use of vindesine. (11) Be alert for signs of bone marrow depression or infection. (12) Maintain adequate hydration. (13) Prophylactic antiemetics may increase patient comfort. (14) Safety and effectiveness for use in children not established.

Contraindications: Hypersensitivity to etoposide or its components.

Incompatible with: All solutions except normal saline or dextrose in water. Consider incompatible with any other drug in syringe or solution because of toxicity and specific use.

Side effects: Usually reversible: alopecia, anaphylactic reactions (bronchospasm, chills, dyspnea, fever, hypotension), anorexia, diarrhea, hypotension, leukopenia (severe), nausea, neuritic pain, oral lacerations, paralytic ileus, peripheral neuropathy, stomatitis, thrombocytopenia (severe), thrombophlebitis, vomiting.

Antidote: Notify the physician of all side effects; symptomatic treatment is often indicated. For extravasation, discontinue the drug immediately and administer into another vein. Consider injection of long-acting dexamethasone (Decadron LA) throughout extravasated tissue. Use a 27- or 25-gauge needle. Elevate extremity, moist heat may be helpful. Hypotension is usually due to a rapid infusion rate. Discontinue infusion. Trendelenburg position and IV fluids should reverse the hypotension; vasopressors (e.g., dopamine [Intropin]) may be required. After recovery, restart at slower rate. Discontinue infusion at first sign of allergic reaction; resuscitate as necessary.

FACTOR IX COMPLEX (HUMAN) pH 7.0 to 7.4

(AlphaNine, Konyne HT, Profinine HT, Proplex T)

Usual dose: Completely individualized based on patient's circumstances, condition, degree of deficiency, and desired blood level percentage. Range is 10 to 60 IU/kg of body weight. May be repeated every 12 hours in some situations, required only every 2 or 3 days in others. Actual number of international units contained shown on each bottle or vial. Units required to raise blood level percentages can be calculated as follows: body weight (kg) × desired increase (% of normal) × 1 unit/kg (70 kg × 40% increase × 1 IU/kg equals 2800 IU]). To maintain levels above 25% calculate each dose to raise level to 40% to 60% of normal.

Minor hemorrhage: a single injection calculated to increase plasma level by 20% to 30%.

Major trauma or surgery: increase plasma level from 25% to 50% and maintain at that level for a minimum of 1 week.

Dental extraction: increase plasma level to 50% before procedure, repeat if indicated.

Reversal of coumarin effect: 15 IU/kg.

Prophylaxis: 10 to 20 IU/kg once or twice a week.

Dilution: Diluent usually provided. Some preparations also supply double-ended needles for dilution and filter needle for aspiration into a syringe. Sterile technique imperative. Confirm expiration date. Factor IX and diluent should be at room temperature. If diluent not provided, use a minimum of 1 ml of sterile water for injection to dilute each 50 units (50 units/ml). This is a maximum concentration for administration, and a more dilute solution is preferred (2 ml of sterile water for injection to dilute each 50 units [25 units/ml]). Direct diluent from above to side of vial to gently moisten all contents. Swirl gently to dissolve, avoid foaming. Do not shake. Should be clear and colorless. Must be used within 3 hours to avoid bacterial contamination. May be given through an IV administration set if multiple vials are required. Discard any unused contents. Discard all administration equipment after single use; do not attempt to resterilize.

Rate of administration: 2 to 3 ml/min. Completely individualized according to patient's condition. Decrease rate of administration for side effects such as chills, fever, flushing, headache, tingling, or changes in blood pressure or pulse. Never exceed 10 ml/min.

Actions: A lyophilized concentrate of human coagulation factors: IX (plasma thromboplastin and antihemophilic factor B, II (prothrombin, VII (proconvertin, X (Stuart-Prower factor). In contrast to older products, AlphaNine is highly purified factor IX and contains only minimal amounts of the other factors. Obtained from fresh human plasma and prepared, irradiated, and dried by a specific process. An additional solvent suspension process is used to prepare AlphaNine. Concentration of 25 units/1 ml is 25 times greater than normal plasma. Also contains total protein in each vial.

Indications and uses: (1) Prevention and control of bleeding in patients with Factor IX deficiency due to hemophilia B. May be required to correct or prevent a dangerous bleeding episode or to perform surgery. Proplex may be used for bleeding episodes in patients with inhibitors to factor VIII. (2) Reversal of coumarin effect. (3) Prophylaxis to prevent spontaneous bleeding in patients with proven specific congenital deficiency (hemophilia B).

Precautions: (1) Used when plasma infusions would result in hypervolemia and/or proteinemia or when blood volume or red blood cell replacement is not indicated.

(2) Monitor the patient's levels of coagulation factors before, after, and between administrations. *Do not overdose.* (see Side effects). (3) Use extreme caution in newborns, infants, and patients with liver disease. AlphaNine would be preferred since studies show no incidence of thrombin generation. (4) AIDS or hepatitis are possible for the recipient. Health professionals should exercise caution in handling. Possibility reduced with additional preparation process of AlphaNine. (5) Observe for signs and symptoms of postoperative thrombosis or DIC. Except for AlphaNine, risk multiplies with repeated administrations. (6) Fresh-frozen plasma may be required in addition to factor IX complex when prompt reversal is required. (7) Safety for use during pregnancy not established, use only if clearly indicated. (8) Store lyophilized powder at 2° to 8° C (36° to 46° F); do not freeze.

Contraindications: Known liver disease with suspicion of intravascular coagulation or fibrinolysis. No known contraindications for AlphaNine.

Incompatible with: All protein precipitants. Sufficient information not available.

Side effects: *Minor:* Changes in blood pressure, chills, fever, flushing, headache, nausea, tingling, urticaria, vomiting.

Major: Anaphylaxis, DIC, hepatitis, myocardial infarction, postoperative thrombosis (except AlphaNine). Consider risk potential of contracting AIDS and hepatitis, reduced with AlphaNine.

Antidote: Temporarily discontinue or decrease rate of administration for minor side effects. If any major symptoms appear, discontinue drug and notify physician. Treat allergic reactions as indicated; a different lot may not cause the reaction. For thrombosis or DIC, anticoagulation with heparin may be indicated.

FAMOTIDINE pH 5.0 to 5.6

(Pepcid IV)

Usual dose: 20 mg (2 ml) every 12 hours. Increase frequency of dose, not amount, if necessary for pain relief.

Dilution: *Direct IV:* Each 20 mg must be diluted with 5 to 10 ml of normal saline or other compatible infusion solutions for injection (e.g., 5% or 10% dextrose in water, lactated Ringer's solution, 5% sodium bicarbonate).

Intermittent infusion: Each 20 mg may be diluted in 100 ml of 5% dextrose in water or other compatible infusion solution and given piggyback.

Rate of administration: *Direct IV:* Each 20 mg or fraction thereof over at least 2 minutes.

Intermittent infusion: Each 20 mg dose over 15 to 30 minutes.

Actions: A histamine H_2 antagonist, it inhibits both daytime and nocturnal basal gastric acid secretion. It also inhibits gastric acid secretion stimulated by food and pentagastrin. Onset of action occurs within 30 minutes and lasts for 10 to 12 hours. No cumulative effect with repeated doses. Eliminated by renal and other metabolic routes. Crosses placental barrier. May be secreted in breast milk.

Indications and uses: Short-term treatment of active duodenal ulcers, active benign gastric ulcers, and pathological hypersecretory conditions in hospitalized patients or in patients unable to take oral medication.

Precautions: (1) Use antacids concomitantly to relieve pain. (2) Gastric malignancy may be present even though patient is asymptomatic. (3) Increase intervals between injections or lower doses to achieve pain relief in impaired renal function. Half-life may exceed 20 hours if creatinine clearance less than 10 ml/min. (4) Stable at room temperature for 48 hours after dilution. (5) Gastric pain and ulceration may recur after medication stopped. (6) Effects maintained with oral dosage. Total treatment usually discontinued after 4 to 8 weeks. (7) No significant drug interactions have been identified as yet. (8) Use during pregnancy only when clearly needed. Advisable to discontinue nursing. (9) Safety for use in children not established.

Contraindications: Known hypersensitivity to famotidine or its components.

Incompatible with: Limited information available. Physically compatible with many drugs for limited time frames; consult pharmacist.

Side effects: Constipation, diarrhea, dizziness, and headache are the most common side effects. Allergic reactions (bronchospasm, fever, pruritus, rash, eosinophilia) can occur. Abdominal discomfort, agitation, alopecia, anorexia, anxiety, arthralgias, confusion, decreased libido, depression, dry mouth, dry skin, elevated SGPT, flushing, grand mal seizure, hallucinations, insomnia, malaise, muscular pain, nausea and vomiting, orbital edema, palpitations, paresthesias, somnolence, taste disorder, thrombocytopenia, and tinnitus have been reported.

Antidote: Notify physician of all side effects. May be treated symptomatically or may respond to decrease in frequency of dosage. Resuscitate as necessary for overdosage. Hemodialysis or peritoneal dialysis may be indicated in overdose.

FENTANYL CITRATE pH 4.0 to 7.5

(Fentanyl, Sublimaze)

Usual dose: *Adjunct to regional anesthesia:* 50 to 100 mcg (0.05 to 0.1 mg).

Low-dose regimen for minor painful surgical procedures: 2 mcg/kg of body weight.

Moderate-dose regimen for major surgical procedures: 2 to 20 mcg/kg.

In all situations, use smallest effective dose at maximum intervals.

Reduce dose to one fourth or one third of usual in patients receiving other CNS depressants, such as narcotic analgesics, general anesthetics, alcohol, anticholinergics, antihistamines, barbiturates, cimetidine (Tagamet), hypnotics, sedatives, and psychotropic agents before, during, and for 24 hours after administration of fentanyl.

Dilution: May be given undiluted by the anesthesiologist. In other situations dilution with at least 5 ml of sterile water or normal saline for injection is preferred to facilitate titration. Other IV solutions may be used. May be given through Y-tube or three-way stopcock of infusion set.

Rate of administration: 0.1 mg or fraction thereof of properly diluted medication over 1 to 2 minutes. Rate must be titrated by desired dose and patient response. If the rate of administration is too slow, delirium and excitement with laryngospasm may occur. If it is too rapid, spasm of the chest wall may completely inhibit respiratory exchange even with a ventilator, and a rapid-acting neuromuscular blocking agent (e.g., succinylcholine [Anectine]) will be required.

Actions: An opium derivative, narcotic analgesic, which is a descending CNS depressant. Approximately 80 times more potent than morphine milligram for milligram. It has definite respiratory depressant actions that outlast its analgesic effect. In healthy individuals, respiratory rate returns to normal more quickly than with other opiates. Effective within one circulation time and lasts about 30 minutes. Effects are cumulative with repeat doses. Has little hypnotic activity, and histamine release rarely occurs. Cardiovascular system remains stable. Depresses many other senses or reflexes. Metabolized in the liver and excreted in the urine. Crosses the placental barrier. Secreted in breast milk.

Indications and uses: (1) Adjunct to general anesthesia when administered by the anesthesiologist; (2) adjunct to regional anesthesia; (3) useful in short-duration minor surgery in outpatients and in diagnostic procedures or treatments that require the patient to be awake or very lightly anesthetized (e.g., bronchoscopy, radiological studies, burn dressings, cystoscopy); (4) prevent or relieve tachypnea and postoperative emergence delirium.

Precautions: (1) Primarily used by or under the direct observation of the anesthesiologist. (2) Oxygen, controlled respiratory equipment, naloxone (Narcan), and neuromuscular blocking agents (e.g., succinylcholine [Anectine]) must always be available. Will cause rigidity of respiratory muscles; may require a muscle relaxant to permit artificial ventilation. (3) Observe patient frequently and monitor vital signs. Patient will appear to be asleep and may forget to breathe unless commanded to do so. Keep patient supine; orthostatic hypotension and fainting may occur. (4) Use caution in the elderly, in patients with impaired hepatic or renal function, and in patients with emphysema; reduced dose may be indicated. (5) Respiratory depression will cause an increased P_{CO_2}, cerebral vasodilation, and increased intracranial pressure. Use extreme caution in craniotomy, head injury, and increased intracranial pressure. (6) May cause apnea in asthmatic patients. (7) Symptoms of acute abdominal conditions may be masked. (8) Use caution in patients with bradyarrhythmias. May increase ventricular response rate in presence of supraventricular tachycardias. (9) Cough reflex is suppressed. (10) A large dose may precipitate seizures in the presence of a history of convulsive disorders. (11) Higher doses may cause prolonged hypotension with diazepam (Valium). (12) Potentiated by phenothiazines (e.g., chlorpromazine [Thorazine]); MAO inhibitors (e.g., isocarboxazid [Marplan]); neuromuscular blocking agents (e.g., tubocurarine); and adrenergic blocking agents (e.g., propranolol [Inderal]). Reduced dosage of both drugs may be indicated. (13) Safety for use in pregnancy not established, has impaired fertility and had embryocidal effects in rats. Postpone breastfeeding for at least 4 to 6 hours after use of fentanyl. (14) Safety for use in children under 2 years not established, has caused methemoglobinemia and hypotension in premature neonates (see Contraindications). (15) Store in refrigerator and protect from light before dilution. Use promptly.

Contraindications: Acute alcoholism, acute bronchial asthma, benign prostatic hypertrophy, biliary tract surgery, diarrhea resulting from poisoning until toxic material is eliminated, hypersensitivity to opiates, premature infants or labor and delivery of premature infants, respiratory depression, surgical anastomosis, upper airway obstruction, patients who are taking or have recently taken MAO inhibitors.

Incompatible with: Diazepam (Valium), methohexitol (Brevitol), pentobarbital (Nembutal), phenytoin (Dilantin), sodium bicarbonate, thiopental (Pentothal). Physically compatible with many other drugs for at least 15 minutes.

Side effects: *Average dose:* Bradycardia, hypersensitivity reactions, hypertension, hypotension, hypothermia, increased intracranial pressure, nausea, orthostatic hypotension, respiratory depression (slight), respiratory muscle rigidity, urinary retention, vomiting.

Overdose: Anaphylaxis, apnea, cardiac arrest, circulatory collapse, coma, excitation, hypotension (severe), inverted T wave on ECG, myocardial depression (severe), pinpoint pupils, respiratory depression (severe), tachycardia, death.

Antidote: With increasing severity of any side effect or onset of symptoms of overdose, discontinue the drug and notify the physician. Naloxone (Narcan) will reverse serious respiratory depression. A patent airway, artificial ventilation, oxygen therapy, and other symptomatic treatment must be instituted promptly. A fast-acting muscle relaxant (e.g., succinylcholine [Anectine]) may be required to facilitate ventilation. Use atropine to treat brachycardia. Resuscitate as necessary.

FENTANYL CITRATE AND DROPERIDOL

pH 3.2 to 3.8

(Innovar)

Usual dose: *Adjunct to regional anesthesia:* 1 to 2 ml. Each milliliter contains 0.5 mg of fentanyl citrate and 2.5 mg of droperidol.

Adjunct to induction of general anesthesia: 0.1 ml/kg of body weight.

After 20 to 30 minutes, supplementary doses of 0.1 mcg/kg of body weight of *fentanyl citrate only* will be required to maintain anesthesia. Increases in pulse rate and blood pressure, sweating, and limb movements are symptoms of sympathetic activity that indicate a need for a supplemental dose.

Reduce dose to one fourth or one third of usual in patients receiving other CNS depressants, such as narcotic analgesics, general anesthetics, alcohol, anticholinergics, antihistamines, barbiturates, cimetidine (Tagamet), hypnotics, sedatives, and psychotropic agents before, during, and for 24 hours after administration of fentanyl and droperidol combination.

Pediatric dose: *Children over 2 years of age as adjunct to induction of general anesthesia:* 0.5 ml/20 lb. 0.25 ml/20 lb is given intramuscularly in most other situations. Decrease dose as above if other CNS depressants have been used.

Dilution: *Adjunct to regional anesthesia:* A single dose may be given undiluted. May be given through Y-tube or three-way stopcock of infusion set.

Adjunct to induction of general anesthesia: 0.1 ml/kg may be diluted with 250 ml of 5% dextrose in water and given as an infusion.

Rate of administration: Each 1 ml of undiluted medication must be given over at least 1 minute. Has been given as an infusion (0.1 ml/kg in 250 ml 5% dextrose in water) administered over 5 to 10 minutes. Rate must be titrated by desired dose and patient response in either situation. If the rate of administration is too slow, delirium and excitement with laryngospasm may occur. If it is too rapid, spasm of chest wall may completely inhibit respiratory exchange even with a ventilator, and a rapid-acting neuromuscular blocking agent (e.g., succinylcholine [Anectine]) will be required.

Actions: A combination of potent narcotic analgesic and a neuroleptic compound. Produces neuroleptic analgesia, a calm state with reduced motor activity, reduced anxiety, and indifference to surroundings. The patient may appear to be asleep but will respond to commands. Fentanyl has definite respiratory depressant actions that outlast its analgesic effect. In healthy individuals, respiratory rate returns to normal more quickly than with other opiates. Effective within one circulation time and lasts about 30 minutes. Droperidol has alpha-adrenergic blocking actions (produces peripheral vascular dilation), and antiemetic, antifibrillatory, and anticonvulsant actions. Effective within 3 to 10 minutes, with maximum results in 30 minutes. Lasts up to 6 or more hours. Both drugs are metabolized in the liver and excreted in the urine. Droperidol crosses the blood-brain barrier; both probably cross the placental barrier and are secreted in breast milk.

Indications and uses: (1) Adjunct to general anesthesia when administered by the anesthesiologist; (2) adjunct to regional anesthesia; (3) useful in short-duration minor surgery in outpatients and in diagnostic procedures or treatments that require the patient to be awake or very lightly anesthetized (e.g., bronchoscopy, radiological studies, burn dressings, cystoscopy).

Precautions: (1) Primarily used by or under the direct observation of the anesthesiologist. (2) Oxygen, controlled respiratory equipment, naloxone (Narcan), and neuromuscular blocking agents (e.g., succinylcholine [Anectine]) must always be available. Will cause rigidity of respiratory muscles; may require a muscle relaxant to permit artifical ventilation. (3) Observe patient frequently, provide oxygen, and monitor vital signs. Patient will appear to be asleep and may forget to breathe unless commanded to do so. (4) Avoid sudden changes in posture, move and position patient with care, severe orthostatic hypotension and fainting may occur. May also occur if the patient is hypovolemic. (5) Reduce dose for elderly, debilitated, and poor-risk patients or those with impaired hepatic or renal function.

Use caution in patients with emphysema. (6) Respiratory depression will cause an increased Pco_2, cerebral vasodilation, and increased intracranial pressure. Use extreme caution in craniotomy, head injury, and increased intracranial pressure. Cerebral blood flow and cerebral metabolism are not altered. (7) May cause apnea in asthmatic patients. (8) Symptoms of acute abdominal conditions may be masked. (9) Use caution in patients with bradyarrhythmias. May increase ventricular response rate in presence of supraventricular tachycardias. (10) Cough reflex is suppressed. (11) A large dose may precipitate seizures in the presence of a history of convulsive disorders. (12) Higher doses may cause prolonged hypotension with diazepam (Valium). (13) Potentiated by phenothiazines (e.g., chlorpromazine [Thorazine]); MAO inhibitors (e.g., isocarboxazid [Marplan]); neuromuscular blocking agents (e.g., tubocurarine); and adrenergic blocking agents (e.g., propranolol [Inderal]). Reduced dosage of both drugs may be indicated. (14) Postpose breastfeeding for at least 4 to 6 hours after use. (15) Store at room temperature and protect from light before opening ampules.

Contraindications: Acute alcoholism, acute bronchial asthma, benign prostatic hypertrophy, biliary tract surgery, children under 2 years, diarrhea resulting from poisoning until toxic material eliminated, hypersensitivity to droperidol or opiates, Parkinson's disease, pregnancy, respiratory depression, surgical anastomosis, upper airway obstruction, patients who are taking or have recently taken MAO inhibitors.

Incompatible with: Diazepam (Valium), methohexitol (Brevitol), nafcillin, pentobarbital (Nembutal), phenytoin (Dilantin), sodium bicarbonate, thiopental (Pentothal). Physically compatible with many other drugs for at least 15 minutes.

Side effect: *Average dose:* Abnormal EEG, bradycardia, chills, confusion, depressed mental state, dizziness, extrapyramidal symptoms, hallucinations, hypersensitivity reactions, hypertension, hypotension, hypothermia, increased intracranial pressure, nausea, orthostatic hypotension, respiratory depression (slight), respiratory muscle rigidity, shivering, tachycardia, urinary retention, vomiting.

Overdose: Anaphylaxis, apnea, cardiac arrest, circulatory collapse, coma, excitation, hypotension (severe), inverted T wave on ECG, myocardial depression (severe), pinpoint pupils, respiratory depression (severe), tachycardia, death.

Antidote: With increasing severity of any side effect or onset of symptoms of overdose, discontinue the drugs and notify the physician immediately. Naloxone (Narcan) will reverse serious respiratory depression. A patent airway, artificial ventilation, oxygen therapy, and other symptomatic treatment must be instituted promptly. A fast-acting muscle relaxant (e.g., succinylcholine [Anectine]) may be required to facilitate ventilation. Use atropine to treat bradycardia. Treat hypotension with fluid therapy (rule out hypovolemia) and vasopressors such as dopamine (Intropin). Some references indicate that epinephrine is contraindicated. Treat extrapyramidal symptoms with benztropine mesylate (Cogentin) or diphenhydramine (Benadryl). Resuscitate as necessary.

FILGRASTIM

pH 4.0

(G-CSF, Human Granulocyte Colony Stimulating Factor, Neupogen)

Usual dose: 5 mcg/kg/day as a single daily dose for up to 2 weeks based on specific chemotherapy protocol and post nadir absolute neutrophil count (ANC). Range may be from 2 to 100 mcg/kg/day. Should not be used 24 hours before to 24 hours after the administration of cytotoxic chemotherapy, because of the potential sensitivity of rapidly dividing myeloid cells to cytotoxic chemotherapy. Expect a transient increase in neutrophil counts in the first several days after initiation of therapy. For a sustained therapeutic response, therapy must be continued until the postnadir ANC is greater than 10,000/mm^3 after the expected chemotherapy nadir (lowest point) has passed. Usually discontinued when this point is reached.

Dilution: Available as a ready to use single dose vial with either 300 mcg/1 ml or 480 mcg/1.6 ml. Remove from refrigerator to allow to warm to room temperature (never longer than 6 hours). Confirm expiration date to ensure valid product. Avoid shaking. Contains no preservatives; use sterile technique, entering vial only once to withdraw a single dose. Discard any unused portion. Should be clear and colorless.

Rate of administration: A single daily dose over 1 minute or less. May be administered through Y-tube or medport of an existing IV.

Actions: Colony-stimulating factors are glycoproteins that bind to specific hematopoietic cell surface receptors and stimulate proliferation, differentiation commitment, and some end-cell functional activation. Endogenous granulocyte colony stimulating factors are produced by monocytes, fibroblasts, and endothelial cells. They are lineage-specific with selectivity for the neutrophil lineage. Utilizing recombinant DNA technology, filgrastim is produced by specifically prepared *Escherichia coli* bacteria inserted with the human G-CSF gene. It regulates the production of neutrophils within the bone marrow. Although not species specific, it mimics the actions of endogenous glycoprotein. By accelerating the recovery of neutrophil counts following a variety of chemotherapy regimens; infection manifested by febrile neutropenia, hospitalization, and IV antibiotic usage are decreased. May also cause some increase in lymphocyte counts. Increase in circulating neutrophils is dose-dependent, and a return to baseline occurs shortly after discontinuation (50% of baseline in 1 to 2 days and to pretreatment levels in 1 to 7 days).

Indications and uses: Decrease the incidence of infection (febrile neutropenia) in patients with nonmyeloid malignancies receiving myelosuppressive anticancer drugs associated with a significant incidence of severe neutropenia with fever.

Precautions: (1) Should be administered under the direction of a physician knowledgeable about appropriate use. (2) Obtain a complete blood count and platelet count before chemotherapy begins and twice weekly thereafter to monitor the neutrophil count and to avoid leukocytosis. Following cytotoxic chemotherapy, the neutrophil nadir occurs earlier during cycles when filgrastim is used, duration of severe neutropenia is reduced, and white blood cell differentials may have a left shift. (3) Instruct patient to promptly report any symptoms of infection (e.g., fever) or allergic reaction (itching, redness, swelling at the injection site). (4) Because higher doses of chemotherapy may be tolerated, side effects associated with the chemotherapeutic drug may be more pronounced, observe carefully. (5) Use caution with any additional drugs known to lower the platelet count. (6) Effective in patients receiving chemotherapy with protocols containing cisplatin, cyclophosphamide, doxorubicin, etoposide, ifosfamide, mesna, methotrexate, vinblastine and similar antineoplastic agents. (7) Effectiveness has not been evaluated in patients receiving chemotherapy associated with delayed myelosuppression (e.g., nitrosoureas [carmustine]), with mitomycin C, or with myelosuppressive doses of antimetabolites (e.g., 5-fluorouracil or cytosine arabinoside). (8) Use extreme caution in any malignancy with myeloid characteristics; can act as a growth factor for any tumor type, particularly myeloid malignancies. (9) Adult respiratory distress syndrome may occur in septic patients. (10) Use caution in patients with preexisting cardiac disease; cardiac events (e.g., myocardial infarction) have occurred but the relationship to filgrastim is unclear. (11) Safety for use during pregnancy not established. Very large doses have caused fetal damage and death in rabbits. Use only if benefit justifies the potential risk to the fetus. (12) Secretion through breast milk not established; use caution during lactation. (13) Has been used in over 100 children from 3 months to 18 years of age with similar experience to the adult population, even though literature says safety not established. (14) Chronic use at varying doses over several years may cause subclinical splenomegaly in adults and children. (15) May be self-injected SC by the patient at home; requires instruction. Literature includes a patient handout. (16) Store in refrigerator before use. Do not allow to freeze. Do not expose to direct sunlight.

Contraindications: Hypersensitivity to *Escherichia coli*–derived proteins.

Incompatible with: Specific information not available. No evidence of interaction with other drugs has been observed.

Side effects: No serious adverse reactions that would limit the use of the product have been reported. Allergic reactions (itching, redness, swelling at the injection site) have occurred; anaphylaxis has not occurred but is possible. Complaints of dose-related bone pain are common and may require analgesics. With doses above 5 mcg/kg/day, leukocytosis (white blood cell counts greater than 100,000/mm^3) has occurred in 5% of patients with no adverse effects reported.

Antidote: Notify physician promptly if any signs of infection (fever) or other potential side effects. Monitor potential leukocytosis with twice weekly complete blood counts. Discontinue therapy after ANC surpasses 10,000/mm^3, and the chemotherapy nadir has occurred. Discontinue filgrastim and notify physician immediately if a generalized allergic reaction should occur. Treat allergic reactions as indicated.

FLUCONAZOLE

pH 4.0 to 8.0

(Diflucan)

Usual dose: IV dose has been used for a maximum of 14 days. Plasma levels are similar with IV or oral, so oral dose can replace IV dose at any time. In all situations the infecting organism and response to therapy may justify increased doses up to 400 mg daily.

Oropharyngeal candidiasis: Initial dose of 200 mg followed by 100 mg daily for a minimum of 14 days. Oral maintenance therapy usually required in patients with AIDS to prevent relapse.

Esophageal candidiasis: Initial dose of 200 mg followed by 100 mg daily for a minimum of 21 days and for at least 2 weeks after symptoms subside. Up to 400 mg/24 hr may be used.

Systemic candiasis: Initial dose of 400 mg followed by 200 mg daily for a minimum of 28 days and for at least 2 weeks after symptoms subside.

Acute cryptococcal meningitis: Initial dose of 400 mg followed by 200 mg daily for a minimum of 10 to 12 weeks after CSF culture becomes negative. Oral maintenance therapy of 200 mg daily usually required in patients with AIDS to prevent relapse.

In impaired renal function, dose should be adjusted according to creatinine clearance and/or dialysis schedule (see literature).

Pediatric dose: *Ages 3 to 13 years:* 3 to 6 mg/kg of body weight daily. Experience with children is limited.

Dilution: Packaged prediluted and ready for use as an isoosmotic solution containing 2 mg/ml in both glass bottles and Viaflex Plus plastic containers. Do not remove moisture barrier overwrap of plastic container until ready for use. Tear overwrap down side at slit to open, and remove sterile inner bag. Plastic may appear somewhat opaque due to sterilization process but will clear. Squeeze inner bag firmly to check for leaks. Discard if leakage noted; sterility is impaired. Do not use if cloudy or precipitated.

Rate of administration: A single dose as a continuous infusion at a rate not to exceed 200 mg/hr. Do not use plastic containers in series connections; air embolism could result.

Actions: A synthetic broad-spectrum bis-triazole antifungal agent. Inhibits fungal growth of *Candida* and *Cryptococcus neoformans* by acting on a key enzyme and depriving the fungus of ergosterol; the cell membrane becomes unstable and can no longer function normally. Human sterol synthesis is not affected. Has shown some effectiveness against *Aspergillus flavus, Aspergillus fumigatus, Blastomyces dermatitidis,* and *Coccidoides immitis* in laboratory mice. Peak action achieved in 1 to 2 hours; half-life extends for 30 hours. Initial double dose results in steady state plasma concentration by day 2 when given IV or orally. Penetrates into all body fluids in similar and effective concentrations and remains constant with daily single dose administration. Eighty percent excreted as unchanged drug through the kidneys.

Indications and uses: Treatment of (1) oropharyngeal and esophageal candidiasis; (2) serious systemic candidal infections including GU tract infections, peritonitis, and pneumonia; (3) cryptococcal meningitis including maintenance to prevent relapse.

Precautions: (1) For IV use only; do not give IM. (2) Specimens for fungal culture, serology, and histopathology should be obtained before therapy to isolate and identify causative organisms. Therapy may begin as soon as all specimens are obtained and before results are known. (3) Inadequate treatment may lead to recurrence of active infection; continuc treatment until clinical parameters or laboratory tests indicate that active fungal infection has subsided. Note specific recommendations in usual dose. (4) Serious hepatotoxicity may occur. Causal relationship uncertain but many patients are taking hepatotoxic drugs for treatment of malignancies and AIDS. Note any increase in liver function tests (e.g., SGOT). If any clinical signs and symptoms that are consistent with liver disease develop, discontinue drug. Has caused deaths. (5) Elevated SGOT noted when used with isoniazid, phenytoin, rifampin, sulfonlyurea hypoglycemic agents, and valproic acid; use extreme caution. (6) Potentiated by hydrochlorothiazide (Hydrodiuril), decreases renal clearance of fluconazole. (7) Potentiates cyclosporine and phenytoin; careful monitoring of their plasma levels is required. Potentiates coumarin-type anticoagulants (e.g., warfarin), monitor prothombin times; and oral hypoglycemic agents (e.g., tolbutamide), monitor blood glucose levels. In all of these situations dose reductions of the above drugs may be indicated. (8) Rifampin increases metabolism; fluconazole dose may need to be increased. (9) Studies have not been completed on interactions with zidovudine (Retrovir) and pentamidine (Pentam 300). (10) Safety for use in pregnancy and lactation and in children not established. Use in pregnancy only if potential benefits outweigh risk to fetus. (11) Store glass bottles between 5° C (41 ° F) and 30° C (86° F); store plastic containers between 5° C (41° F) and 25° C (77° F). Protect both from freezing.

Contraindications: Hypersensitivity to fluconazole or any of its components. Use caution in patients hypersensitive to other azoles (e.g., ketoconazole).

Incompatible with: Manufacturer states "do not add supplementary medication."

Side effects: More frequent in HIV-infected patients.

Average dose: Abdominal pain, diarrhea, dizziness, dry mouth, exfoliative skin disorders, headache, hepatic reactions, increased appetite, increased sweating, nausea, pallor, rash, taste perversion, tremor, vomiting.

Overdose: Cyanosis, decreased motility, decreased respirations, lacrimation, loss of balance, salivation, urinary incontinence. Clonic convulsions preceeded death in experimental animals.

Antidote: Notify physician of all side effects; most will be treated symptomatically. Discontinue drug and notify physician of abnormal liver function tests progressing to clinical signs and symptoms of liver disease. Rash may be the first sign of an exfoliative skin disorder in immunocompromised patients; discontinue drug and notify physician. In overdose a 3 hour dialysis session will decrease plasma levels by 50%. Treat anaplylaxis or resuscitate if indicated.

FLUOROURACIL pH 9.2

(Adrucil, 5-FU, 5-Fluorouracil)

Usual dose: 12 mg/kg of body weight/24 hr for 4 days. Total dose should not exceed 800 mg/24 hr. If no toxicity is observed, one-half dose (6 mg/kg) is given on the even days for 4 doses. No medication is given on the odd days following the initial 4 doses. Dosage regimen is reduced by one half or more throughout a course of therapy for poor-risk patients or those in a poor nutritional state. The most common form of maintenance therapy is to repeat the entire course of therapy beginning 30 days after the previous course is completed or to give a single dose of 10 to 15 mg/kg/week; not to exceed 1 Gm. Adjustments are made depending on side effects and tolerance. Dosage based on average weight in presence of edema or ascites.

Dilution: *Specific techniques required, see Precautions.* May be given undiluted. Do not add to IV solutions. May inject through Y-tube or three-way stopcock of a free-flowing infusion.

Rate of administration: A single dose over 1 to 3 minutes.

Actions: An antimetabolite. A fluorinated pyrimidine antagonist, cell cycle phase nonspecific, that interferes with the synthesis of DNA and RNA. Through various chemical processes this deprivation acts more quickly on rapidly growing cells and causes their death. Complete metabolism occurs within 3 hours. Excretion is through the urine and as respiratory CO_2.

Indications and uses: To suppress or retard neoplastic growth considered incurable by surgery or other means. Response has been experienced in carcinoma of the colon, rectum, breast, ovary, head and neck, urinary bladder, stomach, and pancreas, either alone or in combination with other drugs.

Precautions: (1) Follow guidelines for handling cytotoxic agents. See Appendix, p. 677. (2) Administered by or under the direction of the physician specialist. (3) Confirm patency of vein. Avoid extravasation. Change injection site every 48 hours. (4) Protect from light. May be slightly discolored without affecting safety and potency. Dissolve any precipitate by heating to 60° C (140° F) and shaking vigorously. Cool to body temperature before using. (5) Use caution in patients who have had high-dose pelvic irradiation, previous antimetabolic drugs, metastatic tumor involvement of the bone marrow, and impaired hepatic or renal function. In hepatic insufficiency, omit fluorouracil if serum bilirubin above 5 mg/ml. (6) Not to be considered adjunctive to surgical treatment. (7) May produce teratogenic effects on the fetus. Has a mutagenic potential. Give with caution in men and women capable of conception. (8) Often used with other antineoplastic drugs in reduced doses to achieve tumor remission. (9) Potentiates anticoagulants. (10) Be alert for signs of bone marrow depression or infection. (11) Do not administer any vaccines or chloroquine to patients receiving antineoplastic drugs. (12) Prophylactic antiemetics may reduce nausea and vomiting and increase patient comfort. (13) Toxicity increased by stress, poor nutrition, and bone marrow depression. (14) Obtain a white blood cell count and differential before each dose. (15) May increase alkaline phosphatase, SGOT, serum bilirubin, and lactic dehydrogenase.

Contraindications: Potentially serious infections, depressed bone marrow function, poor nutritional state.

Incompatible with: Do not mix with IV additives or other chemotherapeutic agents; give separately. Cytarabine (ARA-C), diazepam (Valium), doxorubicin (Adriamycin), methotrexate (Folex).

Side effects: Agranulocytosis, alopecia (reversible), anaphylaxsis, anemia, cerebellar syndrome, cramps, dermatitis, diarrhea, disorientation, dry lips, erythema, esophagopharyngitis, euphoria, GI ulceration and bleeding, headache, hemorrhage from any site, increased skin pigmentation, leukopenia, mouth soreness and ulceration, nausea, pancytopenia, photophobia, stomatitis, thrombocytopenia, thrombophlebitis, visual changes, vomiting.

Antidote: Discontinue the drug and notify physician of side effects. Discontinue the drug if the white blood cell count is less than 3,500/mm^3 or platelets are less than 100,000/mm^3; monitor for 4 weeks. Death may occur from the progression of most of these side effects. There is no specific antidote; supportive therapy as indicated will help to sustain patient in toxicity.

FOLIC ACID pH 8.0 to 11.0

(Folvite)

Usual dose: 1 mg daily. Up to 5 mg will be used infrequently.

Dilution: May be given direct IV undiluted or added to most IV solutions and given as an infusion.

Rate of administration: 5 mg or fraction thereof over 1 minute in undiluted form.

Actions: Folic acid (pteroylglutamic acid) is part of the vitamin B complex. It can be synthesized by intestinal bacteria. It is an important growth factor for many cells and is involved in the synthesis of amino acids and DNA. Stimulates the production of red blood cells, white blood cells, and platelets. Crosses the placental barrier. Secreted in breast milk. Excreted in urine.

Indications and uses: Megaloblastic anemias of malnutrition seen in alcoholism, sprue, steatorrhea, celiac disease, pregnancy, developmental or surgical anomalies of the GI tract, and fish tapeworm infestation.

Precautions: (1) Folic acid is not commonly administered by the IV route in adults and *never in children*. Oral or IM administration provides adequate absorption in most cases. (2) Obscures the peripheral blood picture and prevents the diagnosis of pernicious anemia. May actually aggravate the neurological symptoms. (3) Toxic effects of antineoplastic folic acid antagonists are blocked by folinic acid (leucovorin) but not by folic acid IV. (4) Refrigerate and protect from light. (5) Therapeutic dose is higher than actually needed because small doses have not proved effective. (6) Increases hydantoin metabolism (e.g., phenytoin [Dilantin]); seizures may result. (7) Inhibited by antimetabolic agents (e.g., methotrexate, fluorouracil), pyrimethamine, trimethoprim, and triamterene, and by depressed hematopoiesis, alcoholism, and deficiencies of vitamins B_6, B_{12}, C, and E.

Contraindications: IV route contraindicated in children; pernicious anemia unless used in combination with diagnostic testing, liver extracts, etc.; aplastic anemia; iron-deficiency anemia.

Incompatible with: Calcium salts, chlorpromazine (Thorazine), dextrose in 40% or greater concentrations, heavy metal ions, iron sulfate, oxidizing agents, reducing agents, vitamin B complex with C.

Side effects: Almost nonexistent. Some slight flushing or feeling of warmth; anaphylaxis can occur.

Antidote: Discontinue drug, treat anaphylaxis, and notify physician if anaphylaxis occurs. Resuscitate as necessary.

FUROSEMIDE — pH 8.0 to 9.3

(Lasix, ♣ Uritol)

Usual dose: 20 to 40 mg. May be repeated in 1 to 2 hours. If necessary, increase dosage by 20 mg increments (under close medical supervision and no sooner than 2 hours after previous dose) until desired diuresis is obtained. Maximum human dose is 600 mg/24 hr. After the initial diuresis the minimum effective dose may be given once or twice every 24 hours as required for maintenance.

Pediatric dose: 1 mg/kg of body weight. After 2 hours increase by 1 mg/kg increments to effect desired response. Do not exceed 6 mg/kg.

Dilution: May be given undiluted. May be given through Y-tube or three-way stopcock of infusion set. Not usually added to IV solutions, but large doses may be added to 5% dextrose in water or normal saline and given as an infusion. pH of solution must be over 5.5.

Rate of administration: Each 20 mg or fraction thereof should be given over 1 minute. High-dose therapy in an infusion should not exceed a rate of 4 mg/min.

Actions: A sulfonamide diuretic, antihypertensive, and antihypercalcemic agent related to the thiazides. Extremely potent and has a rapid onset of action. Effectiveness is noted within 5 minutes and may last for 2 hours. Apparently acts on the proximal and distal ends of the tubule and the ascending limb of the loop of

Henle to excrete water, sodium, chlorides, and potassium. Will produce diuresis in alkalosis or acidosis. Rapidly absorbed and distributed, it is excreted unchanged in the urine.

Indications and uses: (1) Congestive heart failure; (2) acute pulmonary edema; (3) cirrhosis of the liver with ascites; (4) renal disease including the nephrotic syndrome; (5) edema unresponsive to other diuretic agents; (6) hypercalcemia; (7) hypertension.

Precautions: (1) May be used concurrently with aldosterone antagonists (e.g., spironolactone [Aldactone]) for more effective diuresis and to prevent excessive potassium loss. (2) Discontinue at least 2 days before elective surgery. (3) May precipitate excessive diuresis with water and electrolyte depletion. Routine checks on electrolyte panel, CO_2, and BUN are necessary during therapy. Potassium chloride replacement may be required. (4) Use caution and improve basic condition first in hepatic coma, electrolyte depletion, and advanced cirrhosis of the liver. (5) Causes excessive potassium depletion with corticosteroids and spironolactone hydrochlorothiazide (Aldactazide). (6) Potentiates antihypertensive drugs, propranolol (Inderal), salicylates, muscle relaxants (e.g., curare, tubocurarine), tetracyclines, and hypotensive effect of other diuretics and MAO inhibitors (e.g., pargyline [Eutonyl]). (7) May cause transient deafness in doses exceeding the usual or in conjunction with ototoxic drugs (e.g., cisplatin, dihydrostreptomycin, gentamicin). (8) May increase blood glucose and has precipitated diabetes mellitus and lower serum calcium level, which causes tetany; rarely precipitates an acute attack of gout. (9) Inhibits oral anticoagulants, pressor amines, and sulfonylureas. (10) Inhibited by phenytoin (Dilantin) and indomethacin (Indocin). (11) May increase or decrease effectiveness of theophyllines. (12) May cause cardiac dysrhythmias with digitalis or ethacrynic acid (Edecrin). (13) If diluted in compatible infusion solution (5% dextrose in water, isotonic saline, lactated Ringer's solution), discard after 24 hours. (14) Higher doses may be required in nephrosis or chronic renal failure. Hepatic necrosis may result.

Contraindications: Anuria, severe progressive renal disease with increasing azotemia and oliguria, rarely used in children, pregnancy and lactation, known sulfonamide sensitivity.

Incompatible with: Acidic solutions, ascorbic acid, corticosteroids, diphenhydramine (Benadryl), dobutamine (Dobutrex), esmolol (Brevibloc), epinephrine (Adrenalin), gentamicin (Garamycin), levarterenol (Levophed), meperidine (Demerol), milrione (Primacor), netilmicin (Netromycin), reserpine, spironolactone hydrochlorothiazide (Aldactazide), tetracyclines, any drug in a syringe.

Side effects: Usually occur in prolonged therapy, seriously ill patients, or following large doses.

Minor: Anemia, anorexia, blurring of vision, deafness (reversible), diarrhea, dizziness, hyperglycemia, hyperuricemia, hypokalemia, leg cramps, lethargy, leukopenia, mental confusion, paresthesia, postural hypotension, pruritus, tinnitus, urinary frequency, urticaria, vomiting, weakness.

Major: Anaphylactic shock, blood volume reduction, circulatory collapse, dehydration, excessive diuresis, hypokalemia, metabolic acidosis, vascular thrombosis and embolism.

Antidote: If minor side effects are noted, discontinue the drug and notify the physician, who may treat the side effects symptomatically and continue the drug. If side effects are progressive or any major side effect occurs, discontinue the drug immediately and notify the physician. Treatment of major side effects is symptomatic and aggressive. Resuscitate as necessary.

GALLAMINE TRIETHIODIDE pH 6.5 to 7.5

(Flaxedil)

Usual dose: Must be individualized, depending on previous drugs administered and degree and length of muscle relaxation required. 0.5 to 1.0 mg/kg of body weight initially. Repeat every 30 to 40 minutes as required. Maximum single dose regardless of weight is 100 mg.

Dilution: May be given undiluted.

Rate of administration: A single dose over 30 to 60 seconds.

Actions: A skeletal muscle relaxant. Causes paralysis by interfering with neural transmission at the myoneural junction. Onset of action is immediate and may last up to 60 minutes. Complete recovery from a single dose may take several hours. Duration of action is dose dependent. Excreted in the urine.

Indications and uses: (1) Adjunctive to general anesthesia; (2) management of patients undergoing mechanical ventilation.

Precautions: (1) Administered only by or under the direct observation of the anesthesiologist. (2) This drug produces apnea. Controlled artificial ventilation with oxygen must be continuous and under direct observation at all times. Maintain a patent airway. (3) Repeated doses may produce a cumulative effect. (4) Impaired pulmonary function or respiratory deficiencies can cause critical reactions. Use caution in impaired liver or kidney function. (5) Myasthenia gravis increases sensitivity to drug. Reaction may be fatal (see Contraindications). (6) Potentiated by inhalant anesthetics (e.g., ether), neuromuscular blocking antibiotics (e.g., kanamycin [Kantrex]), calcium and magnesium salts, CO_2, digitalis, diuretics, diazepam (Valium) and other muscle relaxants, lidocaine, MAO inhibitors, propranolol (Inderal), quinidine, tetracyclines, succinylcholine, and others. Markedly reduced dose of gallamine must be used with caution. (7) Antagonized by acetylcholines, anticholinesterases, azathioprine, carbamazepine, and potassium. (8) Hyperkalemia may cause cardiac dysrhythmias and increased paralysis. (9) Patient may be conscious and completely unable to communicate by any means. Gallamine has no analgesic properties. Respiratory depression with narcotics may be preferred in some patients requiring mechanical ventilation. (10) Action altered by dehydration, electrolyte imbalance, body temperature, and some carcinomas. (11) Confirm adequate potassium levels before use. Consider withholding diuretics for at least 4 days before elective surgery. (12) Use a peripheral nerve stimulator to monitor response to gallamine and avoid overdosage. (13) Use extreme caution in infants, especially if under 5 kg.

Contraindications: Myasthenia gravis, known hypersensitivity to gallamine or to iodides, impaired renal function or shock; if tachycardia, would increase the severity of an existing condition.

Incompatible with: Anesthetic agents. Consider incompatible in a syringe with any other drug. Evaluation of predictable results is imperative.

Side effects: Prolonged action resulting in respiratory insufficiency or apnea; airway closure caused by relaxation of epiglottis, pharynx, and tongue muscles; anaphylaxis; tachycardia.

Antidote: All side effects are medical emergencies. Treat symptomatically. Controlled artificial ventilation must be continuous. Edrophonium and neostigmine methylsulfate with atropine may help to reverse muscle relaxation. Not effective in all situations; may aggravate severe overdosage. Treat allergic reactions and resuscitate as necessary.

GALLIUM NITRATE — pH 6.0 to 7.0

(Ganite)

Usual dose: 200 mg/M^2 daily for 5 consecutive days. Must be administered as an IV infusion. Consider reduction to 100 mg/M^2/day for 5 days in patients with mild hypercalcemia (12 mg/dl range, corrected for serum albumin) and few symptoms. Discontinue treatment at any time the serum calcium levels are lowered into the normal range (8.5 to 10.5 mg/dl, corrected for serum albumin). Safety and effectiveness of retreatment not established. Reduced dose may be required in impaired renal function based on creatinine clearance (2.0 to 2.5 mg/dl). See Contraindications.

Dilution: A single daily dose must be diluted in 1,000 ml normal saline (preferred) or 5% dextrose in water. Less diluent may be used if absolutely necessary in patients with compromised cardiovascular status. Stable after dilution for 48 hours at room temperature (15° to 30° C [59° to 86° F]) and for 7 days if refrigerated (2° to 8° C [35.6° to 46.4° F]).

Rate of administration: A single daily dose equally distributed over 24 hours as an IV infusion. Use of a microdrip (60 gtt/ml) or an infusion pump recommended for even distribution.

Actions: A hypocalcemic agent that inhibits calcium resorption from bone. Thought to act by reducing increased bone turnover. Does not have cytotoxic effects on bone cells. Plasma levels achieve a steady state 24 to 48 hours after infusion initiated. In one study it normalized serum calcium in 75% of patients who began treatment with a serum calcium corrected for albumin greater than 12 mg/dl. Maintains duration of normocalcemia/hypocalcemia longer than calcitonin. Route of metabolism is unknown. Significant excretion occurs through the kidneys.

Indications and uses: Treatment of clearly symptomatic cancer-related hypercalcemia that has not responded to adequate hydration. Serum calcium above 12 mg/dl corrected for serum albumin. Symptoms may include anorexia, constipation, depression, fatigue, muscle weakness, and nausca.

Precautions: (1) Baseline measurements of serum calcium corrected for serum albumin, serum phosphorus, electrolytes, plasma pH, serum creatinine and BUN are required. Monitor calcium daily, phosphorus twice weekly, and electrolytes, plasma pH, creatinine, and BUN closely as indicated by baseline results (may be daily). (2) Patients with cancer-related hypercalcemia are frequently dehydrated. Must be adequately hydrated orally and/or intravenously before treatment is initiated. Hydration with saline is preferred to facilitate renal excretion of calcium and correct dehydration. A pretreatment urine output of 2 L/day is recommended.

(3) Avoid overhydration in patients with compromised cardiovascular status. Observe frequently for signs of fluid overload. Correct hypovolemia before using diuretics. (4) Maintain adequate hydration and urine output throughout treatment. (5) Calcium is bound to serum protein, concentration fluctuates with changes in blood volume. Changes in serum calcium (especially during rehydration) may not reflect true plasma levels. All calcium measurement should be corrected for albumin to establish a basis for treatment and evaluation of treatment. (6) Mild or asymptomatic hypercalcemia will be treated with conservative measures (e.g., saline hydration, with or without diuretics). Consider patient's cardiovascular status. Corticosteroids may be indicated if the underlying cancer is sensitive (e.g., hematologic cancers). (7) Nephrotoxicity may be increased with other nephrotoxic drugs (e.g., aminoglycosides [gentamicin], amphotericin B [Fungizone], edecrin). (8) Use in pregnancy has not been studied; use only if clearly needed. (9) Discontinue nursing or do not use gallium nitrate. Consider importance of drug to mother. (10) Safety for use in children not established. (11) Stored at controlled room temperature prior to dilution.

Contraindications: Severe renal impairment (serum creatinine over 2.5 mg/dl).

Incompatible with: Specific information not available. Consider specific use and controlled rate of infusion.

Side effects: *Average dose:* Acute renal failure, anemia, asymptomatic decrease in blood pressure, fluid overload, hearing loss, optic neuritis (acute), respiratory alkalosis, tinnitus. Many other side effects possibly from underlying disease have occurred in less than 1% of patients.

Overdose: Acute renal failure, anemia, hypocalcemia, hypophosphatemia, nausea, vomiting.

Antidote: Discontinue drug if creatinine clearance reaches 2.5 mg/dl at any time during treatment. Discontinue drug for any symptoms of overdose. Monitor serum calcium, use vigorous IV hydration, with or without diuretics for 2 to 3 days. Monitor intake and output to ensure adequacy and balance. For asymptomatic or mild to moderate hypocalcemia (6.5 to 8.0 mg/dl corrected for serum albumin), short-term calcium therapy may be indicated. Oral phosphorus may be required for hypophosphatemia. Red blood cell transfusions may be required in anemia. Keep physician informed. Some side effects may respond to symptomatic treatment. Treat anaphylaxis and resuscitate as indicated.

GANCICLOVIR SODIUM pH 9.0 to 11.0

(Cytovene, DHPG)

Usual dose: 5 mg/kg of body weight every 12 hours for 14 to 21 days. Begin a maintenance dose the next day (day 15 to 22) of 5 mg/kg daily for 7 days each week or 6 mg/kg daily for 5 days each week. If retinitis progresses during the maintenance regimen, initiate the twice-daily program again. Treatment continues as long as the patient is immunocompromised, perhaps months or years. Normal renal function required. Do not exceed recommended dosage or frequency. With impaired renal function and patients receiving dialysis dose may need to be reduced up to 50% or dosing interval may be adjusted. Specific calculation required (see literature).

Dilution: *Specific techniques required, see Precautions.* Initially dissolve the 500 mg vial with 10 ml sterile water for injection (50 mg/ml). Do not use bacteriostatic water containing parabens; will cause precipitation. Shake well to dissolve completely. Discard if particulate matter or discoloration observed. Withdraw the desired dose and further dilute in an amount of solution to provide a concentration less than 10 mg/ml (70 kg adult at 5 mg/kg equals 350 mg, dissolved in 100 ml of solution equals 3.5 mg/ml). Compatible with normal saline, 5% dextrose in water, Ringer's injection, and lactated Ringer's injection for infusion.

Rate of administration: A single dose must be administered at a constant rate over 1 hour as an infusion. Use of an infusion pump or microdrip (60 gtt/ml) recommended. Excessive plasma levels and toxicity will occur with too-rapid rate of injection. Advisable to clear tubing with normal saline if possible before and after administration through Y-tube or three-way stopcock.

Actions: An antiviral agent that stops cytomegalovirus (CMV) from multiplying. Does not destroy existing viruses but stops them from reproducing and invading healthy cells. May allow a weakened immune system to defend the body against the CMV infection. May also be inhibitory against herpes simplex virus 1 and 2, Epstein-Barr virus, and varicella zoster virus, but clinical studies have not been done. Onset of action is prompt, and therapeutic levels are maintained for 3 to 6 hours with some drug remaining 11 hours after infusion. Widely distributed in tissues and body fluids. Probably crosses the placental barrier. Suspected to be secreted in breast milk. Over 90% excreted unchanged in urine by glomerular filtration in patients with normal renal function.

Indications and uses: Treatment of CMV retinitis in immunocompromised individuals including patients with AIDS.

Precautions: (1) Confirm diagnosis of CMV retinitis by indirect ophthalmoscopy. Diagnosis may be supported by cultures of CMV from urine, blood, throat, etc.; negative culture does not rule out CMV retinitis. (2) A nucleoside analog; follow guidelines for handling and disposal of cytotoxic agents. See Appendix, p. 677. (3) Maintain adequate hydration and urine flow before and during infusion. (4) Assess renal function before administration to elderly patients and adjust dose appropriately. (5) For IV use only; IM or SC administration will cause severe tissue irritation. (6) CBC with differential and platelet counts, serum creatinine, and creatinine clearance are required before treatment initiated. Monitor neutrophil and platelet counts every 2 days during twice-daily dosing and weekly thereafter. Monitor daily in patients with previous leukopenia from nucleoside analogs or those with neutrophils less than 1,000 cells/mm^3 at beginning of treatment. Withhold dose if neutrophils less than 500 cells/mm^3 or platelets less than 25,000 cells/mm^3. Monitor serum creatinine or creatinine clearance every 2 weeks. (7) Phlebitis or pain may occur at site of infusion; confirm patency of vein and use small needles and large veins to ensure adequate blood flow for rapid dilution and distribution. (8) Additive toxicity may occur with concomitant use of other drugs that inhibit replication of rapidly dividing cell populations (e.g., dapsone, pentamidine [Pentam 300], flucytosine [Ancobon], vincristine [Oncovin], vinblastine [Velban], vindesine [Eldisine], doxorubicin [Adriamycin], amphotericin B [Fungizone], trimethoprim/sulfamethoxazole [Bactrim]). (9) May cause seizures with imipenem-cilastatin (Primaxin). (10) Potentiated by probenicid and other drugs that may reduce renal clearance. Will increase toxicity. (11) A potential carcinogen. Teratogenic and embryotoxic; will cause birth defects. Do not use during pregnancy unless risk is justified. Both sexes must use effective contraception during treatment, and men should continue barrier contraception for at least 90 days. May cause temporary or permanent infertility. (12) Discontinue nursing during treatment; do not resume until at least 72 hours after final dose of ganciclovir. (13) Use extreme caution in children under 12 years of age. Long-term carcinogenicity and reproductive toxicity are probable. (14) Use reconstituted solution within 12 hours. Do not refrigerate. Solution fully diluted for administration must be refrigerated and used within 24 house to reduce incidence of bacterial contamination.

Contraindications: Hypersensitivity to ganciclovir or acyclovir; patients with a neutrophil count less than 500 cells/mm^3 or a platelet count less than 25,000 cells/mm^3; patients receiving zidovudine (Retrovir), since both drugs cause granulocytopenia.

Incompatible with: Any other drug in syringe or solution because of alkaline pH. Precipitation may occur if pH is altered. Advisable to clear tubing with normal saline if possible before and after administration through Y-tube or three-way stopcock.

Side effects: Granulocytopenia and thrombocytopenia are the most common and are generally reversible if treatment discontinued. Anemia, fever, infection, pain at injection site, phlebitis, rash, and abnormal liver function tests occur in some patients. Fewer than 1% of patients experience abdominal pain, alopecia, ataxia, chills, coma, confusion, daydreaming, diarrhea, dizziness, dreams, dsypnea, dysrhythmias, edema, eosinophilia, headache, hematuria, hemorrhage, hypertension, hypoglyccmia, hypotension, increased BUN and creatinine clearance, malaise, nausea, nervousness, paresthesia, pruritus, psychosis, retinal detachment, somnolence, tremor, and urticaria.

Overdose: Anorexia, bloody diarrhea, cytopenia, hypersalivation, increased BUN and liver function tests, testicular atrophy, vomiting, death.

Antidote: Nofity physician of all side effects; most will be treated symptomatically. Discontinue drug if neutrophils fall below 500 cells/mm^3 or platelets fall below 25,000 cells/mm^3. Hydration and hemodialysis (up to 50% removal) are useful in overdose. Treat anaphylaxis and resuscitate as necessary.

GENTAMICIN SULFATE pH 3.0 to 5.5

(✤ Cidomycin, Garamycin, Jenamicin)

Usual dose: 3 mg/kg of body weight/24 hr equally divided into 3 or 4 doses. Up to 5 mg/kg may be given if indicated. Reduce to usual dose as soon as feasible. Dosage based on ideal weight of lean body mass. Normal renal function is necessary for all recommended doses.

Prevention of bacterial endocarditis in dental, respiratory tract, GI or GU tract surgery or instrumentation: 1.5 mg/kg 30 minutes before procedure. Repeat in 8 hours. Given concurrently with ampicillin or vancomycin.

Pelvic inflammatory disease: 2 mg/kg as an initial dose. Follow with 1.5 mg/kg every 8 hours for 4 days or

48 hours after patient improves. Given concurrently with clindamycin.

Pediatric dose: 6 to 7.5 mg/kg of body weight/24 hr (2 to 2.5 mg/kg every 8 hours).

Newborn dose: *Over 1 week of age:* 7.5 mg/kg of body weight/24 hr (2.5 mg/kg every 8 hours).

Premature infants and neonates less than 1 week: 2.5 mg/kg every 12 hours. Lower doses may be appropriate due to immature kidney function. 2.5 mg/kg every 18 hours or 3 mg/kg every 24 hours has been effective in preterm infants less than 32 weeks gestational age.

Dilution: Prepared solutions equal 10 or 100 mg/ml. Further dilute each single dose in 50 to 200 ml of IV normal saline or 5% dextrose in water. Dilute to a 0.1% solution (1 mg/ml) or less. Decrease volume of diluent for children, but maintain 0.1% solution. Commercially diluted solutions available.

Rate of administration: Each single dose, properly diluted, over 30 to 60 minutes, up to 2 hours in children.

Actions: An aminoglycoside antibiotic with neuromuscular blocking action. Bactericidal against specific gram-positive and gram-negative bacilli, including *Escherichia coli, Klebsiella, Proteus,* and *Pseudomonas.* Not effective for fungi or viral infections. Well distributed throughout all body fluids; serum and urine levels remain adequate for 6 to 12 hours. Usual half-life is 2 hours. Half-life is prolonged in infants, postpartum females, fever, liver disease and ascites, spinal cord injury, cystic fibrosis, and the elderly; shorter in severe burns. Crosses the placental barrier. Excreted through the kidneys.

Indications and uses: (1) Treatment of serious infections of the GI, respiratory and urinary tracts, CNS, skin and soft tissue, and septicemia; (2) primarily used when penicillin and other less toxic antibiotics are ineffective or contraindicated; (3) treat suspected infection in the immunosuppressed patient; (4) prevention of bacterial endocarditis in dental, respiratory tract, GI or GU surgery or instrumentation; (5) used concurrently with clindamycin to treat pelvic inflammatory disease.

Precautions: (1) Narrow range between toxic and therapeutic levels. Monitor peak and trough concentrations to avoid peak serum concentrations above 12 mcg/ml and trough concentrations above 2 mcg/ml. Therapeutic level is between 4 and 8 mcg/ml. (2) Use extreme caution if therapy is required over 7 to 10 days. (3) Sensitivity studies indicated to determine susceptibility of the causative organism to gentamicin. (4) Reduce daily dose commensurate with amount of renal impairment. Intervals between injections should also be increased. (5) Watch for decrease in urine output and rising BUN and serum creatinine. Dosage may require decreasing. Routine serum levels and evaluation of hearing are recommended. (6) Use caution in infants, children, and the elderly. (7) Potentiated by anesthetics, other neuromuscular blocking antibiotics (e.g., kanamycin, streptomycin), anticholinesterases (e.g., edrophonium [Tensilon]), antineoplastics (e.g., nitrogen mustard, cisplatin), barbiturates, cephalosporins, muscle relaxants (e.g., tubocurarine), phenothiazines (e.g., promethazine [Phenergan]), procainamide, quinidine, and sodium citrate (citrate-anticoagulated blood). *Apnea can occur.* (8) Also potentiated by other ototoxic drugs (e.g., ethacrynic acid [Edecrin]) and all potent diuretics. An elevated serum level of gentamicin may occur, increasing nephrotoxicity and neurotoxicity. (9) Superinfection may occur from overgrowth of nonsusceptible organisms. (10) Maintain good hydration. (11) Synergistic when used in combination with penicillins and cephalosporins. Dose adjustment and appropriate spacing required because of physical incompatibilities and interactions. (12) Use in pregnancy and lactation only when absolutely necessary.

Contraindications: Known gentamicin or aminoglycoside sensitivity, renal failure.

Incompatible with: Administer separately. Inactivated in solution with carbenicillin, other penicillins, and most cephalosporins. Incompatible with amphotericin B, ampicillin, cefamandole (Mandol), cephalothin (Keflin), cephapirin (Cefadyl), dopamine (Intropin), furosemide (Lasix), heparin.

Side effects: Occur more frequently with impaired renal function, higher doses, or prolonged administration.

Minor: Anorexia, burning, dizziness, fever, headache, hypertension, hypotension, itching, lethargy, muscle twitching, nausea, numbness, rash, roaring in ears, tingling sensation, tinnitus, urticaria, vomiting, weight loss.

Major: Blood dyscrasias; convulsions; elevated bilirubin, BUN, serum creatinine, SGOT, and SGPT; hearing loss; laryngeal edema; neuromuscular blockade; oliguria; respiratory arrest.

Antidote: Notify the physician of all side effects. If minor side effects persist or any major symptom appears, discontinue the drug and notify the physician. Treatment is symptomatic. In overdose hemodialysis may be indicated. Complexation with ticarcillin or carbenicillin may be as effective as hemodialysis. Consider exchange transfusion in the newborn. Calcium salts or neostigmine may reverse neuromuscular blockade. Resuscitate as necessary.

GLUCAGON HYDROCHLORIDE pH 2.5 to 3.0

Usual dose: *Hypoglycemia:* 0.5 to 1 mg. May be repeated in 20 minutes for 2 doses if indicated. Up to 2 mg has been given as initial dose.

Diagnostic aid: 0.5 mg.

Dilution: Dilute 1 unit (1 mg) of glucagon powder with 1 ml of its own diluting solution. Do not add to IV solutions. May be given through Y-tube or three-way stopcock of infusion set if a dextrose solution is infusing. A 2 mg dose may be diluted with a minimum of 2 ml sterile water for injection. Must be used immediately.

Rate of administration: 1 unit or fraction thereof over 1 minute.

Actions: A pancreatic extract from the alpha cells of the islets of Langerhans. Blood glucose is raised by activating phosphorylase, which converts glycogen to glucose in the liver. Glucagon acts only on liver glycogen. Has a half-life of 3 to 6 minutes. Produces relaxation of the smooth muscle of the stomach, duodenum, small bowel, and colon.

Indications and uses: (1) Treatment of hypoglycemic reactions during insulin therapy in the management of diabetes mellitus and in induced insulin shock during psychiatric therapy; (2) induction of a hypotonic state and smooth muscle relaxation in the radiological examination of the stomach, duodenum, small bowel, and colon.

Investigational uses: May be helpful in reversing adverse effects of β-adrenergic blocking agents (e.g., propranolol [Inderal]), or may be used to enhance digitalis effects in heart failure.

Precautions: (1) Should awaken the patient in 5 to 20 minutes. Prolonged hypoglycemic reactions may result in severe cortical damage. (2) Emesis on awakening is common. Prevent aspiration by turning the patient face down. (3) Dose may be repeated if necessary. Supplement with IV glucose (50%) to precipitate awakening. Utilize oral sugars after awakening to prevent secondary hypoglycemia. (4) Easily absorbed IM or SC. (5) Potentiates oral anticoagulants. (6) If glucagon and glucose do not awaken the patient, coma is probably caused by a condition other than hypoglycemia. (7) Not as effective in the juvenile diabetic patient; supplement with carbohydrate as soon as possible. (8) Use caution in patients with insulinoma and/or pheochromocytoma. (9) As a smooth muscle relaxant, it is as effective as anticholinergic drugs and has fewer side effects. (10) Immediate use after reconstitution is preferred. May refrigerate for up to 48 hours.

Contraindications: Known hypersensitivity to protein compounds.

Incompatible with: Any other drug in the syringe; solutions containing sodium chloride, potassium chloride, or calcium chloride. Not soluble in any solution with a pH range of 3.0 to 9.5.

Side effects: Rare in recommended doses: anaphylaxis, hyperglycemia (excessive dosage), hypersensitivity reactions, hypertension (rare), hypotension (rare), nausea, vomiting.

Antidote: Nausea and vomiting are tolerable and do occur in hypoglycemia. For any other side effects, discontinue the drug and notify the physician. Treat allergic reactions and resuscitate as necessary. Insulin administration may be indicated in acute overdose.

GLYCOPYRROLATE pH 2.0 to 3.0

(Robinul)

Usual dose: *Gastrointestinal disorders:* 0.1 to 0.2 mg at 4-hour intervals 3 or 4 times/day.

Reversal of neuromuscular blockade: 0.2 mg for each 1 mg neostigmine or equivalent dose of pyridostigmine. Administer IV simultaneously. May be mixed in the same syringe.

Intraoperative medication: 0.1 mg as needed, may repeat every 2 to 3 minutes.

Pediatric dose: *Intraoperative medication:* 0.004 mg/kg of body weight. Do not exceed 0.1 mg as a single dose. May repeat every 2 to 3 minutes.

Reversal of neuromuscular blockade: Same as adult dose.

Dilution: May be given undiluted. Administer through Y-tube or three-way stopcock of infusion tubing.

Rate of administration: 0.2 mg or fraction thereof over 1 to 2 minutes.

Actions: A synthetic anticholinergic agent. It inhibits the action of acetylcholine. It reduces the volume and free acidity of gastric secretions and controls excessive pharyngeal, tracheal, and bronchial secretions. Antagonizes cholinergic drugs. Onset of action is within 1 minute. Some effects last 2 to 3 hours.

Indications and uses: (1) Adjunctive therapy in peptic ulcer; (2) reversal of neuromuscular blockade (usually intraoperatively); (3) other intraoperative uses controlled by the anesthesiologist (counteract drug-induced or vagal traction reflexes and associated dysrhythmias).

Precautions: (1) Use IV only when immediate drug effect is essential. (2) Not recommended for peptic ulcer therapy in children. (3) Urinary retention can be avoided if the patient voids just prior to each dose. (4) Use extreme caution in autonomic neuropathy, asthma, pregnancy, lactation, cardiac dysrhythmias, congestive heart failure, coronary artery disease, hepatic or renal disease, hiatal hernia, hypertension, and hyperthyroidism. Toxicity to nursing infants probable. (5) Potentiated by alkalinizing agents, amantadine, synthetic narcotic analgesics, tricyclic antidepressants (e.g., amitryptyline [Elavil]), antihistamines, MAO inhibitors (e.g., pargyline [Eutonyl]), nitrates, phenothiazines (e.g., chlorpromazine [Thorazine]), and many others. Reduced dose of either or both drugs may be indicated. (6) Antagonized by histamine, reserpine, and others. (7) Potentiates atenolol (Tenormin) and digoxin. (8) May produce excitement, agitation, or drowsiness in the elderly.

Contraindications: Known hypersensitivity to glycopyrrolate, glaucoma, obstructive uropathy, obstructive disease of the GI tract, paralytic ileus, unstable cardiovascular status in acute hemorrhage, severe ulcerative colitis, megacolon, myasthenia gravis.

Incompatible with: Alkaline solutions, chloramphenicol, dexamethasone (Decadron), diazepam (Valium), dimenhydrinate (Dramamine), methohexital (Brevital), methylprednisolone (Solu-Medrol), pentazocine (Talwin), pentobarbital (Nembutal), phenothiazines (e.g., Compazine), secobarbital (Seconal), sodium bicarbonate, thiopental (Pentothal).

Side effects: Anaphylaxis, anticholinergic psychosis, blurred vision, constipation, decreased sweating, drowsiness, dry mouth, heat prostration, impotence, increased ocular tension, loss of taste, muscular weakness, nervousness, paralysis, tachycardia, urinary hesitancy and retention.

Antidote: Notify physician of all side effects. May be treated symptomatically or drug may be discontinued. 1 mg of neostigmine for each 1 mg of glycopyrrolate administered may be used for overdose. Resuscitate as necessary.

GONADORELIN ACETATE

(Lutrepulse)

Usual dose: 5 mcg every 90 minutes (range is 1 to 20 mcg). Usually administered over a period of 21 days. Response to Lutrepulse usually occurs within 2 to 3 weeks. When ovulation occurs during this time, therapy is continued for another 2 weeks to maintain the corpus luteum. Dosage adjustments are usually indicated if no ovulation occurs after 3 cycles and may need to be made cautiously in a stepwise fashion based upon response. See manufacturer's literature for specific dose adjustment process.

Dilution: All necessary supplies for administration and dilution provided in Lutrepulse kit and Lutrepulse pump kit. Add 8 ml of provided diluent to both the 0.8 or 3.2 mg vials. Sterile technique essential. Provides 5 mcg/50 mcl with the 0.8 mg vial and 20 mcg/mcl with the 3.2 mg vial. Shake for a few seconds until solution is clear, colorless, and free of particulate matter. Prepare immediately before use and transfer to the plastic reservoir following specific instructions for the Lutrepulse pump. 8 ml of solution provides an adequate supply for 7 days.

Rate of administration: Each dose must be delivered via pulsatile IV injection with the Lutrepulse pump, which delivers a single dose over a pulse period of 1 minute at a pulse frequency of 90 minutes. Pump should be set at 25 or 50 mcl of solution based on desired dose and dilution and is capable of delivering 2.5, 5, 10, or 20 mcg every 90 minutes.

Actions: A sterile lyophilized powder, this synthetic hormone is identical in amino acid sequence to endogenous gonadotropin-releasing hormone (GnRH). When released by pulsatile IV injection through the Lutrepulse pump, it causes normal pulsatile releases of pituitary gonadotropins. Luteinizing and follicle-stimulating hormones are synthesized and released and stimulate the gonads to produce steroids instrumental in regulating reproductive hormonal status. Actually replaces defective hypothalamic secretion of GnRH. Initial and terminal half-life ranges from 2 to 10 minutes to 10 to 40 minutes. Rapidly metabolized to peptide fragments and excreted in urine. Half-life prolonged with renal impairment.

Indications and uses: Induction of ovulation in women with primary hypothalamic amenorrhea.

Investigational use: Treatment of idiopathic hypogonadotropic hypogonadism to stimulate puberty and develop normal virilization.

Precautions: (1) Must be administered under the direction of a physician familiar with pulsatile GnRH delivery and clinical ramifications of ovarian induction. (2) Specific diagnosis of hypothalamic amenorrhea or hypogonadism due to a deficiency in quantity or pulsing of endogenous GnRH must be established. Generally based on the exclusion of other causes of the dysfunction (e.g., disorders of general health, reproductive organs, anterior pituitary, and central nervous system). (3) Ovarian ultrasound is required as a baseline and on therapy day 7 and 14. Obtain a midluteal-phase serum progesterone. At each scheduled visit the infusion site must be observed closely and a physical exam, including a pelvic, performed. (4) Patient education on the use of the pump, signs, and symptoms of infection (e.g., fever, inflammation, or redness at the catheter site), and potential for multiple pregnancy are required. (5) Evidence of ascites, pleural effusion, fluid or electrolyte imbalance, hemoconcentration, or complaints of lower abdominal pain may indicate possible ovarian hyperstimulation; notify physician immediately. Risk of ovarian hyperstimulation may be increased with spontaneous variations in GnRH secretions. (6) IV pulsatile injection results in more pregnancies than SC injection, reduces overall costs, and has a limited risk of infection with appropriate technique and care. (7) Monitoring follicle formation with ovarian ultrasound will minimize multiple pregnancies. (8) Should not be used concomittantly with other ovulation-stimulating drugs (e.g., Follutein). (9) Does not increase risk of abnormalities when administered during the first trimester but should be used during pregnancy only to maintain the corpus luteum in ovulation induction cycles. (10) Spontaneous termination of pregnancy has been reported. (11) Scrupulous aseptic technique in preparation, insertion of catheter, and care of the continuous IV site is required, including changing at 48 hour intervals. (12) Potential for secretion in breast milk unknown; no indication for use in a nursing woman. (13) Safety or efficacy for use in children under the age of 18 not established. (14) Store dry powder between 15° to 30° C (59° to 86° F).

Contraindications: History of sensitivity to gonadorelin acetate or any of its components or to gonadorelin hydrochloride (Factrel); ovarian cysts or other causes of anovulation other than hypothalamic origin; pituitary prolactinoma; hormonally dependent tumors or any other condition that could be exacerbated or worsened by pregnancy or reproductive hormones.

Incompatible with: Specific information not available. Heparin was used in reservoir in some studies. Consider specific use.

Side effects: *Equipment related:* Hematoma, infection, inflammation, or mild phlebitis at IV site; infusion set malfunction; interruption of infusion.

Gonadorelin related: Anaphylaxis (reported with related drug (gonadorelin hydrochloride [Factrel]); multiple pregnancy; ovarian hyperstimulation syndrome (e.g., ascites, cyst rupture, fluid and electrolyte imbalance, hemoconcentration, sudden ovarian enlargement with or without pain and/or pleural effusion); pregnancy termination.

Antidote: Discontinue drug and notify physician immediately for symptoms of ovarian hyperstimulation syndrome. Restart IV in another site for any signs of inflammation. Continuous infusion (versus pulsatile) from pump malfunction or accidental administration of entire dose can temporarily reduce pituitary responsiveness. Keep physician informed, and manage other side effects as indicated by severity. Treat allergic reactions and resuscitate as necessary.

GONADORELIN HYDROCHLORIDE

(Factrel)

Usual dose: 100 mcg. In females administer during the early follicular phase (day 1 through 7 of the menstrual cycle). Specific procedure required (see Precautions and manufacturer's literature).

Dilution: Diluent provided, 1 ml for 100 mcg and 2 ml for 500 mcg. Prepare immediately before use.

Rate of administration: A single dose over 15 to 30 seconds.

Actions: This synthetic hormone is similiar to natural luteinizing hormone–releasing hormone (LH-RH). It has gonadotropin-releasing effects on the anterior pituitary.

Indications and uses: Evaluating hypothalamic-pituitary gonadotropic function (1) in patients with suspected deficiency or (2) following removal of a pituitary tumor by surgery and/or irradiation.

Investigational uses: Ovulation induction, ovulation inhibition, treatment of precocious puberty.

Precautions: (1) Collection and assay methods and thus results vary with each laboratory performing this test. Coordinate process and confirm desired method for collecting blood samples. (2) Draw venous blood samples 15 minutes and immediately before gonadorelin administration. Draw additional blood samples at 15, 30, 45, 60, and 120 minutes after administration. (3) Patient must not be receiving any other drugs that affect pituitary secretion of the gonadotropins (e.g., androgens, estrogens, progestins, or glucocorticoids). (4) Incorrect results may be caused by spironolactone, levodopa, oral contraceptives, digoxin, phenothiazines, and dopamine antagonists. (5) Safety for use during pregnancy not established. (6) May be kept at room temperature but must be used within 1 day of dilution.

Contraindications: Hypersensitivity to gonadorelin or any of its components.

Incompatible with: Specific information not available. Consider specific use.

Side effects: Abdominal discomfort, flushed sensation, headache, lightheadedness, nausea.

Antidote: Notify physician and manage side effects as indicated by severity. Treat allergic reactions and resuscitate as necessary.

HALOPERIDOL LACTATE pH 3.0 to 3.6

(Haldol)

Usual dose: *All IV doses are investigational. Treatment of agitation and delirium:* Initial dose based on degree of agitation. *Mild agitation:* 0.5 to 2 mg. *Moderate agitation:* 5 to 10 mg. *Severe agitation:* 10 mg or more. In all situations observe for effectiveness. If agitation persists in 20 to 30 minutes, either repeat the first dose 1 time or give a second dose double the size of the first dose. Repeat administration of a dose that does not sedate is ineffective. Continue doubling the dose every 20 to 30 minutes until the patient begins to calm down. The dose given when calming begins is the appropriate dose for that particular patient and may be repeated every hour if necessary. 20 to 75 mg has been given every 1 to 4 hours in situations requiring high doses. Titrate repeat doses to beginning signs of agitation; observe carefully and give repeat doses at regular intervals to prevent recurrence of agitation. Up to 150 mg has been given as a single bolus with a cumulative dose of 975 mg in 24 hours. Most patients will be well controlled with much lower doses. On succeeding days the total required daily dose is divided and given at specific intervals for that patient (300 mg in 24 hours may be 12.5 mg every 1 hour or 50 mg every 4 hours). IV dosing has been used for up to several days until the source of agitation subsides or is removed. Most patients can then be treated with lower doses of oral haloperidol at less frequent intervals. IV lorazepam has a synergistic effect with haloperidol and is recommended by some clinicians as the most effective way to control agitation. One regimen recommends 10 mg of haloperidol followed by 0.5 to 10 mg of lorazepam every hour until sedation is achieved. Another recommends 3 mg haloperidol followed by 0.5 to 1 mg lorazepam; if no response in 30 minutes, increase haloperidol to 5 mg and lorazepam to 0.5 to 2 mg. If response is still inadequate, increase haloperidol to 10 mg and lorazepam to 0.5 to 10 mg hourly until adequate sedation is achieved. As in the previous regimen, the successful dose should be repeated as indicated by patient behavior. Morphine has been used instead of lorazepam in some situations.

Alternate regimen for treatment of pain and agitation in cancer patients: Give haloperidol 5 mg, follow with lorazepam 0.5 mg, followed by hydromorphone (Dilaudid) 0.5 mg. Increase haloperidol to 10 mg and gradually increase the lorazepam dose as described above, giving both drugs every 20 to 30 minutes until agitation subsides. Discontinue lorazepam and reduce haloperidol by half while doubling interval between doses. Continue hydromorphone every 3 hours. Morphine may be substituted for the hydromorphine.

Antiemetic or treatment of intractable hiccups: 3 to 5 mg every 2 hours for 5 to 7 doses. May be used in an antiemtic regimen with dexamethasone in chemotherapy.

Dilution: May be given undiluted. Give through Y-tube or three-way stopcock of the infusion set. Flush with at least 2 ml of normal saline before and after administration of haloperidol. A single dose may be added to 30 to 50 ml of most infusion solutions and given as an infusion. According to the literature, a continuous infusion of up to 25 mg/hr has been used to treat an agitated delirium in a cancer patient until the delirium subsided.

Rate of administration: *Direct IV:* A single dose over 1 minute. When using multiple drugs, each individual drug should be given over 1 minute. (Review text of each drug before administration.)

IV piggyback: A single dose over 30 minutes.

Infusion: Up to 25 mg/hr has been used. Must be titrated by desired dose and patient response.

Actions: An antipsychotic agent structurally similar to the neuroleptic droperidol with effects similar to selected phenothiazines (e.g., trifluroperazine [Stelazine], prochlorperazine [Compazine], perphenazine [Trilafon]). A potent dopamine blocker, it produces marked tranquilization and sedation and has a potent antiemetic action. Has minimum effect on cardiac, pulmonary, renal, hepatic, or hematopoietic functions. Effective in 20 to 30 minutes and may last for 1 to 4 hours.

Metabolized in the liver and excreted in urine and feces.

Indications and uses: *All IV uses are investigational.* (1) Control acute delirium especially in emergency situations involving psychotic patients. (2) Control of agitation or acute delirium interfering with appropriate treatment of cancer, cardiac, surgical, respiratory, and medical patients in intensive care units. Common causes of severe agitation may include continuous monitoring of vital signs, use of multiple IV catheters, use of life support devices (e.g., the intraaortic balloon pump), myocardial infarction, uncontrolled dysrhythmia, recent cardiac arrest, feeling of impending doom, coronary artery bypass, cardiotomy, weaning from chronic ventilatory support, and drug overdose. (3) Frequently given concurrently with lorazepam (Ativan). Combination is considered superior to either drug alone. Both haloperidol and lorazepam may be given concurrently with morphine in agitation or hydromorphone (Dilaudid) in cancer patients. (4) Antiemetic in cancer chemotherapy. (5) Treatment of intractable hiccups.

Precautions: (1) *Not FDA approved for IV use* but is being used throughout the United States. (2) Check vial carefully: only haloperidol lactate can be used IV. Haloperidol decanoate contains sesame oil and is for IM use only. (3) Use should be restricted to patients on intensive care units with cardiac monitoring. Primarily used by or under direct observation of the attending physician until adequate sedation and a constant dose is achieved. (4) Rule out other possible causes of agitation (e.g., metabolic and systemic abnormalities, drug toxicity, drug withdrawal) before initiating haloperidol. (5) A potent drug. Monitor the patient constantly. Resuscitation equipment, a narcotic antagonist (if a narcotic has been used concurrently), IV infusion line, and drugs to manage hypotension and extrapyramidal symptoms must be readily available. (6) Reduce dose of narcotics and all CNS depressants to one fourth or one third of usual dose before, during, and for 24 hours after injection of haloperidol. (7) If other CNS depressants (e.g., narcotics) have been given, reduce dose of haloperidol. (8) May cause life-threatening hypotension and bradycardia with propranolol (Inderal). (9) Dose not necessarily reduced for elderly patients. (10) Use caution with known history of seizures or EEG abnormalities; maintain adequate anticonvulsant therapy. (11) Use caution in the presence of severe cardiovascular disorders. (12) May cause severe neurotoxicity in patients with thyrotoxicosis; use caution. (13) May cause increased intraocular pressure with anticholinergic drugs (e.g., atropine), including antiparkinsonian agents. (14) Extrapyramidal side effects rarely occur with IV haloperidol, and abrupt discontinuation does not seem to cause problems with withdrawal dyskinesia. (15) Store in refrigerator, protect from light. Do not freeze.

Contraindications: No specific contraindications except for children under 3 years of age. Risks must be weighed against potential benefits.

Incompatible with: Heparin and phenytoin. IV line must be flushed with 2 ml of normal saline before and after administration. One manufacturer recommends that haloperidol not be mixed in syringe or solution with any other drug.

Side effects: Considered to have a good range of safety, even in large total daily doses.

Minor: Hypotension (mild), muscle twitching, prolongation of corrected QT interval, tremors, tachycardia.

Major: Apnea, cardiac arrest, excessive sedation, extrapyramidal symptoms (rare), hypotension (severe), impaired vision, neuroleptic malignant syndrome, jaundice, respiratory depression. Numerous other side effects common to phenothiazines and neuroleptic drugs are possible but not common with IV use.

Antidote: Notify the physician of any side effect. If minor side effects progress or major side effects occur, discontinue the drug, support the patient, treat symptomatically, and notify the physician. Rule out hypovolemia, other hypotensive agents, low cardiac output, and sepsis as causes of hypotension. Then, if indicated, treat hypotension with fluid therapy or vasopressors such as dopamine hydrochloride (Intropin) or norepinephrine (Levophed). Epinephrine is contraindicated for hypotension. Further hypotension will occur. Treat extrapyramidal symptoms with benztropine mesylate (Congentin) or diphenhydramine hydrochloride (Benadryl). Dialysis is not effective in overdose. Resuscitate as necessary.

HEMIN

(Panhematin)

Usual dose: A single dose of 1 to 4 mg/kg of body weight/24 hr for 3 to 14 days. This dose could be repeated in 12 hours for severe cases. Never exceed a total dose of 6 mg/kg/24 hr. Length of treatment dependent on severity of symptoms and clinical response.

Dilution: Each vial containing 313 mg of hemin must be diluted with 43 ml of sterile water for injection. Shake well for 2 to 3 minutes to ensure dilution. Each 1 ml contains 7 mg hematin. Each 0.14 ml contains 1 mg hematin. May be given directly from vial as an infusion or through Y-tube or three-way stopcock of infusion set. Use of a 0.45 micron or smaller filter recommended.

Rate of administration: A single dose evenly distributed over 10 to 15 minutes.

Actions: An iron-containing metalloporphyrin enzyme inhibitor extracted from red blood cells. Inhibits rate of porphyria/heme biosynthesis in the liver and bone marrow by an unknown mechanism. Induces remission of symptoms only, not curative. Some excretion occurs in urine and feces.

Indications and uses: To control symptoms of recurrent attacks of acute intermittent porphyria in selected patients (often related to the menstrual cycle in susceptible women).

Precautions: (1) Confirm diagnosis of acute porphyria before use (positive Watson-Schwartz or Hoechst test). (2) Alternate therapy of 400 Gm glucose/24 hr for several days should be tried before use of hemin indicated.

(3) Keep frozen until reconstituted immediately before use. Contains no preservatives, decomposes rapidly; discard unused solution. (4) Must be given before irreversible neuronal damage of porphyria has begun. (5) Use of a large arm vein or central venous catheter recommended to avoid phlebitis. (6) Effectiveness monitored by decrease in urine concentration of δ-aminolevulinic acid (ALA), uroporphyrinogen (UPG), or porphobilinogen (PBG). (7) Action inhibited by estrogens, barbiturates, and steroid metabolites. Avoid concurrent use. (8) Potentiates anticoagulants. (9) Use extreme caution in pregnant and lactating women and in children. Safety for use not established.

Contraindications: Hypersensitivity to hemin, porphyria cutanea tarda.

Incompatible with: Specific information not available. Do not mix with other drugs.

Side effects: Almost nonexistent with usual dosage and appropriate technique; fever, phlebitis, reversible renal shutdown.

Antidote: Discontinue temporarily if known or questionable side effect appears, and notify physician. Renal shutdown of overdose has responded to ethacrynic acid (Edecrin) and mannitol. Treat anaphylaxis (antihistamines, epinephrine, corticosteroids) and resuscitate as necessary.

HEPARIN SODIUM — pH 5.0 to 7.5

(✦ Hepalean, Heparin Lock-Flush, Hep-Lock, Hep-Lock PF, Hep-Lock U/P, Liquaemin Sodium, Liquaemin Sodium Preservative Free)

Usual dose: *Intermittent injection:* 10,000 units initially. Dosage is repeated every 4 to 6 hours and adjusted according to clotting time. Usually 5,000 to 10,000 units.

IV infusion: 20,000 to 40,000 units/24 hr in 1,000 ml isotonic saline or other compatible infusion solution. An initial bolus dose of 5,000 units is required.

Open heart surgery: 150 to 400 units/kg of body weight during surgical procedure.

Maintain patency of infusion needle, catheter, or implanted port: 1,000 to 1,500 units to each 1,000 ml IV fluid.

Maintain patency of heparin plug needle, catheter, or implanted port: 10 to 500 units diluted in sufficient milliliters of normal saline to reach the tip of the needle, catheter, or implanted port. Use after each medication injection or every 8 to 24 hours.

Blood transfusion: 400 to 600 units/100 ml whole blood.

Pediatric dose: An initial dose of 50 units/kg of body weight is followed by a maintenance dose of 100 units/kg every 4 hours, or 20,000 units/M^2/24 hr as a continuous infusion.

Dilution: May be given undiluted or diluted in any given amount of isotonic sodium chloride, dextrose, or Ringer's solution for infusion and given direct IV or as an intermittent IV injection or continuous IV infusion. Ensure adequate mixing of heparin with solution in all situations.

Blood transfusion: Add 7,500 units heparin to 100 ml sodium chloride injection. Add 6 to 8 ml of this sterile solution to each 100 ml of whole blood.

Rate of administration: First 1,000 units or fraction thereof over 1 minute. After this test dose, any single injection (5,000 units or fraction thereof) may be given over 1 minute. A continuous IV infusion may be given over 4 to 24 hours, depending on specific dosage of heparin required, amount of heparin added, and amount of infusion fluid used as a diluent. Continuous IV infusion is the preferred method of administration. Use an infusion pump for accuracy.

Actions: An anticoagulant with immediate and predictable effects on the blood. Heparin combines with other factors in the blood to inhibit the conversion of prothrombin to thrombin and fibrinogen to fibrin. Adhesiveness of platelets is reduced. Well-established clots are not dissolved, but growth is prevented and newer clots may be dissolved. Duration of action is short, about 4 to 6 hours. Actual average half-life is 60 to 90 minutes. The half-life is prolonged by higher doses and in liver or kidney disease, and shortened in patients with pulmonary embolism. Does not cross the placental barrier. Metabolized in the liver and excreted in the kidneys. Has a wide margin of safety.

Indications and uses: (1) Prevention and/or treatment of all types of thromboses and emboli; (2) diagnosis and treatment of DIC; (3) prevention of clotting in surgery of the heart or blood vessels, during blood transfusion, and hemodialysis; (4) adjunct in treatment of coronary occlusion with acute myocardial infarction; (5) maintain patency of needle, catheter, or implanted port during prolonged IV infusion; (6) maintain patency of heparin lock needle for intermittent medication injection or vein access.

Precautions: (1) Read label carefully. Comes in many strengths. (2) Unit to milligram conversions are not consistent. (3) Whole blood clotting time or activated PTT must be done before initial injection. Often done before each injection on the first day of treatment. Usually repeated daily thereafter during IV therapy and more often if indicated. Depending on the test chosen the desired therapeutic level is approximately one and one half to three times greater than the control level. Confirm desired control level with physician. Obtain test just before next dose due in intermittent injection. Notify the physician if activated PTT or whole blood clotting time is above therapeutic level. (4) Use with caution during pregnancy. Hemorrhage most likely to occur during the last trimester or postpartum. (5) Use extreme caution in any disease state where risk of hemorrhage may be increased, i.e., subacute bacterial endocarditis; arterial sclerosis; aneurysm; severe hypertension; during or following spinal tap, spinal anesthesia, or major surgery; hemophilia; thrombocytopenia; ulcerative lesions; diverticulitis; ulcerative colitis; continuous tube drainage of the stomach or small intestine; threatened abortion; menstruation; alcohol abuse; tuberculosis; visceral carcinoma; and severe biliary, liver, or renal disease. (6) Decrease dosage gradually. Abrupt withdrawal may precipitate increased coagulability. (7) Monitor platelet count. Discontinue heparin if it falls below 100,000 or a thrombosis forms. May develop white clot syndrome, which may lead to skin necrosis, gangrene, myocardial infarction, pulmonary embolism, and stroke. (8) Monitor hematocrit and occult blood in stool also. (9) May cause an increase in free fatty acid serum levels. (10) Some products contain the preservative benzyl alcohol associated with gasping syndrome in premature infants. (11) May cause hyperkalemia in patients with diabetes or renal insufficiency. (12) Potentiated by chloramphenicol (Chloromycetin), dextran, ibuprofen, indomethacin, hydroxychloroquine, penicillin, phenylbutazone, salicylates, and others. (13) Inhibited by antihistamines, barbiturates, digitalis, calcium disodium edetate, hyaluronidase, hydroxyzine (Vistaril), nicotine, phenothiazines, tetracyclines, and others, some of which may cause increased heparin absorption or result in withdrawal bleeding when discontinued. (14) Potentiates oral anticoagulants, diazepam (Valium), phenytoin (Dilantin), thyroxine, and others. (15) Nitroglycerin IV may cause heparin resistance. (16) To avoid precipitation, irrigate heparin plug catheters with normal saline before and after injecting acidic or incompatible solutions. (17) Use caution if administering ACD converted blood (variable). (18) Use extensive precautionary methods to prevent bleeding if patient requires IM injection, arterial puncture, or venipuncture. (19) Use caution when administered after other anticoagulants. Lab data may not provide an accurate baseline.

Contraindications: Active bleeding, blood dyscrasias, history of bleeding, hypersensitivity to heparin (derived from animal protein), inadequate laboratory facilities, liver disease with hypoprothrombinemia (see Precautions).

Incompatible with: Amikacin (Amikin), ampicillin (Amcill), atropine, cephalothin (Keflin), chlordiazepoxide (Librium), chlorpromazine (Thorazine), chlortetracycline (Aureomycin), codeine, dacarbazine (DTIC), daunorubicin (Cerubidine), dobutamine (Dobutrex), erythromycin (Ilotycin, Erythrocin), ergonovine, gentamicin (Garamycin), hyaluronidase, hydrocortisone (Solu-Cortef), hydroxyzine (Vistaril), insulin (aqueous), kanamycin (Kantrex), levorphanol (Levo-Dromoran), meperidine (Demerol), metaraminol (Aramine), methadone, methicillin (Staphcillin), morphine sulfate, penicillin G, polymyxin B (Aerosporin), procainamide

(Pronestyl), prochlorperazine (Compazine), promazine (Sparine), promethazine (Phenergan), streptomycin, tetracycline (Achromycin), tobramycin (Nebcin), vancomycin (Vancocin).

Side effects: Allergic reactions (rare), alopecia (rare), bruising, epistaxis, hematuria, prolonged coagulation time (in excess of two to three times the control level), tarry stools or any other signs of bleeding, thrombocytopenia, white clot syndrome. Allergic reactions including anaphylaxis do occur. Vasospastic reactions resulting in a painful, ischemic, cyanotic limb may develop. Arthralgias, chest pain, headache, hypertension, and itching on the plantar surface of the feet have been reported.

Antidote: Discontinue the drug and notify the physician of any side effects. Protamine sulfate is a heparin antagonist and specifically indicated in overdose or desired heparin reversal.

HETASTARCH pH 5.5

(Hespan)

Usual dose: *Shock:* Variable, depending on amount of fluid loss and resultant hemoconcentration. Initially 500 ml (30 Gm). Total dose should not exceed 1,500 ml/24 hr or 20 ml/kg of body weight.

Leukapheresis: 250 to 700 ml in continuous flow centrifugation procedures.

Dilution: Available as a 6% solution in 500 ml bottles properly diluted in normal saline and ready for use. Calculated osmolarity is approximately 310 mOsm/L.

Rate of administration: Variable, depending on indication, present blood volume, and patient response. Initial 500 ml may be given at rates approaching 20 ml/kg of body weight/hr. Reduce rate in burns or septic shock. If additional hydroxyethyl starch is required, reduce flow to lowest rate possible to maintain hemodynamic status.

Leukapheresis: Usually infused at a constant ratio to venous whole blood, i.e., 1 to 8.

Actions: A synthetic polymer with properties similar to dextran. Approximates colloidal properties of human albumin. Provides hemodynamically significant plasma volume expansion in excess of the amount infused for about 24 hours. Dilutes total serum protein and hematocrit values. Increases erythrocyte sedimentation rate. Granulocyte collection by centrifuging becomes more efficient. Enzymatically degraded to molecules small enough to be excreted through the kidneys attached to glucose units.

Indications and uses: (1) As an adjunct in treatment of shock due to burns, hemorrhage, sepsis, surgery, or trauma; (2) adjunct in leukapheresis to improve harvesting and increase yield of granulocytes.

Precautions: (1) For IV use only. (2) Not a substitute for whole blood or plasma proteins. (3) Monitor pulse, blood pressure, central venous pressure, and urine output every 5 to 15 minutes for the first hour and hourly thereafter while indicated. (4) Maintain adequate hydration of patient with additional IV fluids. (5) Change IV tubing or flush with normal saline before imposing blood. (6) Use caution in heart disease, renal shutdown, congestive heart failure, pulmonary edema, and liver disease. (7) May reduce coagulability of the circulating blood. Observe patient for increased bleeding and/or circulatory overload. (8) Does not interfere with blood typing or cross-matching. (9) Hemoglobin, hematocrit, electrolyte, and serum protein evaluation are necessary during therapy. During leukapheresis also monitor leukocyte and platelet count, leukocyte differential, PT, and PTT. (10) Observe frequent donors carefully; may have a marked decline in platelet count and hemoglobin levels resulting from hemodilution by hetastarch and saline. Temporary declines in total protein, albumin, calcium, and fibrinogen may also be present.

Contraindications: Severe bleeding disorders, severe congestive heart failure, renal failure with oliguria or anuria. No data available pertaining to use in pregnant women or in children.

Incompatible with: Specific information not available. See Precautions.

Side effects: Chills, fever, headache, itching, muscle pains, peripheral edema, submaxillary and parotid glandular enlargement, urticaria, and vomiting. Anaphylaxis can occur.

Antidote: Notify the physician of any side effect. Discontinue the drug immediately at the first sign of an allergic reaction, provided other means of sustaining the circulation are available. Antihistamines such as diphenhydramine (Benadryl) are helpful. Ephedrine or epinephrine (Adrenalin) may also be indicated. Resuscitate as necessary.

HISTAMINE PHOSPHATE pH 3.0 to 6.0

Usual dose: Must be given in specific sequence to determine validity of test results. 0.01 mg (10 mcg) as initial dose. If no response after 5 minutes, 0.05 mg (50 mcg) may be given.

Dilution: May be given undiluted through tubing of an IV infusion of 5% dextrose in water or normal saline.

Rate of administration: Each single dose may be rapidly injected.

Actions: Histamine is a naturally occurring substance in the body. It acts to dilate even the smallest blood vessels, causing flushing, lowering peripheral resistance, and decreasing blood pressure. It has numerous other effects on the body.

Indications and uses: Presumptive diagnosis of pheochromocytoma. Indicated only for specific patients who have paroxysmal signs of excessive catecholamine secretion but have normal urinary values for assays of catecholamines and metabolites when asymptomatic.

Precautions: (1) Resting blood pressure must be 150/110 or lower. (2) Have epinephrine available for hypotensive reaction and phentolamine (Regitine) available for hypertensive reaction. (3) Withhold antihypertensives, sympathomimetic agents, sedatives, and narcotics for 24 to 72 hours before the test. (4) Place patient on bed rest. Start a slow IV infusion of 5% dextrose in water or normal saline. Record blood pressure until stable. Collect 2-hour urine specimen for catecholamine assay. When completed, give histamine through IV tubing rapidly. Collect another 2-hour urine specimen. Record blood pressure and pulse every 30 seconds for 15 minutes after histamine injection. Expected response includes headache, flushing, and a decrease in blood pressure followed by an increase in blood pressure within 2 minutes. (5) Very small doses can precipitate asthma in patients with bronchial disease. Use extreme caution. (6) Safety during pregnancy and lactation not established.

Contraindications: Hypersensitivity to histamine products; hypotension; severe hypertension; vasomotor instability; history of bronchial asthma; history of urticaria; severe cardiac, pulmonary, or renal disease; the elderly.

Incompatible with: Specific information not available. Consider incompatible in syringe or solution because of specific use.

Side effects: Abdominal cramps, allergic reactions (including anaphylaxis), asthma, bronchial constriction, collapse with convulsions, diarrhea, dizziness, dyspnea, faintness, flushing, headache, hypertension, hypotension, metallic taste, nervousness, palpitations, syncope, tachycardia, urticaria, visual disturbances, vomiting.

Antidote: For accidental overdose, obstruct vein flow with tourniquet, use epinephrine and antihistamines (e.g., diphenhydramine [Benadryl]). Treat anaphylaxis and resuscitate as necessary.

HYDRALAZINE HYDROCHLORIDE

pH 3.4 to 4.0

(Apresoline)

Usual dose: 5 to 40 mg. Begin with a low dose. Increase gradually as indicated. Repeat as necessary. Maximum dose is 300 to 400 mg/24 hr.

Pediatric dose: 1.7 to 3.5 mg/kg of body weight/24 hours, in equally divided doses every 4 to 6 hours.

Dilution: May be given undiluted. Do not add to IV solutions. May be given through Y-tube or three-way stopcock of infusion set.

Rate of administration: Each 10 mg or fraction thereof over 1 minute.

Actions: A potent antihypertensive drug. It lowers blood pressure by direct relaxation of smooth muscle of arteries and arterioles. Peripheral vasodilation results. Stimulation of the carotid sinus reflex increases cardiac output and rate. Action begins 2 to 10 minutes after the drug is given. Renal blood flow increased in some cases, while cerebral blood flow maintained. Well absorbed; 90% bound to plasma protein. Some excretion in urine.

Indications and uses: (1) Severe essential hypertension; (2) vasodilation in cardiogenic shock; (3) pregnancy-induced hypertension.

Precautions: (1) Check blood pressure every 5 minutes until stabilized at the desired level. Check every 15 minutes thereafter throughout crisis. Average maximum decrease occurs in 10 to 80 minutes. (2) IV use recommended only when the oral route is not feasible. (3) Rarely the drug of choice for hypertension unless used in combination (effectiveness increased and side effects decreased) with spironolactone (Aldactone), reserpine (Serpasil), guanethidine (Ismelin), and thiazide diuretics. Sometimes used with a β-adrenergic blocking drug (e.g., propranolol [Inderal]); use caution, may potentiate effects. (4) Tolerance is easily developed but subsides about 7 days after the drug is discontinued. (5) Color changes occur in most 10% dextrose solutions and after drawing through a metal filter. (6) Tricyclic antidepressants (e.g., amitriptyline [Elavil]) may be contraindicated; will require dosage adjustment. (7) Potentiated by anesthetics, ethacrynic acid (Edecrin), MAO inhibitors (e.g., pargyline [Eutonyl]), triamterene (Dyrenium), and other antihypertensive agents. (8) Inhibits epinephrine, levarterenol (Levophed). (9) Use caution in advanced renal damage, cerebrovascular accidents, congestive heart failure, coronary insufficiency, headache, increased intracranial pressure, pregnancy, and tachycardia. (10) Withdraw drug gradually to avoid rebound hypertension.

Contraindications: Hypersensitivity to hydralazine, coronary artery disease, mitral valvular rheumatic heart disease.

Incompatible with: Aminophylline, ampicillin, calcium disodium edetate, chlorothiazide (Diuril), ethacrynic acid (Edecrin), hydrocortisone (Solu-Cortef), mephentermine (Wyamine), methohexital (Brevital), phenobarbital (Luminal), verapamil (Calan), 10% fructose, 10% dextrose in lactated Ringer's injection.

Side effects: *Minor:* Anxiety, depression, dry mouth, flushing, headache, nausea, numbness, palpitations, paresthesia, postural hypotension, tachycardia, tingling, unpleasant taste, vomiting.

Major: Angina, blood dyscrasias, chills, coronary insufficiency, delirium, dependent edema, fever, ileus, lupus erythematosus (simulated), myocardial ischemia and infarction, rheumatoid syndrome (simulated), toxic psychosis.

Antidote: If minor side effects occur, notify the physician, who will probably treat them symptomatically. Ganglionic blocking agents (e.g., trimethaphan camsylate [Arfonad]) will control tachycardia. Pyridoxine will relieve numbness, tingling, and paresthesia. Antihistamines, barbiturates, and salicylates may be required. Treat hypotension with a vasopressor that is least likely to precipitate cardiac dysrhythmias (methoxamine [Vasoxyl]). If side effects are progressive or any major side effects occur, discontinue the drug immediately and notify the physician. Treatment is symptomatic. Resuscitate as necessary. Occasionally methyldopa (Aldomet) will be used as a substitute, since it is effective for the same indications but has fewer side effects.

HYDROCORTISONE SODIUM PHOSPHATE pH 7.5 to 8.5

(Hydrocortone Phosphate)

Usual dose: 25 to 250 mg initially. May repeat as necessary every 4 to 6 hours. Total dose usually does not exceed 1 Gm (20 ml)/24 hr but may be higher in acute disease. Dosage individualized according to the severity of the disease and the response of the patient.

Acute adrenal insufficiency: 100 mg initially. Repeat every 8 hours in IV fluids.

Pediatric dose: 2 to 8 mg/kg of body weight/24 hr. Dose varies with disease.

Acute adrenal insufficiency: 1 to 2 mg/kg direct IV, then 150 to 250 mg/kg/day in divided doses. Maximum of 150 mg/kg/24 hr in divided doses for infants.

Dilution: May be given without mixing or dilution. Always use a separate syringe for hydrocortisone. May be added to sodium chloride or dextrose injection and given by IV infusion. Solution must be used within 24 hours of dilution.

Rate of administration: 25 mg or fraction thereof over 1 minute. Decrease rate of injection if any complaints of burning or tingling along injection site.

Actions: The principal hormone secreted by the adrenal cortex. Very rapidly absorbed adrenocortical steroid with potent metabolic, antiinflammatory, and innumerable other effects. May be used in conjunction with other forms of therapy, such as epinephrine for acute allergic reactions or antibiotics in acute infections. It is absorbed primarily into the lymph stream at extremely high levels and probably excreted in the urine and feces. 75% excretion occurs within 24 hours, allowing the use of very large doses with reasonable safety. Crosses placental barrier. Secreted in breast milk.

Indications and uses: (1) Adrenocortical insufficiency; total, relative, and operative; (2) supplementary therapy for severe allergic reactions; (3) shock unresponsive to conventional therapy; (4) acute exacerbation of disease for patients on steroid therapy; (5) acute life-threatening infections with massive antibiotic therapy; (6) induce remissions of some malignancies; (7) viral hepatitis; (8) thyroid crisis.

Precautions: (1) Sensitive to heat. (2) May cause elevated blood presure and salt and water retention. (3) Salt restriction and potassium and calcium replacement are necessary. (4) May mask signs of infection. (5) To avoid relative adrenocortical insufficiency, do not stop therapy abruptly. Taper off. Patient is observed carefully, especially under stress, for up to 2 years. The exception is very short-term therapy. (6) Maintain on ulcer regimen and antacid prophylactically. (7) May increase insulin needs in diabetes. (8) Inhibited by anticonvulsants, some antihistamines, barbiturates, ephedrine, oral contraceptives, propranolol (Inderal), phenylbutazone (Butazolidin), rifampin, and troleandomycin. (9) Inhibits anticoagulants, aspirin, isoniazid. (10) Potentiates theophyllines and cyclosporine. (11) Monitor serum potassium levels; may cause hypokalemia with digitalis products, amphotericin B, or potassium-depleting diuretics. (12) Dose adjustments may be required with cyclophosphamide. (13) Do not vaccinate with attenuated-virus vaccines (e.g., smallpox) during therapy. (14) Altered protein-binding capacity will impact effectiveness of this drug. (15) Administer before 9 AM to reduce suppression of individual's own adrenocortical activity.

Contraindications: *Absolute contraindications except in life-threatening situations:* Hypersensitivity to any product component including sulfites, systemic fungal infections.

Relative contraindications: Active or latent peptic ulcer, active or healed tuberculosis, acute psychoses, chickenpox, congestive heart failure, diabetes mellitus, diverticulitis, fresh intestinal anastomoses, hypertension, myasthenia gravis, ocular herpes simplex, osteoporosis, pregnancy, psychotic tendencies, renal insufficiency, thromboembolic tendencies, vaccinia.

Incompatible with: Amobarbital (Amytal), calcium gluconate, cephalothin (Keflin), chloramphenicol (Chloromycetin), erythromycin, heparin, kanamycin (Kantrex), metaraminol (Aramine), methicillin (Staphcillin), pentobarbital (Nembutal), phenobarbital (Luminal), phytonadione (Aquamephyton), prochlorperazine (Compazine), promazine (Sparine), tetracycline, vancomycin (Vancocin), vitamin B complex with C, warfarin (Coumadin).

Side effects: Do occur but are usually reversible: alteration of glucose metabolism including hyperglycemia and glycosuria; Cushing's syndrome (moon face, fat pads, etc.); electrolyte and calcium imbalance; euphoria or other psychic disturbances; hypersensitivity reactions including anaphylaxis; increased blood pressure; increased intracranial pressure; masking of infection; menstrual irregularities; perforation and hemorrhage from aggravation of peptic ulcer; protein catabolism with negative nitrogen balance; spontaneous fractures; sweating, headache, or weakness; thromboembolism; transitory burning or tingling; and many others.

Antidote: Notify the physician of any side effect. Will probably treat the side effect if necessary. Resuscitate as necessary for anaphylaxis and notify physician. Keep epinephrine immediately available.

HYDROCORTISONE SODIUM SUCCINATE

pH 7.0 to 8.0

(A-hydrocort, Solu-Cortef)

Usual dose: 100 to 500 mg initially. May be repeated every 1 to 6 hours as necessary. For severe shock, doses up to 2 Gm or more every 2 to 4 hours have been given. These massive doses should not be used longer than 48 to 72 hours. Dosage is individualized according to the severity of the disease and the response of the patient and is not necessarily reduced for children. Never give less than 25 mg/24 hr.

Dilution: Available in a Mix-O-Vial, which is reconstituted by removing the protective cap, turning the rubber stopper a quarter turn, and pressing down, allowing the diluent into the lower chamber. Agitate gently. Using sterile techniques, a needle can be easily inserted through the center of the rubber stopper to withdraw the solution. If a Mix-O-Vial is not available, reconstitute each 250 mg or fraction thereof with 2 ml bacteriostatic water for injection. Agitate gently to mix solution. May be given direct IV, or each 100 mg (250 mg, 500 mg, etc.) may be further diluted in at least 100 ml (250 ml, 500 ml, etc.) but not more than 1,000 ml of suitable IV solution for infusion. Suitable solutions are 5% dextrose in water, isotonic saline, or 5% dextrose in isotonic saline.

Rate of administration: Direct IV each 500 mg or fraction thereof over 1 minute. Direct IV is usually the route of choice and eliminates the possibility of overloading the patient with IV fluids. At the discretion of the physician, a continuous infusion may be given, properly diluted, over the specified time desired.

Actions: The principal hormone secreted by the adrenal cortex. A rapidly absorbed adrenocortical steroid with potent metabolic, antiinflammatory, and innumerable other effects. May be used in conjunction with other forms of therapy, such as epinephrine for acute allergic reactions or antibiotics in acute infections. It is absorbed primarily into the lymph stream at extremely high levels and probably excreted in the urine and feces. 75% excretion occurs within 24 hours, allowing the use of very large doses with reasonable safety. Crosses placental barrier. Secreted in breast milk.

Indications and uses: Situations requiring high doses of hydrocortisone in a small amount of diluent and a need for high blood levels in a short period of time, such as (1) acute adrenocortical insufficiency, (2) acute hypersensitivity reactions, (3) aspiration pneumonitis, (4) bilateral adrenalectomy, (5) overwhelming infections with severe toxicity, (6) severe shock, (7) systemic lupus erythematosus relapse, (8) chemotherapy.

Precautions: (1) Sensitive to heat and light. (2) Discard unused solutions after 3 days. (3) May cause elevated blood pressure and salt and water retention. (4) Salt restriction and potassium and calcium replacement are necessary. (5) May mask signs of infection. (6) To avoid relative adrenocortical insufficiency, do not stop therapy abruptly. Taper off. Patient is observed carefully, especially under stress, for up to 2 years. The exception is very short-term therapy. (7) Maintain on ulcer regimen and antacid prophylactically. (8) May increase insulin needs in diabetes. (9) Inhibited by anticonvulsants, some antihistamines, barbiturates, ephedrine, oral contraceptives, propranolol (Inderal), phenylbutazone (Butazolidin), rifampin, and troleandomycin. (10) Inhibits anticoagulants, aspirin, isoniazid. (11) Potentiates theophyllines and cyclosporine. (12) Monitor serum potassium levels; may cause hypokalemia with digitalis products, amphotericin B, or potassium-depleting diuretics. (13) Dose adjustments may be required with cyclophosphamide. (14) Do not vaccinate with attenuated-virus vaccines (e.g., smallpox) during therapy. (15) Altered protein-binding capacity will impact effectiveness of this drug. (16) Administer before 9 AM to reduce suppression of individual's own adrenocortical activity.

Contraindications: *Absolute contraindications except in life-threatening situations:* Hypersensitivity to any product component including sulfites, systemic fungal infections.

Relative contraindications: Active or latent peptic ulcer, active or healed tuberculosis, acute psychoses, chickenpox, congestive heart failure, diabetes mellitus, diverticulitis, fresh intestinal anastomoses, hypertension, myasthenia gravis, ocular herpes simplex, osteoporosis, pregnancy, psychotic tendencies, renal insufficiency, thromboembolic tendencies, and vaccinia.

Incompatible with: Aminophylline, amobarbital (Amytal), ampicillin, bleomycin (Blenoxane), chlorpromazine (Thorazine), colistimethate (Coly-Mycin M), dimenhydrinate (Dramamine), diphenhydramine (Benadryl), doxorubicin (Adriamycin), ephedrine, heparin, hyaluronidase, hydralazine (Apresoline), hydroxyzine (Vistaril), kanamycin (Kantrex), lidocaine, lobeline, meperidine (Demerol), metaraminol (Aramine), methicillin (Staphcillin), nafcillin, netilmicin (Netromycin), pentobarbital (Nembutal), phenobarbital (Luminal), prochlorperazine (Compazine), promazine (Sparine), promethazine (Phenergan), secobarbital (Seconal), tetracycline, thiamylal (Surital), tolazoline (Priscoline), vancomycin (Vancocin).

Side effects: Do occur but are usually reversible: alteration of glucose metabolism including hyperglycemia and glycosuria; Cushing's syndrome (moon face, fat pads, etc.); electrolyte and calcium imbalance; euphoria or other psychic disturbances; hypersensitivity reactions including anaphylaxis; increased blood pressure; increased intracranial pressure; masking of infection; menstrual irregularities; perforation and hemorrhage from aggravation of peptic ulcer; protein catabolism with negative nitrogen balance; spontaneous fractures; sweating, headache, or weakness; thromboembolism; transitory burning or tingling; and many others.

Antidote: Notify the physician of any side effect. Will probably treat the side effect if necessary. Resuscitate as necessary for anaphylaxis and notify the physician. Keep epinephrine immediately available.

HYDROMORPHONE HYDROCHLORIDE — pH 4.0 to 5.5

(Dilaudid)

Usual dose: *Direct IV*: 2 to 4 mg every 4 to 6 hours. 0.5 mg every 3 hours with specific doses of haloperidol and lorazepam in delirium agitation of critically ill cancer patients.

Reduced dose may be required in impaired renal or hepatic function.

Infusion: In selected critically ill cancer patients hydromorphone may be administered in doses as high as 2 to 9 mg/hr. Must be administered through a controlled infusion device that may be patient activated. The initial loading dose, the continuous background infusion to provide a level of pain relief and maintain patency of the vein, additional patient-activated doses with specific time interval, additional health professional–provided boluses with specific time interval, and the total dose allowed per hour must be determined by the physician specialist and individualized for each patient.

Dilution: *Direct IV:* Each dose should be diluted with 5 ml of sterile water or normal saline for injection. May give through Y-tube or three-way stopcock of infusion set.

Infusion: Each 0.1 to 1 mg is usually diluted in 1 ml normal saline to provide 0.1 to 1 mg/ml for use in a narcotic syringe infusor system. Available in 1, 2, 4, or 10 mg/ml ampoules. Use concentrated preparations for larger doses. May be diluted in larger amounts of 5% dextrose in water or saline, 0.45% or normal saline (concentration is usually 1 mg/ml) for infusion and given through a standard infusion pump (requires very close titration).

Rate of administration: *Direct IV:* 2 mg or fraction thereof properly diluted solution over 2 to 5 minutes. Frequently titrated according to symptom relief and respiratory rate.

Infusion: All parameters (outlined in Usual dose) should be ordered by the physician. Any dose requiring a controlled infusion device requires accurate titration and close monitoring.

Actions: An opium derivative and CNS depressant closely related to morphine. Provides potent analgesia without hypnotic effects. Five times more potent than morphine milligram for milligram. Onset of action is prompt and lasts 3 to 4 hours. Hydromorphone is detoxified in the liver and excreted in the urine. Crosses placental barrier. Secreted in breast milk.

Indications and uses: Moderate to severe, acute or chronic pain, especially in situations in which a hypnotic effect is not desirable, such as postoperatively or in some malignancies.

Precautions: (1) Oxygen, controlled respiratory equipment, and naloxone (Narcan) must be available. (2) Observe patient frequently to continuously based on dose and monitor vital signs. Keep patient supine; orthostatic hypotension and fainting may occur; less likely with continuous low doses, but observe closely during ambulation. (3) Stool softeners and/or laxatives will be required to avoid constipation and fecal impaction, especially with increased doses and extended use. Maintain adequate hydration. (4) Use caution in the elderly and in patients with impaired hepatic or renal function, emphysema, and anticoagulation therapy. (5) Use extreme caution in craniotomy, head injury, and increased intracranial pressure; respiratory depression and intracranial pressure may be further increased. (6) May cause apnea in the asthmatic. (7) Symptoms of acute abdominal conditions may be masked. (8) May increase ventricular response rate in presence of supraventricular tachycardias. (9) Cough reflex is suppressed. (10) Potentiated by phenothiazines and other CNS depressants such as narcotic analgesics, alcohol, anticholinergics, antihistamines, barbiturates, hypnotics, sedatives, MAO inhibitors (e.g., isocarboxazid [Marplan]), neuromuscular blocking agents (e.g., tubocurarine) and psychotropic agents. Reduced dosages of both drugs may be indicated. (11) Tolerance to hydromorphone gradually increases. A marked increase in dose may precipitate seizures in presence of a history of convulsive disorders. (12) Physical dependence can develop but is not a factor in the presence of chronic pain of malignancy. (13) Safety for use during pregnancy or lactation not established.

Contraindications: Acute bronchial asthma, diarrhea caused by poisoning until toxic material eliminated, known hypersensitivity to opiates, obstetric analgesia (premature or term), premature infants, pulmonary edema caused by chemical respiratory irritant, respiratory depression, status asthmaticus, upper airway obstruction.

Incompatible with: Alkalies, bromides, iodides, pentobarbital (Nembutal), prochlorperazine (Compazine), sodium bicarbonate, thiopental (Pentothal).

Side effects: Nausea, vomiting, and drowsiness are less frequent than with morphine.

Minor: Anorexia, constipation, dizziness, skin rash, urinary retention, urticaria.

Major: Anaphylaxis, hypotension, respiratory depression, somnolence.

Antidote: Notify the physician of any side effect. If minor side effects progress or any major side effect occurs, discontinue the drug and notify the physician. Treat anaphylaxis as indicated or resuscitate as necessary. Naloxone (Narcan) will reverse serious respiratory depression.

HYOSCINE HYDROBROMIDE pH 3.5 to 6.5

(Scopolamine hydrobromide)

Usual dose: 0.3 to 0.6 mg (gr 1/200 to 1/100).

Pediatric dose: 6 mcg (0.006 mg)/kg of body weight or 200 mcg/M^2 as a single dose.

Dilution: Dilute desired dose in at least 10 ml of sterile water for injection.

Rate of administration: 0.6 mg or fraction thereof over 1 minute.

Actions: Parasympathetic depressant. Anticholinergic. It dilates the pupils, decreases glandular secretions, relaxes smooth muscle tissue, temporarily increases rate of heartbeat, has a calming, sedative action that produces a partial amnesia, and produces less tenacious sputum postoperatively. It is widely distributed throughout the body. It undergoes changes in the body, but much is excreted unchanged in urine. Crosses the placental barrier. Secreted in breast milk.

Indications and uses: (1) Alone or with sedatives for preanesthetic medication; (2) asthma and rhinitis; (3) biliary or renal colic; (4) gastric hypermotility; (5) motion sickness; (6) combined with analgesic or hypnotics in obstetrics.

Precautions: (1) Most frequently used SC or IM. Rarely given IV. (2) Potentiated by amantadine, antidepressants (e.g., amitriptyline [Elavil]), antihistamines, antiparkinson agents, benzodiazepines (e.g., diazepam [Valium]), buclizine, isoniazid, MAO inhibitors (e.g., pargyline [Eutonyl]), meperidine (Demerol), nitrates, orphenadrine, phenothiazines (e.g., chlorpromazine [Thorazine]), procainamide (Pronestyl), and quinidine. Reduced dose of either or both drugs may be indicated. (3) Antagonized by guanethidine, histamine, reserpine, and others. (4) Use with caution in the elderly, in infants and small children, and in debilitated patients with chronic lung disease. (5) Hyoscine does interact with many drugs and potentiates the effects of both. Sometimes this is a desired interaction, as with morphine. (6) Use caution with cholinergics, digitalis, digoxin, diphenhydramine (Benadryl), levodopa, and neostigmine. May cause adverse effects. (7) Potentiates atenolol (Tenormin), sympathomimetics (e.g., terbutaline), nitrofurantoin, and thiazide diuretics. (8) Use with methotrimeprazine (Levoprome) may cause a drop in blood pressure and tachycardia. (9) May cause respiratory depression and hemorrhage in the neonate. Do not use during pregnancy or labor. (10) Inhibits lactation. Toxicity to nursing infants probable. (11) May produce excitement, agitation, or drowsiness in the elderly.

Contraindications: Known sensitivity to hyoscine, acute glaucoma, acute hemorrhage with unstable cardiovascular status, asthma, hepatic disease, intestinal atony of the elderly or debilitated, myasthenia gravis, myocardial ischemia, obstructive disease of the GI or GU tracts, paralytic ileus, renal disease, pyloric stenosis, prostatic hypertrophy, severe ulcerative colitis, tachycardia, toxic megacolon.

Incompatible with: Alkalies. Limited information available. Incompatibilities listed under atropine should be considered.

Side effects: Mild in therapeutic doses, aggravated with overdosage; anticholinergic psychosis, delirium, dry mouth, excitement, fever (heat loss by evaporation is inhibited), flushing, hallucination, hypertension, restlessness, slow reaction of pupils to light, tachycardia, thirst, urinary retention.

Overdose: Coma, respiratory failure, and unconsciousness do occur.

Antidote: Wide margin of safety between therapeutic and lethal dosage. Notify physician of aggravated side effects. Neostigmine methylsulfate, 0.5 to 1 mg IV, may be used for symptomatic treatment, as may sedatives and barbiturates.

IDARUBINCIN HYDROCHLORIDE

(Idamycin, IDR)

Usual dose: *Adult acute myeloid leukemia (AML) induction therapy:* 12 mg/M^2 daily for 3 days. Used in combination with cytarabine (ARA-C) as an infusion of 100 mg/M^2 daily for 7 days. An alternate schedule is 25 mg/M^{2}daily for 2 days in combination with an infusion of cytarabine 200 mg/M^2 daily for 5 days. If unequivocal evidence of leukemia remains after the first course a second course may be given. Delay second course until full recovery if mucositis has occurred and reduce dose by 25%. Maintenance with idarubicin not recommended because of toxcity.

Consider dose reductions in impaired liver and kidney function based on bilirubin and/or creatinine levels above the normal range. Do not administer if bilirubin above 5 mg/dl.

Dilution: *Specific techniques required, see Precautions.* Each 5mg must be diluted with 5 ml of nonbacteriostatic normal saline for injection (1 mg/ml). Use extreme caution inserting the needle; vial contents are under negative pressure. Avoid any possibility of inhalation from aerosol or any skin contamination. Stable after reconstitution for 7 days under refrigeration (2° to 8° C, 36° to 46° F) or 3 days (72 hours) at room temperature (15° to 30° C, 59° to 86° F). Discard unused solution appropriately.

Rate of administration: A single dose of properly diluted medication over 10 to 15 minutes through Y-tube or three-way stopcock of free-flowing infusion of 5% dextrose or normal saline.

Actions: A highly toxic synthetic antibiotic antineoplastic agent. An analog of daunorubicin. Rapidly cleared from plasma and has an increased rate of cellular uptake compared to other anthracyclines. It inhibits synthesis of DNA and interacts with the enzyme topoisomerase II. Results in a greater number of remissions and longer survival than previous protocols (daunorubin and cytarabine). Extensive extrahepatic metabolism. It is severely immunosuppressive. Half-life averages 20 to 22 hours. Slowly excreted in bile and urine.

Indications and uses: (1) Treatment of acute myeloid leukemia (AML) in adults in combination with other approved antileukemic drugs.

Precautions: (1) Follow guidelines for handling cytotoxic agents. See Appendix, p. 677. (2) Administered by or under the direction of the physician specialist, with facilities for monitoring the patient and responding to any medical emergency. (3) For IV use only. Do not give IM or SC. (4) Determine absolute patency of vein. A stinging or burning sensation indicates extravasation, but extravasation may occur without stinging or burning; severe cellulitis and tissue necrosis will result. Discontinue injection; use another vein. (5) Monitoring of white blood cells, red blood cells, platelet count, liver function, kidney function, ECG, chest x-ray, echocardiography, and systolic ejection fraction indicated before and during therapy. (6) Severe myelosuppression occurs with effective therapeutic doses. Observe closely for all signs of infection or bleeding. (7) Use extreme caution in preexisting drug-induced bone marrow suppression, existing heart disease, previous treatment with other anthracyclines (e.g., daunorubicin), other cardiotoxic agents (e.g., bleomycin), or radiation therapy encompassing the heart. (8) Myocardial toxicity may cause potentially fatal acute congestive heart failure, acute life-threatening dysrhythmias, or other cardiomyopathies. (9) Prophylactic antiemetics may reduce nausea and vomiting and increase patient comfort. (10) Monitor uric acid levels; maintain hydration; allopurinol may be indicated. (11) May produce teratogenic effects on the fetus. Contraceptive measures indicated during childbearing years. (12) Discontinue nursing before taking idarubicin. (13) Safety and efficacy for use in children not established. (16) Do not administer any vaccines or chloroquine to patients receiving antineoplastic drugs.

Contraindications: Not absolute; preexisting bone marrow suppression, impaired cardiac function, preexisting infection (see Precautions).

Incompatible with: Heparin. Should be considered incompatible with any other drug because of toxicity and specific use. Prolonged contact with solution of an alkaline pH (e.g., sodium lactate, sodium bicarbonate) will result in degradation of idarubicin.

Side effects: Acute congestive heart failure, alopecia (reversible), bone marrow suppression (marked with average doses), cramping, decrease in systolic ejection fraction, depressed QRS voltage, diarrhea, dysrhythmias, erythema and tissue necrosis (if extravasation occurs), fever, headache, hemorrhage (severe), hepatic function changes, mucositis, myocarditis, nausea, pericarditis, renal function changes, skin rash, urticaria (local), vomiting.

Antidote: Most side effects will be tolerated or treated symptomatically. Keep physician informed. Close monitoring of bone marrow, ECG, chest x-ray, echocardiography, and systolic ejection fraction may prevent most serious and potentially fatal side effects. There is no specific antidote, but adequate supportive care including platelet transfusions, antibiotics and symptomatic treatment of mucositis is required. For extravasation, elevate the extremity and apply intermittent ice packs over the area immediately and 4 times a day for ½ hour. Continue for 3 days. Consider aspiration of as much infiltrated drug as possible, flooding of the site with normal saline, and injection of hydrocortisone sodium succinate (Solu-Cortef) or hyaluronidase (Wydase) throughout extravasated tissue. Use a 27- or 25-gauge needle. Site should be observed promptly by a reconstructive surgeon. If ulceration begins or there is severe persistent pain at the site, early wide excision of the involved area will be considered. Hemodialysis or peritoneal dialysis probably not effective in overdose.

IFOSFAMIDE pH 6.0

(IFEX)

Usual dose: 1.2 Gm/M^2/day for 5 consecutive days. Repeat every 3 weeks as hematological recovery permits. To initiate this protocol, platelets must be above 100,000/mm^3 and white blood cells above 4,000/mm^3.

To prevent hemorrhagic cystitis, a protector such as mesna should be administered with every dose. Ifosfamide dose has been mixed with the initial mesna dose every day in the same solution. Appears to be compatible. Dosage adjustment may be required for adrenalectomized patients and in renal or hepatic impairment. Adequate data not available.

Dilution: *Specific techniques required, see Precautions.* Each 1 Gm must be diluted with 20 ml sterile water or bacteriostatic water for injection (parabens or benzyl alcohol preserved only). Shake solution to dissolve. May be further diluted with 5% dextrose in water, normal saline, lactated Ringer's injection, or sterile water for injection. 1 Gm in 20 ml equals 50 mg/ml, 1 Gm in 50 ml equals 20 mg/ml, 1 Gm in 200 ml equals 5 mg/ml (additional diluent recommended by some researchers to reduce side effects).

Rate of administration: A single dose over a minimum of 30 minutes as an infusion. Extend administration time based on amount of diluent and patient condition.

Actions: An alkylating agent. A synthetic analog of cyclophosphamide chemically related to the nitrogen mustard group. An inert compound, metabolic activation by microsomal liver enzymes is required to produce biologically active metabolites. These alkylated metabolites interact with DNA to effect regression in the size of malignant tumors. Half-life for a usual dose is 6 to 7 hours. Larger doses extend half-life. Extensively metabolized (considerable individual variation), this drug or its metabolites are excreted in urine. Secreted in breast milk.

Indications and uses: In combination with other specific antineoplastic agents to suppress or retard neoplastic growth in germ cell testicular cancer. Usually used after other chemotherapy protocols have failed.

Unlabeled uses: Lung, breast, ovarian, pancreatic, and gastric cancer; sarcomas; acute leukemias (except acute myelogenous); malignant lymphomas.

Precautions: (1) Follow guidelines for handling cytotoxic agents. See Appendix, p. 677. (2) Usually administered by or under the direction of the physician specialist. (3) Urinalysis before each dose recommended. Withhold drug if red blood cells in urine exceed 10 per high-powered field. Reinstitute after complete resolution. Mesna given concurrently should prevent hemorrhagic cystitis. (4) Severe myelosuppression is frequent, especially when ifosfamide is given with other chemotherapeutic agents. Dose adjustments of all agents may be required. (5) Differential white blood cell count, platelet count, and hemoglobin are recommended before each daily dose and as clinically indicated. White blood cells must be above 2,000/mm^3 and platelet count above 50,000/mm^3. (6) Use caution in impaired renal function; may increase CNS toxicity. Use caution in patients with compromised bone marrow reserve (e.g., leukopenia, granulocytopenia, extensive bone marrow metastases, prior radiation therapy, treatment with other cytotoxic agents) and patients with severe hepatic or renal disease. (7) Dosage based on average weight in presence of edema or ascites. (8) Observe constantly for signs of infection (e.g., fever, sore throat, tiredness) or unusual bleeding or bruising. (9) May interfere with normal wound healing. Consider waiting 5 to 7 days or more after a major surgical procedure before beginning treatment. (10) Because it is a synthetic analog of cyclophosphamide, ifosfamide may share similar interactions with numerous drugs, including allopurinol, antidiabetics, barbiturates, chloramphenicol, corticosteroids, succinylcholine (Anectine), thiazide diuretics, and other alkylating agents to produce potentially serious reactions. (11) Discontinue breast feeding. Use extreme caution in men and women capable of conception. Embryotoxic and teratogenic to the fetus. (12) Safety and effectiveness for use in children not established. (13) Adequate hydration required; encourage fluid intake (minimum of 2 L/day) and frequent voiding to prevent cystitis. Bladder irrigation with acetylcysteine (2,000 ml/day) has also been used to prevent hematuria. (14) Do not administer any live vaccine to patients receiving antineoplastic drugs. (15) Prophylactic administration of antiemetics recommended. (16) Store dry powder at room temperature, never above 40° C (104° F). Diluted solution may be stored at room temperature up to 1 week except solutions prepared with sterile water for injection without preservatives. These must be refrigerated and used within 6 hours.

Contraindications: Hypersensitivity to ifosfamide, patients with severely depressed bone marrow function.

Incompatible with: Limited information available. Note Precautions. Give separately except as indicated in usual dose.

Side effects: Hematuria, hemorrhagic cystitis, and myelosuppression are dose-limiting side effects. Alopecia, anorexia, confusion, constipation, diarrhea, depressive psychosis with hallucinations, nausea, somnolence, and vomiting occur frequently. Allergic reactions, cardiotoxicity, coagulopathy, coma, cranial nerve dysfunction, dermatitis, dizziness, disorientation, fatigue, fever of unknown origin, hematuria, hemorrhagic cystitis, hypertension, hypotension, infection, liver dysfunction, leukopenia, malaise, neutropenia, phlebitis, polyneuropathy, pulmonary symptoms, thrombocytopenia, or seizures may occur.

Antidote: Minor side effects will be treated symptomatically if necessary. Discontinue ifosfamide and notify physician immediately if hematuria, hemorrhagic cystitis, confusion, coma, white blood cells below 2,000/mm^3, or platelets below 50,000/mm^3 occur. There is no specific antidote. Supportive therapy as indicated will help sustain the patient in toxicity. May respond to hemodialysis.

IMIPENEM-CILASTATIN pH 6.5 to 7.5

(Primaxin)

Usual dose: Range is from 250 mg to 1 Gm every 6 to 8 hours. Dosage based on severity of disease, susceptibility of pathogens, condition of the patient, age, weight, and creatinine clearance. Do not exceed the lower of 50 mg/kg of body weight/24 hr or 4 Gm/24 hr. Normal renal function required. Continue for at least 2 days after all symptoms of infection subside.

Dilution: Dilute each single dose with 10 ml of compatible infusion solutions (e.g., 5% or 10% dextrose in water, normal saline [see literature]). Must be further diluted in 100 ml of the same infusion solution and given as an intermittent infusion. Agitate until clear. Also available in 120 ml infusion bottles for one-step dilution.

Rate of administration: *Intermittent IV:* Each 500 mg or fraction thereof over 20 to 30 minutes. Slow infusion rate if patient develops nausea. May be given through Y-tube or three-way stopcock of infusion set.

Actions: A potent broad-spectrum antibacterial agent. Imipenem is a thienamycin antibiotic, and cilastatin sodium inhibits its renal metabolism. Both components are present in equal amounts. Bactericidal to many gram-negative, gram-positive, and anaerobic organisms. Effective against many otherwise resistant organisms. Therapeutic levels absorbed into many body fluids and tissues. Excreted in the urine. May cross the placental barrier.

Indications and uses: Treatment of serious lower respiratory tract, urinary tract, skin and skin structure, bone and joint, gynecological, intraabdominal, and polymicrobic infections; bacterial septicemia and endocarditis. Most effective against specific organisms (see literature).

Precautions: (1) Specific sensitivity studies are indicated to determine susceptibility of the causative organism to imipenem-cilastatin. (2) Use extreme caution in patients with a history of allergic reactions. (3) Reduce total daily dose if renal function impaired. Calculated according to degree of impairment (see literature). (4) Avoid prolonged use of drug; superinfection caused by overgrowth of nonsusceptible organisms may result. (5) Stable for 4 hours after preparation at room temperature or refrigerated for 24 hours. Do not freeze. (6) May be used concomitantly with aminoglycosides and other antibiotics, but these drugs must never be mixed in the same infusion or given concurrently. (7) Use only if absolutely necessary in pregnancy and lactation. (8) Safety for use in infants and children under 12 years of age not established. (9) May cause thrombophlebitis. Use small needles and large veins, and rotate infusion sites. (10) Electrolyte imbalance and cardiac irregularities resulting from sodium content are possible. Contains 3.2 mEq of sodium/Gm. (11) Monitor renal, hepatic, and hemopoietic systems in prolonged therapy.

(12) Use extreme caution in patients with a history of CNS disorders and/or seizures. Continue administration of anticonvulsants (13) Use with ganciclovir (Cytovene) may cause generalized seizures. Use only if benefit outweighs risk. (14) Half-life and plasma levels slightly increased by probenecid. Avoid concurrent use.

Contraindications: Known sensitivity to any component of this product.

Incompatible with: All aminoglycosides (e.g., kanamycin [Kantrex]), all solutions except those recommended for dilution by manufacturer, sodium bicarbonate. Should be considered incompatible in syringe or solution with any other bacteriostatic agent.

Side effects: Full scope of allergic reactions including anaphylaxis. Abdominal pain; abnormal clotting time; altered CBC and electrolytes; anuria; burning, discomfort, and pain at injection site; confusion; diarrhea; dizziness; dyspnea; elevated alkaline phosphatase, SGOT, SGPT, bilirubin, creatinine, BUN, and LDH; fever; gastroenteritis; glossitis; headache; heartburn; hemorrhagic colitis; hyperventilation; hypotension; increased salivation; myoclonus; nausea and vomiting; paresthesia; pharyngeal pain; polyarthralgia; polyuria; positive direct Coombs' test; presence of white or red blood cells, protein, casts, bilirubin, or urobilinogen in urine; pseudomembranous colitis; seizures; somnolence; thrombophlebitis; tinnitus; tongue papillar hypertrophy; transient hearing loss in the hearing impaired; vertigo; and many others.

Antidote: Notify physician of any side effects. Discontinue the drug if indicated. Treat allergic reaction as indicated and resuscitate as necessary. Begin anticonvulsants if focal tremors, myoclonus, or seizures occur. If symptoms continue, decrease dose or discontinue the drug. Mild cases of colitis may respond to discontinuation of drug. Oral vancomycin is the treatment of choice for antibiotic-related pseudomembranous colitis. Hemodialysis may be useful in overdose.

IMMUNE GLOBULIN INTRAVENOUS

pH 4.0 to 7.2

(Gamimune N, Gammagard, Gammar-IV, IGIV, Iveegam, Sandoglobulin, Venoglobulin-1)

Usual dose: ***Immunodeficiency syndrome:***

Gamimune N: 100 to 200 mg/kg (2 to 4 ml/kg) as a single dose IV infusion. May be repeated monthly if indicated. If adequate IgG levels in the circulation or clinical response not achieved, may be increased to 400 mg/kg (8 ml/kg), or a lesser dose may be given more frequently.

Gammagard: 200 to 400 mg/kg of body weight as a single-dose IV infusion. Repeat at least 100 mg/kg monthly.

Gammar-IV: 100 to 200 mg/kg as a single-dose IV infusion every 3 to 4 weeks. A loading dose of 200 mg/kg may be given initially and for several doses at more frequent intervals based on individual patient response and adequate IgG levels. Resume standard dose and interval when therapeutic IgG levels are achieved.

Iveegam: 200 mg/kg/month as a single-dose IV infusion. If adequate IgG levels in the circulation or clinical response not achieved, may be increased up to 800 mg/kg or intervals shortened. Do not exceed 800 mg/kg/month.

Sandoglobulin: 200 mg/kg as a single-dose IV infusion. May be repeated monthly if indicated. If adequate IgG levels in the circulation or clinical response not achieved, may be increased to 300 mg/kg or a lesser dose may be given more frequently.

Venoglobulin-1: 200 mg/kg monthly. If adequate IgG levels in the circulation or clinical response not achieved, increase to 300 to 400 mg/kg monthly, or a lesser dose may be given more frequently.

Idiopathic thrombocytopenic purpura:

Gamimune N: 400 mg/kg for 5 consecutive days.

Gammagard: 1,000 mg/kg. Up to 3 doses can be given on alternate days based on clinical response and platelet count.

Sandoglobulin: 400 mg/kg for 2 to 5 consecutive days.

Venoglobulin-1: 500 mg/kg for 2 to 7 consecutive days. If clinically significant bleeding occurs or the platelet count falls below 30,000/mm^3, 500 to 2000 mg/kg may be given as a single IV infusion every 2 weeks or less. Maintain platelet count above 20,000/mm^3 in adults and 30,000/mm^3 in children.

B-cell chronic lymphocytic leukemia (CLL):

Gammagard: 400 mg/kg every 3 to 4 weeks.

Dilution: Absolute sterile technique required at all steps of reconstitution process for each formulation. Complete dilution may take up to 20 minutes. For all preparations, filtration is required as drawn into a syringe for administration or as administered through IV tubing.

Gamimune N: May be given undiluted (a 5% solution) or may be further diluted with a given amount of 5% dextrose for injection to facilitate slow and accurate rate of infusion. Available in 10, 50, and 100 ml single-dose vials. pH 4.0 to 4.5.

Gammagard: Must be at room temperature prior to dilution. Diluent (sterile water for injection), transfer device, administration set with integral airway, and filter provided with each single-use vial. Available as a 2.5 gm single-dose vial with 50 ml diluent (50 mg/ml). Must be used within 2 hours of dilution. pH 6.4 to 7.2.

Gammar IV: Must be at room temperature prior to dilution. Diluent (sterile water for injection), transfer device (plastic piercing pin to diluent vial; metal needle to product vial), administration set with integral airway, and filter provided with each single-use vial. Available as a 2.5 gm single-dose vial with 50 ml diluent (50 mg/ml). Do not shake to dissolve; rotate or agitate vial. Must be used within 2 hours of dilution. pH 6.4 to 7.2.

Iveegam: Diluent (sterile water for injection), transfer device, administration set with integral airway, and filter provided with each single-use vial. Available as 500 mg, 1, 2.5, and 5 Gm vials with 10, 20, 50, or 100 ml diluent providing 50 mg/ml. Do not shake to dissolve; rotate or agitate vial. Use immediately after dilution. May be further diluted with a given amount of 5% dextrose in water or saline.

Sandoglobulin: Dilute with normal saline diluent provided. Makes a 3% solution. Invert so that diluent flows into the IV bottle. Available as 1 (3 or 6) Gm with 33 (100 or 200) ml diluent. For a 6% solution use one-half diluent provided. pH 6.4 to 6.8.

Venoglobulin-1: Must be at room temperature prior to dilution. Diluent (sterile water for injection), reconstitution kit, and transfer device usually provided. If not, dilute 2.5 Gm vial with 50 ml sterile water for injection and 5 Gm vial with 100 ml (50 mg/ml). Use promptly. pH 6.8.

Rate of administration: In all situations, slow rate of infusion at onset of patient discomfort or any adverse reactions. Administer via a separate IV tubing with filter or filter needle (provided by some manufacturers). Do not mix with other drugs or IV solutions. An infusion pump will facilitate an accurate rate of administration.

Gamimune N: 0.01 to 0.02 ml/kg/min for the first 30 minutes (0.7 to 1.4 ml/min of undiluted drug for a 70 kg individual). If no discomfort or adverse effects, may be increased to 0.08 ml/kg/min.

Gammagard: 0.5 ml/kg/hr. May be gradually increased to 4 ml/kg/hr if no discomfort or adverse effects. Do not exceed 4 ml/kg/hr.

Gammar-IV: 0.01 ml/kg/min. May be increased to 0.02 ml/kg/min after 15 to 30 min. May be gradually increased to 0.03 to 0.06 ml/kg/min if no discomfort or adverse effects.

Iveegam: 1 ml/min. May be increased to a maximum of 2 ml/min in the standard 5% solution. Rate may be adjusted proportionately with further dilution.

Sandoglobulin: 0.5 to 1 ml/min for 15 to 30 minutes. May then be increased to 1.5 to 2.5 ml/min. After the first infusion, the rate may be initiated at 2 to 2.5 ml/min. After the first dose a 6% solution may be used to facilitate the administration of larger doses. Begin at 1 to 1.5 ml/min and increase in 15 to 30 minutes to 2 to 2.5 ml/min.

Venoglobulin-1: 0.01 to 0.02 ml/kg/min for 30 minutes. May be gradually increased to 0.04 ml/kg/min if no discomfort or adverse effects. Subsequent infusions may be given at the higher rate.

Actions: An immune serum containing immune globulin. Obtained, purified, and standardized from human serum or plasma. Provides immediate antibody levels that last for about 3 weeks.

Indications and uses: (1) Maintenance and treatment of individuals unable to produce adequate amounts of IgG antibodies, especially in the following situations: need for immediate increase in intravascular immunoglobulin levels, small muscle mass or bleeding tendencies that contraindicate IM injection, and selected disease states (congenital agammaglobulinemia, common variable hypogammaglobulinemia, or combined immunodeficiency); (2) temporary increase in platelet counts in patients with idiopathic thrombocytopenic purpura and with thrombocytopenia associated with bone marrow transplant; (3) Gammagard only is used to prevent bacterial infections in patients with hypogammaglobulinemia or recurrent bacterial infection associated with B-cell CLL.

Precautions: (1) Check label; must state for IV use. (2) Do not use IM or SC. Do not skin test. Will cause a localized chemical skin reaction. (3) Monitor vital signs and observe patient continuously during infusion. A precipitous drop in blood pressure or anaphylaxis can occur at any time. Emergency equipment and supplies must be at bedside. (4) Minimum serum level of IgG after infusion should exceed 300 mg/dl. (5) Store Gammagard and Sandoglobulin at room temperature not exceeding 25° C (77° F). Store Gamimune-N and Iveegam at 2° to 8° C (35° to 46° F). Store Gammar-IV and Venoglobulin-1 at room temperature not exceeding 30° C (86° F). Discard partially used vials. Do not use if turbid or has been frozen. (6) Use extreme caution in individuals with isolated IgA deficiency or a history of prior systemic allergic reactions. Incidence of anaphylaxis may be increased, especially with repeated injections. (7) Use with caution in pregnancy; no adverse effects documented, but adequate studies are not available. (8) Do not administer live virus vaccines from 2 weeks before to at least 3 months after immune globulin IV.

Contraindications: Individuals known to have allergic response to gamma globulin or thiomerosol; patients with isolated IgA deficiency or preexisting anti-IgA antibodies.

Incompatible with: Should be considered incompatible in syringe or solution with any other drug or solution because of specific use, potential for anaphylaxis, and manufacturer's recommendation.

Side effects: Full range of allergic symptoms including anaphylaxis is possible. Angioedema, erythema, fever, and urticaria are most frequently observed. Flushing, headache, hypertension, nausea, rash, and vomiting have been reported. Is made from human plasma, process attempts to eliminate risk of hepatitis or HIV infection. A precipitous hypotensive reaction can occur and is most frequently associated with too-rapid rate of injection.

Antidote: Reduce rate immediately for patient discomfort or any sign of adverse reaction. Discontinue the drug if symptoms persist and notify the physician. May be treated symptomatically, and infusion resumed at slower rate if symptoms subside. Treat anaphylaxis immediately. Epinephrine (Adrenalin), diphenhydramine (Benadryl), oxygen, vasopressors (e.g., dopamine [Intropin]), corticosteroids, and ventilation equipment must always be available. Resuscitate as necessary.

INDOMETHACIN SODIUM TRIHYDRATE

pH 6.0 to 7.5

(Indocin IV)

Neonatal dose: Three IV doses, specific to age at first dose, given at 12- to 24-hour intervals, constitute a course of therapy.

Less than 48 hours of age: First dose (0.2 mg/kg of body weight), second dose (0.1 mg/kg), third dose (0.1 mg/kg).

2 to 7 days of age: 0.2 mg/kg for each of 3 doses.

Over 7 days of age: First dose (0.2 mg/kg), then 0.25 mg/kg for the next 2 doses.

If urinary output is less than 0.6 ml/hr at any time a dose is to be given, withhold dose until lab studies confirm normal renal function. A second course of 1 to 3 doses may be repeated one time at 12- to 24-hour intervals as above if the ductus arteriosus reopens.

Dilution: Each 1 mg must be diluted with at least 1 ml normal saline or sterile water for injection without preservatives (0.1 mg/0.1 ml); may be diluted with 2 ml diluent (0.05 mg/0.1 ml). The preservative benzyl alcohol is toxic in neonates.

Rate of administration: A single dose properly diluted direct IV over 5 to 10 seconds.

Actions: A potent inhibitor of prostaglandin synthesis. Through an unconfirmed method of action (thought to be inhibition of prostaglandin synthesis), it causes closure of a patent ductus arteriosus 75% to 80% of the time, eliminating the need for surgical intervention. Plasma half-life varies inversely with postnatal age and weight and ranges from 12 to 20 hours. Circulated through the liver and eventually excreted in urine.

Indications and uses: Closure of a hemodynamically significant patent ductus arteriosus in premature infants weighing between 500 and 1,750 Gm if usual medical management (e.g., fluid restriction, diuretics, digitalis, respiratory support) has not been effective after 48 hours.

Precautions: (1) Clinical evidence of a hemodynamically significant patent ductus arteriosus (respiratory distress, a continuous murmur, a hyperactive precordium, cardiomegaly and pulmonary plethora on chest x-ray) should be present before use is considered. (2) For use only in a highly supervised setting such as an intensive care nursery. Vital signs, oxygenation, acid-base status, fluid and electrolyte balance, and kidney function must be monitored and maintained. (3) Prepare a fresh solution for each dose. Discard any unused portion. (4) May increase potential for intraventricular bleeding by inhibiting platelet aggregation. (5) Can cause marked reduction in urine output (over 50%), increase BUN and creatinine, and reduce glomerular filtration rate and creatinine clearance. These symptoms usually disappear when therapy completed but may cause acute renal failure, especially in infants with impaired renal function from other causes. (6) Use caution in presence of existing controlled infection; may mask signs and symptoms of exacerbation. (7) Discontinue drug if signs of impaired liver function appear. (8) Confirm absolute patency of vein. Avoid extravasation; will irritate tissue. (9) Will potentiate aminoglycosides (e.g., gentamicin [Garamycin]) and digitalis. (10) Use with furosemide (Lasix) may help to maintain renal function. (11) For IV use only. (12) Surgery is indicated if condition is not responsive to two courses of therapy.

Contraindications: Bleeding, especially active intracranial hemorrhage or GI bleeding; coagulation defects; necrotizing enterocolitis; patients with congenital heart disease (e.g., pulmonary atresia, severe coarctation of the aorta, severe tetralogy of Fallot) who require patency of the ductus arteriosus for satisfactory pulmonary or systemic blood flow; proven or suspected untreated infection; significant renal impairment; thrombocytopenia.

Incompatible with: Any other drug in a syringe. Dilute only with stated preparations. Further dilution with IV infusion solutions not recommended.

Side effects: Abdominal distention; acidosis; alkalosis; apnea; bleeding into the GI tract (gross or microscopic); bradycardia; DIC; elevated BUN or creatinine; exacerbation of preexisting pulmonary infection; fluid retention; hyperkalemia; hypoglycemia; hyponatremia; intracranial bleeding; necrotizing enterocolitis; oliguria; oozing from needle puncture sites; pulmonary hemorrhage; pulmonary hypertension; reduced urine sodium, chloride, potassium, urine osmolality, free water clearance, or glomerular filtration rate; retrolental fibroplasia; uremia; transient ileus; vomiting.

Antidote: Discontinue the drug and notify the physician of all side effects. Based on severity, side effects may be treated symptomatically or drug will be completely discontinued in favor of surgical intervention. Resuscitate as necessary.

INSULIN INJECTION (REGULAR) pH 7.0 to 7.8

(Actrapid, ✱ Actrapid McPork, Beef Regular Iletin II, Humulin R, ✱ Insulin-Toronto, Novolin R, ✱ Novolin-Toronto, Pork Regular Iletin II, Purified Pork Insulin, Regular Iletin I, Velosulin)

Usual dose: Varies greatly. Range is from 2 to 100 units/hr as indicated by patient's condition and response.

Low-dose treatment in ketoacidosis or diabetic coma is preferred: 10 to 30 units initially, then 2 to 12 units/hr.

Dilution: May be given undiluted either directly into the vein or through a Y-tube or three-way stopcock. Insulin is compatible with commonly used IV solutions and may be given as an infusion. Usually diluted in 0.9% (normal) or 0.45% saline for infusion. Fifty units of insulin added to 500 ml of infusion solution given at a rate of 1 ml/min will deliver 6 units/hr. Another regimen adds 100 units of insulin to 100 ml of normal saline. This solution is given at a rate of 0.1 unit/kg of body weight/hr.

Rate of administration: Each 50 units or fraction thereof over 1 minute. When given in an IV infusion, the rate should be ordered by the physician and will depend on insulin and fluid needs (see Dilution for example).

Actions: An aqueous solution that acts as a catalyst in carbohydrate metabolism in combination with adrenal, anterior pituitary, and thyroid hormones. This action is thought to occur at the cell membrane, facilitating glucose entry into peripheral tissues and lowering the blood glucose level. Also affected is the transport and incorporation of amino acids into protein. Release of free fatty acids from adipose tissue is inhibited. Insulin promotes storage of carbohydrate in liver and muscle cells and reduces the liver's capacity to put glucose into the blood. Potassium is also deposited in the liver with lower blood levels. Rapidly absorbed and readily distributed throughout the body; excretion, if any, is in changed form in the urine. Not found in breast milk.

Indications and uses: (1) Diabetic coma; (2) ketoacidosis; (3) in combination with glucose to treat hyperkalemia; (4) induction of insulin shock for psychotherapy.

Precautions: (1) *Regular insulin only may be given IV.* Humulin R is one of the newest products (recombinant DNA origin). All insulin is standardized at 100 units/ml. (2) Use only if water clear. (3) Insulin potency may be reduced by at least 20% and possibly up to 80% via the glass or plastic infusion container and plastic IV tubing before it actually reaches the venous system in an infusion. The percentage absorbed is inversely proportional to the concentration of insulin (the larger the dose, the less absorption) and takes place within 30 to 60 minutes. Albumin is sometimes added to reduce this absorption. (4) Response to insulin measured by blood glucose, blood pH, acetone, BUN, sodium, potassium, chloride, and CO_2 levels. Monitor patient carefully in all situations. Use frequent blood glucose and ketone monitoring. (5) In low-dose treatment of diabetic coma or ketoacidosis, an initial priming dose of 10 units followed by 2 to 12 units/hr has achieved normal plasma levels of 100 to 200 microunits/ml of blood more quickly than previously used large doses. (6) Hypovolemia is a common complication of diabetic acidosis. (7) Insulin is inactivated at pH above 7.5. (8) Store in refrigerator (preferred); may be stored in a cool, dark room. Discard any open vial not used for several weeks. (9) Combination of insulin and MAO inhibitors (e.g., pargyline [Eutonyl]) or alcohol is hazardous and may be lethal. (10) Hypoglycemic effect is potentiated by β-adrenergic blockers (e.g., propranolol [Inderal]), anabolic steroids (e.g., nandrolone [Durabolin]), anticoagulants (e.g., warfarin [Coumadin]), antineoplastics (e.g., methotrexate), guanethidine, isoniazid, pyrazolone compounds (e.g., phenylbutazone [Butazolidin]), salicylates, sulfonamides, tetracyclines, and many others. (11) Inhibited by corticosteroids, thiazide diuretics, dobutamine (Dobutrex), epinephrine (Adrenalin), furosemide (Lasix), oral contraceptives, smoking, thyroid preparations, and others. (12) Will affect serum potassium levels; use caution in patients taking digitalis products.

Contraindications: There are no contraindications when insulin is indicated as a lifesaving measure.

Incompatible with: Aminophylline, amobarbital (Amytal), chlorothiazide (Diuril), dobutamine (Dobutrex), heparin, penicillin G potassium, pentobarbital (Nembutal), phenobarbital (Luminal), phenytoin (Dilantin), secobarbital (Seconal), sodium bicarbonate, thiopental (Pentothal).

Side effects: Hypoglycemia with overdose.

Early: Ashen color, clammy skin, drowsiness, faintness, fatigue, headache, hunger, nausea, nervousness, sweating, tremors, weakness.

Advanced: Coma, convulsions, disorientation, hypokalemia (with ECG changes), psychic disturbances, unconsciousness, hypersensitivity reactions including anaphylaxis; death is rare.

Antidote: Discontinue the drug immediately and notify the physician. *Glucagon* is the specific antidote for insulin overdose. It may be supplemented by glucose 50% IV and/or oral carbohydrates such as orange juice. Oral carbohydrates may be sufficient to combat the early symptoms of hypoglycemia. Allergic reactions will usually respond to symptomatic treatment.

20% INTRAVASCULAR PERFLUOROCHEMICAL EMULSION pH 7.3

(Fluosol)

Usual dose: *Test dose:* Administration of a 0.5 ml test dose with or without prior oxygenation of fluosol directly IV into a peripheral vein is advisable before intracoronary use.

Intracoronary perfusion: 3 to 5 ml/kg of body weight. Administer only via intracoronary perfusion during balloon angioplasty, using an angiographic power injector. Verify proper position of balloon catheter. Should not be administered more than one time in 6 months.

Dilution: *A specific and sequential process using aseptic technique throughout. Absolute adherence is required.* The complete process will take over 1 hour. Complete continuous oxygenation kit for dilution of fluosol (except for carbogen) is supplied. Literature in kit contains illustrated step-by-step procedure. Follow carefully.

Rate of administration: 60 to 90 ml/min at a constant temperature of 37° C (98.6° F). Use of an angiographic power injector with a heating jacket required. Must be administered within 8 hours of thawing. Filters are used in the dilution and oxygenation process, but do not use filters during administration. Discontinue adminstration if any evidence of emulsion instability.

Actions: A stable emulsion of perfluorochemicals in water. After oxygen is preferentially dissolved in the emulsion and injected through a PTCA catheter during an angioplasty procedure, it will deliver oxygen to the myocardium distal to the point of balloon inflation. A cardioprotective agent with a greater oxygen affinity than blood; a particle size 1⁄900 the volume of red blood cells; and a viscosity one-half that of blood. Protects the heart from ischemia manifested by decreased ventricular wall motion and decreased global ejection fraction. Half-life is dose dependent. Primary route of elimination is through the lungs in expiratory gases. One component is readily excreted by the kidneys. The specific perfluorochemicals are taken up primarily by the liver, speen, and bone marrow (reticuloendothelial system); their molecules are eventually excreted intact. Process may take several months.

Indications and uses: To prevent or diminish myocardial ischemia during coronary angioplasty. Especially useful in high-risk patients with low baseline ejection fraction; large areas of the myocardium at risk; recent myocardial infarction; or unstable or refractory angina requiring hospitalization.

Precautions: (1) Administered by or under the direction of the physician specialist knowledgeable in its use and with facilities for emergency coronary bypass graft surgery as well as other emergency, diagnostic, and laboratory facilities available. (2) Do not administer if mild back pain, mild chills, mild generalized pruritus, nausea, vomiting, or urticaria occur after the test dose. (3) Monitor ECG continuously for signs of ischemia. Ischemic ST segment changes, angina, and creatinine kinase elevation may occur if the position of the balloon catheter occludes side branches, which will not receive perfusion from oxygenated fluosol. (4) ST segment elevation reaching a plateau at 30 to 45 seconds of balloon inflation with an amplitude of 1 to 2 mm is seen in many patients. Thought to be a nonischemic mechanical artifact of perfusion. (5) Thaw in warming water bath only. Do not use microwave; will damage emulsion. Do not allow fluosol bag to come into direct contact with water in warming bath (plastic protective bag provided). (6) Use carbogen (95% 0_2/5% CO_2) only. 100% oxygen will adversely affect pH of the emulsion. (7) Do not use filters in the direct line during administration; will disturb the emulsion. (8) Fluosol (400 ml) must be kept frozen (between −5° and −30° C [23° and −22° F] until thawed. Do not use if appears to have thawed in storage. Do not refreeze; discard. Solutions #1 and #2 must be stored at room temperature not exceeding 30° C (86° F). (9) After thawing, fluosol must be kept and administered at a constant 37° C (98.6° F) temperature. Cooler temperatures at time of administration may cause ventricular fibrillation and require cardioversion. (10) Half-life may be extended in asplenic patients because of increased absorption in liver and bone marrow. (11) May potentiate action of lipid-soluble anesthetics (e.g., short-acting barbiturates [thiopental]). (12) Centrifuged samples of blood containing fluosol may have a packed layer of perfluorochemicals at the bottom of the tube, called fluorocrit. High concentration in blood (well above those seen with usual dose) may interfere with some spectrophotometric tests due to turbidity. (13) Use in pregnancy only if clearly needed. Discontinue breast feeding. (14) Safety and effectiveness for use in children not established.

Contraindications: Known hypersensitivity to any components of fluosol, patients with a functionally critical secondary stenosis in the dilated and perfused vessel distal to the treated lesion.

Incompatible with: Manufacturer states "do not add any additives other than solution #1, solution #2 and carbogen."

Side effects: Difficult to separate from the complications of the procedure itself, but may include angina, bradycardia, chest discomfort after procedure, coughing, dyspnea, hypotension, increase in pulmonary artery wedge pressure, increased respiratory rate, pruritus (mild), ST segment elevation, ventricular fibrillation, and ventricular tachycardia.

Antidote: Physician is present during entire procedure. Some side effects (ST segment elevation of 1 to 2 mm amplitude reaching a plateau at 30 to 45 seconds of balloon inflation) will be tolerated. Others will be treated symptomatically. Treat allergic reaction with diphenhydramine (Benadryl) and/or methylprednisolone. Cardioversion may be required for ventricular dysrhythmias. Procedure may need to be discontinued and angioplasty without distal perfusion or coronary artery bypass surgery may be appropriate.

INTRAVENOUS FAT EMULSION — pH 6.0 to 9.0

(Intralipid 10% & 20%, Liposyn II 10% & 20%, Liposyn III 10% & 20%, Nutrilipid 10% & 20%, Soyacal 10% & 20%, Travamulsion 10% & 20%)

Usual dose: *Total parenteral nutrition component:* 500 ml of 10% or 250 ml of 20% on the first day. (Exception is Soyacal; give only 250 ml the first day.)Increase dose gradually each day. Do not exceed 60% of the patient's total caloric intake or 2.5 Gm/kg of body weight.

Fatty acid deficiency: Supply 8% to 10% of the total caloric intake each 24 hours.

Pediatric dose: *Total parenteral nutrition component:* Up to 1 Gm/kg of body weight. Increase dose gradually each day. Do not exceed 60% of total caloric intake or 4 Gm/kg.

Dilution: Must be given as prepared by manufacturer.

Rate of administration: *Adult:* 10%, 1 ml/min for the first 15 to 30 minutes. If no untoward effects, increase rate to administer 500 ml equally distributed over 4 to 6 hours. 20%, 0.5 ml/min for the first 15 to 30 minutes. If no untoward effects, increase rate to administer 250 ml equally distributed over 4 to 6 hours.

Pediatric: 10%, 0.1 ml/min for the first 10 to 15 minutes. Reduce initial rate to 0.05 ml/min for a 20% solution. If no untoward effects, increase rate to administer 1 Gm/kg of body weight (total usual dose) equally distributed over 4 hours. An infusion pump is recommended. Do not exceed a rate of 50 ml/hr (20%) or 100 ml/hr (10%).

Actions: A parenteral nutrient. Has an osmolarity of 280 mOsm/L and contains emulsified fat particles about 0.5 micron in size. Total caloric value (fat, phospholipid, and glycerol) is 1.1 cal/ml. Metabolized and used as a source of energy. Increases heat production and oxygen consumption. Decreases respiratory quotient. Cleared from the bloodstream by a process not fully understood.

Indications and uses: (1) To provide additional calories and essential fatty acids for patients requiring parenteral nutrition whose caloric requirements cannot be met by glucose or who will be receiving parenteral nutrition over extended periods (over 5 days usually); (2) to prevent essential fatty acid deficiency.

Precautions: (1) Isotonic; may be administered by a peripheral vein or central venous infusion. (2) Infuse separately from any other IV solution or medication. Do not disturb emulsion. Heparin 1 to 2 units/ml is the exception. It may be added before administration (activates lipoprotein lipase). (3) May be administered via a Y-tube or three-way stopcock near the infusion site. Rates of both solutions (fat emulsion and amino acid products) should be controlled by infusion pumps. Keep fat emulsion line higher than all other lines (has low specific gravity and could run up into other lines). (4) Do not use filters; will disturb emulsion. (5) Use only freshly opened solutions; discard remainder of partial dose. (6) May be stored at 25° to 30° C (77° to 86° F) or refrigerated. Specific storage conditions required (see literature). Do not freeze. (7) Do not use if there appears to be an oiling out of the emulsion. (8) Normal liver function required. (9) Monitor lipids before each infusion; lipemia should clear daily. (10) Monitor hemogram, blood coagulation, liver function tests, plasma lipid profile, and platelet count, especially in neonates; Discontinue use for significant abnormality. (11) Use extreme caution in neonates; death from intravascular fat accumulation in the lungs has occurred. (12) Fatty acids displace bilirubin bound to albumin. Use caution in jaundiced or premature infants. (13) Use caution in pulmonary disease, anemia, or blood coagulation disorders, or when there is any danger of fat embolism. (14) Use in pregnancy only when clearly needed.

Contraindications: Any condition that disturbs normal fat metabolism, such as pathological hyperlipemia, lipoid nephrosis, and acute pancreatitis with hyperlipemia; severe egg allergies.

Incompatible with: Manufacturer recommends not to mix with any electrolyte or other nutrient solution. No additives or medications are to be placed in bottle or tubing (see Precautions). In actual practice carbohydrates, amino acids, and fat emulsion are being mixed in specific percentages and in a specific order to meet individual total parenteral nutritional needs (consult with pharmacist).

Side effects: Anaphylaxis, back pain, chest pain, cyanosis, dizziness, dyspnea, elevated temperature, flushing, head ache, hypercoagulability, hyperlipemia, nausea and vomiting, pressure over eyes, sepsis (from contamination of IV catheter), sleepiness, sweating, thrombophlebitis (from concurrent hyperalimentation fluids), a delayed overloading syndrome (focal seizures, fever, leukocytosis, splenomegaly, shock), and many others.

Antidote: Notify physician of all side effects. Many will be treated symptomatically. Treat allergic reaction promptly and resuscitate as necessary. For accidental overdose, stop the infusion. Obtain blood sample for inspection of plasma, triglyceride concentration, and measurement of plasma light-scattering activity by nephelometry. Repeat blood samples until the lipid has cleared.

IRON DEXTRAN INJECTION pH 5.2 to 6.5

(Imferon IM/IV)

Usual dose: 0.5 ml (25 mg) on the first day as a test dose. Wait 1 hour. If no adverse reactions, may be increased gradually to 2 ml (100 mg)/24 hr and repeated daily until results achieved or maximum calculated dosage reached (see literature). A total calculated dose has been given as an infusion. Though not FDA approved, this method is preferred to multiple small-dose infusions or injections by some.

Pediatric dose: 0.5 ml (25 mg) on the first day as a test dose. Wait 1 hour. If no adverse reactions, may be increased gradually to 1 ml (50 mg)/24 hr for children from 5 to 10 kg (over 4 months of age) and repeated daily until results achieved or maximum calculated dosage reached (see literature).

Dilution: Given undiluted, or up to the total desired dose may be further diluted in 50 to 250 ml normal saline for infusion.

Rate of administration: 1 ml (50 mg) or fraction thereof over 1 minute or more.

Infusion: Test dose of 25 mg over 5 minutes. If no adverse reactions, infuse remaining dose over 1 to 2 hours. Discontinue IV infusion solutions during administration of iron dextran injection.

Actions: The iron-dextran complex is separated into smaller molecules by cellular systems in the bone marrow, liver, spleen, etc. By chemical processes usable iron can then be absorbed into the hemoglobin. After hemoglobin needs of the blood are met, iron is stored in the body for reserve use. Small amounts of unabsorbed iron are excreted in the urine, feces, and bile. Crosses the placental barrier.

Indications and uses: (1) Iron-deficiency anemia only, identify and treat the cause; (2) insufficient muscle to allow repeated deep IM injection, or oral therapy is not possible or practical; (3) impaired muscle absorption; (4) hemophilia; (5) intermittent or repetitive substantial blood loss (familial telangiectasia, renal hemodialysis).

Precautions: (1) Check vial carefully; must state "for IV use." (2) Discontinue oral iron before starting iron dextran. (3) Use only when truly indicated to avoid excess storage of iron. (4) Increases joint pain and swelling in patients with rheumatoid arthritis. (5) Keep patient lying down after injection to prevent postural hypotension. (6) Use caution with history of asthma or allergies. (7) Use only if absolutely necessary in liver disease, lactation, pregnancy, or childbearing years. Known hazard to fetus. (8) Monitor serum ferritin assays in prolonged therapy. Consider possibility of false results for months after injection caused by delayed utilization. (9) Inhibits doxycycline (Vibramycin). (10) Inhibited by chloramphenicol.

Contraindications: Manifestation of allergic reaction, any anemia other than iron deficiency, infants younger than 4 months of age.

Incompatible with: Any other drug in syringe or solution.

Side effects: *Minor:* Headache, itching, nausea, rash, shivering, transitory paresthesias.

Major: Anaphylaxis; arthritic reactivation; chest pain; hypotension; leukocytosis; local phlebitis; lymphadenopathy; peripheral vascular flushing, especially with too-rapid injection; PVCs; tachycardia; shock.

Antidote: Discontinue the drug and notify the physician of early symptoms. For severe symptoms, discontinue drug, treat allergic reactions or resuscitate as necessary, and notify physician. Epinephrine (Adrenalin) and diphenhydramine (Benadryl) should always be available. In acute poisoning, an iron-chelating drug (deferoxamine), 1 to 2 Gm in 5% dextrose solution, may be given by slow IV drip over 24 hours. Deferoxamine can remove the iron from transferrin but not from the hemoglobin itself.

ISOPROTERENOL HYDROCHLORIDE

pH 3.5 to 4.5

(Isuprel Hydrochloride)

Usual dose: *Infusion:* 1 to 5 mcg/min of a 1:250,000 solution.

Direct IV: 0.02 to 0.06 mg (1 to 3 ml of a 1:50,000 solution) as initial dose. Repeat as necessary.

Intracardiac: 0.02 mg (0.1 ml) of a 1:5,000 solution (rarely used).

Bronchospasm: 0.01 to 0.02 mg (0.5 to 1 ml) of a 1:50,000 solution as initial dose. Repeat as necessary.

Pediatric dose: One tenth to one half of the adult dose. Adjust to patient response.

Dilution: *Infusion:* 2 mg (10 ml) of a 1:5,000 solution in 500 ml of 5% dextrose in water. 4 mcg equals 1 ml in this 1:250,000 solution. Use an infusion pump or microdrip (60 gtt equals 1 ml) to administer. Less diluent may be used to reduce fluid intake.

Direct IV or bronchospasm: Dilute 0.2 mg (1 ml) of a 1:5,000 solution with 10 ml normal saline for injection to make a 1:50,000 solution.

Intracardiac: 1:5,000 solution undiluted.

Rate of administration: *Infusion:* Each 1 ml of a 1:250,000 (4 mcg) solution over 1 minute. May be increased if necessary. Adjust to patient response.

Direct IV: Each 1 ml of a 1:50,000 (0.02 mg) solution or fraction thereof over 1 minute.

Intracardiac: Each 0.1 ml of a 1:5,000 solution over 1 second.

Actions: A synthetic cardiac β-receptor stimulant (sympathomimetic amine) similar to epinephrine and norepinephrine. Has positive inotropic and chronotropic actions more potent than those of epinephrine. It increases stroke volume, cardiac output, cardiac work, coronary flow, and venous return. Improves atrioventricular conduction. Stimulates only the higher ventricular foci, allowing a more normal cardiac pacemaker to take over, thus suppressing ectopic pacemaker activity. Decreases peripheral vascular resistance by relaxing arterial smooth muscle and is a most effective bronchial smooth muscle relaxant. Onset of action is immediate and lasts 1 to 2 hours. Excreted in the urine.

Indications and uses: (1) Atrioventricular heart block (Stokes-Adams syndrome) and cardiac standstill; (2) some ventricular dysrhythmias, including ventricular tachycardia if increased inotropic activity is required for treatment; (3) bronchospasm during anesthesia; (4) management of shock (effective only with normal or elevated central venous pressure); (5) cardiac catheterization to simulate exercise; (6) on occasion as an antidote to reverse severe hypotension caused by tricyclic antidepressants (e.g., amitriptyline [Elavil].

Precautions: (1) Decrease rate of infusion as necessary. Ventricular rate generally should not exceed 110 beats/min. Maintain adequate blood volume and correct acidosis. (2) Intracardiac or IV injection in cardiac standstill must be accompanied by cardiac massage to perfuse drug into the myocardium. (3) Continuous cardiac monitoring, central venous pressure readings, blood pressure, and urine flow measurements are advisable during therapy with isoproterenol. (4) *May be used alternately with epinephrine (Adrenalin), but they may not be used together.* Both are direct cardiac stimulants, and death will result. An adequate interval between doses must be maintained. (5) Use extreme caution when inhalant anesthetics (e.g., cyclopropane) are being administered and supplementary to digitalis administration. (6) Use caution in coronary insufficiency, diabetes, hyperthyroidism, known sensitivity to sympathomimetic amines, and preexisting cardiac dysrhythmias with tachycardia. (7) Simultaneous use with oxytoxics or MAO inhibitors (e.g., pargyline [Eutonyl]) may cause hypertensive crisis. (8) Antagonized by propranolol (Inderal). Tachycardia and hypotension secondary to peripheral vasodilation may occur. (9) Potentiated by tricyclic antidepressants. (10) Severe hypotension and bradycardia may occur with hydantoins (e.g., phenytoin [Dilantin]). (11) Do not use if pink or brown in color or contains a precipitate.

Contraindications: Patients with tachycardia caused by digitalis intoxication.

Incompatible with: Aminophylline, barbiturates, carbenicillin (Geopen), diazepam (Valium), epinephrine (Adrenalin), sodium bicarbonate.

Side effects: Anginal pain, cardiac dysrhythmias, flushing, headache, nausea, nervousness, palpitations, sweating, tachycardia, vomiting. Cardiac dilation, marked hypotension, pulmonary edema, and death occur with prolonged use or overdose.

Antidote: Notify the physician of any side effect. Treatment will probably be symptomatic. For ventricular rate over 110 beats/min, decrease rate of infusion or discontinue drug. For accidental overdose, discontinue drug immediately, resuscitate and sustain patient, and notify physician.

KANAMYCIN SULFATE pH 4.5

(✤ Anamid, Kantrex)

Usual dose: Up to 15 mg/kg of body weight/24 hr equally divided into 2 to 4 doses. Dosage based on ideal weight of lean body mass. Do not exceed a total adult dose of 1.5 Gm by all routes in 24 hours.

Dilution: Each 500 mg or fraction thereof must be diluted with at least 100 ml of 5% dextrose in water, 5% dextrose in normal saline, or normal saline for infusion.

Rate of administration: Do not exceed a rate of 3 to 4 ml/min diluted solution. Give total dose over 30 to 60 minutes.

Actions: An aminoglycoside antibiotic with neuromuscular blocking action. Bactericidal against many gram-negative organisms resistant to other antibiotics. Well distributed through all body fluids; crosses the placental barrier. Usual half-life is 2 to 3 hours. Half-life is prolonged in infants, postpartum females, fever, liver disease and ascites, spinal cord injury, cystic fibrosis, and the elderly; shorter in severe burns. Excreted in high concentrations through the kidneys. Secreted in breast milk. Cross-allergenicity does occur between aminoglycosides.

Indications and uses: Short-term treatment of serious infections caused by susceptible organisms. Concurrent therapy with a penicillin or cephalosporin sometimes indicated. Primarily used when penicillin and other less toxic antibiotics are ineffective or contraindicated.

Precautions: (1) Most frequently given IM. (2) Discard partially used vials after 48 hours. (3) Use extreme caution if therapy is required over 7 to 10 days. (4) Sensitivity studies necessary to determine susceptibility of the causative organism to kanamycin. (5) Reduce daily dose for renal impairment; intervals between injections should also be increased. (6) Routine evaluation of hearing is necessary. Watch for decrease in urine output, rising BUN and serum creatinine, and declining creatinine clearance levels. Dosage may need to be decreased. (7) Narrow range between toxic and therapeutic levels. Monitor peak and trough concentrations to avoid peak serum concentrations above 30 mcg/ml and trough concentrations above 5 mcg/ ml. The therapeutic level is between 8 and 16 mcg/ml. (8) Use caution in children and the elderly, and during pregnancy and lactation. Rarely used IV in infants; use extreme caution, lower doses may be appropriate due to immature renal function. (9) Potentiated by anesthetics, other neuromuscular blocking antibiotics (e.g., gentamicin, streptomycin), anticholinesterases (e.g., edrophonium [Tensilon]), antineoplastics (e.g., cisplatin, nitrogen mustard), barbiturates, cephalosporins, muscle relaxants (e.g., tubocurarine), phenothiazines (e.g., promethazine [Phenergan]), procainamide, quinidine, and sodium citrate (citrate-anticoagulated blood). *Apnea can occur.* (10) Ototoxicity may be potentiated by loop diuretics (e.g., furosemide [Lasix]). Concurrent use not recommended. (11) Synergistic when used in combination with penicillins and cephalosporins. Dose adjustment and appropriate spacing required because of physical incompatibilities and interactions. Inhibited by penicillins. (12) Digoxin dose may need adjustment. (13) Superinfection may occur from overgrowth of nonsusceptible organisms. (14) Maintain good hydration.

Contraindications: Known kanamycin or aminoglycoside

sensitivity, prior hearing damage by kanamycin or other ototoxic agents unless infection is life threatening.

Incompatible with: Administer separately. Incompatible with amphotericin B, ampicillin, carbenicillin (Geopen), cefoxitin (Mefoxin), cephalothin (Keflin), cephapirin (Cefadyl), chlorpheniramine (Chlor-Trimeton), colistimethate (Coly-Mycin M), heparin, hydrocortisone (Solu-Cortef), methohexital (Brevital), penicillins.

Side effects: *Minor:* Fever, headache, paresthesias, skin rash, thrombophlebitis.

Major: Apnea; azotemia; elevated BUN, nonprotein nitrogen, creatinine; hearing loss; neuromuscular blockade; oliguria; proteinuria; tinnitus; vertigo.

Antidote: Notify the physician of all side effects. If minor symptoms persist or any major symptom appears, discontinue the drug and notify the physician. Treatment is symptomatic, or a reduction in dose may be required. In overdose hemodialysis may be indicated. Complexation with ticarcillin or carbenicillin may be as effective as hemodialysis. Consider exchange transfusion in the newborn. Calcium salts or neostigmine may reverse neuromuscular blockade. Resuscitate as necessary.

L-HYOSCYAMINE SULFATE pH 3.0 to 6.5

(Levsin)

Usual dose: *GI disorders:* 0.25 to 0.5 mg (0.5 to 1.0 ml) at 4-hour intervals 3 or 4 times/day.

Hypotonic duodenography: 0.25 to 0.5 mg 5 to 10 minutes prior to the diagnostic procedure.

Reversal of neuromuscular blockade: 0.2 mg for each 1 mg of neostigmine or equivalent dose of physostigmine and pyridostigmine.

Dilution: May be given undiluted. Administer through Y-tube or three-way stopcock of infusion tubing.

Rate of administration: A single dose over at least 1 minute.

Actions: A chemically pure anticholinergic/antispasmodic component of belladonna alkaloids. Affects peripheral cholinergic receptors in autonomic effector cells of smooth muscle, cardiac muscle, sinoatrial node, atrioventricular node, and exocrine glands. Does not affect autonomic ganglia. Inhibits GI motility, reduces gastric secretions, and controls excessive pharyngeal, tracheal, and bronchial secretions. Onset of action is prompt and lasts 4 to 6 hours. Metabolized in the liver and excreted in urine. Traces occur in breast milk.

Indications and uses: (1) Adjunctive therapy in peptic ulcer, spastic colitis, cystitis, pylorospasm, dysentery, diverticulitis, irritable bowel syndrome, and neurogenic bowel disturbances; (2) biliary and renal colic; (3) hypotonic duodenography; (4) antidote for overdose of anticholinesterase agents (reversal of neuromuscular blockade).

Precautions: (1) Urinary retention can be avoided if the patient voids just before each dose. (2) Use caution in autonomic neuropathy, cardiac dysrhythmias (especially tachycardia), congestive heart failure, coronary artery disease, dehydration, hypertension, and hyperthyroidism. (3) Potentiated by alkalinizing agents, amantadine, synthetic narcotic analgesics, tricyclic antidepressants (e.g., amitryptyline [Elavil]), antihistamines, MAO inhibitors (e.g., pargyline [Eutonyl]), nitrates, phenothiazines (e.g., chlorpromazine [Thorazine]), and many others. Reduced dose of either or both drugs may be indicated. (4) Antagonized by histamine, reserpine, and others. (5) Use caution with digoxin, cholinergics, diphenhydramine (Benadryl), levodopa, and neostigmine. May cause adverse effects. (6) Will cause cardiac dysrhythmias with cyclopropane anesthesia.

Contraindications: Glaucoma, hypersensitivity, intestinal atony of the elderly or debilitated, megacolon, myasthenia gravis, obstructive disease of the GI tract, obstructive uropathy, paralytic ileus, ulcerative colitis, unstable cardiovascular status in acute hemorrhage.

Incompatible with: Specific information not available.

Side effects: Anaphylaxis, blurred vision, cycloplegia, decreased sweating, drowsiness, dry mouth, headache, heat prostration, increased ocular tension, mydriasis, nervousness, palpitations, suppression of lactation, tachycardia, urinary hesitancy and retention, urticaria, weakness.

Antidote: Notify the physician of all side effects. May be treated symptomatically or the drug may be discontinued. For overdose, physostigmine 0.5 to 2 mg IV up to 4 mg may be used; however, it may cause profound bradycardia, seizures, or asystole. Thiopental sodium 2% may be required to decrease excitement. Mechanical ventilation equipment must be available. Treat fever with cooling measures. Treat anaphylaxis and resuscitate as necessary.

LABETALOL HYDROCHLORIDE pH 3.0 to 4.0

(Normodyne, Trandate)

Usual dose: 20 mg as an initial dose direct IV. May repeat with injections of 40 to 80 mg at 10-minute intervals until desired blood pressure is achieved, or may be diluted and given as a continuous infusion. Usually effective with 50 to 200 mg. Do not exceed a total dose of 300 mg.

Dilution: *Direct IV:* May be given undiluted.

Continuous infusion: May be diluted in most commonly used IV solutions; i.e., Ringer's injection; lactated Ringer's injection; 5% dextrose in water; normal saline; 5% dextrose in 0.2%, 0.9%, or 0.33% sodium chloride; and 2.5% dextrose in 0.45% sodium chloride. Addition of 200 mg (40 ml) to 160 ml solution yields 1 mg/ml, 300 mg (60 ml) to 240 ml yields 1 mg/ml, or 200 mg (40 ml) to 250 ml yields 2 mg/3 ml. Amount of solution may be decreased if required by fluid restrictions of the patient.

Rate of administration: *Direct IV:* Each 20 mg or fraction thereof over at least 2 minutes.

Continuous infusion: Adjust according to orders of physician and blood pressure response. Use of a microdrip (60 gtt/ml) or an infusion pump may be helpful.

Actions: Labetalol is an α/β-adrenergic blocking agent. Causes dose-related falls in blood pressure without reflex tachycardia or significant reduction in heart rate. Maximum effect of each dose is reached in 5 minutes. Half-life is about 5 hours, but some effects last up to 16 hours. Metabolized and excreted as metabolites in urine and through bile to feces. Crosses the placental barrier. Present in small amounts in breast milk.

Indications and uses: Control of blood pressure in severe hypertension.

Precautions: (1) Keep patient supine. Postural hypotension can occur for several hours after administration. Ambulate with care and assistance. (2) Monitor blood pressure before and 5 and 10 minutes after each direct IV injection. Monitor at least every 5 minutes during infusion. Avoid rapid or excessive falls in either systolic or diastolic blood pressure. When severely elevated blood pressure drops too rapidly, catastrophic reactions can occur (e.g., cerebral infarction, optic nerve infarction, angina, ischemic ECG changes). (3) Initiate oral labetalol after desired blood pressure has been achieved and the supine diastolic pressure starts to rise. See literature for dosing regimen. (4) Use extreme caution in patients with any degree of cardiac failure; may further depress myocardial contractility. Does not alter effectiveness of digitalis on heart muscle. (5) Effective in lowering blood pressure in pheochromocytoma, but may cause a paradoxical hypertensive response. (6) While it has not been a problem with labetalol, it is recommended that the dose of β-adrenergic blockers be reduced gradually to avoid rebound angina, myocardial infarction, or ventricular dysrhythmias. (7) May potentiate tricyclic antidepressants (e.g., imipramine [Tofranil]). (8) Inhibits β-agonist bronchodilators (e.g., epinephrine); increased doses may be required, especially in asthmatics. (9) Synergistic with halothane anesthesia. Notify anesthesiologist that patient is receiving labetalol. (10) Potentiated by cimetidine (Tagamet). (11) May cause further hypotension with nitroglycerin. (12) Use with extreme caution in diabetics or patients with a history of hypoglycemia. May mask the symptoms of hypoglycemia. May decrease insulin availability; dosage of antidiabetics may need to be adjusted.

(13) May interfere with lab tests in diagnosis of pheochromocytoma. (14) Some authorities recommend that drugs with β-adrenergic properties be discontinued 48 hours before major surgery (β-blockade interferes with cardiac response to reflex stimuli). (15) Use in pregnancy only when clearly indicated and benefit outweighs risk. Use caution during lactation. Safety for use in children not established. (16) Use caution in impaired liver function. (17) Stable after dilution at room temperature for 24 hours.

Contraindications: Bronchial asthma, cardiogenic shock, greater than first-degree heart block, overt cardiac failure, and severe bradycardia.

Incompatible with: Cefoperazone (Cefobid), nafcillin (Unipen), sodium bicarbonate. Mixing with any other drug in syringe or solution not recommended. Consider special use and need for adjustment of rate.

Side effects: Diaphoresis, dizziness, flushing, moderate hypotension, numbness, severe postural hypotension, somnolence, tingling of scalp and ventricular dysrhythmias (e.g., intensified atrioventricular block) occur most frequently.

Antidote: Notify the physician of all side effects. Decrease rate or discontinue drug if hypotension occurs. Notify physician immediately. Trendelenburg position may be appropriate. May require treatment with IV fluids or vasopressors (e.g., norepinephrine [Levarterenol], dopamine [Intropin]). Use atropine for severe bradycardia, digitalis and diuretics for cardiac failure. Unresponsive hypotension and bradycardia may be reversed by glucagon 5 to 10 mg over 30 seconds followed by a continuous infusion of 5 mg/hr. Reduce rate as condition improves. Treat other side effects symptomatically and resuscitate as necessary.

LEUCOVORIN CALCIUM pH 6.0 to 8.0

(Citrovorum Factor, Folinic Acid)

Usual dose: *Overdose of methotrexate:* Milligram for milligram or greater than dose of methotrexate. Administer within first hour, or up to 75 mg as an IV infusion within 12 hours of methotrexate dose. Follow with 12 mg IV every 6 hours for 4 doses. After 24 hours of treatment obtain a serum creatinine. If it is more than 50% above pretreatment serum creatinines, increase the leucovorin dose to 100 mg/M^2 every 3 hours until the serum methotrexate level is satisfactory (see literature).

Folinic acid rescue: For high-dose methotrexate, an IV infusion of leucovorin is initiated anywhere up to 36 hours after methotrexate and continued for 36 to 96 hours, depending on the dose of methotrexate, serum levels, and creatinine clearance of patient. Many schedules have been used. Examples are (a) 10 to 40 mg/M^2 IV 24 hours after methotrexate followed by 10 to 25 mg/M^2 IM or IV every 6 hours for 72 hours; (b) 6 to 15 mg/M^2 every 6 hours for 72 hours beginning 2 hours after methotrexate. Dose regimen depends on methotrexate dose. Usually started within 24 hours. See recommendation in overdose above about obtaining a serum creatinine.

Dilution: The 50 mg vial (powder) must be diluted initially with 50 ml of sterile water for injection with benzyl alcohol. A single dose of the above or the 5 mg/ml prepared solution should then be diluted in 100 to 500 ml of any common IV infusion solution. 1 ml (3 mg) ampoules may be given undiluted.

Rate of administration: A single dose equally distributed over 15 minutes to 1 hour. May be given more rapidly if patient's condition warrants. For massive-dose folinic acid rescue, total dose may be infused equally distributed over a 6-hour period.

Actions: Potent agent for neutralizing immediate toxic effects of methotrexate (and folic acid antagonists) on the hematopoietic system. Preferentially rescues normal cells without reversing the oncolytic effect of methotrexate.

Indications and uses: Treatment of accidental methotrexate overdose.

Investigational (not FDA approved but in common use): Folinic acid rescue to prevent or decrease the toxicity of massive doses of methotrexate used to treat resistant neoplasms.

Precautions: (1) Usually administered in the hospital by or under the direction of the physician specialist. (2) Permits use of massive doses of methotrexate. (3) Do not discontinue leucovorin until methotrexate serum levels fall below toxic levels. (4) Monitor serum blood levels of methotrexate and serum creatinine levels. Death can occur in 5 to 10 days if methotrexate remains at toxic levels longer than 48 hours. (5) Minimum fluid intake of 3 L/24 hr and alkalinization of urine with oral sodium bicarbonate recommended. Begin 12 hours before methotrexate dose administered and continue for 48 hours after final dose in each sequence. (6) Much less effective in accidental overdose after a 1-hour delay. (7) May inhibit phenytoins (e.g., Dilantin). (8) Safety for use in pregnancy and lactation not established. Use only if clearly indicated. (9) Toxicity of fluorouracil increased. (10) All doses over 25 mg should be given IM or IV. (11) Use freshly prepared initial solution immediately if prepared without a preservative; with a preservative may be used for up to 7 days.

Contraindications: None when used as indicated.

Incompatible with: Specific information not available. Consider incompatible in solution with any other drug because of specific use.

Side effects: Almost nonexistent. Some slight flushing or feeling of warmth may occur.

Antidote: Keep physician informed of patient's condition. Symptomatic treatment indicated.

LEVORPHANOL TARTRATE pH 4.3

(Levo-Dromoran)

Usual dose: 2 to 3 mg every 4 to 6 hours. Reduced dose may be required with hepatic or renal disease.

Dilution: Each dose should be diluted with 5 ml of sterile water or normal saline for injection. Do not add to IV solutions. May give through Y-tube or three-way stopcock of infusion set.

Rate of administration: 3 mg or fraction thereof properly diluted solution over 4 to 5 minutes.

Actions: A synthetic narcotic analgesic and CNS depressant closely related to morphine. Five times more potent than morphine milligram for milligram. Onset of action is immediate and lasts 6 to 8 hours. Levorphanol is detoxified in the liver and excreted in the urine. Crosses the placental barrier. Secreted in breast milk.

Indications and uses: (1) Relief of moderate to severe, acute or chronic pain such as pain of biliary or renal colic, cancer, myocardial infarction, severe trauma, or postoperatively; (2) preanesthetic sedation.

Precautions: (1) Oxygen, controlled respiratory equipment, and naloxone (Narcan) must be available. (2) Observe patient frequently and monitor vital signs. Keep patient supine; orthostatic hypotension and fainting may occur. (3) Tolerance to levorphanol gradually increases. A marked increase in dose may precipitate seizures in presence of a history of convulsive disorders. (4) Use caution in the elderly, in patients with impaired hepatic or renal function, emphysema, anticoagulation therapy, and during pregnancy or delivery. (5) Use extreme caution in craniotomy, head injury, and increased intracranial pressure; respiratory depression and intracranial pressure may be further increased. (6) May cause apnea in the asthmatic. (7) Symptoms of acute abdominal conditions may be masked. (8) May increase ventricular response rate in presence of supraventricular tachycardias. (9) Cough reflex is suppressed. (10) Potentiated by phenothiazines (e.g., chlorpromazine [Thorazine]) and other CNS depressants such as narcotic analgesics, alcohol, anticholinergics, antihistamines, barbiturates, hypnotics, sedatives,

MAO inhibitors (e.g., isocarboxazid [Marplan]), neuromuscular blocking agents (e.g., tubocurarine), and psychotropic agents. Reduced dosage of both drugs may be indicated. (11) IV is not the route of choice. Usually given SC. (12) Physical dependence can develop with abuse. (13) Safety for use in pregnancy or lactation not established.

Contraindications: Acute alcoholism, anoxia, bronchial asthma, diarrhea caused by poisoning until toxic material eliminated, increased intracranial pressure, known hypersensitivity to levorphanol, premature infants or labor and delivery of premature infants, respiratory depression, upper airway obstruction.

Incompatible with: Aminophylline, ammonium chloride, amobarbital (Amytal), chlorothiazide (Diuril), heparin, methicillin (Staphcillin), pentobarbital (Nembutal), phenobarbital (Luminal), phenytoin (Dilantin), secobarbital (Seconal), sodium bicarbonate, sodium iodide, thiopental (Pentothal).

Side effects: Nausea, vomiting, and constipation are less frequent than with morphine.

Minor: Dizziness, skin rash, urinary retention, urticaria.

Major: Anaphylaxis, cardiac dysrhythmias, hypotension, respiratory depression.

Antidote: With increasing severity of any side effect or onset of symptoms of overdose, discontinue the drug and notify the physician. Naloxone (Narcan) will reverse serious respiratory depression. A patent airway, artificial ventilation, oxygen therapy, and other symptomatic treatment must be instituted promptly. Resuscitate as necessary.

LEVOTHYROXINE SODIUM

(Levothroid, Synthroid, Synthrox)

Usual dose: 0.2 to 0.5 mg as initial dose. 0.1 to 0.2 mg/24 hr may be repeated as indicated by patient response or serum protein-bound iodine levels. 0.1 mg equals approximately 65 mg (gr 1) thyroid hormone. Maintain with oral medication.

Pediatric dose: *Under 1 year:* 18 to 37 mcg as a single daily dose.

Over 1 year: 2 to 3.5 mcg/kg of body weight as a single daily dose. Do not exceed adult dose.

Dilution: Diluent usually provided. Each 0.5 mg of lyophilized powder is diluted with 5 ml of sodium chloride for injection (without preservatives). Shake well to dissolve completely. 1 ml equals 0.1 mg. Do not add to IV solutions. May be given through Y-tube or three-way stopcock of infusion set.

Rate of administration: 0.1 mg or fraction thereof over 1 minute.

Actions: A synthetic thyroid hormone. Effective replacement for decreased or absent thyroid function. Onset of action is slow. Up to 5 or 6 hours is required before any noticeable improvements occur, and 24 hours may be required to note full benefits. Thyroid hormone is essential to many body functions, including rate of metabolism.

Indications and uses: (1) Hypothyroid states due to any cause; (2) an emergency measure in myxedematous coma.

Precautions: (1) Must be used immediately after dilution; any remaining solution is discarded. (2) Correct adrenocortical insufficiency before administration or acute adrenal crisis and death will result. Corticosteroid therapy is also required concomitantly to prevent acute adrenal insufficiency in myxedematous coma or any preexisting manifestation of adrenal insufficiency. (3) Observe patient continuously and monitor vital signs. (4) Use caution in diabetes and cardiovascular disease. (5) Increases rate of metabolism and requires dosage adjustment for anticoagulants, antidepressants, oral antidiabetics, barbiturates, digitalis, catecholamines (e.g., epinephrine), β-adrenergic blockers (e.g., propranolol), insulin, and others. Cardiac dysrhythmias, hypoglycemia, and bleeding can occur with unadjusted dosage of some of these drugs.

Contraindications: Hypersensitivity to levothyroxine, myocardial infarction, thyrotoxicosis.

Incompatible with: No specific references available. Should be considered incompatible in the syringe with any other drug.

Side effects: Chest pain, diarrhea, heart palpitations, muscle cramps, nervousness, perspiration, tachycardia, vomiting.

Antidote: Notify the physician of any side effect. A reduction in dosage will usually decrease symptoms.

LIDOCAINE HYDROCHLORIDE pH 5.0 to 7.0

(Xylocaine, ✦Xylocard)

Usual dose: 1 mg/kg of body weight. May repeat 0.5 mg/kg every 8 to 10 minutes up to a total of 3 mg/kg if indicated. Follow with 1 to 4 mg/min as an IV infusion. *Do not exceed 4 mg/min rate.*

Prophylactic dose: Initiate a keep-open IV of 5% dextrose in water. 75 mg as a bolus dose independent of weight, height, or age. Repeat 50 mg bolus every 5 minutes if ventricular ectopic activity is present up to a maximum dose of 325 mg, or every 10 minutes if no ectopic activity up to a maximum of 275 mg while en route to hospital.

Pediatric dose: 0.5 to 1 mg/kg of body weight as a bolus dose. Follow with an infusion of 20 to 50 mcg/kg/min.

Dilution: Bolus dose may be given undiluted.

Infusion: Add 1 Gm of lidocaine to 500 or 250 ml of 5% dextrose in water. Solution gives 2 or 4 mg/ml of lidocaine.

Pediatric infusion: Add 120 mg of lidocaine to 100 ml of 5% dextrose in water. 1 to 2.5 ml/kg/hr will deliver 20 to 50 mcg/kg/min.

Rate of administration: *Bolus dose:* 50 mg or fraction thereof over 1 minute. Too-rapid injection may cause seizures.

Infusion: Using a microdrip (60 gtt/ml) or an infusion pump delivers lidocaine in recommended doses. Adjust as indicated by progress in patient's condition.

Actions: A local anesthetic agent. Exerts an antiarrhythmic effect similar to procainamide, but is more potent. Decreases ventricular excitability without depressing the force of ventricular contractions by increasing the stimulation threshold of the ventricle during diastole. Decreases cell membrane permeability and prevents loss of sodium and potassium ions. Onset of action should occur within 2 minutes and last approximately 10 to 20 minutes. Crosses placental barrier. Metabolized in the liver and excreted in the urine.

Indications and uses: Ventricular dysrhythmias such as PVCs or ventricular tachycardia occurring during acute myocardial infarction and during cardiac and other surgery.

Precautions: (1) Label must state "for IV use." (2) Monitor flow rate and the patient's ECG continuously. Therapeutic serum levels range from 1.5 to 5 mcg/ml; above 6 mcg/ml is usually toxic. (3) Discontinue lidocaine when patient's cardiac condition is stable or any signs of toxicity become apparent. (4) Oral antiarrhythmic drugs are preferred for maintenance. (5) Keep a bolus dose, 100 mg (5 ml), available at all times for emergency use in myocardial infarction. (6) Cross-sensitivity and/or potentiation may occur with procainamide or quinidine. (7) Use caution in severe liver or renal disease, hypovolemia, shock, all forms of heart block, and untreated bradycardia. (8) Reduce dose in congestive heart failure, reduced cardiac output, digitalis toxicity with AV block, and the elderly. (9) Discard diluted solution after 24 hours. (10) Do not add lidocaine to blood transfusion tubings. (11) Potentiates succinylcholine (Anectine). (12) Potentiated by β-adrenergic blockers (e.g., propranolol [Inderal]) and cimetidine (Tagamet). (13) May produce excessive cardiac depression with phenytoin (Dilantin). (14) Will potentiate neuromuscular blockade of muscle relaxants (e.g., tubocurarine) and aminoglycoside antibiotics (e.g., polymyxin B).

Contraindications: Known sensitivity to lidocaine or any other local anesthetic of the amide type; Stokes-Adams syndrome or any other severe first-, second-, or third-degree heart block without an artificial pacemaker in place.

Incompatible with: Ampicillin, cefazolin (Kefzol), methohexital (Brevital), phenytoin (Dilantin). Physically compatible with many drugs. However, combination is not practical because of extensive individualized rate adjustments to achieve desired effects.

Side effects: Transient because of short duration of action of lidocaine.

Minor: Apprehension; blurred vision; confusion; dizziness; drowsiness; euphoria; lightheadedness; sensations of heat, cold, and numbness; slurred speech; tinnitus; vomiting.

Major: Anaphylaxis, bradycardia, cardiac arrest, cardiovascular collapse, convulsions, hypotension, malignant hyperthermia (tachycardia, tachypnea, metabolic acidosis, fever), PR interval prolonged, QRS complex widening, respiratory depression, tremors, twitching, unconsciousness.

Antidote: Notify the physician of any side effects. For major side effects, discontinue the drug immediately and institute appropriate measures. For anaphylactic shock use epinephrine and corticosteroids, etc. To correct CNS stimulation use diazepam (Valium), rapid ultrashort-acting barbiturates (e.g., pentobarbital [Nembutal]), or short-acting muscle relaxants (e.g., succinylcholine [Anectine]). Use vasopresssors (e.g., dopamine [Intropin]) to correct hypotension. Maintain and support patient; resuscitate as necessary.

LINCOMYCIN HYDROCHLORIDE pH 3.0 to 5.5

(Lincocin)

Usual dose: 600 mg to 1 Gm every 8 to 12 hours. Total doses from 4 to 8 Gm/24 hr have been given in life-threatening infections.

Pediatric dose: *Children over 1 month of age:* 10 to 20 mg/kg of body weight/24 hr divided into 2 or 3 doses.

Dilution: Add 1 Gm or fraction thereof to a minimum of 100 ml of 5% glucose in water, normal saline, or other compatible solutions. If 4 Gm or more is to be given, add to 500 ml of solution.

Rate of administration: Give properly diluted solution as an infusion. Infusion rate must not exceed 100 ml/hr (1 Gm/hr).

Actions: Interferes with protein synthesis of bacterial organism. It may be bactericidal or bacteriostatic. Well distributed in most body tissues, including spinal fluid if the meninges are inflamed. Actively excreted in bile and urine. Crosses placental barrier. Secreted in breast milk.

Indications and uses: Rarely used. (1) Infections caused by life-threatening susceptible gram-positive and anaerobic organisms that do not respond or are resistant to other less toxic antibiotics such as penicillins or cephalosporins; (2) patients allergic to penicillin.

Precautions: (1) Sensitivity studies necessary to determine susceptibility of the causative organism to lincomycin. (2) Keep patient lying down after injection to prevent hypotension. (3) Avoid prolonged use of drug; superinfection caused by overgrowth of nonsusceptible organisms may result. (4) Periodic blood cell counts and liver function studies are indicated in prolonged therapy. (5) Capable of causing severe, even fatal, colitis; observe for symptoms of diarrhea. (6) May potentiate other neuromuscular blocking agents (e.g., kanamycin, streptomycin, tubocurarine); *apnea can result.* (7) Severe hypotension and cardiac arrest can occur with too-rapid injection. (8) Keep epinephrine immediately available. (9) Use caution in patients with allergic tendencies and in the elderly. Reduce dose to 30% in severe renal impairment. (10) Discard diluted solution after 24 hours. (11) Dilution with other antibiotics in infusion solution may be possible. Consult pharmacist. Adhere to minimum rate of administration.

Contraindications: Colitis; known lincomycin, clindamycin, or erythromycin sensitivity; known candidal infections unless they are being treated concurrently; minor bacterial or viral infections; preexisting liver disease; lactation and pregnancy; newborns.

Incompatible with: Ampicillin, carbenicillin (Geopen), kanamycin (Kantrex), novobiocin (Albamycin), phenytoin (Dilantin). Compatible in solution with penicillin for 4 hours only.

Side effects: Agranulocytosis, anaphylaxis, cardiac arrest, diarrhea, enterocolitis, hypotension, jaundice and elevated SGOT, leukopenia, neutropenia, pruritus ani, skin rashes, thrombocytopenic purpura, urticaria, vaginitis.

Antidote: Notify the physician of early symptoms. For severe symptoms, including significant diarrhea, discontinue the drug. Do not treat diarrhea with opiates or diphenoxylate with atropine (Lomotil); condition will worsen. Treatment will be symptomatic. Fluids, antihistamines, corticosteroids, and vasopressors (e.g., dopamine [Intropin]) may be required. Treat allergic reaction or resuscitate as necessary, and notify the physician. Consider vancomycin as an alternate choice for antibiotic treatment. Hemodialysis or CAPD will not decrease blood levels in toxicity.

LORAZEPAM

(Ativan)

Usual dose: 2 mg or 0.044 mg/kg of body weight, whichever is smaller, 15 to 20 minutes before procedure. For greater lack of recall 0.05 mg/kg up to 4 mg may be given. 2 mg is usually the maximum dose for patients over 50 years of age.

Control of acute agitated delirium in combination with haloperidol: Range is from 0.5 to 10 mg lorazepam every hour until agitation subsides. Repeat successful dose as needed for agitation. Consult haloperidol monograph.

Treatment of pain and agitation in critically ill cancer patients in combination with haloperidol and hydromorphone (Dilaudid): Range is from 0.5 to 10 mg lorazepam every 20 to 30 minutes. Begin with a small dose and increase gradually until agitation subsides, then discontinue lorazepam. Consult haloperidol monograph and hydromorphone monograph.

Management of emetic-inducing chemotherapy: One protocol calls for 1.5 mg/M^2 35 minutes before administration of antineoplastic agent. Given in combination with metoclopramide and dexamethasone.

Dilution: Must be diluted immediately before use with an equal volume of sterile water, 5% dextrose, or 0.9% sodium chloride for injection. Most soluble in dextrose solution. May be given direct IV or through the Y-tube or three-way stopcock of infusion tubing.

Rate of administration: Each 2 mg or fraction thereof over 1 minute.

Actions: A benzodiazepine that relieves anxiety, produces sedation, and inhibits ability to recall events. Effective in 15 to 20 minutes. Lasts up to 16 hours. Widely distributed in body fluids, some is slowly excreted in urine. Crosses the placental barrier. Secreted in breast milk.

Indications and uses: Preanesthetic medication for adult patients.

Investigational uses: Management of status epilepticus especially in children; (2) treatment of severe agitation concurrently with haloperidol; (3) treatment of pain and agitation in critically ill cancer patients concurrently with haloperidol and hydromorphone or morphine sulfate.

Precautions: (1) Bed rest required for a minimum of 3 hours after IV injection and assistance required for up to 8 hours. (2) To reduce incidence of thrombophlebitis, avoid smaller veins. Extravasation or arterial administration is hazardous. (3) Maintain patent airway. Respiratory assistance must be available. (4) Potentiates narcotics, phenothiazines (e.g., prochlorperazine [Compazine]), antihistamines, barbiturates, MAO inhibitors (e.g., pargyline [Eutonyl]), and tricyclic antidepressants (e.g., imipramine [Tofranil-PM]) for up to 48 hours. Potentiated by alcohol and other CNS depressants. (5) Reduce dosages for the elderly and debilitated and in those with impaired liver or renal function. (6) Scopolamine increases sedation, hallucinations, and irrational behavior. (7) Inhibits antiparkinson effectiveness of levodopa. (8) Rarely given IV. Rapidly and completely absorbed IM. (9) Refrigerate, use only freshly prepared solutions, discard if discolored or precipitate forms. (10) Patient is able to respond to simple instructions.

Contraindications: Hypersensitivity to benzodiazepines (e.g., diazepam [Valium], chlordiazepoxide [Librium]), glycols, or benzyl alcohol; acute narrow-angle glaucoma; psychoses; pregnancy, labor, delivery, and lactation; children.

Incompatible with: Limited information available. Specific incompatibilities not documented.

Side effects: Airway obstruction, apnea, blurred vision, confusion, crying, delirium, depression, excessive drowsiness, hallucinations, restlessness.

Antidote: Notify physician of all symptoms. Treatment if indicated will be supportive. In overdose, maintain an adequate airway and ventilation. Promote excretion through fluid and electrolyte administration and osmotic diuretics (e.g., mannitol). Consider hemodialysis. Physostigmine 0.5 to 4 mg at 1 mg/min may reverse symptoms of anticholinergic overdose (e.g., confusion), but may also cause seizures.

LYMPHOCYTE IMMUNE GLOBULIN pH 6.8

(Anti-thymocyte Globulin [Equine], Atgam)

Usual dose: Range is 10 to 30 mg/kg of body weight/24 hr. Actual potency and activity may vary from lot to lot. Given concomitantly with other immunosuppressive therapy (antimetabolites such as azathioprine [Imuran] and corticosteroids). Skin test required (see Precautions).

Delay onset of renal allograft rejection: 15 mg/kg/24 hr for 14 days, then every other day for 7 more doses. Initial dose should be given 24 hours before or after the transplant.

Treat allograft rejection: 10 to 15 mg/kg/24 hr for 14 days, then every other day for 7 more doses (optional). Initial dose should be given when first rejection episode is diagnosed.

Pediatric dose: Range is 5 to 25 mg/kg/24 hr.

Dilution: Total daily dose must be further diluted with 0.45% to 0.9% saline for infusion. Invert saline while injecting drug so contact is not made with air in infusion bottle. Preferred minimum concentration is 1 mg drug/1 ml saline infusion solution. May be infused into a vascular shunt, AV fistula, or high-flow central vein. Use of a 0.2 to 1.0 micron filter recommended.

Rate of administration: A total daily dose equally distributed over a minimum of 4 hours.

Actions: A lymphocyte-selective immunosuppressant. Reduces the number of thymus-dependent lymphocytes and contains low concentrations of antibodies against other formed elements in blood. Effective without causing severe lymphopenia. Supports an increase in the frequency of resolution of an acute rejection episode. Has a serum half-life of 5 to 8 days.

Indications and uses: (1) Management of allograft rejection in renal transplant patients; (2) adjunctive to other immunosuppressive therapy to delay onset of initial rejection episode.

Precautions: (1) Administered only under the direction of a physician experienced in immunosuppressive therapy and management of renal transplant patients in a facility with adequate laboratory and supportive medical resources. (2) Intradermal skin test required before administration. Use 0.1 ml of a 1:1,000 dilution in normal saline and a saline control. If a systemic reaction (rash, dyspnea) occurs, do not administer. If a limited reaction (10 mm wheal or erythema) occurs, proceed with extreme caution. Anaphylaxis can occur even if skin test is negative. (3) Will cause chemical phlebitis in peripheral veins. (4) Keep refrigerated before and after dilution. Discard diluted solution after 12 hours. (5) Monitor carefully for signs of leukopenia, thrombocytopenia, or infection. Notify physician immediately so prompt treatment can be instituted and/or drug discontinued. (6) Masked reactions may occur as dosage of corticosteroids and antimetabolites is decreased. Observe carefully. (7) Anaphylaxis can occur at any time. Emergency equipment and supplies must be at bedside. (8) Safety for use in pregnancy and lactation not established. Limited experience on use in children. (9) Use caution in repeat courses of therapy.

Contraindications: Systemic hypersensitivity reaction to previous injection of lymphocyte immune globulin or any other equine gamma globulin preparation.

Incompatible with: Should be considered incompatible in syringe or solution with any other drug or solution (except 0.45% or 0.9% saline) because of specific use. Will precipitate with 5% dextrose in water or other acid infusion solutions.

Side effects: Full range of allergic symptoms including anaphylaxis is possible. Arthralgia, back pain, chest pain, chills, clotted AV fistula, diarrhea, dyspnea, fever, headache, hypotension, infusion site pain, leukopenia, nausea, night sweats, pruritus, rash, stomatitis, thrombocytopenia, thrombophlebitis, urticaria, vomiting, wheal and flare.

Antidote: Notify physician of all side effects. Discontinue if anaphylaxis, severe and unremitting thrombocytopenia, and/or severe and unremitting leukopenia occur. May be discontinued if infection or hemolysis present even if appropriately treated. Clinically significant hemolysis may require erythrocyte transfusion, IV mannitol, furosemide, sodium bicarbonate, and fluids. Prophylactic or therapeutic antihistamines (e.g., diphenhydramine [Benadryl]) or corticosteroids should control chills caused by release of endogenous leukocyte pyrogens. Treat anaphylaxis immediately. Epinephrine (Adrenalin), diphenhydramine (Benadryl), oxygen, vasopressors (e.g., dopamine [Intropin]), corticosteroids, and ventilation equipment must always be available. Resuscitate as necessary.

MAGNESIUM SULFATE

pH 5.5 to 7.0

Usual dose: *Convulsive states:* 1 to 4 Gm (10 to 40 ml) of a 10% solution. Repeat as indicated, observing all necessary precautions.

Hypomagnesemia (severe): 5 Gm (40 mEq) to 1,000 ml 5% dextrose in water or saline as an infusion.

Hyperalimentation: Adults, 8 to 24 mEq/24 hr. Infants, 2 to 10 mEq/24 hr.

Dilution: May be given undiluted. May be added to IV solutions; dilute to at least a 20% solution. May be given through Y-tube or three-way stopcock of infusion set.

Rate of administration: *Direct IV:* 1.5 ml of a 10% solution or its equivalent over at least 1 minute.

IV infusion in hypomagnesemia: A single dose infused over 3 hours. Do not exceed 3 ml/min.

Actions: A CNS depressant and a depressant of smooth, skeletal, and cardiac muscle. It also possesses a mild diuretic effect and vasodilating effect. Onset of action is immediate and effective for about 30 minutes. Excreted in the urine. Crosses the placental barrier.

Indications and uses: (1) Convulsive states (eclampsia, glomerulonephritis, hypoparathyroidism); (2) severe hypomagnesemia; (3) nutritional supplementation in hyperalimentation; (4) cerebral edema; (5) uterine tetany, especially after large doses of oxytocin.

Investigational uses: Inhibit premature labor; counteract postinfarction hypomagnesemia (given on admission to patient with suspected myocardial infarction); treatment of alcohol withdrawal; bronchodilator in asthma.

Precautions: (1) Discontinue IV administration when the desired therapeutic effect is obtained. (2) Test knee jerks and observe respirations before each additional dose. If the knee jerk is absent or respirations are less than 16/min, do not give additional magnesium sulfate. (3) Equipment to maintain artificial respiration must be available at all times. Patient must be continuously observed. Maintain minimum of 100 ml of urine output every 4 hours. (4) Each 1 Gm contains 8.12 mEq of magnesium. A normal adult body contains 20 to 30 Gm of magnesium. (5) Use caution in impaired renal function and in patients receiving digitalis. (6) Inhibits tetracycline absorption. (7) Reduce dosage of other CNS depressants (e.g., narcotics, barbiturates) when given in conjunction with magnesium sulfate. (8) Potentiates neuromuscular blocking agents (e.g., tubocurarine [Curare]). (9) Do not administer during the 2 hours preceding delivery of the toxemic patient. May cause magnesium toxicity in the newborn requiring assisted ventilation and calcium administration. (10) Can harm fetus during pregnancy if mother is not toxic. Use caution during lactation. Safety for children not established.

Contraindications: Presence of heart block or myocardial damage; within 2 hours of delivery.

Incompatible with: Alcohol, alkalies (bicarbonates, carbonates, hydroxides), arsenates, calcium gluconate, calcium gluceptate, chlorpromazine (Thorazine), clindamycin (Cleocin), dobutamine (Dobutrex), hydrocortisone (Solu-Cortef), IV fat emulsion 10%, phosphates, polymyxin B (Aerosporin), phytonadione (Aquamephyton), procaine (Novocaine), salicylates, sodium bicarbonate, strontium, tartrates, tobramycin (Nebcin), vitamin B complex.

Side effects: Usually the result of magnesium intoxication; absence of knee jerk reflex, cardiac arrest, circulatory collapse, complete heart block, flaccid paralysis, flushing, hypocalcemia with signs of tetany, hypotension, hypothermia, increased PR interval, increased QRS complex, prolonged QT interval, respiratory depression and failure, sweating.

Antidote: Discontinue the drug and notify the physician of the occurrence of any side effect. Calcium gluconate and calcium gluceptate are specific antidotes; 5 to 10 mEq should reverse respiratory depression and heart block. Treat hypotension with dopamine (Intropin). Employ artificial respiration as necessary and resuscitate as necessary. Peritoneal dialysis or hemodialysis are effective in overdose.

MANNITOL

pH 4.5 to 7.0

(Osmitrol)

Usual dose: Very flexible. 1 to 2 Gm/kg of body weight or 50 to 200 Gm/24 hr. 1 Gm equal to approximately 5.5 mOsm. Available as:

25% solution (12.5 Gm/50ml) (1,375 mOsm/L)

20% solution (50 Gm/250 ml, 100 Gm/500 ml) (1,100 mOsm/L)

15% solution (22.5 Gm/150 ml, 75 Gm/500 ml) (825 mOsm/L)

10% solution (50 Gm/500 ml, 100 Gm/L) (550 mOsm/L)

5% solution (50 Gm/L) (275 mOsm/L)

Prevention of oliguric phase of acute renal failure: 50 to 100 Gm as a 5% to 25% solution.

Treatment of oliguria: 300 to 400 mg/kg of body weight of a 20% or 25% solution, or up to 100 Gm of a 15% or 20% solution.

Reduction of intracranial pressure and brain mass: 1.5 to 2.0 Gm/kg of body weight as a 15% to 25% solution.

Reduction of intraocular pressure: 1.5 to 2 Gm/kg of body weight as a 15%, 20%, or 25% solution. May be used 60 to 90 minutes before surgery.

Promote diuresis in intoxication: Up to 200 Gm. Discontinue if no benefit derived from this dose.

Pediatric dose: 1 to 2 Gm/kg of body weight or 30 to 60 Gm/M^2 of body surface as a 15% to 20% solution. Start with low dose and increase gradually based on clinical situation.

Dilution: No further dilution is necessary; however, if there are any crystals present in the solution, they must be completely dissolved before administration. Warm ampoule or bottle in hot water (to 50° C [122° F]) and shake vigorously at intervals. Cool to at least body temperature before administraton. Use an in-line filter for 15%, 20%, and 25% solutions.

Rate of administration: A single dose should be given over 30 to 90 minutes. Up to 3 Gm/kg has been given over this time span. A test dose (see Precautions) or loading doses may be given over 3 to 5 minutes.

Oliguria: A single dose over 90 minutes to several hours.

Reduction of intracranial pressure and brain mass: A single dose over 30 to 60 minutes.

Glomerular filtration rate: 100 ml of a 20% solution (20 Gm) diluted with 180 ml of normal saline should be infused at a rate of 20 ml/min. Collect urine samples as ordered.

Actions: A sugar alcohol and most effective osmotic diuretic. It is a stable, inert, nontoxic solution. Distribution in the body is limited to extracellular compartments. Mannitol is not reabsorbed by the tubules of the kidneys. It is excreted almost completely in the urine along with water. Reduction in cerebrospinal and intraocular fluid occurs within 15 minutes and lasts 4 to 8 hours. Rebound may occur within 12 hours.

Indications and uses: (1) Prophylaxis of acute renal failure (cardiovascular procedures, severe trauma, surgery in presence of jaundice, hemolytic transfusion reactions); (2) reduction of intracranial pressure and brain mass before and after surgery; (3) reduction of extremely high intraocular pressure; (4) promotion of excretion of toxic substances from sedative overdose; (5) kidney function test (glomerular filtration); (6) reduction of generalized edema and ascites; (7) oliguric phase of acute renal failure.

Precautions: (1) Use only freshly prepared solutions. Discard unused portions. (2) Test dose should be used in patients with marked oliguria or impaired renal functions. Give 200 mg/kg of body weight over 3 to 5 minutes. 40 ml of urine should be produced in 1 hour. (3) Observe urine output continuously; should exceed 30 to 50 ml/hr. Insert Foley catheter if necessary. (4) Electrolyte depletion may occur. Check with laboratory studies and replace as necessary. (5) Observe infusion site to prevent infiltration. (6) May cause deafness with kanamycin (Kantrex). (7) Calcium disodium edetate will increase the amount of mannitol absorbed, an undesirable effect. (8) Maintain hydration; may obscure signs of inadequate hydration or hypovolemia. (9) Reduce dose by one half for small or debilitated patients. (10) Evaluate cardiac status to avoid fulminating congestive heart failure. (11) Mixing with whole blood may cause agglutination and irreversible crenation.

Contraindications: Anuria, edema associated with capillary fragility of membrane permeability, fluid and electrolyte depletion, intracranial bleeding except during craniotomy, some cases of metabolic edema, pregnancy, severe congestive heart failure, severe dehydration, severe renal impairment.

Incompatible with: Potassium chloride, sodium chloride, whole blood.

Side effects: Rare when used as directed but may include backache, blurred vision, chest pain, chills, convulsions, decreased chloride levels, decreased sodium levels, dehydration, diuresis, dizziness, dryness of mouth, edema, fever, fulminating congestive heart failure, headache, hyperosmolality, hypertension, hypotension, nausea, polyuria then oliguria, pulmonary edema, rhinitis, tachycardia, thirst, thrombophlebitis, and urinary retention.

Antidote: If minor side effects persist, notify the physician. For all major side effects or if urine output is under 30 to 50 ml/hr, discontinue the drug and notify the physician. Treatment will be supportive to correct fluid and electrolyte imbalances. Hemodialysis may be used to clear mannitol and reduce serum osmolality.

MECHLORETHAMINE HYDROCHLORIDE

pH 3.0 to 5.0

(HN_2, Mustargen, Nitrogen mustard)

Usual dose: 0.4 mg/kg of body weight as a single dose is preferred, or may be divided into 2 to 4 equal doses and given daily for 2 to 4 days. Allow about 3 to 6 weeks between courses of therapy. Confirm bone marrow recovery. Results with subsequent courses are rarely as satisfactory as the initial course. Dosage based on average weight in presence of ascites or edema.

Dilution: *Specific techniques required, see Precautions.* Wear disposable mask, gown, and gloves for mixing. Safety glasses are appropriate. Dilute each 10 mg vial with 10 ml of sterile water or sodium chloride for injection. Do not remove needle and syringe. Hold securely and shake vial to dissolve completely. Withdraw desired dose. Contains 1 mg/ml. May be given direct IV, but administration through a Y-tube or three-way stopcock of a free-flowing infusion is preferred.

Rate of administration: Total daily dose equally distributed over 3 to 5 minutes.

Actions: An alkylating agent, cell cycle phase nonspecific, with antitumor activity. It has a selective cytotoxic effect on rapidly growing cells. Palliative, not curative, in its effects; regression in the size of malignant tumor may occur; pain and fever subside; appetite, strength, and a sense of well-being are increased. Immediately absorbed and metabolized, it is excreted in changed form in the urine.

Indications and uses: To suppress or retard neoplastic growth. Good response is inconsistent but has been experienced in Hodgkin's disease, lymphosarcoma, bronchogenic carcinoma, specific types of chronic leukemia, polycythemia vera, and mycosis fungoides. Used in generalized metastasis and in patients refractory to radiation therapy.

Precautions: (1) Follow guidelines for handling cytotoxic agents recommended. See Appendix, p. 677. (2) Administered by or under the direction of the physician specialist. (3) Highly toxic; must not be inhaled or come into contact with skin or any mucous membrane, especially the eyes, at any stage of mixing, administration, or destruction. For accidental contact, copious irrigation with water for at least 15 minutes is indicated. Follow with rinse of 2% sodium thiosulfate. Use an isotonic ophthalmic irrigation solution if eye contamination occurs. (4) Mix solution immediately before use. Very unstable. Neutralize unused portion with equal volume sodium thiosulfate–sodium bicarbonate solution and let stand 45 minutes. Then discard. (5) Do not use if solution is discolored or if droplets of water remain isolated in the vial. (6) Extremely narrow margin of safety; dosage is individual, and frequent blood examinations are mandatory. (7) Use precaution with radiation therapy, other chemotherapy, severe leukopenia, thrombocytopenia, anemia, and bone marrow infiltrated with malignant cells. (8) May produce teratogenic effects on the fetus. Has mutagenic potential. Give with caution in men and women capable of conception. Discontinue breast feeding. (9) Alkalating agents interact with numerous drugs such as amphotericin B (Fungizone), radiation therapy, other antineoplastics, and many others to produce serious reaction. (10) Extravasation into surrounding tissue can cause sloughing and possible necrosis. (11) Often given in the late evening with antiemetics and sedatives to promote patient comfort. (12) Used in reduced doses with other chemotherapeutic agents to produce tumor remission. (13) Maintain adequate hydration. (14) Allopurinol may prevent formation of uric acid crystals. (15) Do not administer any vaccine or chloroquine to patients receiving antineoplastic drugs. (16) Observe closely for all signs of infection. (17) Specific tissue can be protected from the effects of this agent by temporary interruption of its blood supply during and immediately after injection. (18) In the presence of acute or chronic suppurative inflammation, do not use nitrogen mustard. May cause rapid development of amyloidosis.

Contraindications: Not recommended in patients with infectious disease, previous anaphylactic reactions, or in terminal stages of malignancy.

Incompatible with: Any other drug in syringe or solution.

Side effects: Alopecia, anaphylaxis, anorexia, bleeding, bone marrow depression, cerebrovascular accidents, delayed menses, depression of formed elements in circulating blood, diarrhea, hemolytic anemia, hyperuricemia, jaundice, leukopenia, nausea, petechiae, sloughing, susceptibility to infection, tinnitus, thrombophlebitis, vertigo, vomiting, weakness, death.

Antidote: (1) For external contact and cleaning purposes, use a 2% sodium thiosulfate solution. (2) To prevent sloughing and necrosis in areas where extravasation has occurred, inject isotonic sodium thiosulfate with a fine hypodermic needle into the indurated area. Apply ice compress, elevate extremity. (3) Use chlorpromazine (Thorazine) or other phenothiazides to control nausea and sodium pentobarbital (Nembutal) to produce sedation. (4) Notify physician of any side effect. Discontinue the drug and use supportive therapy, including blood transfusion, as necessary to sustain the patient in toxicity.

MENADIOL SODIUM DIPHOSPHATE pH 8.0

(✤ Synkavite, Synkayvite, vitamin K_4)

Usual dose: 5 to 15 mg once or twice every 24 hours.

Pediatric dose: 5 to 10 mg once or twice every 24 hours.

Dilution: May be given undiluted or added to most infusion solutions.

Rate of administration: Each dose over 1 minute in undiluted form.

Actions: Menadiol is a synthetic, water-soluble vitamin essential for the production of prothrombin by the liver. Hemorrhage will occur in its absence. Rapidly absorbed and utilized; PT should be elevated within 12 to 18 hours. One third as potent as menadione. Metabolized completely by the body. Crosses the placental barrier. Secreted in breast milk.

Indications and uses: (1) Prevention and treatment of hypoprothrombinemia secondary to deficient absorption from biliary disease, intestinal disease, surgical resection, or after large doses or long-term use of some medications such as salicylates, quinine, sulfonamides, arsenicals, barbiturates, dicumarol, and many antibiotics including cephalosporins and penicillins; (2) liver function test.

Precautions: (1) Phytonadione is the drug of choice for impending or actual hemorrhage because of its rapid action. (2) Menadiol is not commonly administered by the IV route. IM or SC administration provides adequate absorption at a slower rate. (3) Dosage and effects are determined by PTs. Keep physician informed. (4) Do not use for premature infants or neonates or during the last trimester of pregnancy; bilirubinemia, hemolytic anemia, hemoglobinuria, kernicterus, brain damage, and death may occur. (5) Supplement with whole blood transfusion if necessary. (6) Protect from light. (7) May promote temporary resistance to prothrombin-depressing anticoagulants. (8) Use caution in asthmatics; contains sulfites.

Contraindications: Hemorrhagic disease not caused by prothrombin deficiency and severe nonfunctioning liver disease; last trimester of pregnancy; newborns and premature infants.

Incompatible with: Alkaloids, codeine, levarterenol (Levophed), levorphanol (Levo-Dromoran), meperidine (Demerol), metals, methadone, mineral acids, procaine (Novocain).

Side effects: Rare when used as recommended: allergic reactions such as skin rash; anaphylaxis; cyanosis; depressed liver function; diaphoresis; dizziness; dyspnea; erythrocyte hemolysis; flushing sensation; hypotension; shock; tachycardia.

Antidote: Discontinue the drug and notify the physician of any side effects. Physician may choose to continue drug at a decreased rate of administration. Treat allergic reactions as necessary.

MEPERIDINE HYDROCHLORIDE pH 3.5 to 6.0

(Demerol, Demerol Hydrochloride)

Usual dose: *Direct IV:* 10 to 50 mg. Repeat every 2 to 4 hours as necessary.

Reduced dose may be required in hepatic or renal disease.

Infusion: Must be administered through a controlled infusion device. May be patient activated. Based on a 10 mg/ml dilution an initial loading dose of 20 to 25 mg (2 to 2.5 ml) is average. The continuous background infusion to provide a level of pain relief and maintain patency of the vein may range from 10 to 15 mg/hr (1 to 1.5 ml/hr). Additional doses of 5 to 10 mg (0.5 to 1.0 ml) may be activated by the patient at selected intervals every 3 to 60 minutes (averaging 10 to 15 minutes). Additional boluses (averaging 5 to 10 mg [0.5 to 1.0 ml]) may be given by health care professionals (e.g., every 30 min prn). In selected patients all of these doses may be somewhat higher.

Pediatric dose: Not recommended for IV use in children.

Dilution: *Direct IV:* Must be diluted. Use at least 5 ml of sterile water or normal saline for injection or other IV solutions.

Infusion: Each 10 mg must be diluted in at least 1 ml of normal saline, 5% dextrose in water or saline or other compatible infusion solution. Usually diluted in normal saline for use in narcotic syringe infusor systems. Sometimes diluted in IV fluids to a dilution of 1 mg/ml and given as a continuous infusion under the direct observation and control of the anesthesiologist.

Rate of administration: *Direct IV:* A single dose over 4 to 5 minutes. Frequently titrated according to symptom relief and respiratory rate.

Infusion: Must be administered through a controlled infusion device. May be patient activated. Initial loading dose, basal rate (continuous rate of infusion), patient self-adminstered dose and interval, additional boluses permitted, and total dose for 1 hour should be ordered by physician. Do not exceed direct IV rate. For continuous infusion note range of mg/hr under Usual dose; distribute evenly via infusion device.

Actions: A synthetic narcotic analgesic and descending CNS depressant, similar to but slightly less potent than morphine. Onset of action occurs in about 5 minutes and lasts for about 2 hours. Pain threshold is elevated, and the reaction of the individual to the painful experience is altered. Crosses the placental barrier. Readily absorbed and distributed throughout the body. Metabolized to normeperidine in the liver, its extended half-life (15 to 30 hours) may lead to cumulative effects. Excreted in the urine. Secreted in breast milk.

Indications and uses: (1) Relief of most moderate to severe pain; (2) preoperative medication; (3) support of anesthesia; (4) obstetrical analgesia; (5) restore uterine tone and contractions in a uterus made hyperactive by oxytocics.

Precautions: (1) Oxygen, controlled respiratory equipment, and naloxone (Narcan) must always be available. (2) Observe patient frequently to continuously based on dose and monitor vital signs. Keep patient supine; orthostatic hypotension and fainting may occur; less likely with continuous low doses, but observe closely during ambulation. (3) Stool softeners and/or laxatives may be required to avoid constipation and fecal impaction. Maintain adequate hydration. (4) Use with caution in glaucoma, head injuries, increased intracranial pressure (elevates spinal fluid pressure), asthma, chronic obstructive pulmonary disease, decreased respiratory reserve or respiratory depression, supraventricular tachycardia, convulsions, acute abdominal conditions before diagnosis, the elderly and debilitated, and hepatic or renal insufficiency. (5) Cough reflex is suppressed. (6) Morphine is usually preferred for pain during cardiac dysrhythmias. (7) Physical dependence can develop with abuse. (8) IM route frequently used. (9) Potentiated by antacids, anticholinergics, cimetidine (Tagamet), tricyclic antidepressants (e.g., amitriptyline [Elavil]), MAO inhibitors (e.g., isocarboxazid [Marplan]), isoniazid (Nydrazid), neostigmine (Prostigmin), neuromuscular blocking agents (e.g., tubocurarine), oral contraceptives, phenothiazines (e.g., promazine [Sparine]), general anesthetics, other narcotic analgesics, and CNS depressants including alcohol. Reduced dosage of both drugs may be indicated. (10) Inhibited by hydantoins (e.g., phenytoin [Dilantin]).

Contraindications: Acute bronchial asthma, hypersensitivity to meperidine, patients who have received MAO inhibitors (e.g., isocarboxazid [Marplan]) in the previous 2 weeks, diarrhea resulting from poisoning until toxic material eliminated, pregnancy before labor, lactation, premature infants or labor and delivery of premature infants, pulmonary edema caused by chemical respiratory irritant, upper airway obstruction.

Incompatible with: Aminophylline, amobarbital (Amytal), furosemide (Lasix), heparin, hydrocortisone sodium succinate (Solu-Cortef), methicillin (Staphcillin), methylprednisolone (Solu-Medrol), morphine, pentobarbital (Nembutal), phenobarbital (Luminal), phenytoin (Dilantin), secobarbital (Seconal), sodium bicarbonate, sodium iodide, thiopental (Pentothal).

Side effects: *Minor:* Dizziness, flushing, lightheadedness, nausea, postural hypotension, rash, restlessness, sedation, sweating, syncope, vomiting.

Major: Allergic reactions, apnea, cardiac arrest, cardiovascular collapse, cold and clammy skin, convulsions, dilated pupils, respiratory depression, shock, tremor.

Antidote: With increasing severity of minor side effects or onset of any major side effect, discontinue the drug and notify the physician. Naloxone hydrochloride (Narcan) will reverse serious respiratory depression. A patent airway, artificial respiration, oxygen therapy, and other symptomatic treatment must be instituted promptly. Resuscitate as necessary.

MEPHENTERMINE SULFATE pH 4.0 to 6.5

(Wyamine)

Usual dose: 15 to 60 mg as the initial dose. May be followed by repeat doses of 15 to 45 mg as indicated. At the same time a continuous infusion of 1 mg/ml may be given. Dosage requirements are dependent on patient response. 0.5 to 1 mg/kg of body weight should effect response in most hypotensive states. Up to 3 mg/kg of body weight may be required.

Dilution: May be given undiluted or may be diluted in 5% dextrose in water and given as an infusion. Add 600 mg to 500 ml of diluent to deliver approximately 1 mg/ml.

Rate of administration: Undiluted, each 30 mg or fraction thereof over 1 minute. Infusion rate is more easily regulated with a microdrip (60 gtt/ml) or an infusion pump. Rate will be determined by patient response.

Actions: A potent vasopressor similar to ephedrine. Has positive inotropic and chronotropic effects. Initial pressor effect results from increased myocardial contractility and enhancement by increased peripheral vasoconstriction and resistance. Its use in cardiac arrhythmias results from a decreased atrioventricular conduction time, a decreased refractory period of the atrium, and a decreased conduction time in ventricular muscle. It has some CNS stimulation similar to that of amphetamines and increases cerebral oxygen utilization. Effective within 1 to 2 minutes for a period of 1 to 2 hours. After metabolism, it is excreted in the urine.

Indications and uses: (1) May be used prophylactically or as a treatment for hypotensive states not associated with hemorrhage, such as myocardial infarction; (2) surgical, postoperative, obstetrical, and spinal anesthesia; (3) hypotension secondary to ganglionic blockade.

Precautions: (1) Check blood pressure every 2 minutes until stabilized at the desired level. Check every 5 minutes thereafter during therapy. (2) Discontinue the medication temporarily after patient's condition and blood pressure are stabilized. Restart as necessary until stabilization occurs. (3) If pressor action is not effective, short-term therapy with norepinephrine (Levarterenol) may restore the catecholamine sites necessary to make it effective. (4) Diluted infusion may be used to maintain blood pressure in shock caused by hemorrhage until whole blood replacement is begun. (5) Use with care in known hypertensive patients and with cyclopropane or halothane anesthesia. (6) Potentiated or inhibited depending on timing of interaction by guanethidine (Ismelin), methyldopa (Aldomet), rauwolfia alkaloids (e.g., Reserpine), and others. (7) Potentiated by MAO inhibitors (e.g., pargyline [Eutonyl]). Hypertensive crisis may result. (8) May cause severe hypertension or stroke with ergot alkaloids. (9) May cause hypotension and bradycardia with hydantoins (e.g., phenytoin [Dilantin]).

Contraindications: Do not use to treat overdosage of phenothiazines (e.g., chlorpromazine [Thorazine]). A further drop in blood pressure will occur, and irreversible shock may result. Known sensitivity to mephentermine.

Incompatible with: Epinephrine (Adrenalin), hydralazine (Apresoline).

Side effects: Usually minimal: anorexia, anxiety, hypertension, nervousness. Cardiac arrhythmias are possible.

Antidote: No reports of toxic reactions. Notify the physician if CNS stimulation seems excessive. Discontinue drug and notify the physician for hypertension.

MESNA pH 6.5 to 8.5

(Mesnex, ♣ Uromitexan)

Usual dose: Total daily dose is 60% of the ifosfamide dose equally divided into 3 doses. A single dose of mesna equal to 20% of the ifosfamide dose is given at the time of the ifosfamide injection and repeated 4 hours and 8 hours later (e.g., ifosfamide 1.2 Gm/M^2 would require mesna 240 mg/M^2 with the ifosfamide, 240 mg/M^2 in 4 hours, and again at 8 hours). The initial mesna dose each day may be mixed with the ifosfamide. Appears to be compatible.

Dosage of mesna must be repeated each day ifosfamide is administered and adjusted with each increase or decrease of the ifosfamide dose.

Dilution: Each 100 mg (1 ml) must be diluted in a minimum of 4 ml 5% dextrose in water or normal saline, normal saline, or lactated Ringer's injection. Desired concentration is 20 mg/ml.

Rate of administration: A single dose over a minimum of 1 minute given as a single agent. Administer at rate for ifosfamide if given together.

Actions: A detoxifying agent. Reacts chemically in the kidney with urotoxic ifosfamide metabolites to detoxify them and inhibit hemorrhagic cystitis. Remains in the intravascular compartment, and much of a single dose is excreted within 4 hours in the urine.

Indications and uses: A prophylactic agent used to reduce the incidence of hemorrhagic cystitis caused by ifosfamide.

Unlabeled uses: May reduce the incidence of hemorrhagic cystitis caused by cyclophosphamide.

Precautions: (1) Repeated doses are required to maintain adequate levels of mesna in the kidneys and bladder to detoxify urotoxic ifosfamide metabolites. (2) Hemorrhagic cystitis caused by ifosfamide is dose dependent. Mesna is most effective when ifosfamide dose is less than 1.2 Gm/M^2/24 hr. Somewhat less effective when ifosfamide dose 2 to 4 gm/M^2/24 hr. If hematuria develops with appropriate doses of mesna, ifosfamide dose may need to be reduced or discontinued. (3) Does not inhibit any other side effects or toxicities caused by ifosfamide therapy. (4) Not effective in preventing hematuria caused by other conditions (e.g., thrombocytopenia). (5) May cause a false positive reaction for urinary ketones. If a red-violet color develops, glacial acetic acid returns the coloring to violet. (6) Use during pregnancy only if benefits clearly outweigh risks. Discontinue nursing. (7) Discard any unused drug from the ampoule. Mesna oxidizes to the disulfide dimesna when exposed to oxygen. Refrigerate diluted solutions and use within 6 hours.

Contraindications: Hypersensitivity to mesna or other thiol compounds.

Incompatible with: Cisplatin.

Side effects: *Average dose:* Bad taste in the mouth, diarrhea, nausea, soft stool, vomiting.

Overdose: Allergic reactions, diarrhea, fatigue, headache, hematuria, hypotension, limb pain, nausea.

Antidote: No specific antidote. Keep physician informed of all side effects. Notify promptly if signs of overdose occur. Resuscitate as necessary.

METARAMINOL BITARTRATE pH 3.5 to 4.5

(Aramine)

Usual dose: 0.5 to 5 mg direct IV only in an extreme emergency. 15 to 100 mg in 500 ml of specific infusion solution. 150 to 500 mg/500 ml of infusion solution has been used at an extremely slow rate. Adjust to desired clinical fluid volume. Allow at least 10 minutes before increasing any dose.

Pediatric dose: 0.01 mg/kg of body weight as a single dose or as a solution of 1 mg/25 ml in dextrose or saline for infusion.

Dilution: Single dose up to 5 mg may be given undiluted. Should be diluted in at least 500 ml of sodium chloride or 5% dextrose and administered as an IV infusion.

Rate of administration: Direct IV administration, 5 mg or fraction thereof over 1 minute. In solution use slowest possible flow rate to correct hypotension gradually and maintain adequate or preset blood pressure. Use of a microdrip (60 gtt/ml) or an infusion pump helpful.

Actions: A potent vasopressor but less potent than norepinephrine. Produces gradual action with long effect. It constricts blood vessels, increases peripheral resistance, and elevates systolic and diastolic pressure. Increases cardiac contractility and cerebral, coronary, and renal blood flow. May cause reflex bradycardia. Inactivated in the body and excreted in the urine. Effective within 1 to 2 minutes. Maximum effect may take 10 minutes and lasts 20 minutes to 1 hour.

Indications and uses: Acute hypotensive states resulting from anesthesia, hemorrhage, medication reaction, cardiogenic shock, surgical complications, trauma, septicemia, and shock, with brain damage owing to trauma or tumor.

Precautions: (1) Check blood pressure every 5 minutes until stabilized at the desired level. Check every 15 minutes thereafter throughout therapy. (2) Hypovolemia must be corrected to receive adequate response. (3) Whole blood or plasma should be given in a separate IV site. (4) Avoid hypertension; cardiac arrest may result. (5) Use a large vein and confirm patency. Discontinue IV administration if vein infiltrates or is thrombosed; can result in tissue necrosis and sloughing. (6) Cumulative effect is possible. Hypertension may remain even after drug is discontinued. (7) MAO inhibitors and tricyclic antidepressants potentiate metaraminol and can cause an acute hypertensive crisis with brain hemorrhage. (8) Use care in liver, heart, and thyroid disease and in hypertension or diabetes. (9) May cause a relapse of malaria. (10) May cause severe hypertension and stroke with ergot alkaloids. (11) May cause dysrhythmias with digitalis. (12) May cause hypotension and bradycardia with hydantoins (e.g., phenytoin [Dilantin]). (13) Discontinue slowly; rebound effect may occur if stopped abruptly.

Contraindications: Do not use with cyclopropane or halothane anesthesia.

Incompatible with: Amphotericin B (Fungizone), ampicillin, cephalothin (Keflin), dexamethasone (Decadron), erythromycin (Erythrocin), heparin, hydrocortisone phosphate, hydrocortisone sodium succinate (Solu-

Cortef), invert sugar, lactated Ringer's injection, levarterenol (Levophed), methicillin (Staphcillin), methylprednisolone (Solu-Medrol), oxacillin (Prostaphlin), oxytetracycline (Terramycin), penicillin G potassium or sodium, pentobarbital (Nembutal), phenytoin (Dilantin), prednisolone (Hydeltrasol), Ringer's injection, sodium bicarbonate, sodium lactate injection, thiopental (Pentothal), warfarin (Coumadin), whole blood.

Side effects: May occur with average doses; cardiac arrest, cardiac dysrhythmias, dizziness, headache, hypertension, nervousness, tachycardia.

Antidote: Notify the physician of any side effects. Most will be treated symptomatically or dosage of metaraminol will be decreased. Should a sudden or uncontrolled hypertensive state occur, discontinue metaraminol, notify the physician, and treat with antihypertensive agents such as nitroprusside (Nipride) or phentolamine (Regitine). Resuscitate as necessary. To prevent sloughing and necrosis in areas where extravasation has occurred, with a fine hypodermic needle inject 5 to 10 mg of phentolamine diluted in 10 to 15 ml of normal saline liberally throughout the tissue in the extravasated area.

METHICILLIN SODIUM pH 6.0 to 8.5

(Staphcillin)

Usual dose: 4 to 12 Gm/24 hr in equally divided doses every 4 to 6 hours. If creatinine clearance is less than 10 ml/min, do not exceed 2 Gm/12 hr.

Pediatric dose: 100 to 300 mg/kg of body weight/24 hr in equally divided doses every 4 to 6 hours.

Neonatal dose: *Under 2,000 Gm; age up to 7 days:* 50 mg/kg of body weight/24 hr in equally divided doses every 12 hours (meningitis, 100 mg/kg/24 hr). *Over 7 days of age:* 75 mg/kg/24 hr in equally divided doses every 8 hours (meningitis, 150 mg/kg/24 hr).

Over 2,000 Gm; age up to 7 days: 75 mg/kg/24 hr in equally divided doses every 8 hours (meningitis, 150 mg/kg/24 hr). *Over 7 days:* 100 mg/kg/24 hr in equally divided doses every 6 hours (meningitis, 150 to 200 mg/kg/24 hr).

Dilution: Each 1 Gm vial is diluted with 1.8 ml of sterile water for injection (4 Gm vial with 5.7 ml, 6 Gm vial with 8.6 ml). Each 1 ml equals 500 mg. Further dilute each 500 mg (1 ml) with a minimum of 25 ml of sodium chloride for injection. May be administered directly IV, through an additive infusion set, or added to specific IV solutions such as isotonic sodium chloride, 5% dextrose in water or normal saline, lactated Ringer's injection, and others (see literature) and given as an infusion over not more than 8 hours. Diluted concentrations of 2 mg/ml are stable for 4 hours, 10 to 30 mg/ml for 8 hours.

Rate of administration: Each 10 ml properly diluted medication or fraction thereof over 1 minute or longer to avoid vein irritation. Infusion rate of a single dose can be from 30 minutes to 8 hours.

Actions: A semisynthetic penicillin used for its bactericidal action against gram-positive organisms, primarily penicillinase-producing staphylococci. Appears in all body fluids. Absorption into spinal fluid is minimal unless inflammation is present. Crosses the placental barrier. Excreted in the urine. Secreted in breast milk.

Indications and uses: Severe infections caused by penicillinase-producing staphylococci.

Precautions: (1) Sensitivity studies necessary to determine susceptibility of the causative organism to methicillin sodium. Sometimes difficult to determine accurately. (2) Watch for early symptoms of allergic reaction. Individuals with a history of allergic problems are more susceptible to untoward reactions. (3) Avoid prolonged use of this drug; superinfection caused by overgrowth of nonsusceptible organisms may result. (4) Initial solution stable for 24 hours; stable for 4 days if refrigerated. (5) Renal, hepatic, and hematopoietic function should be checked during long-term therapy. (6) Use caution for infants. Abnormal blood levels may appear because of undeveloped renal function. (7) Inhibited by chloramphenicol, erythromycin, and tetracyclines. Bactericidal action actually negated by these drugs. (8) Potentiated by aminohippuric acid and probenecid (Benemid). Toxicity may result. (9) May cause thrombophlebitis, especially with too-rapid injection. (10) Inactivates aminoglycosides (e.g., gentamicin). Do not mix in same IV container. (11) Concomitant use with β-adrenergic blockers (e.g., propranolol [Inderal]) may increase risk of anaphylaxis and inhibit treatment. (12) Risk of bleeding with anticoagulants (e.g., heparin) is increased. (13) Neuromuscular excitability or convulsions may be caused by higher than normal doses. (14) Inhibits effectiveness of oral contraceptives. Breakthrough bleeding or pregnancy could result.

Contraindications: Known hypersensitivity to any penicillin or cephalothin, pregnancy.

Incompatible with: Manufacturer recommends: do not use as an additive with any other drug. Do not mix in any solutions other than those specifically recommended. Do not administer into IV tubing if solution is not recommended. Incompatible with aminophylline, ascorbic acid, cephalothin (Keflin), chloramphenicol, chlorpromazine (Thorazine), codeine, hydrocortisone sodium succinate (Solu-Cortef), levorphanol (Levo-Dromoran), lincomycin (Lincocin), metaraminol (Aramine), methadone, methohexital (Brevital), morphine, promethazine (Phenergan), sodium bicarbonate, tetracycline (Achromycin), vancomycin, vitamin B complex.

Side effects: Primarily hypersensitivity reactions such as anaphylaxis, serum sickness, skin rashes, urticaria. Anemia, eosinophilia, fever, glossitis, candidiasis (oral and rectal), neutropenia, nephrotoxicity (interstitial nephritis), and stomatitis have been reported.

Antidote: Notify the physician immediately of any adverse symptoms. For severe symptoms, discontinue the drug, treat allergic reaction (antihistamines, epinephrine, corticosteroids), and resuscitate as necessary. Hemodialysis or peritoneal dialysis is effective in overdose.

METHOCARBAMOL **pH 4.0 to 5.0**

(Robaxin)

Usual dose: 1 Gm (10 ml) every 8 hours for no more than 3 days. Not recommended for children under 12 years of age except in tetanus. In tetanus treatment, dosage may be as high as 3 Gm every 6 hours. Initiate with 1 to 2 Gm direct IV. Give balance of dose by infusion.

Pediatric dose: *In tetanus:* 15 mg/kg of body weight initially. Repeat every 6 hours as indicated.

Dilution: May be given undiluted, or a single dose may be given as an IV infusion diluted in no more than 250 ml of isotonic sodium chloride or 5% dextrose solution.

Rate of administration: 300 mg (3 ml) or fraction thereof over 1 minute or longer. Adjust infusion rate for patient comfort.

Actions: A skeletal muscle depressant that acts as an interneuronal blocking agent. Diminishes skeletal muscle hyperactivity without altering normal muscle tone. Well absorbed and distributed throughout the body. Concentration of the drug is higher in the brain than in plasma. Metabolized in the liver and excreted in the urine.

Indications and uses: (1) Acute neuromusculoskeletal injury; (2) acute exacerbation of chronic musculoskeletal disorders; (3) acute exacerbation of chronic neurological disorders; (4) orthopedic, gynecological, and dental surgery; (5) convulsive states caused by strychnine poisoning, tetanus, black widow spider bite, lead poisoning, opiate withdrawal, acute alcoholism, and phenothiazine reactions.

Precautions: (1) Observe site of injection continuously. A hypertonic solution; extravasation may cause thrombophlebitis or sloughing. (2) Blood aspirated into syringe will not mix with medication; an expected phenomenon. (3) Keep patient in recumbent position for at least 15 minutes to avoid postural hypotension. (4) Do not refrigerate after dilution. (5) Use caution in known or suspected epileptic patients. (6) Maintenance doses should be oral even if the pills are crushed and given through a nasogastric tube. (7) Potentiated by alcohol, CNS depressants, MAO inhibitors (e.g., paragyline [Eutonyl]), and phenothiazines (e.g., chlorpromazine [Thorazine]). (8) May interfere with some laboratory tests (5-HIAA, VMA). (9) Use caution in pregnancy and lactation. Safety for use not established. (10) Urine may discolor to very dark green.

Contraindications: Hypersensitivity to methocarbamol, known or suspected renal pathology. Do not use in conjunction with propoxyphene (Darvon).

Incompatible with: Physically compatible with many drugs. Sufficient information not available. Note Precautions and Contraindications.

Side effects: Infrequent but more often associated with too-rapid injection or an acute alcoholic state.

Minor: Blurred vision, conjunctivitis, diplopia, dizziness, drowsiness, fainting, fever, flushing, headache, hypotension, GI upset, lightheadedness, metallic taste, muscular incoordination, nystagmus, pruritus, rash, urticaria, vertigo.

Major: Anaphylactic reaction, bradycardia, convulsions, pain at injection site, sloughing at injection site, syncope, thrombophlebitis.

Antidote: Notify the physician of minor side effects. If these side effects progress or major side effects occur, discontinue the drug, notify the physician, and treat symptomatically. Epinephrine, steroids, and antihistamines should be readily available. Resuscitate as necessary.

METHOTREXATE SODIUM pH 8.5

(Abitrexate, Folex, Folex PFS, Methotrexate LPF, MTX)

Usual dose: Many dose limitations based on patient condition, renal and hepatic function, and concomitant drugs, see Precautions. 15 to 30 mg/24 hr for 5 days. Repeat course of therapy 3 to 5 times with rest periods of 7 to 12 days unless toxicity contraindicates it. Usually given orally.

Leukemia: 3.3 mg/M^2 with prednisone 60 mg/M^2. Give daily if tolerated, and continue for up to 8 weeks or until satisfactory response (usually 4 to 6 weeks). Maintenance dose individualized; 2.5 mg/kg every 14 days has been used IV or orally.

Psoriasis: 10 to 25 mg once a week. Do not exceed 50 mg. Use smallest effective dose. Usually given orally.

Mycosis fungoides: 2.5 to 10 mg daily. Weeks to months may be required to produce clinical remission. Usually given orally.

Osteosarcoma: One regimen recommends 12 Gm/M^2 as a single dose. Begin the 4th week after surgery and repeat weekly at weeks 5, 6, 7, 11, 12, 15, 16, 29, 30, 44, and 45. A peak serum concentration of 1,000 micromolars/L at the end of the infusion is desired. Dose may be increased to 15 Gm/M^2 if required. Must be accompanied by leucovorin rescue; begin 24 hours after start of methotrexate infusion and give 15 mg every 6 hours times 10 doses. Usually given orally. Osteosarcoma also requires combination chemotherapy. Protocols vary but may include doxorubicin, cisplatin, bleomycin, cyclophosphamide, and dactinomycin. These massive doses are highly individualized, require exacting calculations, and constant patient monitoring (see Precautions).

Dilution: *Specific techniques required, see Precautions.* 25 mg/ml is the maximum concentration that can be given IV. Reconstitution of each 5 mg with 2 ml of preservative-free 5% dextrose in water or 0.9% sodium chloride is preferred. Each milliliter equals 2.5 mg of methotrexate. Available in preservative-free solutions. Do not use formulations or diluents with preservatives (e.g., bacteriostatic) for experimental high-dose therapy or intrathecal injection. Not usually added to IV solutions when given in standard doses. May be given through Y-tube or three-way stopcock of a free-flowing IV. A single dose may be further diluted with 5% dextrose solution or normal saline immediately before use as an infusion with high methotrexate doses.

Rate of administration: *Direct IV:* Each 10 mg or fraction thereof over 1 minute.

Infusion: A single dose equally distributed over 4 hours.

Actions: An antimetabolite and folic acid antagonist. Cell cycle specific for the S phase, it interrupts the mitotic process during nucleic acid synthesis. Rapidly proliferating malignant cells are inhibited by a cytostatic effect. Readily absorbed and widely distributed, average doses of methotrexate are excreted unchanged in the urine within 24 hours. Clearance rates decrease with higher doses. Does not cross blood-brain barrier. Secreted in breast milk.

Indications and uses: (1) To suppress or retard neoplastic growth in uterine choriocarcinoma, acute lymphocytic leukemia, lymphosarcoma, mycosis fungoides, osteogenic sarcoma, and malignancies of the breast, testis, head, neck, and lung; (2) severe disabling psoriasis unresponsive to other treatment; (3) given orally for other diagnoses and intrathecally for meningeal leukemia.

Unlabeled use: High-dose regimen for treatment of osteosarcoma.

Precautions: (1) Follow guidelines for handling cytotoxic agents recommended. See Appendix, p. 677. (2) Administered by or under the direction of the physician specialist. Close patient observation is mandatory. Course of therapy is not repeated until all signs of toxicity from the previous course subside. (3) Complete blood cell counts, bone marrow biopsies, chest x-ray, and renal and liver function tests before, during, and after therapy are essential to comprehensive treatment. Liver biopsy and bone marrow studies are indicated in high-dose or long-term therapy. (4) Monitor renal function closely; verify by creatinine clearance levels. Maintain adequate hydration and urine alkalinization.

Monitor serum methotrexate levels. (5) Evacuate excess fluid from ascites and pleural effusions before treatment. (6) Use with extreme caution in patients with infection, impaired renal or liver function, peptic ulcer, or ulcerative colitis; in debilitated patients; and in the very young or very elderly. (7) The following drugs may be toxic when administered concomitantly with methotrexate: alcohol, antibacterials (e.g., tetracycline, chloramphenicol), nonsteroidal antiinflammatory drugs (NSAIDS) (e.g., indomethacin, ketoprofen, naproxen), probenecid, salicylates, barbiturates, any hepatotoxic drug, sulfonamides, tranquilizers, para-aminobenzoic acid (PABA), phenylbutazone, phenytoin (Dilantin), and pyrimethamine. (8) Vitamins with folic acid may alter response to methothrexate. (9) Methotrexate interacts with many drugs such as antidiabetics, barbiturates, charcoal, corticosteroids, etretinate (Tegison), other antineoplastics, (e.g., procarbazine), thiopurines (e.g., azathioprine [Imuran]), and others to produce potentially serious reactions. (10) Often used with other antineoplastic drugs in reduced doses to achieve tumor remission. (11) Do not administer any live vaccine to patients receiving antineoplastic drugs. (12) Use prophylactic antiemetics to reduce nausea and vomiting and increase patient comfort. (13) Has caused fetal death and congenital anomalies. Discontinue breast feeding. (14) Administration of high-dose methotrexate requires a white blood cell count above 1,500/mm^3; neutrophil count above 200/mm^3; platelet count above 75,000/mm^3; serum bilirubin less than 1.2 mg/dl; alanine aminotransferase (ALT) level less than 450 units; any mucositis must be healing; ascites or pleural effusion must be drained dry; serum creatinine must be normal ($>$ 60 ml/min); 1 L/M^2 of IV fluid over 6 hours before dosing and 3 L/M^2 on day of infusion and for 2 days after; alkalinization of urine with sodium bicarbonate; and repeat serum methotrexate and serum creatinine levels at least daily until methotrexate level is below 0.05 micromolar. Reduce dose by 25% if bilirubin is between 4 and 5 or alanine aminotransferase (ALT) above 180; if bilirubin above 5, omit dose. (15) Discard solution if a precipitate forms. (16)

Stable at room temperature for up to 2 weeks. (17) Safety for use in children is limited to chemotherapy.

Contraindications: Hypersensitivity to methotrexate, nursing mothers. Not absolute, but methotrexate is not recommended during pregnancy or with hepatic, renal, or bone marrow damage.

Incompatible with: Limited information available. Note Precautions and Contraindications. Bleomycin (Blenoxane), fluorouracil, metoclopramide (Reglan), prednisolone (Hydeltrasol).

Side effects: Toxicity usually dose related. Death can occur from average doses, high doses, drug interactions (NSAIDS), bone marrow toxicity, and GI toxicity. Acne, alopecia (occasional), chills, cystitis, dehydration, depigmentation, diabetes, diarrhea, edema, enteritis, fever, GI ulceration, gingivitis, hematological depression, hemorrhage from any site, hepatotoxicity, leukoencephalopathy, menstrual dysfunction, nausea, oral ulceration, pharyngitis, pruritus, pulmonary disease (dry nonproductive cough), rash, septicemia, stomatitis, urticaria, vomiting.

Antidote: Citovorum factor, folinic acid (leucovorin), may be given orally, IM, or IV promptly to counteract inadvertent overdose (IV route is not FDA approved but in common use). Citrovorum factor is also indicated as a planned rescue mechanism for large doses of methotrexate required to treat some malignancies. Doses equal to dose of methotrexate are frequently required. Should be given within 1 hour. Repeat every 4 to 6 hours for up to 72 hours. Doses up to 100 to 150 mg/M^2 every 3 hours may be required if serum creatinine is 50% or greater than before methotrexate administration. Serum methotrexate must come down to below 0.05 micromolar. Hydration and urinary alkalinization are mandatory to prevent precipitation in renal tubules. Discontinue methotrexate and notify the physician of any side effects. Death may occur from the progression of most of these side effects. Symptomatic and supportive therapy is indicated.

METHOXAMINE HYDROCHLORIDE

pH 3.0 to 5.0

(Vasoxyl)

Usual dose: 3 to 5 mg initially. May repeat after at least 15 minutes. Follow with continuous or intermittent IV drip or administer IM. One dose of 10 mg is indicated in paroxysmal supraventricular tachycardia.

Dilution: May be given undiluted or may be given as IV infusion by diluting 40 mg of methoxamine in 250 ml of 5% dextrose in water.

Rate of administration: Each 5 mg or fraction thereof over 1 minute. Begin with 5 ml of infusion/min (approximately 1 mg of methoxamine/6 ml). Use the slowest possible flow rate to correct hypotension gradually and maintain adequate or preset blood pressure. Use of a microdrip (60 gtt/ml) or an infusion pump will aid correct evaluation of dosage.

Actions: A potent vasopressor because of peripheral vasoconstriction. Unique in that it does not produce undesired cardiac or CNS stimulation. Cardiac output is slightly reduced because of reflex bradycardia, but central venous pressure and both systolic and diastolic blood pressure are elevated. Renal vessels will be constricted. Onset of action of a single dose is instantaneous and lasts about 1 hour. Widely distributed in body fluids, excreted in the urine.

Indications and uses: (1) Prevention and treatment of hypotension during anesthesia. May be used during most anesthesia including inhalant anesthesia (e.g., cyclopropane) and spinal anesthesia. (2) Shock caused by traumatic, surgical, or medical conditions including myocardial infarction, and drug reactions when cardiac stimulus is contraindicated. (3) Prompt termination of episodes of paroxysmal supraventricular tachycardia.

Precautions: (1) IM injection preferred. IV administration is for emergencies only and indicated only if systolic blood pressure is 60 mm Hg or less. (2) Discontinue IV administration if vein infiltrates or is thrombosed; can result in tissue necrosis and sloughing. (3) Keep in refrigerator. (4) Check blood pressure every 2 minutes until stabilized at the desired level. Check every 5 minutes thereafter during therapy. Avoid hypertension. (5) Replace blood, plasma, fluids, and electrolytes as necessary in hypovolemic shock. Use Y-tube or three-way stopcock with blood. (6) May cause severe hypertension after administration of ergot alkaloids. (7) Use care in hyperthyroidism, with known hypertensive patients, and during halothane anesthesia. (8) Potentiated by MAO inhibitors (e.g., isocarboxazid [Marplan]), thyroid preparations, and tricyclic antidepressants (e.g., amitriptyline [Elavil]). (9) Capable of many interactions with other drugs; however, these may be slightly less serious because of lack of myocardial stimulation.

Contraindications: Do not use in combination with local anesthetics for tissue infiltration to prolong action.

Incompatible with: Alkaline compounds. Limited information available. Note precautions and contraindications. Chemical composition similar to that of ephedrine, metaraminol (Aramine), and mephentermine (Wyamine).

Side effects: Rare unless very high dosage is used; bradycardia, headache, hypertension, projectile vomiting, urinary urgency.

Antidote: Atropine may be used to counteract the bradycardia. Notify the physician of any side effect. Should a sudden or uncontrolled hypertensive state occur, discontinue methoxamine, notify the physician, and treat with antihypertensive agents such as nitroprusside (Nipride) or phentolamine (Regitine). Resuscitate as necessary. To prevent sloughing and necrosis in areas where extravasation has occurred, with a fine hypodermic needle inject 5 to 10 mg of phentolamine diluted in 10 to 15 ml of normal saline liberally throughout the tissue in the extravasated area.

METHYLDOPATE HYDROCHLORIDE pH 3.0 to 4.2

(Aldomet)

Usual dose: 250 to 500 mg every 6 hours. Up to 1 Gm every 6 hours is acceptable. Maintain with oral medication in same dosage as soon as practical.

Pediatric dose: 20 to 40 mg/kg of body weight/24 hr in divided doses every 6 hours. Maximum dose is 65 mg/kg or 3 Gm, whichever is less.

Dilution: Single dose is diluted in 100 to 200 ml of 5% dextrose in water and given as an infusion.

Rate of administration: Each dose as an infusion is given over 30 to 60 minutes.

Actions: A moderate antihypertensive drug, it lowers the blood pressure by replacing norepinephrine in the body with methylnorepinephrine, thus producing decreased sympathetic activity. Lowers peripheral and renal vascular resistance. Readily permeates brain tissue but does not affect cardiac output. Maximum action does not occur for 2 to 3 hours but lasts 10 hours. Some excretion through the urine. Crosses placental barrier and is secreted in breast milk.

Indications and uses: Hypertensive crises, especially for patients with renal or coronary insufficiency.

Precautions: (1) Check blood pressure every 30 minutes until stabilized at desired level. Slow response lessens usefulness. (2) More effective combined with diuretics. (3) Liver function tests and complete blood cell count indicated. (4) Causes false elevated urinary catecholamine response. (5) Observe for adequate urine output. Use caution in impaired liver and renal function, pregnancy, and lactation. (6) Potentiated by MAO inhibitors (e.g., isocarboxazid [Marplan]), CNS depressants (e.g., alcohol, anesthesia, narcotics), and verapamil. Combination may cause death. (7) Inhibited by tricyclic antidepressants (e.g., amitriptyline [Elavil]), amphetamines, and others. (8) Potentiates oral anticoagulants, oral antidiabetics, levodopa, levarterenol (Levophed), and all antihypertensive drugs (e.g., hydralazine [Apresoline]). May produce adverse mental symptoms with haloperidol. (9) Capable of paradoxical reactions with adrenergics, amphetamines, antidepressants, and sympathomimetics. Severe hypertension can occur.

Contraindications: Hypersensitivity to any component, liver disease.

Incompatible with: Amphotericin B (Fungizone), methohexital (Brevital), tetracycline (Achromycin). Physically compatible with many drugs. Consider specific use and precautions above.

Side effects: Anaphylaxis, apprehension, depression, dizziness, dry mouth, edema, elevated alkaline phosphatase, elevated SGOT, fever, hemolytic anemia, nasal congestion, nightmares, paradoxical hypertension, positive Coombs' test, postural hypotension (mild), sedation.

Antidote: Notify the physican of all side effects. Most can be decreased in severity by reducing dosage. Drug may be discontinued. Dopamine (Intropin) or levarterenol (Levophed) should reverse hypotension of overdose. Hemodialysis may be used in acute overdose.

METHYLERGONOVINE MALEATE pH 2.7 to 3.5

(Methergine)

Usual dose: 1 ml (0.2 mg or gr 1/320); may be repeated in 2 to 4 hours as necessary.

Dilution: May be given undiluted. Do not add to IV solutions. May be given through Y-tube or three-way stopcock of infusion set.

Rate of administration: 0.2 mg or fraction thereof over 1 minute.

Actions: A synthetic oxytocic, more potent and with a more prolonged action than ergonovine. It exerts a direct stimulation on the smooth muscle of the uterus, causing contraction of the uterus itself and vasoconstriction of uterine vessels, which reduces blood loss. In therapeutic doses the prolonged initial contraction is followed by periods of relaxation and contraction. Preferred because it is less likely to cause hypertension. Effective within 1 minute for up to 3 hours. It is probably detoxified in the liver and excreted in bile and urine.

Indications and uses: (1) Routine management after delivery of the placenta; (2) postpartum atony; (3) hemorrhage; (4) subinvolution.

Precautions: (1) Occasionally given after the anterior shoulder is delivered if the obstetrician directs and is present. (2) IV administration is for emergency use only. IM or oral routes are preferred and should be used after the initial IV dose. Monitor the blood pressure. (3) Should be refrigerated; may not be stored at room temperature more than 60 days. (4) Check expiration date on vial; methylergonovine deteriorates with age. (5) Uterine response may be poor in calcium-deficient patients; calcium replacement may be required for effective response. (6) Use caution in presence of sepsis, obliterative vascular disease, and cardiac, hepatic, or renal involvement. (7) Severe hypertension and cerebrovascular accidents can result in the presence of regional anesthesia (caudal or spinal) and with ephedrine, methoxamine (Vasoxyl), and other vasopressors. Chlorpromazine (Thorazine) IV will reduce this hypertension.

Contraindications: Hypersensitivity, hypertension, pregnancy before third stage of labor, toxemia.

Incompatible with: Specific information not available. Do not mix in a syringe with any other drug.

Side effects: Rare in therapeutic doses but may include:

Average dose: Allergic phenomena, chest pain (temporary), diaphoresis, dilated pupils, dizziness, dyspnea, headache, hypertension (transient), hypotension, nausea, tinnitus, vomiting, weakness.

Overdose: Abortion, blindness, cerebrovascular accident, convulsions, excitement, gangrene, hypercoagulability, palpitations, shock, tachycardia, thirst, tremor, uterine bleeding.

Antidote: Discontinue the drug immediately at the onset of any side effect and notify the physician. Most side effects are transient unless there is severe toxicity and will be treated symptomatically. Severe poisoning is treated with vasodilator drugs, sedatives, calcium gluconate to relieve muscular pain, and other supportive treatment. Heparin is used to control hypercoagulability.

METHYLPREDNISOLONE SODIUM SUCCINATE pH 7.0 to 8.0

(A-MethaPred, Solu-Medrol)

Usual dose: 10 to 250 mg initially. May be repeated every 2 to 6 hours as necessary. 30 mg/kg of body weight in high-dose therapy. In acute conditions such as severe shock, doses up to 1,000 mg or more every 4 hours have been given. These massive doses should not be used longer than 48 to 72 hours. Dosage is individualized according to the severity of the disease and the response of the patient and is not necessarily reduced for children. Available in vials containing 40 mg, 125 mg, 500 mg, 1,000 mg, and 2,000 mg. Each vial has an appropriate amount of diluent.

Pediatric dose: See adult dose. Do not give less than 0.5 mg/kg of body weight every 24 hours.

Dilution: Available in a Mix-O-Vial, which is reconstituted by removing the protective cap, turning the rubber stopper a quarter turn, and pressing down, allowing the diluent into the lower chamber. Agitate gently. Using sterile technique, insert a needle through the center of the rubber stopper to withdraw diluted solution. To be diluted only with diluent supplied in Mix-O-Vial. May be given direct IV, as an infusion, or further diluted in desired amounts of 5% dextrose in water or normal saline and isotonic saline solution (see incompatibilities).

Rate of administration: Direct IV administration, each 500 mg or fraction thereof over 1 minute or longer. Direct IV administration is usually route of choice and eliminates possibility of overloading the patient with IV fluids. May be given as an infusion in its own diluent over 10 to 20 minutes. At the discretion of the physician, a continuous infusion may be given, properly diluted, over a specified time.

Actions: An adrenocortical steroid with potent metabolic, antiinflammatory actions and innumerable other effects. Has a greater antiinflammatory potency than prednisolone and less tendency to cause excessive potassium and calcium excretion and sodium and water retention. Has four times the potency of hydrocortisone sodium succinate. May be used in conjunction with other forms of therapy, such as epinephrine, for acute allergic reactions or antibiotics in acute infections. Primarily excreted in the urine and feces. 75% excretion occurs within 24 hours, allowing use of very large doses with reasonable safety. Crosses the placental barrier. Will appear in breast milk.

Indications and uses: (1) Hypersensitivity and dermatological conditions; (2) supplementary therapy for severe allergic reaction (use epinephrine first); (3) to initiate therapy in acute gout, acute systemic lupus erythematosus, and acute rheumatic fever; (4) severe shock, whether hemorrhagic, traumatic, or surgical; (5) overwhelming infections with severe toxicity; (6) ulcerative colitis; (7) esophageal burns; (8) adjunctive therapy in croup and other respiratory problems; (9) chemotherapy; (10) antiemetic; (11) spinal cord injury.

Precautions: (1) Discard unused solutions after 48 hours. (2) May cause elevated blood pressure and salt and water retention. (3) Salt restriction and potassium and calcium replacement may be necessary. (4) May mask signs of infection. (5) To avoid relative adrenocortical insufficiency, do not stop therapy abruptly, taper off. Patient is observed carefully, especially under stress, for up to 2 years; exception is very short-term therapy. (6) Maintain on ulcer regimen and antacid prophylactically. (7) May increase insulin needs in diabetics. (8) Inhibited by anticonvulsants, some antihistamines, barbiturates, ephedrine, oral contraceptives, propranolol (Inderal), phenylbutazone (Butazolidin), rifampin, and troleandomycin. (9) Not the drug of choice to treat acute adrenocortical insufficiency. (10) Use caution in patients with renal transplants; large doses may cause circulatory collapse. (11) Inhibits anticoagulants, isoniazid, and salicylates. (12) Potentiates theophyllines and cyclosporine. (13) May cause hypokalemia with digitalis products, amphotericin B, or potassium-depleting diuretics. (14) Dose adjustment may be required with cyclophosphamide. (15) Do not vaccinate with attenuated-virus vaccines (e.g., smallpox) during therapy. (16) Altered protein-binding capacity will impact effectiveness of this drug.

Contraindications: *Absolute contraindications in long-term therapy, except in life-threatening situations:* Hypersensitivity to any product component, including sulfites; newborns; systemic fungal infections.

Relative contraindications: Active or latent peptic ulcer, active or healed tuberculosis, acute psychoses, chickenpox, congestive heart failure, diabetes mellitus, diverticulitis, fresh intestinal anastomoses, hypertension, myasthenia gravis, ocular herpes simplex, osteoporosis, pregnancy, psychotic tendencies, renal insufficiency, septic shock, thromboembolic tendencies, vaccinia.

Incompatible with: Aminophylline, calcium gluconate, cephalothin (Keflin), chlorpromazine (Thorazine), cytarabine (ARA-C), dextrose 5% in 0.45% normal saline, digitoxin (Crystodigin), diphenhydramine (Benadryl), glycopyrrolate (Robinul), insulin, meperidine (Demerol), metaraminol (Aramine), nafcillin (Unipen), penicillin G sodium and potassium, promethazine (Phenergan), tetracycline (Achromycin), thiamylal (Surital), thiopental (Pentothal), tolazoline (Priscoline), vitamin B complex and vitamin B complex with C. Doses above 80 mg have compatibility problems with most infusion solutions. Consult pharmacist.

Side effects: Do occur but are usually reversible: Cushing's syndrome; electrolyte and calcium imbalance; euphoria; glycosuria; hyperglycemia; hypersensitivity reactions, including anaphylaxis; hypertension; increased intracranial pressure; menstrual irregularities; peptic ulcer perforation and hemorrhage; protein catabolism; spontaneous fractures; transitory burning or tingling; sweating, headache, or weakness; thromboembolism; and many others.

Antidote: Notify the physician of any side effect. Will probably treat the side effect if necessary. Resuscitate as necessary for anaphylaxis and notify physician. Keep epinephrine immediately available.

METHYLTHIONINE CHLORIDE pH 3.0 to 4.5
(Methylene Blue)

Usual dose: 1% methylene blue, 1 ml equals 10 mg. 0.1 to 0.2 ml/kg of body weight is recommended dose.

Dilution: Usually given undiluted.

Rate of administration: 1 ml (10 mg) or fraction thereof over 5 minutes.

Actions: Low concentrations will convert methemoglobin to hemoglobin (methemoglobin is toxic and gives the blood a chocolate-brown color; it does not carry oxygen). High concentrations convert ferrous iron of hemoglobin to ferric iron and forms methemoglobin. Will stain tissue and turn urine or feces blue-green. Excreted in urine and bile.

Indications and uses: (1) Drug-induced methemoglobinemia; (2) antidote for cyanide poisoning; (3) diagnostic dye; (4) to identify body structures and fistulas.

Precautions: (1) Inject very slowly over several minutes to prevent toxic effects of local high concentration of the compound. (2) Do not exceed recommended dosage. (3) May cause cyanosis or cardiac irregularities. (4) May induce hemolysis in patients deficient in glucose 6-phosphate dehydrogenase. (5) Check hemoglobin; may cause a marked anemia resulting from accelerated destruction of erythrocytes. (6) May discolor urine and stool blue-green.

Contraindications: Hypersensitivity to methylene blue, intraspinal injection, renal insufficiency.

Incompatible with: Do not mix with any other drug.

Side effects: *Minor:* Nausea, vomiting, bladder irritation, diarrhea, headache.

Major: Abdominal pain, anemia, dizziness, fever, precordial pain, profuse diaphoresis, mental confusion, methemoglobin.

Antidote: Discontinue the drug upon appearance of any side effect. Remove skin stains with hypochlorite solution.

METOCLOPRAMIDE HYDROCHLORIDE

pH 3.0 to 6.5

(✤ Maxeran, Octamide PFS, Reglan)

Usual dose: *Radiologic examination of the small bowel:* 10 mg (2 ml) as a single dose.

Antiemetic: 2 mg/kg of body weight 30 minutes before giving emetogenic cancer chemotherapy (e.g., cisplatin, dacarbazine). Repeat every 2 hours for 2 doses, then every 3 hours for 3 doses. Dose may be reduced to 1 mg/kg if initial doses suppress vomiting. Initial doses may be reduced to 1 mg/kg for less emetogenic regimens. Another regimen calls for 3mg/kg 30 minutes before and 90 minutes after emetogenic chemotherapy. Given in combination with dexamethasone and lorazepam or diphenhydramine.

Pediatric dose: *Radiologic examination of the small bowel: 6 to 14 years:* 2.5 to 5 mg.

Under 6 years: 0.1 mg/kg of body weight.

Dilution: May be given undiluted if dose does not exceed 10 mg. For doses exceeding 10 mg dilute in at least 50 ml of 5% dextrose in water, sodium chloride, Ringer's injection, or lactated Ringer's injection, and give as an infusion.

Rate of administration: 10 mg or fraction thereof over 2 minutes.

Infusion: Administer over a minimum of 15 minutes.

Actions: A dopamine antagonist that stimulates tone and amplitude of gastric contractions and increases peristalsis of the duodenum and jejunum. It relaxes the lower esophageal sphincter, pyloric sphincter, and duodenal bulb. Does not stimulate gastric, biliary, or pancreatic secretions. Acts even if vagal innervation not present. Action negated by anticholinergic drugs. Onset of action occurs in 1 to 3 minutes and lasts 1 to 2 hours.

Indications and uses: (1) Facilitate small bowel intubation; (2) stimulate gastric and intestinal emptying of barium to permit radiological examination of the stomach and small intestine; (3) prevention of nausea and vomiting associated with emetogenic cancer chemotherapy.

Precautions: (1) A phenothiazine-related drug, may produce sedation and extrapyramidal symptoms. (2) Use caution in pregnancy and lactation. May increase milk production during lactation. (3) Antagonized by anticholinergic drugs (atropine) and narcotic analgesics (morphine). (4) Potentiated by alcohol, sedatives, hypnotics, narcotics, and tranquilizers. (5) Drugs ingested orally may be absorbed more slowly or more rapidly depending on the absorption site. (6) A prolactin-elevating compound, may be carcinogenic. Risk with a single dose almost nonexistent. (7) May cause methemoglobinemia in premature and full-term neonates at doses exceeding 0.5 mg/kg/24 hr. (8) Insulin reactions may result from gastric stasis, making diabetic control difficult. Dosage or timing of insulin may need adjustment. (9) Extrapyramidal effects may be potentiated with concomitant use of phenothiazines, butyrophenones, and thioxanthines (antipsychotic drugs). (10) Too rapid IV injection will cause intense anxiety, restlessness, and then drowsiness.

Contraindications: Situations in which gastric motility is contraindicated, i.e., gastric hemorrhage, obstruction, or perforation; known hypersensitivity to metoclopramide; patients with epilepsy or patients taking drugs that may also cause extrapyramidal reactions; pheochromocytoma.

Incompatible with: Ampicillin, calcium gluconate, cephalothin (Keflin), chloramphenicol (Chloromycetin), cisplatin (Platinol), erythromycin (Erythrocin), methotrexate (Folex), penicillin G potassium, sodium bicarbonate, tetracycline (Achromycin).

Side effects: *Average dose:* Bowel disturbances, dizziness, drowsiness, fatigue, headache, insomnia, methemoglobinemia in neonates, nausea, restlessness.

Overdose: Disorientation, drowsiness, and extrapyramidal reactions.

Antidote: Notify physician of all side effects. Treat overdose or extrapyramidal reactions with diphenhydramine (Benadryl) or benzotropine (Cogentin). Symptoms should disappear within 24 hours. Treat methemoglobinemia with IV methylene blue. Resuscitate as necessary.

METOPROLOL TARTRATE

(Lopressor)

Usual dose: 5 mg as an IV bolus dose. Initiate as soon as the patient's hemodynamic condition has stabilized. Repeat at 2-minute intervals for 2 more doses (total of three 5 mg doses). If IV doses are well tolerated, give 50 mg orally every 6 hours for 48 hours beginning 15 minutes after the last bolus. Follow with an oral maintenance dose of 100 mg twice daily. In patients who do not tolerate the full IV dose start 25 to 50 mg orally within 15 minutes of the last IV dose. Dosage based on degree of intolerance. May have to discontinue metoprolol.

Dilution: May be given undiluted.

Rate of administration: A single dose over 1 minute. Monitor ECG, heart rate, and blood pressure and discontinue metoprolol if adverse symptoms occur (bradycardia less than 45 beats/min, heart block greater than first degree, systolic blood pressure less than 90 mm Hg, or moderate to severe cardiac failure).

Actions: Metoprolol is a cardioselective (β_1-) adrenergic blocking agent. Its mechanism of action in patients with suspected or definite myocardial infarction is not known. It reduces the incidence of recurrent myocardial infarctions and reduces the size of the infarct and the incidence of fatal dysrhythmias. Well distributed throughout the body, it acts within 1 to 2 minutes and lasts about 3 to 4 hours. Metabolized in the liver and throughout the body. Excreted as metabolites in the urine.

Indications and uses: (1) To reduce cardiac mortality in hemodynamically stable individuals with suspected or definite myocardial infarction; (2) antihypertensive in oral dosage form.

Investigational use: To suppress atrial ectopy in patients with chronic obstructive pulmonary disease.

Precautions: (1) Continuous ECG, heart rate, and blood pressure monitoring is mandatory during administration of IV metoprolol. (2) Use caution in the presence of heart failure controlled by digitalis. Both drugs slow atrioventricular conduction. (3) May mask tachycardia occurring with hypoglycemia in diabetes and tachycardia of hyperthyroidism. (4) β-Adrenergic blocking agents antagonize antihistamines, antiinflammatory agents, isoproterenol (Isuprel), ritodrine, and others. (5) Potentiated by general anesthetics, cimetidine (Tagamet), furosemide, phenothiazines (e.g., promethazine [Phenergan]), phenytoin (Dilantin), and urethane. Death can occur. (6) Potentiates antidiabetics, barbiturates, catecholamine-depleting drugs (e.g., reserpine), insulin, lidocaine, narcotics, muscle relaxants, theophyllines, and thyroid agents; dosage adjustment may be required. Increased CNS depression may cause death. (7) Used concurrently with digitalis or α-adrenergic blockers (e.g., phentolamine [Regitine]), as indicated. (8) Use with extreme caution in asthmatics. (9) Use with clonidine may precipitate acute hypertension. May aggravate rebound hypertension if clonidine stopped abruptly. (10) Use with verapamil may potentiate both drugs and result in severe depression of myocardium and AV conduction. (11) No adustment in dose is required in patients with impaired renal function. (12) Some authorities recommend that β-adrenergic blockers be discontinued 48 hours before major surgery (β-blockade interferes with cardiac response to reflex stimuli). (13) May cause severe bradycardia in patients with Wolff-Parkinson-White syndrome. (14) Reduce dose gradually to avoid rebound angina, myocardial infarction, or ventricular dysrhythmias. (15) Safety for use in pregnancy and lactation and in children not established.

Contraindications: Heart rate below 45 beats/min, second or third degree heart block, significant first degree heart block (PR interval greater than 0.24 second), systolic blood pressure below 100 mm Hg, moderate to severe cardiac failure.

Incompatible with: Any other drug in a syringe because of specific use.

Side effects: Bradycardia, bronchospasm, cardiac failure, confusion, dizziness, dyspnea, first degree heart block, headache, nightmares, hypotension, pruritus, rash, respiratory distress, second or third degree heart block, syncopal attacks, tiredness, visual disturbances, vertigo.

Antidote: For any side effect, discontinue the drug and notify the physician immediately. Patients with myocardial infarction may be more hemodynamically unstable; treat with caution. Use atropine for bradycardia; use isoproterenol with caution if atropine is not effective. Glucagon 5 to 10 mg IV may be effective if atropine and isoproterenol are not (investigational use). Transvenous cardiac pacing may be needed. Treat hypotension with IV fluids if indicated or vasopressors (dopamine [Intropin] or norepinephrine [Levarterenol]), treat cause of hypotension (e.g., bradycardia). Use all vasopressors with extreme caution, severe hypotension can result. Use digitalis and diuretics at first sign of cardiac failure; dobutamine, isoproterenol, or glucagon may be required. Use aminophylline or isoproterenol (with extreme care) for bronchospasm, glucagon for hypoglycemia. Treat other side effects symptomatically and resuscitate as necessary.

METRONIDAZOLE HYDROCHLORIDE

pH 5.0 to 7.0

(Flagyl IV, Flagyl IV RTU, Metro IV, Metronidazole Redi-infusion, Metryl IV)

Usual dose: Begin with an initial loading dose of 15 mg/kg of body weight. Follow with 7.5 mg/kg in 6 hours and every 6 hours thereafter for 7 to 10 days or longer if indicated. Do not exceed 4 Gm in 24 hours.

Pseudomembranous colitis: 1 to 2 Gm/day for 7 to 10 days.

Perioperative prophylaxis: 15 mg/kg infused over 30 to 60 minutes and completed 1 hour before surgery. Follow with 7.5 mg/kg in 6 hours and again in 12 hours.

Dilution: All solutions are prediluted and ready to use (5 mg/ml), except Flagyl IV. Do not use plastic containers in series connections. Risk of air embolism is present. Avoid all contact with aluminum in needles and syringes in all situations. Color change will occur. Flagyl IV requires a specific dilution process; initially add 4.4 ml sterile water or 0.9% sodium chloride for injection (100 mg/ml). Solution must be clear. Will be yellow to yellow-green in color with a pH of 0.5 to 2.0. Must be further diluted to at least 8 mg/ml with 0.9% sodium chloride, 5% dextrose in water, or lactated Ringer's for infusion. Must be neutralized before infusion with 5 mEq of sodium bicarbonate per 500 mg. CO_2 gas will be generated and may require venting.

Rate of administration: Must be given as a slow IV infusion, each single dose over 1 hour. Discontinue primary IV during administration. May be given as a continuous infusion. Rate should be ordered by physician.

Actions: A bactericidal agent with cytotoxic effects, active against specific anaerobic bacteria and protozoa. Widely distributed in therapeutic levels to all body fluids (including abscesses). Levels are directly proportional to dose given. Onset of action is prompt and lasts about 8 hours. Crosses placental and blood-brain barriers. Excreted in urine, some in feces. Secreted in breast milk.

Indications and uses: (1) Treatment of serious intraabdominal, skin and skin structure, gynecologic, bone and joint, CNS, and lower respiratory tract infections; bacterial septicemia; and endocarditis caused by susceptible anaerobic bacteria; (2) perioperative prophylaxis to reduce infection rates in gynecologic, abdominal, and colorectal surgery; (3) hepatic encephalopathy; (4) as a radiosensitizer to make resistant tumors more susceptible to radiation therapy; (5) Crohn's disease; (6) antibiotic-related pseudomembranous colitis.

Precautions: (1) A mixed (anaerobic/aerobic) infection will require use of additional appropriate antibiotics. (2) Sensitivity studies indicated to determine susceptibility of the causative organism to metronidazole. (3) Avoid prolonged use of the drug; superinfection caused by overgrowth of nonsusceptible organisms may result. (4) Rotate IV site frequently to avoid thrombophlebitis. Avoid extravasation. (5) Store at room temperature before and after dilution. Discard diluted and neutralized solutions in 24 hours. Do not refrigerate; a precipitate will result. Protect from light when storing. (6) Symptoms of candidiasis may be exacerbated and require treatment. (7) May cause decreased SGOT levels. (8) Use caution in patients predisposed to edema and/or taking corticosteroids, impaired cardiac function (contains 5 to 14 mEq/ml sodium), CNS disease, or a history of blood dyscrasias. (9) Avoid alcohol and disulfiram; toxic reactions will occur. (10) Inhibited by barbiturates (e.g., phenobarbital), cimetedine (Tagamet), and hydantoins (e.g., phenytoin [Dilantin]). (11) Carcinogenic in rodents; use only when necessary. (12) Potentiates oral anticoagulants (e.g., warfarin). (13) Safety for use in pregnancy and lactation, children, and neonates not established. Newborns are unable to eliminate metronidazole. (14) Reduce dose in patients with hepatic disease, monitor serum levels, and observe for toxicity.

Contraindications: Hypersensitivity to metronidazole or nitroimidazole derivatives, first trimester of pregnancy.

Incompatible with: Administer separately per manufacturer's recommendation. Discontinue primary infusion during administration.

Side effects: Abdominal discomfort, convulsions, diarrhea, dizziness, fever, headache, metallic taste (expected), nausea, neutropenia (reversible), peripheral neuropathy, pruritus, rash, syncope, thrombophlebitis, vomiting.

Antidote: Notify physician of all side effects. Treatment will be symptomatic and supportive. Benefit/risk of therapy must be reconsidered with onset of convulsions or peripheral neuropathy. Rapidly removed by hemodialysis or peritoneal dialysis. Treat anaphylaxis and resuscitate as necessary.

MEZLOCILLIN SODIUM pH 4.5 to 8.0

(Mezlin)

Usual dose: 200 to 300 mg/kg of body weight/24 hr equally divided in 4 to 6 doses. (3 Gm every 4 hours equals 18 Gm/24 hr). Do not exceed 24 Gm/24 hr.

Perioperative prophylaxis: Give a single dose specific for the adult, child, or neonate 30 to 90 minutes before incision.

Pediatric dose: *Infants 1 month to children 12 years:* 50 mg/kg of body weight every 4 hours (300 mg/kg/24 hr). Limited data available on use in children.

Neonatal dose: *Less than 7 days of age:* 75 mg/kg of body weight every 12 hours (150 mg/kg/24 hr).

Over 7 days of age and less than 2,000 Gm: 75 mg/kg every 8 hours (225 mg/kg/24 hr).

Over 7 days of age and more than 2,000 Gm: 75 mg/kg every 6 hours (300 mg/kg/24 hr).

Dilution: Each 1 Gm or fraction thereof should be diluted with at least 10 ml of sterile water, 5% dextrose, or 0.9% sodium chloride for injection. Shake vigorously to dissolve. Must be diluted to a minimum 10% concentration for direct IV use. Should be further diluted to the desired volume (50 to 100 ml) with 5% dextrose in water or 0.45% normal saline or other compatible infusion solutions (see literature) and given as an intermittent infusion.

Rate of administration: *Direct IV:* A single dose properly diluted over 3 to 5 minutes.

Intermittent infusion: A single dose properly diluted over 30 minutes. Discontinue primary IV infusion during administration. Pediatric dose must be given over 30 minutes.

Actions: An extended-spectrum penicillin. Bactericidal against a variety of gram-negative and gram-positive bacteria including aerobic and anaerobic strains. Especially effective against *Klebsiella* and *Pseudomonas*. Well distributed in all body fluids, tissue, bone, and through inflamed meninges. Onset of action is prompt. Excreted in the urine. Crosses placental barrier. Secreted in breast milk.

Indications and uses: (1) Treatment of serious lower respiratory tract, intraabdominal, urinary tract, gynecologic, and skin and skin structure infections and septicemia caused by susceptible organisms; (2) perioperative prophylaxis in surgical procedures classified as contaminated.

Precautions: (1) Stable at room temperature for up to 72 hours depending on solution used for admixture. (2) Warm to 37° C (98.6° F) in a water bath for 20 minutes if precipitation occurs on refrigeration. Shake vigorously. (3) Slightly darkened color does not affect potency. (4) Frequently used concurrently with aminoglycosides (e.g., gentamicin [Garamycin]), but must be administered in separate infusions; inactivates aminoglycosides. (5) Sensitivity studies indicated to determine susceptibility of the causative organism to mezlocillin. (6) Oral probenecid will achieve higher and more prolonged blood levels. May be desirable or may cause toxicity. (7) Watch for early symptoms of allergic reaction. (8) Avoid prolonged use of drug; superinfection caused by overgrowth of nonsusceptible organisms may result. (9) Periodic evaluation of renal, hepatic, and hematopoietic systems and serum potassium is recommended in prolonged therapy. (10) Electrolyte imbalance and cardiac irregularities resulting from sodium content are very possible. Contains 1.85 mEq sodium/Gm. (11) Confirm patency of vein; avoid extravasation or intraarterial injection. Slow infusion rate for pain along venipuncture site. (12) Usual duration of therapy is 7 to 10 days. Continue at least 2 days after symptoms of infection disappear. (13) Reduce dose only in severe renal impairment with creatinine clearance temporarily below 30 ml/min. May be given to patients undergoing hemodialysis and peritoneal dialysis (see literature for dose). (14) Test for syphilis also before treating gonorrhea. (15) Concomitant use with β-adrenergic blockers (e.g., propranolol [Inderal]) may increase risk of anaphylaxis and inhibit treatment. (16) Risk of bleeding with anticoagulants (e.g., heparin) is increased. (17) Inhibits effectiveness of oral contraceptives; breakthrough bleeding or pregnancy may result. (18) Inactivated by chloramphenicol, erythromycin, and tetracyclines. Bactericidal action is actually negated by these drugs. (19) Neuromuscular excitability or convulsions may be caused by higher than normal doses. (20) Elimination rate markedly reduced in neonates.

Contraindications: History of sensitivity to multiple allergens, penicillin sensitivity.

Incompatible with: Aminoglycosides (amikacin, colistimethate, gentamicin, kanamycin, streptomycin, tobramycin), amphotericin B (Fungizone), chloramphenicol, lincomycin, oxytetracycline, polymyxin B, promethazine (Phenergan), tetracycline (Achromycin), verapamil (Calan), vitamin B with C.

Side effects: Anaphylaxis; bleeding abnormalities (with severe renal impairment); convulsions; decreased hemoglobin or hematocrit; diarrhea; elevated SGOT, SGPT, and BUN; eosinophilia; fever; hypokalemia; interstitial nephritis; leukopenia; nausea; neuromuscular excitability; neutropenia; pruritus; pseudoproteinuria; skin rash; taste sensation (abnormal); thrombocytopenia; thrombophlebitis; urticaria; vomiting.

Antidote: Notify the physician immediately of any adverse symptoms. For severe symptoms, discontinue the drug, treat allergic reaction (antihistamines, epinephrine, corticosteroids), and resuscitate as necessary. Hemodialysis is effective in overdose.

MICONAZOLE

pH 3.7 to 5.7

(Monistat IV)

Usual dose: Initial dose of 200 mg with the physician in attendance, then 600 to 3,600 mg/24 hr equally divided into three infusions and given every 8 hours.

Pediatric dose: 20 to 40 mg/kg of body weight as a total daily dose equally divided into three infusions. Do not exceed 15 mg/kg/infusion.

Dilution: A single dose (200 to 1,200 mg in the adult) must be diluted in 200 ml of normal saline. May use 5% dextrose in water if necessary.

Rate of administration: A single dose over 30 to 60 minutes.

Actions: An antifungal agent. Alters the permeability of the fungal cell membrane. Only effective against specific organisms. Metabolized in the liver with some excretion in the urine.

Indications and uses: Severe systemic fungal infections such as coccidioidomycosis, candidiasis, cryptococcosis, paracoccidioidomycosis, and chronic mucocutaneous candidiasis.

Precautions: (1) Hospitalize patient for at least several days to initiate treatment. (2) Monitor blood counts, electrolytes, and lipids during therapy. (3) Rapid injection may produce tachycardia or dysrhythmias. (4) Supplemented in some situations with intrathecal injection and bladder irrigation. (5) Monitor plasma levels of both drugs when given concomitantly with phenytoin (Dilantin). (6) Potentiates coumarin drugs; reduction of anticoagulant dose may be indicated. (7) May potentiate cyclosporine (Sandimmune). (8) May antagonize amphotericin B. Inhibited by rifampin. (9) Use caution in pregnancy. (10) Lengthy treatment (up to 20 weeks) may be required for cure. (11) Antiemetics before each dose will reduce nausea and vomiting. (12) Pruritus is a common side effect and is most uncomfortable. (13) Discard solution that darkens in color.

Contraindications: Known sensitivity to miconazole. Safety for children under 1 year not established.

Incompatible with: Specific information not available. Should be considered incompatible in syringe or solution with any other drug.

Side effects: Allergic reactions including anaphylaxis; anorexia; cardiac dysrhythmias; diarrhea; drowsiness; fever; flushing; nausea; phlebitis; pruritus; rash; tachycardia; vomiting.

Antidote: Notify the physician of all side effects. Most will respond to symptomatic treatment or reduction of infusion rate and are reversible when the drug is discontinued. Treat allergic reaction as necessary and resuscitate as indicated.

MIDAZOLAM HYDROCHLORIDE pH 3.0

(Versed)

Usual dose: *Conscious sedation for endoscopic or cardiovascular procedures in healthy adults less than 60 years of age:* 1 to 2.5 mg immediately before the procedure. Begin with 1 mg and titrate slowly up to slurred speech or 2.5 mg. If additional medication is needed wait a full 2 minutes, then titrate additional dosage slowly in small increments (no more than 1 mg). Wait a full 2 minutes between each increment. A total dose exceeding 5 mg is rarely necessary. Reduce dose by 30% in the presence of narcotic premedication or other CNS depressants. 25% of the sedating dose can be used for maintenance only when clearly indicated by clinical evaluation.

Conscious sedation for endoscopic or cardiovascular procedures in patients over 60 years of age or debilitated or chronically ill patients: 0.5 to 1.5 mg. Begin with 0.5 mg and titrate slowly up to slurred speech or 1.5 mg. If additional medication is needed wait a full 2 minutes, then titrate additional dosage in small increments, i.e., 0.5 to 1 mg. Wait a full 2 minutes between each increment. A total dose exceeding 3.5 mg is rarely necessary. Reduce dose by 50% in the presence of narcotic premedication or other CNS depressants. 25% of the sedating dose can be used for maintenance only when clearly indicated by clinical evaluation.

Induction of anesthesia: 0.15 to 0.35 mg/kg of body weight depending on age, condition, and premedication. Allow a full 2 minutes to evaluate effect. Rarely, up to 0.6 mg/kg may be required; titrate in increments as above. 25% of the initial dose may be used for maintenance, or other anesthetic agents may be used.

Dilution: May be diluted with normal saline or 5% dextrose in water for injection. Dilute in a sufficient amount to permit slow titration, i.e., 1 mg in 4 ml or 5 mg in 20 ml (0.25 mg/ml).

Rate of administration: *Conscious sedation:* Any single increment of a total dose titrated slowly over at least 2 minutes. Stop at any point that the speech becomes slurred.

Induction of anesthesia: Any single increment of a total dose over 20 to 30 seconds.

Rapid injection in any situation may cause respiratory depression or apnea.

Actions: A short-acting benzodiazepine CNS depressant. Depressant effects are dependent on dose, route of administration, and the presence or absence of other premedications. Can depress the ventilatory response to CO_2 stimulation. Mechanics of respiration are not adversely affected with usual doses. Mean arterial pressure, cardiac output, stroke volume, and systemic vascular resistance may be slightly decreased. May cause heart rates of less than 65/min to rise and of more than 85/min to fall. Produces sleepiness and relief of apprehension, and diminishes patient recall very effectively. Onset of action occurs within 3 to 5 minutes. Half-life ranges from 1.2 to 12.3 hours, shorter than that of diazepam (Valium). Metabolized and excreted as metabolites in urine. Crosses the placental barrier.

Indications and uses: To produce sedation, relieve anxiety, and impair memory of perioperative events. May be used with or without narcotic sedation for (1) conscious sedation before short diagnostic or endoscopic procedures (e.g., bronchoscopy, gastroscopy, cystoscopy, coronary angiography, cardiac catheterization), (2) induction of anesthesia before administration of other anesthetic agents.

Precautions: (1) A topical anesthetic agent should be used with midazolam during peroral endoscopy, and premedication with a narcotic is recommended in bronchoscopy since increased cough reflex and laryngospasm frequently occur. (2) Monitor respiration and cardiac function continuously. Has caused apnea and cardiac arrest. Resuscitative drugs and equipment must be immediately available. Maintain a patent airway and support adequate ventilation. (3) Extravasation or arterial administration hazardous. (4) Bed rest required for a minimum of 3 hours after IV injection. Do not drive or operate hazardous machinery until the day after surgery or longer. All effects must have subsided. (5) Use extreme caution in patients with chronic obstructive pulmonary disease; may have increased risks of apnea. (6) Reduce doses in congestive heart failure, chronic renal failure, the debilitated, and patients over 55 years of age. Half-life is extended and depressant effects will be potentiated. (7) Potentiated by narcotics, alcohol, barbiturates, fentanyl, droperidol, and other CNS depressants, including phenothiazines (e.g., prochlorperazine [Compazine]); antihistamines; MAO inhibitors (e.g., pargyline [Eutonyl]); and tricyclic antidepressants (e.g., imipramine [Tofranil-PM]). May produce apnea or prolonged effect, depress ventilatory response to CO_2, or cause hypotension. Reduce dose of midazolam as suggested. (8) Potentiates halothane, inhalation anesthetics, and thiopental. Reduce doses of these agents. (9) Does not protect against increased intracranial pressure or circulatory changes noted with succinylcholine or pancuronium. (10) Compatible in syringe with morphine, meperidine, atropine, or scopolamine. (11) Some clinicians prefer midazolam over diazepam because of effectiveness, minimum pain if any on injection, and miscibility with many drugs and solutions.

Contraindications: Acute narrow-angle glaucoma, infants and children under 18 years, known hypersensitivity to midazolam, open-angle glaucoma unless receiving appropriate treatment, pregnancy, childbirth, lactation, shock, coma, acute alcohol intoxication with depression of vital signs.

Incompatible with: Dimenhydrinate (Dramamine), pentobarbital (Nembutal), perphenazine (Trilafon), prochlorperazine (Compazine), ranitidine (Zantac).

Side effects: Airway obstruction; apnea; ataxia; blurred vision; bradycardia; bronchospasm; cardiac arrest; cardiac dysrhythmias including bigeminy, PVCs, nodal rhythm, and tachycardia; coma; confusion; coughing; depressed respiration; depression; diminished reflexes; dreaming during emergence from anesthesia; drowsiness; dyspnea; fluctuation in vital signs; headache; hiccups; hyperexcited states; hyperventilation; hypotension; laryngospasm; nausea and vomiting; nightmares; nystagmus; pain; prolonged emergence from anesthesia; induration; redness or phlebitis at injection site; shallow respirations; slurred speech; somnolence; syncope; tachypnea; vasovagal episode; vertigo; wheezing; and many others. Has caused death and hypoxic encephalopathy.

Antidote: Notify the physician of all side effects. Reduction of dosage may be required or will be treated symptomatically. Discontinue the drug for major side effects or paradoxical reactions. In overdose maintain an adequate airway and ventilation, promote excretion through fluid and electrolyte administration and osmotic diuretics (e.g., mannitol). Effectiveness of hemodialysis is not confirmed. Use dopamine (Intropin), levarterenol (Levophed), or metaraminol (Aramine) for hypotension. Treat allergic reaction and resuscitate as necessary.

MILRINONE LACTATE*

(Primacor*)

Usual dose: 50 mcg/kg (0.05 mg/kg) of body weight as the initial loading dose (3.5 mg [3.5 ml] for a 70 kg person). Follow with a maintenance infusion of 0.5 mcg/kg/min (35 mcg/min for a 70 kg person). Titrate the infusion dose between 0.375 mcg/kg/min to 0.75 mcg/kg/min (26 mcg/min to 52 mcg/min for a 70 kg person) based on hemodynamic effect. Do not exceed a total dose of 1.13 mg/kg/24 hr, including boluses. Duration of infusion usually does not exceed 48 to 72 hours but has been used for up to 5 days.

Reduced dose required in impaired renal function based on creatinine clearance (see literature).

Dilution: *Loading dose:* may be given undiluted, or each 1 mg (1 ml) may be diluted in 1 ml normal saline or 0.45% saline for injection.

Infusion: dilute each 10 mg (10 ml) in 40 ml normal saline, 0.45% saline, or 5% dextrose. 1 ml equals 200 mcg/ml. Amount of diluent may be increased or

*Available in the United Kingdom, France, the Netherlands. It has been approved by the FDA and will be available in the United States later. Available as Corotrope in Europe and South America.

decreased based on patient fluid requirements. May be given through Y tube or three-way stopcock of IV infusion set but should never come in contact with furosemide (Lasix) or bumetanide (Bumex). Use only freshly prepared solutions. Store at room temperature before dilution, avoid freezing.

Rate of administration: *Loading dose:* A single dose over 10 minutes.

Infusion: Use a microdrip (60 gtt/ml) or an infusion pump to deliver milrinone in recommended doses. Manufacturer includes a dosage chart defining selected dose in mcg/kg/min in infusion rate of ml/kg/hr (e.g., dose: 0.500 mcg/kg/min, infusion rate: 0.15 ml/kg/hr). Adjust as indicated by physician's orders and progress in pateint's condition.

Actions: A new class of cardiac inotropic agent different in chemical structure and mode of action from digitalis glycosides and catecholemines. Similar to amrinone (Inocor), with fewer side effects. With a loading dose, peak effect occurs within 10 minutes. Continuous administration is required to maintain serum levels. It has positive inotropic action with vasodilator activity. Reduces afterload and preload by direct relaxant effect on vascular smooth muscle. Produces slight enhancement of AV node conduction. Cardiac output is improved without significant increases in heart rate or myocardial oxygen consumption or changes in arteriovenous oxygen difference. Pulmonary capillary wedge pressure, total peripheral resistance, diastolic blood pressure, and mean arterial pressure are decreased. Heart rate generally remains the same. Metabolized by conjugated pathways, it is primarily excreted in urine.

Indications and uses: Short-term management of congestive heart failure in patients who have not responded adequately to digitalis, diuretics, or vasodilators.

Precautions: (1) Observe patient continuously; monitoring of ECG, blood pressure, urine output, fluid and electrolyte changes (especially potassium), and body weight are recommended. Monitoring of cardiac index, pulmonary capillary wedge pressure, central venous pressure, and plasma concentration is very useful. Observe for orthopnea, dyspnea, and fatigue. Reduce rate or stop infusion for excessive drop in blood pressure.

(2) Use caution in impaired renal function; serum levels may increase considerably. (3) May be given to digitalized patients without causing signs of digitalis toxicity. (4) May increase ventricular response in atrial flutter/fibrillation. Consider pretreatment with digitalis. (5) Additional fluids and electrolytes may be required to facilitate appropriate response in patients who have been vigorously diuresed and may have insufficient cardiac filling pressure. Use caution. (6) Safety for use in the acute phase of myocardial infarction not established. (7) Monitor electrolytes; hypokalemia due to diuretics may cause dysrhythmias. Reduction of diureteic dose may be indicated. (8) Theoretical potential for interaction with calcium channel blockers (e.g., verapamil [Calan]), no clinical evidence to date. (9) Safety for use during pregnancy, lactation, and in children not established. Use during pregnancy only if potential benefit justifies potential risk. (10) May aggravate outflow tract obstruction in hypertrophic subaortic stenosis or severe obstructive aortic or pulmonary valvular disease (see Contraindications).

Contraindications: Hypersensitivity to milrinone, severe aortic or pulmonic valvular disease in lieu of surgical relief of the obstruction.

Incompatible with: Bumetanide (Bumex), furosemide (Lasix). Should not be mixed with other drugs until further compatibility data are available.

Side effects: Supraventricular and ventricular dysrhythmias including nonsustained ventricular tachycardia do occur. Angina, chest pain, headaches, hypokalemia, hypotension, thrombocytopenia, and tremor have been reported.

Antidote: Notify the physician of any side effect. Based on degree of severity and condition of the patient, may be treated symptomatically, and dose may remain the same, be decreased, or the milrinone may be discontinued. Reduce rate or discontinue the drug at the first sign of marked hypotension and notify the physician. May be resolved by these measures alone or vasopressors (e.g., dopamine [Intropin]) may be required. Treat dysrhythmias with the appropriate drug. Resuscitate as necessary.

MINOCYCLINE HYDROCHLORIDE

pH 2.0 to 2.8

(Minocin)

Usual dose: 200 mg initially, then 100 mg every 12 hours. Maximum dose is 400 mg/24 hr. Normal renal function required.

Pediatric dose: *Over 8 years of age:* 4 mg/kg of body weight as initial dose, followed by 2 mg/kg every 12 hours.

Dilution: Reconstitute each 100 mg vial with 5 ml of sterile water for injection. Must be further diluted in 500 to 1,000 ml of compatible infusion fluids such as sodium chloride, dextrose solutions, Ringer's injection, or lactated Ringer's injection.

Rate of administration: Each 100 mg properly diluted at prescribed rate of infusion (e.g., 500 ml 5% dextrose in water with minocycline 100 mg every 6 hours).

Actions: A broad-spectrum antibiotic that is bacteriostatic against many gram-positive and gram-negative organisms. Well distributed in most body tissues, tetracyclines are concentrated in the liver and excreted through bile to urine and feces in a biologically active state. Minocycline may penetrate normal meninges, the eye, and the prostate more easily than other tetracyclines. Crosses the placental barrier. Secreted in breast milk.

Indications and uses: (1) Infections caused by susceptible organisms; (2) to substitute for contraindicated penicillin or sulfonamide therapy; (3) adjunct to amebicides in acute intestinal amebiasis.

Precautions: (1) Stable at room temperature for 24 hours. (2) Sensitivity studies necessary to determine susceptibility of causative organism to minocycline. (3) Avoid prolonged use; superinfection due to overgrowth of nonsusceptible organisms may result. (4) Use extreme caution in impaired liver or renal function, pregnancy, postpartum, and lactation. Minocycline serum concentrations and liver and kidney function tests are indicated. (5) May cause skeletal retardation in the fetus and infants and permanent tooth discoloration in children under 8 years of age, either by direct administration or by transmission through placenta or mother's milk. Do not use during pregnancy; discontinue breast feeding. (6) Inhibits oral contraceptives; may result in pregnancy or breakthrough bleeding. (7) Monitor blood glucose; may reduce insulin requirements. (8) May alter lithium levels. (9) Inhibits bactericidal action of penicillin, ampicillin, oxacillin, methicillin, etc. May be toxic with sulfonamides. (10) Potentiates digoxin and anticoagulants; reduced dosage of these drugs may be necessary. (11) Inhibited by alkalizing agents, calcium, cimetidine (Tagamet), iron and magnesium salts, riboflavin, sodium bicarbonate, and others. (12) Alert patient to possibility of photosensitive skin reaction. (13) Determine absolute patency of vein and avoid extravasation; thrombophlebitis is not infrequent. (14) Organisms resistant to one tetracycline are usually resistant to others. (15) Check expiration date. Outdated ampoules may cause nephrotoxicity. (16) If syphilis is suspected, perform a dark-field examination before initiating tetracyclines. (17) Potentiated by alcohol and hepatotoxic drugs (e.g., methoxyflurane [Penthrane]); severe liver damage may result.

Contraindications: Known hypersensitivity to tetracyclines, pregnancy, lactation. Not recommended in children under 8 years.

Incompatible with: Sufficient information not available. See tetracycline hydrochloride; same incompatibilities may exist. Forms a precipitate with calcium.

Side effects: Relatively nontoxic in average doses, more toxic in larger doses or if given too rapidly.

Minor: Anogenital lesions, anorexia, blood dyscrasias, diarrhea, dizziness, dysphagia, enterocolitis, nausea, skin rashes, vertigo, vomiting.

Major: Hypersensitivity reactions, including anaphylaxis; blurred vision and headache (benign intracranial hypertension); bulging fontanels in infants; liver damage; photosensitivity; systemic candidiasis; thrombophlebitis.

Antidote: Notify the physician of all side effects. If minor side effects are progressive or any major side effect occurs, discontinue drug, treat allergic reactions, and resuscitate as necessary.

MITOMYCIN pH 6.0 to 8.0

(Mitomycin-C, Mutamycin, MTC)

Usual dose: 20 mg/M^2 as a single dose or 2 mg/M^2 daily for 5 days. After 2-day rest period, repeat 2 mg/M^2 daily for 5 additional days (total dose equals 20 mg/M^2). Entire schedule may be repeated in 6 to 8 weeks if no bone marrow toxicity occurs.

Dilution: *Specific techniques required, see Precautions.* Each 5 mg must be diluted with 10 ml sterile water for injection. Allow to stand at room temperature until completely in solution. May be given through the Y-tube or three-way stopcock of a free-flowing infusion of normal saline or 5% dextrose in water or further diluted in either of the same solutions and given as an infusion. Stable in 5% dextrose in water for only 3 hours.

Rate of administration: A single dose over 5 to 10 minutes. Infusion rate determined by amount and type of solution. Will maintain potency in 5% dextrose in water for 3 hours.

Actions: A highly toxic antibiotic, antineoplastic agent. Cell cycle phase nonspecific, it is most useful in G and S phases. Interferes with cell division by binding with DNA to slow production of RNA. Metabolized in the liver. Some excreted in urine.

Indications and uses: A palliative treatment, adjunct to surgery, radiation, or patients resistant to other chemotherapeutic agents. May be useful in pancreatic, gastric, cervical, breast, bronchogenic, and head and neck carcinoma and malignant melanoma.

Precautions: (1) Follow guidelines for handling cytotoxic agents recommended. See Appendix, p. 677. (2) Administered by or under the direction of the physician specialist. (3) Determine absolute patency of vein; use of an IV catheter is preferred because severe cellulitis and tissue necrosis will result from extravasation. If extravasation occurs, discontinue injection and use another vein. Elevate extremity, apply cold compresses to extravasated area. (4) Monitor white blood cells, red blood cells, platelet count, prothrombin time, bleeding time, differential, and hemoglobin before, during, and

7 to 10 weeks after therapy. (5) Monitor all patients receiving any dose (initial or cumulative) of 60 mg or more for unexplained anemia with fragmented cells on peripheral blood smear, thrombocytopenia, and decreased renal function. Use extreme caution in impaired renal function. (6) May precipitate adult respiratory distress syndrome. Oxygen can be toxic to the lungs; monitor intake carefully and use only enough to provide adequate arterial saturation. Monitor fluid balance, avoid overhydration. (7) May produce teratogenic effects on the fetus; use caution in men and women capable of conception. (8) Do not administer vaccines or chloroquine to patients receiving antineoplastic drugs. (9) Be alert for signs of bone marrow depression or infection. (10) Used with other antineoplastic drugs and radiation in reduced doses to achieve tumor remission. (11) Prophylactic antiemetics may reduce nausea and vomiting and increase patient comfort. (12) Discontinue drug if no response after two courses of treatment. (13) Stable after initial dilution at room temperature for 7 days, up to 14 days if refrigerated.

Contraindications: Not recommended as single-agent primary therapy. Known hypersensitivity to mitomycin, thrombocytopenia, coagulation disorders, increased bleeding from other causes, white blood cell count below 4,000, platelet count below 150,000, potentially serious infections, serum creatinine above 1.7 mg/100 ml.

Incompatible with: Bleomycin (Blenoxane).

Side effects: Alopecia, anaphylaxis, anorexia, bleeding, blurring of vision, cellulitis at injection site, confusion, coughing, diarrhea, drowsiness, dyspnea with nonproductive cough, edema, elevated BUN or serum creatinine, fatigue, fever, headache, hematemesis, hemolytic uremic syndrome (microangiopathic hemolytic anemia [hematocrit less than 25%], irreversible renal failure [serum creatinine greater than 16 mg/dl], and thrombocytopenia [less tham 100,000 mm^3]), hemoptysis, hypertension, leukopenia, mouth ulcers, nausea, paresthesias, pneumonia, pruritus, pulmonary edema, purple discoloration of vein, radiographic evidence of pulmonary infiltrates, renal failure, respiratory distress syndrome (adult), skin toxicity, stomatitis, syncope, thrombophlebitis, vomiting.

Antidote: Most side effects will be treated symptomatically. Keep the physician informed. All are potentially serious, and many can be life threatening. Hematopoietic depression requires cessation of therapy until recovery occurs. Discontinue drug if dyspnea, nonproductive cough, or radiographic evidence of pulmonary infiltrates are present. Discontinue drug for any symptoms of hemolytic uremic syndrome. There is no specific antidote. Supportive therapy as indicated will help sustain the patient in toxicity. If extravasation has occurred, L.A. dexamethasone injected into the indurated area with a fine hypodermic needle may be helpful; elevate extremity.

MITOXANTRONE HYDROCHLORIDE — pH 3.0 to 4.5

(Novantrone)

Usual dose: *Combination initial therapy in acute nonlymphocytic leukemia:* 12 mg/M^2/day of mitoxantrone on days 1 through 3 and cytosine arabinoside 100 mg/M^2/day as a continuous 24-hour infusion on days 1 through 7. Should a complete remission not be achieved, repeat mitoxantrone, 12 mg/M^2/day for only 2 days, and cytosine arabinoside 100 mg/M^2/day for 5 days after all signs or symptoms of severe or life-threatening nonhematologic toxicity have cleared. After full hematologic recovery, some consolidation therapy trials have repeated the second course doses in approximately 6 weeks and again in 4 weeks. Severe myelosuppression occurred in these subsequent courses.

Dilution: *Specific techniques required, see Precautions.* A single dose must be diluted with at least 50 ml of normal saline or 5% dextrose in water. May be further diluted in normal saline or 5% dextrose in water or normal saline. Do not add to IV solutions. Must be given through Y-tube or three-way stopcock of a free-flowing infusion of 5% dextrose in water or normal saline.

Rate of administration: A single dose of properly diluted medication over at least 3 to 5 minutes. Titrate infusion based on total amount of solution used.

Actions: The first of a new class of synthetic antineoplastic agents called anthracenediones. Has achieved complete remissions with a single course of combination therapy. Extensive distribution to tissue occurs rapidly. Has a cytocidal effect on proliferating and nonproliferating cells. Probably not cell cycle specific. Half-life varies from 3 hours to 12 days. Slowly excreted in bile and urine.

Indications and uses: (1) To induce remission of acute nonlymphocytic leukemia in adults, including myelogenous, promyelocytic, monocytic, and erythroid acute leukemias.

Investigational uses: Treatment of solid tumors, including advanced breast cancers, and treatment of malignant lymphomas.

Precautions: (1) Follow guidelines for handling cytotoxic agents recommended. See Appendix, p. 677. (2) Administered by or under the direction of the physician specialist. (3) Will cause severe myelosuppression; use extreme caution in preexisting drug-induced bone marrow suppression. (4) Monitoring of white blood cells, red blood cells, platelet count, liver function, and kidney function indicated before and during therapy. (5) Use extreme caution and monitor ECG, chest x-ray, echocardiography, and systolic ejection fraction in patients with preexisting heart disease, previous treatment with daunorubicin (Cerubidine), doxorubicin (Adriamycin), or radiation therapy encompassing the heart. (6) May cause acute congestive heart failure. (7) Because of rapid lysis of cancer cells, initiate hypouricemic therapy with allopurinol or similar agents before beginning treatment. Monitor uric acid levels and maintain hydration. (8) Use caution if liver or renal function impaired. (9) Observe closely and frequently for all signs of bleeding or infection. (10) Urine and sclera may turn bluish in color. (11) Has nonvesicant properties, but extravasation must be avoided. Should extravasation occur, discontinue injection, use another vein. (12) Diluted solution should be used immediately; do not freeze. (13) May produce teratogenic effects on the fetus; avoid pregnancy. Discontinue breast feeding. (14) Safety for use in children not established. (15) Prophylactic antiemetics may reduce nausea and vomiting and increase patient comfort. (16) Dosage based on average weight if edema or ascites present. (17) Do not administer any vaccines or chloroquine to patients receiving antineoplastic drugs. (18) Use of goggles, gloves, and protective gown recommended. Flush skin copiously with warm water should any contact occur. Irrigate eyes immediately in case of contact. Clean spills with 5.5 parts calcium hypochlorite to 13 parts by weight of water for each 1 part of mitoxantrone.

Contraindications: Hypersensitivity to mitoxantrone or other anthracyclines.

Incompatible with: Heparin, hydrocortisone sodium phosphate (Hydrocortone) in a PVC container. Should be considered incompatible with any other drug in syringe or solution until further data available because of toxicity and specific use.

Side effects: Abdominal pain, acute congestive heart failure, alopecia (reversible), bone marrow suppression (severe with standard doses), bleeding, cough, decrease in systolic ejection fraction, diarrhea, dyspnea, fever, headache, infections, jaundice, mucosities, nausea, renal failure, seizures, stomatitis, vomiting.

Antidote: There is no specific antidote. Notify physician of all side effects. Most will be treated symptomatically. Blood and blood products, antibiotics, and other adjunctive therapies must be available. Overdose has resulted in death. Peritoneal dialysis or hemodialysis not effective. Supportive therapy as indicated will help sustain the patient in toxicity.

MORPHINE SULFATE pH 3.0 to 6.0

Astramorph PF, Duramorph)

Usual dose: *Direct IV:* 2.5 to 15 mg (gr 1⁄16 to 1⁄4). Repeat every 2 to 4 hours as necessary. May be titrated to achieve pain relief with lowest dose (e.g., pain relief in myocardial infarction). 10 mg (gr 1⁄6) is adequate for all but exceptional needs. Dose must be individualized based on response and tolerance. Cancer patients suffering with severe chronic pain often require higher doses because of increased tolerance (up to 150 mg/hr has been given). Extremely high doses (275 to 440 mg/hr) are occasionally used for short periods of time (hours to days) for extreme exacerbations of pain in these drug-tolerant individuals. 1 to 3 mg/kg over 15 to 20 minutes will induce unconsciousness.

Reduced dose may be required in hepatic or renal disease.

Infusion: 1 mg/ml (range is 0.1 to 1 mg/ml) in sterile water for injection, normal saline or 5% dextrose in water per controlled infusion device (may be patient activated). Based on a 1 mg/ml dilution an initial loading dose may range from 3 to 5 mg (3 to 5 ml). The continuous background infusion to provide a level of pain relief and maintain patency of the vein may range from 1 to 2.5 mg/hr (1 to 2.5 ml). Additional doses averaging 0.5 to 1.5 mg (0.5 to 1.5 ml) may be activated by the patient at selected intervals every 3 to 60 minutes (averaging 10 to 15 min). Additional boluses (averaging 1 to 2 mg (1 to 2 ml) may be given by health care professionals (e.g., every 30 min prn). In selected cancer patients all of these doses may be considerably higher.

Pediatric dose: *Selected children with severe chronic pain from cancer:* 0.025 to 2.6 mg/kg/hr (averaging 0.04 to 0.07 mg/kg/hr).

Selected children with severe pain during sickle cell crisis: 0.03 to 0.15 mg/kg/hr.

Selected children requiring postoperative analgesia: 0.01 to 0.04 mg/kg/hr. Reduce to 0.015 ot 0.02 mg/kg/hr in neonates because of reduced elimination and susceptibility to CNS side effects.

Dilution: *Direct IV:* Should be diluted. Use at least 5 ml of sterile water or normal saline for injection or other IV solutions. May be given through Y-tube or three-way stopcock of infusion set.

Infusion: Each 0.1 to 1 mg is usually diluted in 1 ml sterile water for injection, normal saline, or 5% dextrose in water and administered via a controlled infusion device that may be patient activated (e.g., a narcotic syringe infuser system). Available in 60 ml amps containing 1 to 2 mg/ml for direct transfer to syringe infuser systems (Astramorph PF and Duramorph are preservative free, can be used IV, but are the only choice for intrathecal injection; see drug literature). Fluid restriction or high doses may require more concentrated solutions. Concentrations above 5 mg/ml are rarely exceeded. Available in vials containing 25 mg/ml, which must be further diluted before infusion. Is sometimes added to larger amounts (500 ml to 1 L) of IV solution in selected situations and infused via a large volume-controlled infusion pump (requires close titration).

Rate of administration: *Direct IV:* 15 mg or fraction thereof of properly diluted medication over 4 to 5 minutes. Frequently titrated according to symptom relief and respiratory rate. Side effects markedly increased if rate of injection too rapid.

Infusion: Initial loading dose, basal rate (continuous rate of infusion), patient self-administered dose and interval, additional boluses permitted, and total dose for 1 hour should be ordered by physician. Administer initial dose and boluses at rate for direct IV. For continuous infusion and self-administered dose and interval, note range of ml/hr under Usual dose.

Actions: An opium-derivative narcotic analgesic, which is a descending CNS depressant. It has definite respiratory depressant actions. Pain relief is effected almost immediately and lasts about 2 hours. Morphine induces sleep and inhibits perception of pain by binding to opiate receptors, decreasing sodium permeability, and inhibiting transmission of pain impulses. Depresses many other senses or reflexes. Readily absorbed, detoxified in the liver, and excreted in the urine. Crosses the placental barrier. Secreted in breast milk.

Indications and uses: (1) Relief of severe to excruciating pain and apprehension from coronary occlusion, malignancies, traumatic injury, renal or biliary colic, and painful manipulation or instrumentation (e.g., cystoscopy, burn dressing changes, fracture reduction), dyspnea, seizures of acute left ventricular failure, and pulmonary edema; (2) postoperative relief of severe pain; (3) restore uterine tone and contractions in a uterus made hyperactive by oxytocics.

Precautions: (1) Oxygen, controlled respiratory equipment, and naloxone (Narcan) must always be available. (3) Observe patient frequently to continuously based on dose and monitor vital signs. Keep patient supine; orthostatic hypotension and fainting may occur; less likely with continuous low doses, but observe closely during ambulation. (3) Stool softeners and/or laxatives will be required to avoid constipation and fecal impaction, especially with increased doses and extended use. Maintain adequate hydration. (4) Use caution in the elderly, in patients with impaired hepatic or renal function, emphysema, and anticoagulation therapy. (5) Use extreme caution in craniotomy, head injury, and increased intracranial pressure; respiratory depression and intracranial pressure may be further increased. (6) May cause apnea in asthmatic patients. (7) Symptoms of acute abdominal conditions may be masked. (8) May increase ventricular response rate in presence of supraventricular tachycardias. (9) Cough reflex is suppressed. (10) Tolerance for the drug gradually increases, but abstinence for 1 to 2 weeks will restore effectiveness. (11) Physical dependence can develop with abuse. (12) A marked increase in dose may precipitate seizures in presence of a history of convulsive disorders. (13) Potentiated by phenothiazines (e.g., chlorpromazine [Thorazine]); other CNS depressants such as narcotic analgesics, general anesthetics, alcohol, anticholinergics, antihistamines, barbiturates, cimetidine (Tagamet), methocarbamol (Robaxin), hypnotics, sedatives, and psychotropic agents; MAO inhibitors (e.g., isocarboxazid [Marplan]); neuromuscular blocking agents (e.g., tubocurarine); and adrenergic blocking agents (e.g., propranolol [Inderal]). Reduced dosage of both drugs may be indicated. (14) Safety for use in pregnancy or lactation not established.

Contraindications: Acute alcoholism, acute bronchial asthma, benign prostatic hypertrophy, biliary tract surgery, diarrhea caused by poisoning until toxic material eliminated, hypersensitivity to opiates, premature infants or labor and delivery of premature infants, pulmonary edema caused by a chemical respiratory irritant, respiratory depression, surgical anastomosis, upper airway obstruction, patients who are taking or have recently taken MAO inhibitors.

Incompatible with: Aminophylline, amobarbital (Amytal), chlorothiazide (Diuril), heparin, meperidine (Demerol), methicillin (Staphcillin), pentobarbital (Nembutal), phenobarbital (Luminal), phenytoin (Dilantin), sodium bicarbonate, sodium iodide, thiopental (Pentothal).

Side effects: *Average dose:* Constipation, delayed absorption of oral medications, hypersensitivity reactions, hypothermia, increased intracranial pressure, nausea, neonatal apnea, orthostatic hypotension, respiratory depression (slight), urinary retention, vomiting.

Overdose: Anaphylaxis, Cheyne-Stokes respiration, coma, excitation, hypotension (severe), inverted T wave on ECG, myocardial depression (severe), pinpoint pupils, respiratory depression (severe), tachycardia, death.

Antidote: With increasing severity of any side effect or onset of symptoms of overdose, discontinue the drug and notify the physician. Naloxone (Narcan) will reverse serious respiratory depression. A patent airway, artificial ventilation, oxygen therapy, and other symptomatic treatment must be instituted promptly. Resuscitate as necessary.

MOXALACTAM DISODIUM ph 5.5 to 6.5

(Moxam)

Usual dose: 2 to 6 Gm/24 hr in equally divided doses every 8 hours for 5 to 10 days. Range is 250 mg every 12 hours to 4 Gm every 8 hours.

Pediatric dose: *Up to 1 week:* 50 mg/kg of body weight every 12 hours.

1 to 4 weeks: 50 mg/kg every 8 hours.

Infants: 50 mg/kg every 6 hours.

Children: 50 mg/kg every 6 or 8 hours. Up to 200 mg/kg/day may be needed. In gram-negative meningitis use an initial loading dose of 100 mg/kg.

Dilution: Each 1 Gm must be diluted with 10 ml sterile water, 5% dextrose, or 0.9% sodium chloride.

Direct IV: May be given through tubing port of free-flowing IV solutions of compatible fluid (see literature).

Intermittent IV: Must be further diluted to at least 20 ml/Gm with 5% dextrose, 0.9% saline, or other compatible infusion solutions. May be added to 500 to 1,000 ml compatible infusion fluids and given as a continuous infusion.

Rate of administration: *Direct IV:* A single dose equally distributed over 3 to 5 minutes. May be given through Y-tube or three-way stopcock of infusion set.

Intermittent IV: A single dose over 30 minutes. Discontinue primary infusion during administration.

Continuous infusion: 500 to 1,000 ml over 6 to 24 hours, depending on total dose and concentration.

Actions: A broad-spectrum third-generation cephalosporin antibiotic. Bactericidal to many gram-negative, gram-positive, and anaerobic organisms. Effective against many otherwise resistant organisms. Absorbed by most body fluids including inflamed meninges. Excreted in the urine. Crosses placental barrier. Secreted in breast milk.

Indications and uses: Treatment of serious lower respiratory tract, urinary tract, intraabdominal, CNS, skin and skin structure, and bone and joint infections and bacterial septicemia.

Precautions: (1) Sensitivity studies indicated to determine susceptibility of the causative organism to moxalactam. (2) Watch for early symptoms of allergic reaction. (3) Reduce total daily dose if renal function impaired. Calculated according to degree of impairment. (4) Continue for at least 2 to 3 days after all symptoms of infection subside. Avoid prolonged use of drug; superinfection caused by overgrowth of nonsusceptible organisms may result. (5) Administer within 24 hours of preparation. Selected solutions may be preserved 96 hours with refrigeration. (6) Use extreme caution in the penicillin-sensitive patient; cross-sensitivity may occur. (7) Adverse interaction may occur with promethazine (Phenergan), procainamide (Pronestyl), quinidine, muscle relaxants, potent diuretics, and aminoglycosides. Will produce symptoms of acute alcohol intolerance with alcohol. Abstain until at least 72 hours after discontinued. (8) Frequently used concomitantly with aminoglycosides in severe infections, but these drugs must never be mixed in the same infusion or given concurrently. Nephrotoxicity markedly increased when both drugs utilized. (9) Use only if absolutely necessary in pregnancy. (10) Use caution in patients with liver impairment. (11) *Pseudomonas* infections may require higher doses. Choose another drug if response not prompt. (12) Avoid concurrent administration of bacteriostatic agents. Will inhibit bactericidal action. (13) May cause thrombophlebitis. Use small needles and large veins, and rotate infusion sites. (14) Electrolyte imbalance and cardiac irregularities resulting from high sodium content are very possible. Contains 3.8 mEq sodium/Gm. (15) Will cause hypoprothrombinemia; 10 mg/week of prophylactic vitamin K is recommended. Platelet dysfunction can be avoided by limiting dose to 4 Gm/24 hr and using vitamin K. (16) Bleeding tendency increased with heparin and oral anticoagulants (warfarin [Coumadin]).

Contraindications: Known sensitivity to cephalosporins or related antibiotics (penicillins).

Incompatible with: All aminoglycosides (e.g., kanamycin [Kantrex]). Limited information available. Should be considered incompatible in syringe or solution with any other bacteriostatic agent.

Side effects: Full scope of allergic reactions including anaphylaxis. Bleeding episodes (severe); decreased hemoglobin, hematocrit, PT, or platelet functions; diarrhea; dyspnea; eosinophilia; elevation of SGOT, SGPT, total bilirubin, alkaline phosphatase, LDH, and BUN (transient); false positive reaction for urine glucose except with Tes-Tape or Keto-Diastix; fever; leukopenia; local site pain; platelet dysfunction; pseudomembranous colitis; seizures (large doses); thrombocytopenia; thrombophlebitis; transient neutropenia; vaginitis; vomiting.

Antidote: Notify the physician of any side effect. Discontinue the drug if indicated. Treat allergic reaction as indicated and resuscitate as necessary. Hemodialysis may be useful in overdose. Vitamin K, fresh frozen plasma, packed red cells, or platelet concentrates may be indicated in abnormal bleeding tendencies confirmed by lab evaluations. If bleeding results from platelet dysfunction, discontinue and use cefamandole or cefoperazone with caution.

MULTIVITAMIN INFUSION

(M.V.C. 9 + 3, M.V.C. 9 + 4 Pediatric, M.V.I.-12, M.V.I. Pediatric)

Usual dose: One 5 to 10 ml dose every 24 hours.

Dilution: Each dose must be diluted in at least 500 ml but preferably 1,000 ml of IV fluids. Soluble in all commonly used infusion fluids, including dextrose, saline, electrolyte replacement fluids, plasma, and most protein amino acid products.

Rate of administration: Give at prescribed rate of infusion fluids.

Actions: A multiple vitamin solution containing fat-soluble and water-soluble vitamins in an aqueous solution. Provides B complex and vitamins A, D, and E. Readily absorbed, it provides daily requirements or corrects an existing deficiency.

Indications and uses: Need of optimum vitamin intake to

maintain the body's normal resistance and repair processes, such as after surgery, extensive burns, trauma, severe infectious diseases, and comatose states.

Precautions: (1) Never use undiluted. (2) Do not use if any crystals have formed. (3) Should be refrigerated.

Contraindications: Known hypersensitivity to thiamine hydrochloride.

Incompatible with: Alkaline solutions, bleomycin (Blenoxane), doxycycline (Vibramycin), erythromycin (Erythrocin), FreAmine III (8.5% amino acids), kanamycin (Kantrex), lincomycin (Lincocin), sodium bicarbonate, tetracycline (Achromycin).

Side effects: Rare when administered as recommended: anaphylaxis, dizziness, fainting.

Antidote: With onset of any side effect, discontinue administration immediately and notify the physician. Treat anaphylaxis or resuscitate as necessary.

MUROMONAB-CD3

(Orthoclone OKT3)

Usual dose: 5 mg/24 hr for 10 to 14 days. Initiate on diagnosis of acute renal rejection. Do not give initial or subsequent doses unless patient temperature is less than 37.8° C (100° F). Administration of IV methylprednisolone sodium succinate 1 mg/kg of body weight before muromonab-CD3 and IV hydrocortisone sodium succinate 100 mg 30 minutes after muromonab-CD3 is recommended to reduce side effects associated with the first dose. Acetaminophen and antihistamines may also be used concomitantly.

Dilution: May be given undiluted. Must be withdrawn from vial through a low protein-binding 0.2 or 0.22 micron filter. Discard filter and attach needle for direct IV administration.

Rate of administration: A single dose as an IV bolus in 1 minute.

Actions: A murine monoclonal antibody to the T3 (CD3) antigen of human T cells. An immunosuppressive agent that reverses graft rejection by blocking all known T-cell functions. Onset of action is within minutes. CD3 positive cells reappear within several days and reach pretreatment levels in 1 week after daily injections are stopped.

Indications and uses: Treatment of acute allograft rejection in renal transplant patients.

Precautions: (1) Usually administered in the hospital by or under the direction of a physician experienced in immunosuppressive therapy and management of organ transplant patients. Adequate laboratory and supportive medical resources must be available. (2) To reduce incidence of serious side effects, evaluate patients for fluid overload. Must have a clear chest x-ray within 24 hours and have gained no more than 3% above minimum weight present 7 days before injection. (3) Monitor white blood cell count and differential, circulating T cells as CD3 antigen, and 24-hour trough values of muromonab-CD3 (rise rapidly for the first 3 days of treatment and then average 0.9 mcg/ml thereafter during treatment). (4) Observe for fever, chills, dyspnea, and malaise, which frequently occur 30 minutes to 6 hours after first dose. (5) Increased susceptibility to infection; observe closely. (6) Treat any fever over 37.8° C (100° F) with antipyretics to lower before giving any single dose. (7) Dosage of concomitant immunosuppressive therapy must be reduced during muromonab-CD3 therapy (prednisone to 0.5 mg/kg daily, azathioprine to 25 mg daily; reduce or discontinue cyclosporine). Resume maintenance doses 3 days before completion of muromonab-CD3 therapy. (8) Contains polysorbate 80, not for use in the in vitro treatment of bone marrow. (9) A protein substance that induces antibodies; use extreme caution if a second course of therapy is needed. (10) Safety for use in pregnancy and men and women capable of conception not established. Use only when absolutely necessary. Has been used in children over 2 years of age, but safety not established. (11) May cause lymphomas. (12) Keep unopened vials under refrigeration. May have some fine translucent particles. Will not affect potency, and use of filter will clear.

Contraindications: Hypersensitivity to muromonab-CD3 or any product of murine origin, patients in fluid overload as evidenced by chest x-ray or greater than 3% weight gain within the week before treatment.

Incompatible with: Manufacturer states, "Do not give by IV infusion or in conjunction with other drug solutions."

Side effects: Chills, dyspnea, fever, and malaise are very common with the first dose; incidence lessens with subsequent doses. Anaphylaxis, chest pain, diarrhea, infections (e.g., cytomegalovirus, herpes simplex, *Staphylococcus epidermidis, Pneumocystis carinii, Legionella, Cryptococcus, Serratia),* lymphomas, nausea, serum sickness, severe pulmonary edema, tremors, vomiting, and wheezing have occurred. A disorder similar to Epstein-Barr occurred in one patient.

Antidote: Notify the physician of all side effects. Most can be treated symptomatically. Pretreat as indicated in usual dose to reduce side effects with first dose. Use antipyretics and antihistamines as indicated. Proper patient screening should reduce incidence of pulmonary edema. Drug may be decreased or discontinued or other immunosuppressive agents used. Resuscitate as necessary.

NAFCILLIN SODIUM — pH 6.0 to 6.5

(Nafcill, Nallpen, Unipen)

Usual dose: 500 mg to 1 Gm every 4 hours.

Pediatric dose: *Over 1 month of age:* 50 to 100 mg/24 hr in equally divided doses every 6 hours in moderate infections. 100 to 200 mg/kg/24 hr in equally divided doses every 4 to 6 hours has been used in serious infections. IM route preferred; rarely used IV in children.

Dilution: Each 500 mg vial is diluted with 1.7 ml of of sterile water for injection (1 Gm vial with 3.4 ml, 2 Gm vial with 6.8 ml). Each 1 ml equals 250 mg. Further dilute each 500 mg with a minimum of 15 to 30 ml of 5% dextrose in water, isotonic sodium chloride, or other compatible IV solutions (see literature). May be given through Y-tube, three-way stopcock, or with additive tubing, or may be added to larger volume of compatible solutions and given over 24 hours or less.

Rate of administration: Each 500 mg or fraction thereof properly diluted over 5 to 10 minutes. When diluted in large volumes of infusion fluids, give at rate prescribed.

Actions: A semisynthetic penicillin, bactericidal against penicillin G–sensitive and resistant strains of *Staphylococcus aureus* as well as other specific gram-positive organisms. Readily absorbed into most body fluids and tissues except spinal fluid. Crosses the placental barrier. Primarily excreted through bile; a small amount is excreted in the urine. Secreted in breast milk.

Indications and uses: Treatment of infections caused by penicillinase-producing staphylococci.

Precautions: (1) Refrigerate unused medication after initial dilution, and discard after 7 days. Stable in specific solutions at concentrations of 2 to 40 mg/ml for 24 hours at room temperature and 96 hours if refrigerated. (2) Sensitivity studies necessary to determine susceptibility of the causative organism to nafcillin; sometimes difficult to determine accurately. (3) Watch for early symptoms of allergic reaction. Individuals with a history of allergic problems are more susceptible to untoward reactions. (4) Avoid prolonged use of the drug; superinfection caused by overgrowth of nonsusceptible organisms may result. (5) Renal, hepatic, and hematopoietic function should be checked during long-term therapy. (6) Inactivated by chloramphenicol, erythromycin, and tetracyclines. Bactericidal action is negated by these drugs. (7) Potentiated by aminohippuric acid and probenecid (Benemid); toxicity may result. (8) May cause thrombophlebitis, especially in the elderly or with too-rapid injection. Change to oral therapy as soon as practical. (9) Inhibits aminoglycosides (e.g., gentamicin). Do not mix in same IV container. (10) Concomitant use with β-adrenergic blockers (e.g., propranolol [Inderal]) may increase risk of ana phylaxis and inhibit treatment. (11) Risk of bleeding with anticoagulants (e.g., heparin) is increased. (12) Inhibits effectiveness of oral contraceptives; breakthrough bleeding or pregnancy could result. (13) Neuromuscular excitability or convulsions may be caused by higher than normal doses. (14) Elimination rate markedly reduced in neonates.

Contraindications: Known hypersensitivity to any penicillin, infants under 1 month of age.

Incompatible with: Aminoglycosides (e.g., gentamicin, kanamycin), aminophylline, ascorbic acid, bleomycin (Blenoxane), hydrocortisone sodium succinate (Solu-Cortef), labetalol (Trandate), methylprednisolone (Solu-Medrol), promazine (Sparine), solutions with a pH below 5.0 or over 8.0, verapamil (Calan), vitamin B complex with C.

Side effects: Relatively infrequent except for sensitivity reactions such as anaphylaxis, skin rashes, and urticaria. Bleeding abnormalities, diarrhea, nausea, pruritus, and vomiting have been reported.

Antidote: Notify the physician immediately of any adverse symptoms. For severe symptoms discontinue the drug, treat allergic reaction (antihistamines, epinephrine, corticosteroids), and resuscitate as necessary. Hemodialysis or peritoneal dialysis is minimally effective in overdose.

NALBUPHINE HYDROCHLORIDE pH 3.5

(Nubain)

Usual dose: 10 mg. Repeat every 3 to 6 hours as necessary. Up to 20 mg can be given in a single dose if required. Maximum total daily dose is 160 mg.

Reduce dose to one fourth if previous medication a narcotic. Observe for symptoms of withdrawal. Increase to effective dose gradually.

Reduced dose may be required in hepatic or renal disease.

Dilution: May be given undiluted.

Rate of administration: Each 10 mg or fraction thereof over 3 to 5 minutes. Frequently titrated according to symptom relief and respiratory rate.

Actions: A synthetic narcotic agonist-antagonist analgesic. It equals morphine in analgesic effect and has one-fourth the antagonist effect of naloxone. Does produce respiratory depression, but this does not increase markedly with increased doses. Pain relief is effected in 2 to 3 minutes and lasts about 3 to 5 hours. Metabolized in the liver. Some excretion in urine. Crosses the placental barrier. Secreted in breast milk.

Indications and uses: (1) Relief of moderate to severe pain; (2) preoperative analgesia; (3) surgical anesthesia supplement; (4) obstetrical analgesia during labor.

Precautions: (1) May precipitate withdrawal symptoms if stopped too quickly after prolonged use or if patient has been on opiates. (2) Oxygen and controlled respiratory equipment must be available. (3) Observe patient frequently and monitor vital signs. (4) Physical dependence can develop with abuse. (5) Potentiated by phenothiazines (e.g., chlorpromazine [Thorazine]), by other CNS depressants such as narcotic analgesics, general anesthetics, alcohol, anticholinergics, antihistamines, barbiturates, cimetidine (Tagamet), hypnotics, neuromuscular blocking agents (e.g., tubocurarine), psychotropic agents, and sedatives. Reduced doses of both drugs may be indicated. (6) Use caution in asthma, respiratory depression or difficulty from any source, impaired renal or hepatic function, and myocardial infarction with nausea and vomiting. (7) Safety for use in pregnancy or lactation not established.

Contraindications: Acute bronchial asthma, hypersensitivity to nalbuphine, upper airway obstruction. Biliary surgery, head injury, pregnancy, lactation, and children under 18 years are probable contraindications.

Incompatible with: Diazepam (Valium), pentobarbital (Nembutal).

Side effects: Anaphylaxis, blurred vision, bradycardia, clammy skin, dizziness, dry mouth, headache, hypertension, hypotension, nausea, respiratory depression, sedation, tachycardia, urinary urgency, vertigo, vomiting.

Antidote: With increasing severity of any side effect or onset of symptoms of overdose, discontinue the drug and notify the physician. Naloxone hydrochloride (Narcan) will reverse respiratory depression. A patent airway, artificial ventilation, oxygen therapy, and other symptomatic treatment must be instituted promptly.

NALOXONE HYDROCHLORIDE pH 3.0 to 4.5

(Narcan)

Usual dose: *Narcotic overdose:* 0.4 to 2 mg. Repeat in 2 to 3 minutes for 3 doses if indicated. If effective, dosage may be repeated as necessary for recurrence of symptoms.

Postoperative narcotic depression: 0.1 to 0.2 mg at 2- to 3-minute intervals to desired response. Titrate to avoid excessive reduction of narcotic analgesic action.

Pediatric dose: Ampoules containing 0.02 mg/ml are available, but larger doses are frequently required. Adult strength is often used to reduce amount of injection and to effect desired response.

Narcotic overdose: 0.01 mg/kg of body weight initially. May repeat as in adult dose. May dilute with sterile water for injection. A single dose of 0.1 mg/kg may be indicated if above dose ineffective.

Postoperative narcotic depression: 0.005 to 0.01 mg IV at 2- to 3-minute intervals to desired response.

Neonatal dose: 0.01 mg/kg of body weight into umbilical vein.

Dilution: May be given undiluted, diluted with sterile water for injection, or further diluted with normal saline or 5% dextrose solution and given as an infusion (2 mg in 500 ml equals a concentration of 0.004 mg/ml).

Rate of administration: Each 0.4 mg or fraction thereof over 15 seconds. Titrate infusion to patient response.

Actions: A potent narcotic antagonist. Overcomes narcotic-induced respiratory depression and other effects of narcotic overdose. Unlike other narcotic antagonists, it does not have any narcotic effect itself. Onset of action is prompt and lasts 1 to 4 hours. Excreted in urine.

Indications and uses: (1) Reversal of narcotic depression; (2) antidote for natural and synthetic narcotics, butorphanol, methadone, nalbuphine, pentazocine, and propoxyphene; (3) diagnosis of acute opiate overdose.

Investigational use: Reversal of alcoholic coma and improvement of circulation in refractory shock.

Precautions: (1) Does not produce respiratory depression with nonnarcotic drug overdose, a beneficial action. (2) It is ineffective against respiratory depression caused by barbiturates, anesthetics, other nonnarcotic agents, or pathological conditions. (3) Symptomatic treatment with oxygen and artificial ventilation as necessary should be continued until naloxone is effective. Observe patient continuously. Duration of narcotic action may exceed that of naloxone. (4) Will precipitate acute withdrawal symptoms in narcotic addicts; use caution, especially with newborns of narcotic-dependent mothers. (5) Use in lactation and pregnancy only when clearly needed. Safety for use not established. (6) Use caution in patients with cardiac disease or those receiving cardiotoxic drugs. (7) Discard infusions after 24 hours.

Contraindications: Known hypersensitivity to naloxone, pregnancy (except during labor).

Incompatible with: Limited information available. Preparations containing bisulfite, sulfite, long chain or high molecular weight anions, solutions with an alkaline pH. Confirm physical and chemical stability before mixing with any drug or agent.

Side effects: Elevated PTT (occasional), hypertension, irritability and increased crying in the newborn, nausea and vomiting, sweating, tachycardia, tremulousness. Overdose postoperatively may result in excitement, hypertension, hypotension, reversal of analgesia, pulmonary edema, ventricular tachycardia and fibrillation.

Antidote: Notify the physician of any side effect. Treatment will probably be symptomatic. Resuscitate as necessary.

NEOSTIGMINE METHYLSULFATE pH 5.9

(Prostigmin)

Usual dose: 0.5 to 2 mg as antidote for tubocurarine and other skeletal relaxants. Repeat as required to restore voluntary respiration. 5 mg is the normal maximum total dose.

Myasthenia gravis: 0.5 mg; titrate carefully; usually given IM.

Pediatric dose: 40 mcg (0.04 mg)/kg of body weight with 20 mcg (0.02 mg)/kg of atropine as antidote for tubocurarine, etc.

Dilution: May be given undiluted. Do not add to IV solutions. May be given through Y-tube or three-way stopcock of infusion set.

Rate of administration: 0.5 mg or fraction thereof over 1 minute.

Actions: An anticholinesterase and antagonist of skeletal muscle relaxants. Inhibits the enzyme cholinesterase, allowing acetylcholine to accumulate at the myoneural junction. Restores normal transmission of nerve impulses and makes muscle contraction stronger and more prolonged.

Indications and uses: (1) Antidote for tubocurarine, atropine, hyoscine; (2) treatment of myasthenia gravis.

Precautions: (1) A physician should be present when this drug is used IV. Confirm ampoule or vial is for IV use. (2) A peripheral nerve stimulator device should be used to monitor effectiveness. (3) Has many additional uses given IM or orally. (4) When used as an antidote for tubocurarine, administer atropine sulfate, 0.6 to 1.2 mg, before IV neostigmine. Pulse rate must be at least 80 beats/min. *Caution:* atropine may mask symptoms of neostigmine overdose. (5) Epinephrine should always be available. (6) Hyperventilate the patient. (7) Use extreme caution and minimum effective dose in small children, cardiac disease, asthma, epilepsy, hypothyroidism, vagotonia, peptic ulcer, and severely ill patients. Titrate exact dose, evaluate response with a peripheral stimulator device. (8) Edrophonium (Tensilon) can differentiate between increased symptoms of myasthenia and cholinergic crisis. (9) Potentiates narcotic analgesics (e.g., morphine, codeine, meperidine) and succinylcholine (Anectine). (10) Antagonizes ganglionic blocking agents (e.g., trimethaphan [Arfonad]) and aminoglycoside antibiotics (e.g., gentamycin [Garamycin]). (11) May be inhibited by corticosteroids and magnesium. (12) May induce premature labor in pregnancy near term. Transient muscular weakness in swallowing, sucking, and breathing has been observed in neonates of myasthenic mothers. Confirm distinction between cholinergic or myasthenic crisis in neonate with edrophonium test. Treat neonate with IM pyridostigmine 0.05 to 0.15 mg/kg of body weight if indicated.

Contraindications: High concentrations of inhalant anesthesia (e.g., halothane, cyclopropane), known sensitivity to bromides and neostigmine, mechanical intestinal or urinary obstruction, patients taking mecamylamine, peritonitis.

Incompatible with: Limited information available. Because of specific use and potential toxicity, neostigmine should not be mixed with any other drug.

Side effects: Usually caused by overdose: abdominal cramps, anorexia, anxiety, bradycardia, cardiac dysrhythmias and arrest, cholinergic crises, cold moist skin, convulsion, diaphoresis, diarrhea, hypotension, increased bronchial secretions, increased lacrimation, increased salivation, miosis, muscle cramps, muscle weakness, nausea, pulmonary edema, vomiting.

Antidote: *Atropine sulfate.* If side effects occur, discontinue drug and notify the physician. Atropine sulfate in doses of 0.6 mg IV will counteract most side effects and may be repeated every 3 to 10 minutes. Endotracheal intubation or tracheostomy is considered prophylactic in anesthesia or crises. Artificial ventilation, oxygen therapy, cardiac monitoring, adequate suctioning, and treatment of shock or convulsions must be instituted and maintained as necessary. Treat allergic reactions with epinephrine. Pralidoxime chloride (PAM) 2 gm IV followed by 250 mg every 5 minutes may be required to reactivate cholinesterase and reverse paralysis.

NETILMICIN SULFATE pH 3.5 to 6.0

(Netromycin)

Usual dose: 1.5 to 3.25 mg/kg of body weight every 12 hours. 1.3 to 2.2 mg/kg every 8 hours in serious systemic infections. Dosage based on ideal weight of lean body mass. Adjust according to severity of infection and to peak and trough concentrations. Normal renal function necessary.

Pediatric dose: *6 weeks to 12 years:* 1.8 to 2.7 mg/kg of body weight every 8 hours or 2.7 to 4 mg/kg every 12 hours. Note caution in Dilution.

Neonatal dose: 2 to 3.25 mg/kg of body weight every 12 hours. Lower doses may be appropriate because of immature kidney function. Note caution in Dilution.

Dilution: Pediatric and Neonatal concentrations have been discontinued. Use extreme caution to ensure correct dose for neonates and children. Begin with 100 mg/ml concentration for adults. Further dilute each single dose in 50 to 200 ml of 0.9% normal saline, 5% dextrose in water, saline, or other compatible solutions (see literature). Decrease volume of diluent for neonates and children based on fluid requirements. Concentrations of 2 to 3 mg/ml acceptable.

Rate of administration: Each single dose over 30 minutes to 2 hours.

Actions: An aminoglycoside antibiotic with neuromuscular blocking action. Bactericidal against specific gram-positive and gram-negative bacilli by interfering with protein synthesis. Well distributed throughout all body fluids. Usual half-life is 2 to 3 hours, half-life prolonged in infants, postpartum females, fever, liver disease and ascites, spinal cord injury, cystic fibrosis, and the elderly; shorter in severe burns. Crosses the placental barrier. Excreted through the kidneys. Secreted in breast milk.

Indications and uses: (1) Short-term treatment of serious infections caused by specific organisms; (2) primarily used when penicillin and other less toxic antibiotics are ineffective or contraindicated; (3) to treat suspected infection in the immunosuppressed patient.

Precautions: (1) Narrow range between toxic and therapeutic levels. Monitor peak and trough concentrations to avoid peak serum concentrations above 16 mcg/ml and trough concentrations above 4 mcg/ml. Desired range is 6 to 10 and 0.5 to 2 mcg/ml, respectively. (2) Synergistic when used in combination with penicillins and cephalosporins. Dose adjustment and appropriate spacing required because of physical incompatibilities and interactions. (3) Use extreme caution if therapy is required over 7 to 10 days; ototoxic and nephrotoxic. (4) Sensitivity studies indicated to determine susceptibility of the causative organism to netilmicin. (5) Reduce daily dose commensurate with amount of renal impairment. Intervals between injections should also be increased. See manufacturer's specific recommendations. (6) Watch for decrease in urine output and rising BUN and serum creatinine. Dosage may require decreasing. Routine serum levels and evaluation of hearing are recommended. (7) Use caution in infants, children, the elderly, and severely burned patients. (8) Potentiated by anesthetics, citrate-anticoagulated blood, other neuromuscular blocking antibiotics (e.g., kanamycin, streptomycin), anticholinesterases (e.g., edrophonium [Tensilon]), antineoplastics (e.g., nitrogen mustard, cisplatin), barbiturates, muscle relaxants (e.g., tubocurarine), phenothiazines (e.g., promethazine [Phenergan]), procainamide, quinidine, and sodium citrate. *Apnea can occur.* (9) Also potentiated by other ototoxic drugs (e.g., cephalosporins, ethacrynic acid [Edecrin]), and all potent diuretics. An elevated serum level of netilmicin may occur, increasing nephrotoxicity and neurotoxicity. (10) Superinfection may occur from overgrowth of nonsusceptible organisms. (11) Maintain good hydration. (12) Stable for up to 72 hours. (13) Use only if absolutely necessary in pregnancy and lactation.

Contraindications: Known netilmicin or aminoglycoside sensitivity, renal failure.

Incompatible with: Administer separately. Inactivated in solution with carbenicillin, other penicillins, and most cephalosporins. Amphotericin B, cefamandole (Mandol), cephalothin (Keflin), dopamine (Intropin), furosemide (Lasix), heparin, vitamin B complex.

Side effects: Occur more frequently with impaired renal function, higher doses, or prolonged administration.

Minor: Anorexia, burning, dizziness, fever, headache, hypertension, hypotension, itching, lethargy, muscle twitching, nausea, numbness, rash, roaring in ears, tingling sensation, tinnitus, urticaria, vomiting, weight loss.

Major: Blood dyscrasias; convulsions; elevated bilirubin, BUN, serum creatinine, SGOT, and SGPT; hearing loss; laryngeal edema; neuromuscular blockade; oliguria; respiratory arrest.

Antidote: Notify the physician of all side effects. If minor side effects persist or any major symptom appears, discontinue the drug and notify physician. Treatment is symptomatic. In overdose, hemodialysis may be indicated. Complexation with ticarcillin or carbenicillin may be as effective as hemodialysis. Consider exchange transfusion in the newborn. Calcium salts or neostigmine may reverse neuromuscular blockade. Resuscitate as necessary.

NICOTINAMIDE AND NICOTINIC ACID — pH 6.0 to 6.5

(Niacin, Niacinamide)

Usual dose: 25 to 100 mg 2 or more times in 24 hours may be given. Up to 3 Gm/24 hr is unusual but acceptable. Dosage determined by response. Maintain with oral dosage as soon as feasible.

Dilution: 50 to 100 mg or more may be diluted in 500 ml of isotonic sodium chloride. May be given undiluted.

Rate of administration: IV infusion may be given at a prescribed rate not to exceed the recommended rate for undiluted solution. Larger doses may extend over 12 to 24 hours. Undiluted nicotinic acid should be given at a rate not to exceed 2 mg or fraction thereof over 1 minute.

Actions: Nicotinic acid is a water-soluble vitamin that is converted to niacinamide in the body. It is essential to the metabolic activity of all living cells. Nicotinic acid produces marked peripheral vasodilation; nicotinamide does not. Metabolized in the liver, excess is excreted in the urine.

Indications and uses: Treatment of acute pellagra, which usually occurs secondary to an underlying disease.

Precautions: (1) Other B vitamins are also indicated. (2) Use caution in patients with severe diabetes, history of peptic ulcer, impaired liver function, gallbladder disease, gout, pregnancy, lactation, women of childbearing age, and aspirin sensitivity. (3) Large doses may increase blood glucose levels. (4) Begin therapy with small doses and increase gradually. (5) Potentiates some antihypertensive drugs. (6) May potentiate vasodilation with adrenergic blocking drugs (e.g., isoproterenol, dopamine). (7) Inhibits probenecid and sulfinpyrazone.

Contraindications: Active acute peptic ulcer, arterial bleeding, hemorrhage, hepatic dysfunction, hypersensitivity, serious hypotension.

Incompatible with: Alkalies, erythromycin, kanamycin (Kantrex).

Side effects: Expected to occur with nicotinic acid but not with nicotinamide; sometimes violent flushing with tingling, burning, and itching of the skin accompanied by an overwhelming sensation of heat is most uncomfortable for the patient. Occasionally dizziness, faintness, nausea, and vomiting occur. These symptoms are transient and subside without ill effects. With large doses, activation of peptic ulcer, abnormal liver function tests, hyperuricemia, hypotension, skin rash, or dryness may occur. Anaphylaxis is rare but may occur.

Antidote: Discontinue the drug and notify the physician of severe side effects. Treat anaphylaxis and resuscitate as necessary.

NITROGLYCERIN IV pH 3.0 to 6.5

(Nitro-Bid IV, Nitrostat IV, Tridil)

Usual dose: 5 mcg/min initially. Increase by 5 mcg/min increments every 3 to 5 minutes until some blood pressure response is noted. Reduce increments and/or increase time to fine-tune to desired hemodynamic response. If no response at 20 mcg/min, 10 mcg/min increases may be used. No fixed optimum dose.

Dilution: Available premixed in 250 ml 5% dextrose in water with 25, 50, or 100 mg nitroglycerin. All other preparations must be diluted and administered as an infusion. Use only glass infusion bottles and specific (non-polyvinyl chloride) infusion tubing (provided by manufacturer). Do not use filters. Dilute in a given amount of 5% dextrose or 0.9% normal saline for infusion. Concentration dependent on initial preparation (0.8 mg/ml or 5 mg/ml) and patient fluid tolerances. 10 ml of 0.8 mg/ml in 250 ml diluent equals 32 mcg/ml (in 1,000 ml, 8 mcg/ml). 10 ml of 5 mg/ml in 250 ml diluent equals 200 mcg/ml (in 1,000 ml, 50 mcg/ml). May be used in dilutions from 25 to 500 mcg/ml.

Rate of administration: Dependent on patient response and effective dose. Specific adjustments required, see Usual dose. Use extreme caution in patients responsive to initial 5 mcg/min dose. Decrease adjustments and increase time between doses as patient begins to respond. Use of an infusion pump or microdrip (60 gtt/ml) required. Exact and constant delivery mandatory.

Actions: A smooth muscle relaxant and vasodilator. Affects arterial and venous beds. Reduces myocardial oxygen consumption, preload, and afterload by reducing systolic, diastolic, and mean arterial blood pressure; central venous and pulmonary capillary wedge pressures; and pulmonary and systemic vascular resistance. Effective coronary perfusion is usually maintained. Widely distributed throughout the body. Onset of action occurs in 1 to 2 minutes and lasts 3 to 5 minutes. Some excretion in urine.

Indications and uses: (1) Control of blood pressure in perioperative hypertension (especially cardiovascular procedures); (2) congestive heart failure in presence of acute myocardial infarction; (3) treatment of angina pectoris if patient unresponsive to therapeutic doses of organic nitrates and/or a β-blocker; (4) controlled hypotension during surgical procedures.

Precautions: (1) Special tubing causes problems with infusion pump control. Patient may still be receiving nitroglycerin even though pump is off or tubing clamped. Low flow rates may actually be higher and not deliver accurate dosage. (2) Plastic (polyvinyl chloride) tubing or containers will absorb up to 80% of diluted nitroglycerin. Use extreme caution and adjust dosage if changing tubing, using extension tubings, etc. Absorption greatest with slowest rate. (3) If changing preparations from 0.8 mg/ml to 5.0 mg/ml, use new tubing or clear tubing with a minimum of 15 ml, adjust dosage carefully, and observe effects. (4) Protect vials from light. Solution stable for up to 48 hours. (5) Maintain adequate systemic blood pressure and coronary perfusion pressure. Heart rate and blood pressure measurements mandatory, pulmonary wedge pressure recommended. (6) Use caution in patients with low left ventricular filling pressure or low pulmonary capillary wedge pressure. May have exaggerated response to low dosage. (7) Observe for tachycardia, which can decrease diastolic filling time. (8) Observe for fall in pulmonary wedge pressure. Precedes arterial hypotension and impending shock. Reduce or discontinue drug temporarily. (9) Reduce dose gradually to prevent rebound symptoms. (10) Potentiated by alcohol, antihypertensives, β-adrenergic blockers (e.g., propranolol [Inderal]), other vasodilators, phenothiazines (e.g., prochlorperazine [Compazine]), and tricyclic antidepressants. (11) Inhibited by sympathomimetics (phenylephrine, epinephrine). (12) Inhibits acetylcholine, histamine, norepinephrine (e.g., dopamine [Intropin]). (13) Potentiates nondepolarizing muscle relaxants (e.g., tubocurarine [Curare]), may cause apnea. (14) Use caution in hepatic or renal disease, pericarditis, or postural hypotension. (15) May cause marked orthostatic hypotension with calcium channel blockers (e.g., verapamil [Isoptin]).

Contraindications: Hypersensitivity to nitrates, hypotension or uncorrected hypovolemia, cerebral hemorrhage, head trauma, increased intracranial pressure, pericardial tamponade, constrictive pericarditis. Safety for use in pregnancy and lactation and in children not established.

Incompatible with: Manufacturer states, "Do not admix with any other drug."

Side effects: Abdominal pain, angina, apprehension, dizziness, headache, hypotension, methemoglobinemia, muscle twitching, nausea, palpitations, postural hypotension, restlessness, retrosternal discomfort, tachycardia, vomiting. Severe hypotension may result in shock, reflex paradoxical bradycardia, inadequate cerebral circulation, constrictive pericarditis, pericardial tamponade, decreased organ perfusion, and death.

Antidote: Notify physician of all side effects. For accidental overdose with severe hypotension and reflex tachycardia and/or fall in pulmonary wedge pressure, reduce rate or temporarily discontinue until condition stabilizes. Lower head of bed (Trendelenburg position). Administer IV fluids. An α-adrenergic agonist (methoxamine [Vasoxyl] or phenylephrine [Neo-Synephrine]) is rarely required. Epinephrine and related compounds (dopamine) are contraindicated. Treat methemoglobinemia with methylene blue 0.2 ml/kg of body weight (1 to 2 mg/kg) IV and high flow oxygen. Treat anaphylaxis and resuscitate as necessary.

NITROPRUSSIDE SODIUM — pH 3.5 to 6.0

(Nipride, Nitropress)

Usual dose: 3 mcg/kg of body weight/min. Reduce dose to as little as 0.5 mcg/kg/min in patients who are receiving other antihypertensive agents by any route. Do not exceed 10 mcg/kg/min. If 10 mcg/kg/min does not promote adequate blood pressure reduction in 10 minutes, discontinue administration and use another antihypertensive agent.

Pediatric dose: 1.4 mcg (0.0014 mg)/kg/min, adjusted slowly to individual response.

Dilution: Each 50 mg must be dissolved with 2 to 3 ml of 5% dextrose in water. Further dilute this stock solution in a minimum of 250 ml of 5% dextrose in water. Must be administered as an infusion. Larger amounts of solution may be used. 50 mg in 250 ml equals 200 mcg/ml. 50 mg in 500 ml equals 100 mcg/ml. No other diluent may be used. Immediately after mixing, wrap infusion bottle in aluminum foil to protect from light.

Rate of administration: Use flow rate required to reduce blood pressure gradually to preset or desired levels. Do not exceed maximum dose. Response should be noted almost immediately. Use an infusion pump or a microdrip (60 gtt/ml) to regulate dosage accurately.

Actions: A potent, rapid-acting antihypertensive agent. Produces peripheral vasodilation through direct action on smooth muscle of the blood vessels. Effective almost immediately. Will lower diastolic blood pressure 30% to 40% or more below pretreatment levels. Increases cardiac output. Effectiveness ends when IV infusion is stopped. Blood pressure will return to pretreatment levels in 1 to 10 minutes. Rapidly converted to thiocyanate and eventually excreted in the urine.

Indications and uses: Drug of choice for hypertensive emergencies, cardiogenic shock, controlled hypotension during anesthesia.

Investigational uses: (1) Alone or in combination with dopamine to reduce afterload in hypertensive patient with myocardial infarction, persistent chest pain, or left ventricular failure and in severe refractory congestive heart failure; (2) to treat lactic acidosis due to impaired peripheral perfusion and to attenuate vasoconstrictor effects of dopamine and norepinephrine.

Precautions: (1) Use only freshly prepared solutions; usually discard infusion within 4 hours of mixing. (Literature now states "stable to 24 hours.") Avoid use of filters; some absorb nitroglycerin. (2) Solution has a faint brownish tint; discard immediately if highly colored, blue, green, or dark red. (3) Determine patency of vein, avoid extravasation. (4) Check blood pressure every 1 minute until stabilized at the desired level and every 5 to

15 minutes thereafter during therapy. Continuous monitoring is preferred. Never allow systolic blood pressure to fall below 60 mm Hg. (5) Monitor pulmonary wedge pressure in patients with myocardial infarction or severe congestive heart failure. (6) Oral hypertensive agents may be given concomitantly to maintain ongoing blood pressure regulation. Reduced nitroprusside dosage may be indicated. (7) Use caution in hypothyroidism, liver or renal impairment, and the elderly. (8) Safety for use in pregnancy and in children not yet established. Discontinue breast feeding. (9) In long-term use, measure blood thiocyanate levels daily. Must not exceed 10 mg/dl. Cyanide toxicity may be prevented with hydroxocobalamin. (10) Potentiated by ganglionic blocking agents (e.g., pentolinium [Ansolysen]), volatile liquid anesthesia (e.g., halothane), and circulatory depressants. (11) In controlled hypotension, monitor blood loss and correct hypovolemia before and during surgery.

Contraindications: Compensatory hypertension, e.g., arteriovenous shunt or coarctation of the aorta; known inadequate cerebral circulation; emergency surgery on moribund patients.

Incompatible with: Consider incompatible in solution with any other drug.

Side effects: Usually occur with too rapid rate of infusion and are reversible: abdominal pain, apprehension, coma, diaphoresis, dizziness, dyspnea, headache, muscle twitching, nausea, palpitations, profound hypotension, restlessness, retching, retrosternal discomfort, tachyphylaxis. With prolonged therapy or overdose, hypothyroidism and/or cyanide intoxication can occur.

Antidote: At first sign of side effects, decrease rate of administration. If blood pressure begins to rise or side effects persist, notify the physician. Hemodialysis or peritoneal dialysis may be indicated for thiocyanate levels over 10 mg/dl. For massive overdose with signs of cyanide toxicity or tachyphylaxis, discontinue nitroprusside. Administer amyl nitrite inhalations for 15 to 30 seconds each minute until 3% sodium nitrite solution can be initiated as an IV infusion. Do not exceed a rate of 2.5 to 5 ml 3% sodium nitrite solution/min to a total dose of 10 to 15 ml. Monitor blood pressure carefully. Next, inject sodium thiosulfate 12.5 Gm in

50 ml of 5% dextrose in water IV over 10 minutes. Observe patient. If signs of overdose reappear, repeat the above process but use one-half the dosage. Correct hypotension with vasopressors (e.g., dopamine [Intropin]).

NOREPINEPHRINE pH 3.0 to 4.5

(Levarterenol bitartrate, Levophed)

Usual dose: 8 to 12 mcg/min initially, then adjust to maintain desired blood pressure range, usually 2 to 4 mcg/min. Larger doses may be given safely as long as the patient remins hypotensive and blood volume depletion is corrected.

Pediatric dose: 1 to 2 mcg/min adjusted to maintain desired blood pressure.

Dilution: Must bc diluted in 500 to 1,000 ml of 5% dextrose in water or saline and given as an IV infusion. Average dose dilution is 4 ml (8 mg of 0.2% solution) to each 1 L of diluent. This dilution equals 8 mcg/ml. More or less may be added to each 1 L of diluent, depending on clinical fluid volume requirements. Administration in a dextrose solution reduces loss of potency resulting from oxidation. Normal saline without dextrose is not recommended.

Rate of administration: Begin with 2 to 3 ml/min of infusion. Use the slowest possible flow rate to correct hypotension gradually and maintain adequate or preset blood pressure. Some response should be noted within 1 to 2 minutes of IV administration. Use of an infusion pump or microdrip (60 gtt/ml) is an aid to correct evaluation of dosage.

Actions: Levarterenol is the levo isomer of norepinephrine, a sympathomimetic drug and powerful vasoconstrictor. Greatly increases blood flow to all vital organs without increasing the workload or output of the heart. Dilates the coronary arteries more than twice as much as epinephrine can. It is rapidly inactivated in the body by various enzymes and excreted in changed form in the urine.

Indications and uses: All hypotensive states, including anesthesia, blood reactions, drug reactions, hemorrhage, myocardial infarction, pheochromocytomectomy, septicemia, surgery, sympathectomy, and trauma.

Precautions: (1) Check blood pressure every 2 minutes until stabilized at the desired level. Check every 5 minutes thereafter during therapy. Avoid hypertension. (2) Observe for hypovolemia and replace fluids immediately. In an emergency, levarterenol can be effective in a hypovolemic state before fluid replacement has been accomplished. (3) Check flow rate and injection site constantly. (4) Infusion should be through a large vein, preferably the antecubital vein, to prevent complications of prolonged peripheral vasoconstriction. Avoid veins in the hands, ankles, and legs. Use of the femoral vein may be considered. (5) Causes severe tissue necrosis, sloughing, and gangrene. Insert a plastic IV catheter or similar intravascular device at least 6 inches long well into the large vein chosen to prevent extravasation into any surrounding tissue. (6) Blanching along the vein pathway is a preliminary sign of extravasation. Change the injection site. (7) Whole blood or plasma should be given in a separate IV site. May be given through Y-tube connection. (8) Use caution in the elderly and in those with peripheral vascular disease. (9) Phentolamine (Regitine) 5 to 10 mg and/or heparin sodium 10 mg have been recommended by some authorities to prevent any sloughing, necrosis, and/or thrombosis from slight leakage along the vein pathway. These are added with the levarterenol to 500 ml of the diluent. (10) Therapy may be continued until the patient can maintain his own blood pressure. Decrease dosage gradually. (11) Hazardous when potentiated by amphetamines, antihistamines, tricyclic antidepressants (e.g., desipramine [Norpramine]), MAO inhibitors (e.g., isocarboxazid [Marplan]), Rauwolfia alkaloids (e.g., reserpine), thyroid preparations, and methylphenidate (Ritalin). (12) Interacts in numerous and sometimes contradictory ways with many drugs. (13) May cause severe hypertension with ergot alkaloids. (14) Will cause hypotension and bradycardia with hydantoins (e.g., phenytoin [Dilantin]).

Contraindications: Do not use in hypotension from blood

loss unless an emergency, in mesenteric or peripheral vascular thrombosis, or with cyclopropane or halothane (inhalant) anesthesias.

Incompatible with: Aminophylline, amobarbital (Amytal), ampicillin (Polycillin), ascorbic acid, cephalothin (Keflin), cephapirin (Cefadyl), chlorpheniramine (ChlorTrimeton), chlorothiazide (Diuril), diazepam (Valium), heparin, metaraminol (Aramine), methicillin (Staphcillin), oxytocin (Pitocin, Syntocinon), pentobarbital (Nembutal), phenobarbital (Luminal), phenytoin (Dilantin), secobarbital (Seconal), sodium bicarbonate, sodium iodide, streptomycin, tetracycline (Achromycin), thiopental (Pentothal), warfarin (Coumadin), whole blood.

Side effects: Rare when used as directed; bradycardia, chest pain, decreased cardiac output, headache, ischemia, necrosis caused by extravasation, pallor, photophobia, seizures, ventricular tachycardia, vomiting.

Antidote: To prevent sloughing and necrosis in areas where extravasation has occurred, with a fine hypodermic needle inject 5 to 10 mg of phentolamine (Regitine) diluted in 10 to 15 ml of normal saline liberally throughout the tissue in the extravasated area. Treatment should be started as soon as extravasation is recognized. Atropine may be used to counteract the bradycardia. Notify physician of any side effect. Should a sudden or uncontrolled hypertensive state occur, discontinue levarterenol, notify the physician, and treat with antihypertensive agents such as phentolamine (Regitine) or phenoxybenzamine (Dibenzyline).

NORMAL SERUM ALBUMIN (HUMAN)

pH 6.4 to 7.4

(Albuminar-5 & -25, Albutein 5% & 25%, Buminate 5% & 25% Plasbumin-5 & -25)

Usual dose: Variable, depending on hemoglobin and hematocrit and amount of pulmonary or venous congestion present. Range is from 5 to 75 Gm/24 hr. Available as 5% solution (5 Gm/dl) in 50 ml, 250 ml, 500 ml, and 1,000 ml vials, or 25% solution (25 Gm/dl) in 20 ml, 50 ml, and 100 ml vials. Maximum dose is 250 Gm in 48 hours.

Hypoproteinemia: 1 ml/lb of body weight/24 hr of 25% solution. Up to 75 Gm may be used.

Burns: Maintain albumin level from 2.5 to just below 4 Gm/dl.

Shock: Initial dose determined by patient's condition.

Pediatric dose: 5 to 25 Gm/24 hr. 25% solution is usually used in infants and children.

Erythroblastosis fetalis: 1 Gm/kg of body weight 1 to 2 hours before blood transfusion or with transfusion (exchange 50 ml of albumin 25% for 50 ml plasma).

Hypoproteinemia in premature infants: 3 to 4 ml/lb of body weight.

Dilution: May be given undiluted in solution (preferred) or further diluted with normal saline or 5% glucose for infusion.

Rate of administration: Variable, depending on indication, present blood volume, patient response, and concentration of solution. Any rate greater than 10 ml/min may cause hypotension. Averages are:

Normal blood volume: 1 to 2 ml/min.

Deficient blood volume: 25 to 50 Gm as rapidly as tolerated. 25 Gm may be repeated in 15 to 30 minutes.

Hypoproteinemia: 2 to 3 ml/min.

Shock: 1 ml/min if normal blood volume present. A more rapid rate may be utilized in hypovolemia.

Rate of administration in infants and children should be about one-fourth to one-half the adult rate.

Actions: A sterile natural plasma protein substance prepared by a specific process, which makes it free from the danger of serum hepatitis. Expands blood volume proportionately to amount of circulating blood, prevents marked hemoconcentration, aids in reduction of edema, and raises serum protein levels. Low sodium content helps to maintain electrolyte balance and should promote diuresis in presence of edema (contains 130 to 160 mEq sodium/L).

Indications and uses: (1) Shock, actual or impending (5% or 25%); (2) burns (5% or 25%); (3) hypoproteinemia with or without edema until cause determined and corrected (5% or 25%); (4) nephrosis (25); (5) hepatic cirrhosis (5% or 25%); (6) cerebral edema (5% or 25%); (7) erythrocyte resuspension (25%); (8) adult respiratory distress syndrome (25%); (9) cardiopulmonary bypass (25%); (10) hyperbilirubinemia or erythroblastosis fetalis as adjunct to exchange transfusion (25%); (11) sequestration of protein-rich fluids in conditions such as peritonitis, pancreatitis, mediastinitis, and extensive cellulitis (5% or 25%).

Precautions: (1) Use only clear solutions. (2) Store at room temperature below 37° C (98.6° F). Use promptly after opening. (3) Whole blood or packed cells are adjunctive to use of large amounts of serum albumin to prevent anemia. (4) Monitor blood pressure. (5) Hemoglobin, hematocrit, electrolyte, and serum protein evaluations are mandatory during therapy. Alkaline phosphatase may be elevated. (6) Observe patient carefully for increased bleeding resulting from more normal blood pressure, circulatory embarrassment, pulmonary edema, or lack of diuresis. Central venous pressure readings are most helpful. (7) Use caution in hypertension, low cardiac reserve, hepatic or renal failure, or lack of albumin deficiency. (8) The 5% product is isotonic and osmotically approximates human plasma. One volume of 25% to four volumes of diluent is isotonic. 25 Gm of albumin is the osmotic equivalent of 2 units of fresh frozen plasma. 25 Gm of albumin provides as much plasma protein as 500 ml of plasma or 2 units of whole blood. (9) Maintain hydration with additional fluids. (10) Albumin is not a source of nutrition.

Contraindications: Anemia (severe), cardiac failure, history of allergic reaction to albumin, normal or increased intravascular volume

Incompatible with: Ionosol D-CM, Ionosol G with dextrose 10%.

Side effects: *Minor:* Fever, nausea, salivation, vomiting.

Major: Circulatory failure, dyspnea, elevated central venous pressure, precipitous hypotension, pulmonary edema.

Antidote: Notify the physician of all side effects. Minor side effects are generally tolerated and treated symptomatically. For major side effects, discontinue albumin and treat symptomatically. Resuscitate as necessary.

OCTREOTIDE ACETATE

(Sandostatin)

Usual dose: Usually given SC (see Precautions). Initial dose is 50 mcg once or twice daily. In all situations begin with this lower dose and increase gradually based on patient response and tolerance.

Carcinoid tumors: 100 to 600 mcg/24 hr in equally divided doses 2 to 4 times daily during first 2 weeks of therapy. Average total daily dose ranges from 300 to 450 mcg, but therapeutic response is obtained with ranges from 50 to 750 mcg. Up to 1,500 mcg/day has been used in selected patients.

Vasoactive intestinal peptide tumors: 200 to 300 mcg/24 hr in equally divided doses 2 to 4 times daily during first 2 weeks of therapy. Average total daily dose ranges from 150 to 750 mcg but therapeutic response usually achieved with doses under 450 mcg/24 hr.

In all situations dosage adjustment may be required on a daily basis to maintain symptomatic control. After initial 2 weeks of therapy, gradually decrease dose to achieve therapeutically effective maintenance dose.

Pediatric dose: 1 to 10 mcg/kg of body weight/24 hr. Experience is limited, but seems to be well tolerated in infants and young children.

Dilution: May be given undiluted.

Rate of administration: A single dose over at least 1 minute.

Actions: A long-acting octapeptide. Mimics the actions of the natural hormone somatostatin, suppressing secretion of serotonin, gastroenteropancreatic peptides (e.g., gastrin, vasoactive intestinal peptide, insulin, glucagon, secretin, motilin, pancreatic polypeptide), and growth hormone. Decreases splanchnic blood flow. Readily absorbed, and about 65% bound to plasma protein. Half-life longer than the natural hormone (1.5 hours compared to 1 to 3 minutes). Action may extend to 12 hours. Some excreted unchanged in urine.

Indications and uses: (1) To suppress or inhibit the severe diarrhea and flushing episodes associated with carcinoid tumors; (2) treatment of profuse watery diarrhea associated with vasoactive intestinal peptide tumors (VIPomas).

Precautions: (1) IV use is limited to emergency situations. SC injection with rotation of injection sites is preferred route of administration. (2) Can alter fat absorption and decrease gallbladder motility; observe for gallbladder disease. Baseline and periodic ultrasound of gallbladder and bile ducts indicated in long-term SC therapy. Periodic fecal fat and carotene studies also indicated. (3) Half-life markedly extended in severe renal failure requiring dialysis. Reduction of maintenance dose indicated. (4) May decrease size of tumors and slow rate of growth and metastases. Data not definitive. (5) Observe for transient hyper- or hypoglycemia during induction and dosage changes because of changes in balance of hormones (e.g., insulin, glucagon, growth hormone). (6) Use caution in patients with diabetes; requirements for insulin, sulfonylureas, and diazoxide may be reduced. (7) Monitor fluids and electrolytes carefully. (8) Use caution in patients receiving concomitant β-blockers (e.g., atenolol [Tenormin], propranolol [Inderal] or any agents used for fluid and electrolyte balance. Will require adjustment in these therapies as symptoms are controlled by octreotide. (9) 5-HIAA, plasma serotonin, and plasma substance P may be useful laboratory studies to evaluate patient response with carcinoid tumor. Measurement of plasma vasoactive intestinal peptide will be helpful in VIPoma. (10) May inhibit effectiveness of cyclosporine and may result in transplant rejection. (11) Monitor baseline and periodic thryoid function tests, especially in long-term SC therapy. (12) Although studies do not indicate harm to the fetus, use in pregnancy and lactation only if clearly needed. (13) Store in refrigerator (2° to 8° C [36° to 46° F]); may store at room temperature on day of use.

Contraindications: Sensitivity to octreotide acetate or any of its components.

Incompatible with: Specific information not available. Consider specific use.

Side effects: Most side effects are of mild to moderate severity and of short duration. Abdominal pain/discomfort, abnormal stools, anxiety, anorexia, cholelithiasis, constipation, convulsions, depression, diarrhea, dizziness, drowsiness, fatigue, fat malabsorption, flatulence, fluttering sensation, GI bleeding, headache, heartburn, hepatitis, hyperesthesia, hyperglycemia, hypoglycemia, increase in liver enzymes, insomnia, irritability, jaundice, nausea, pounding in the head, rectal spasm, swollen stomach, vomiting. Many other side effects occur in less than 1% of patients.

Antidote: Keep physician informed of all side effects. A dose adjustment of either octreotide or other concomitant therapies may be required. Symptomatic and supportive treatment may be indicated. Overdose will cause hyperglycemia or hypoglycemia depending on tumor involved and endocrine status of patient. Discontinue ostreotide temporarily, notify the physician, and monitor the patient carefully. Symptomatic treatment should be sufficient.

ONDANSETRON HYDROCHLORIDE pH 3.3 to 4.0

(Zofran)

Usual dose: 0.15 mg/kg of body weight 30 minutes before giving emetogenic cancer chemotherapy (e.g., cisplatin, methotrexate). Repeat at 4 and 8 hours after the first dose. No dose adjustment required for the elderly or in renal or hepatic disease.

Pediatric dose: *Children 4 to 18 years of age:* Identical to adult dose.

Dilution: A single dose should be diluted in 50 ml of normal saline or 5% dextrose in water, 0.45%, or normal saline.

Rate of administration: A single dose equally distributed over 15 minutes.

Actions: A selective antagonist of serotonin receptors. Chemotherapeutic agents such as cisplatin increase the release of serotonin from specific cells in the GI tract causing emesis. By antagonizing these receptors, chemotherapy-induced nausea and vomiting are prevented. Lacks the activity at dopamine receptors of metoclopramide (Reglan), so it does not cause sedation. No correlation between plasma levels and antiemetic activity. Metabolized by specific hepatic enzymes; onset of action is prompt and lasts about 4 hours. May last only 2 to 3 hours in children under 15 years of age. Excreted in feces and urine. May be secreted in breast milk.

Indications and uses: Prevention of nausea and vomiting associated with initial and repeat courses of emetogenic cancer chemotherapy, including high-dose cisplatin, nonplatinum agents, and radiation. Has been shown to be effective with cyclophosphamide (Cytoxan), doxorubicin (Adriamycin), etoposide (VePesid), fluorouracil (Adrucil), ifosfamide (Ifex), methotrexate (Folex), mitoxantrone (Novantrone), and vincristine (Oncovin).

Experimental use: (1) As an antianxiety agent. Thought to be as effective as diazepam (Valium) with no rebound anxiety or sedation; (2) treatment of schizophrenia.

Precautions: (1) Even though metabolized in the liver and changes in clearance rates do occur, no specific drug interactions requiring dose adjustments have been identified. (2) No evidence of impaired fertility or harm to fetus. Use in pregnancy only if potential benefit justifies potential risk. (3) Use caution if required during lactation. (4) Safety for use in children under 3 years of age not established. (5) Stool softeners or laxatives may be required to prevent constipation.

Contraindications: Hypersensitivity to ondansetron.

Incompatible with: Specific information not available. Consider specific use.

Side effects: Abdominal pain or discomfort, constipation, cramps, dizziness, faintness, headache, lightheadedness, transient elevation of AST or ALT. Other side effects have occurred (e.g., bronchospasm, extrapyramidal reaction, rash) in fewer than 1% of patients.

Antidote: Most side effects will be treated symptomatically. Keep physician informed as indicated. Overdose of 10 times the usual dose has not caused significant problems. Treat anaphylaxis and resuscitate as necessary.

ORPHENADRINE CITRATE — pH 5.0 to 6.0

(Banflex, Flexoject, Flexon, Myolin, Neocyten, Norflex, O-Flex, Orphenate)

Usual dose: 60 mg (2 ml) every 12 hours.

Dilution: May be given undiluted, or a single dose may be diluted in 5 to 10 ml of sterile water for injection.

Rate of administration: 60 mg or fraction thereof over 5 minutes.

Actions: A diphenhydramine derivative with anticholinergic effects. Produces long-acting muscle relaxation through interneuronal blocking activity, with minimum toxic effects. Excreted in feces and urine.

Indications and uses: (1) Acute spasm of voluntary muscle, especially posttraumatic, discogenic, and tension spasms; (2) treatment of nicotine-induced convulsions.

Precautions: (1) Equal effectiveness produced by IM or oral route. Use IV only when necessary for rapid onset of action. (2) Keep patient in recumbent position for at least 15 minutes to avoid postural hypotension. (3) Use caution in tachycardia, cardiac dysrhythmias, cardiac decompensation, coronary insufficiency, pregnancy, and lactation. (4) Not recommended for concomitant use with propoxyphene (Darvon) or perphenazine (Trilafon). (5) Potentiates anticholinergic drugs and thiazide diuretics. (6) Absorption of many oral drugs inhibited or potentiated due to decreased GI motility. (7) Inhibits haloperidol and phenothiazines (e.g., prochlorperazine [Compazine]). (8) Not recommended for children.

Contraindications: Achalasia, bladder neck obstruction, cardiospasm, glaucoma, hypersensitivity to orphenadrine citrate, myasthenia gravis, pregnancy and lactation, prostatic hypertrophy, pyloric or duodenal obstruction, stenosing peptic ulcer.

Incompatible with: No specific information available. Note Precautions and Contraindications.

Side effects: Usually associated with higher doses or too rapid administration: blurred vision, dizziness, drowsiness, dryness of mouth, excitation, headache, lightheadedness, nausea, palpitations, pupil dilation, tachycardia, urinary retention, urticaria, vomiting, weakness.

Overdose: Deep coma, tonic and clonic seizures, shock, respiratory arrest, death.

Antidote: Notify the physician of any side effects. Reduction of dosage will probably relieve them. For symptoms of hypersensitivity, discontinue the drug, notify the physician, and treat symptomatically. Treat overdose promptly. Resuscitate as necessary.

OXACILLIN SODIUM pH 8.0

(Bactocill, Prostaphlin)

Usual dose: *Over 40 kg (88 lb):* 250 mg to 1 Gm or more every 4 to 6 hours. Maximum dose is 12 Gm/24 hr.
Under 40 kg: 50 to 100 mg/kg of body weight/24 hr in equally divided doses every 6 hours. Maximum dose is 200 mg/kg/24 hr.

Infant dose: *Premature infants and neonates:* 25 mg/kg of body weight/24 hr in equally divided doses every 6 hours.

Dilution: Each 500 mg or fraction thereof should be diluted in 5 ml of sterile water or sodium chloride for injection. May be further diluted in 5% dextrose in water or saline, normal saline, lactated Ringer's solution, or other compatible IV solutions (see literature).

Rate of administration: 1 Gm (10 ml) or fraction thereof slowly over 10 minutes. May be administered in specific IV solutions (check literature) over a 6-hour period. Concentration should be about 2 mg/ml.

Actions: A semisynthetic penicillin with bactericidal effect against penicillinase-producing organisms. Easily absorbed. Evidenced in most body fluids, including trace amounts in spinal fluid. Crosses the placental barrier. Excreted primarily in the urine. Secreted in breast milk.

Indications and uses: Infection caused by penicillinase-producing staphylococci.

Precautions: (1) Sensitivity studies necessary to determine susceptibility of the causative organism to oxacillin. (2) Superinfection caused by overgrowth of nonsusceptible organisms is a possibility. (3) Periodic liver, kidney, and hematopoietic studies are advised. (4) Limited experience in use on premature infants and neonates. Use with caution. Elimination rate markedly reduced in neonates. (5) Diluted solution stable for no more than 6 hours. (6) May be used concurrently with aminoglycosides (e.g., gentamicin [Garamycin]) but must be administered in separate infusions; inactivates aminoglycosides. (7) Inactivated by chloramphenicol, erythromycin, and tetracyclines. Bactericidal action is actually negated by these drugs. (8) Potentiated by probenecid (Benemid); toxicity may result. (9) May potentiate heparin. (10) Concomitant use with β-adrenergic blockers (e.g., propranolol [Inderal]) may increase risk of anaphylaxis and inhibit treatment. (11) Neuromuscular excitability or convulsions may be caused by higher than normal doses. (12) May inhibit effectiveness of oral contraceptives; breakthrough bleeding or pregnancy could result. (13) Change to oral therapy as soon as practical.

Contraindications: Known sensitivity to any penicillin or cephalothin.

Incompatible with: Amikacin (Amikin), levarterenol (Levophed), metaraminol (Aramine), tetracycline (Achromycin), verapamil (Calan).

Side effects: Relatively infrequent: diarrhea, hepatic dysfunction, elevated SGOT, hypersensitivity with anaphylaxis, nausea, pruritus, skin rash, thrombophlebitis, transient hematuria in newborns, urticaria, vomiting.

Antidote: Notify the physician of any adverse symptoms. For severe symptoms, discontinue the drug, treat allergic reaction (antihistamines, epinephrine, corticosteroids), and resuscitate as necessary. Hemodialysis or peritoneal dialysis is minimally effective in overdose.

OXYMORPHONE HYDROCHLORIDE

pH 2.7 to 4.5

(Numorphan)

Usual dose: 0.5 mg initially. May repeat every 2 to 4 hours. Up to 1.5 mg may be required. Reduced dose may be required in hepatic or renal disease.

Dilution: Each dose should be diluted with 5 ml of sterile water or normal saline for injection. May give through Y-tube or three-way stopcock of infusion set.

Rate of administration: A single dose properly diluted over 2 to 5 minutes. Usually titrated according to symptom relief and respiratory rate.

Actions: An opium derivative and CNS depressant closely related to morphine. Ten times more potent than morphine milligram for milligram. Onset of action is prompt and lasts 3 to 4 hours. Detoxified in the liver and excreted in the urine. Crosses placental barrier. Secreted in breast milk.

Indications and uses: (1) Relief of moderate to severe pain; (2) support of anesthesia; (3) obstetrical analgesia; (4) relief of anxiety in dyspnea of acute left ventricular failure and pulmonary edema.

Precautions: (1) Oxygen, controlled respiratory equipment, and naloxone (Narcan) must be available. (2) Observe patient frequently and monitor vital signs. Keep patient supine; orthostatic hypotension and fainting may occur. (3) Use caution in the elderly and in patients with impaired hepatic or renal function and emphysema. (4) Use extreme caution in craniotomy, head injury, and increased intracranial pressure; respiratory depression and intracranial pressure may be further increased. (5) May cause apnea in the asthmatic. (6) Symptoms of acute abdominal conditions may be masked. (7) May increase ventricular response rate in presence of supraventricular tachycardias. (8) Cough reflex is suppressed. (9) Potentiated by phenothiazines and other CNS depressants such as narcotic analgesics, alcohol, antihistamines, barbiturates, cimetidine (Tagamet), hypnotics, sedatives, MAO inhibitors (e.g., isocarboxazid [Marplan]), neuromuscular blocking agents (e.g., tubocurarine), and psychotropic agents. Reduced dosages of both drugs may be indicated. (10) Tolerance to oxymorphone gradually increases. A marked increase in dose may precipitate seizures in presence of a history of convulsive disorders. (11) With chronic use, physical dependence develops quickly. (12) Safety for use in pregnancy or lactation not estblished.

Contraindications: Acute bronchial asthma, children under 12 years of age, diarrhea caused by poisoning until toxic material eliminated, known hypersensitivity to opiates, premature infants and labor and delivery of premature infants, pulmonary edema caused by chemical respiratory irritant, upper airway obstruction.

Incompatible with: Specific information not available (consider similarity to morphine).

Side effects: Nausea, vomiting, and drowsiness are less frequent than with morphine.

Minor: Anorexia, constipation, dizziness, skin rash, urinary retention, urticaria.

Major: Anaphylaxis, hypotension, respiratory depression, somnolence.

Antidote: Notify the physician of any side effect. If minor side effects progress or any major side effect occurs, discontinue the drug and notify the physician. Treat anaphylaxis as indicated or resuscitate as necessary. Naloxone hydrochloride (Narcan) will reverse serious respiratory depression.

OXYTOCIN INJECTION

pH 2.5 to 4.5

(Pitocin, Syntocinon)

Usual dose: Determined by intended use, dilution, and rate of administration.

Dilution: *Induction of labor:* Dilute 1 ml (10 units) in 1 liter of 0.9% normal saline or 5% dextrose in normal saline for infusion (10 mU/ml).

Control of postpartum bleeding: Dilute 1 to 4 ml (10 to 40 units) in 1 liter of above infusion fluids (10 to 40 mU/ml).

Incomplete or inevitable abortion: Dilute 1 ml (10 units) in 500 ml of above infusion fluids (20 mU/ml).

Rotate gently to distribute medication through solution in all situations.

Rate of administration: Given only as an IV infusion. Use of an infusion pump or other accurate control device is required. In all situations, use the minimum effective rate and monitor strength, frequency, and duration of contractions; resting uterine tone; fetal heart rate; and maternal blood pressure at least every 15 minutes or more often if indicated.

Induction of labor: Begin with 1 to 2 mU/min (0.1 to 0.2 ml), increase in increments of 1 to 2 mU/min at 15- to 30-minute intervals until contractions simulate normal labor. Maximum dose rarely exceeds 20 mU/min.

Control of postpartum bleeding: Rate of infusion must control uterine atony. Begin with 10 to 20 mU/min.

Increase or decrease rate as indicated. Proceed quickly but with caution because of strength of solution.

Incomplete or inevitable abortion: 10 to 20 mU/min.

Actions: A synthetic posterior pituitary derivative that will produce rhythmic contraction of uterine smooth muscle. Its effectiveness depends on the level of uterine excitability, which usually increases as a pregnancy progresses. Very rapid acting, it has a shorter duration of action than ergot derivatives (half-life of 1 to 6 minutes) and is the drug of choice for induction of delivery. Probably detoxified in the liver and excreted in the urine. Has a weak antidiuretic effect.

Indications and uses: (1) After selective patient evaluation by the physician, it is used to induce or stimulate labor at term or before; (2) to control postpartum bleeding; (3) to treat incomplete or inevitable abortion.

Investigational use: Oxytocin challenge test.

Precautions: (1) An IV of 0.9% normal saline without oxytocins must be hung, connected by Y-tube or three-way stopcock, ready for use in adverse reactions. (2) Should be administered only in the hospital; the physician must be immediately available. (3) Monitor blood pressure, fetal heart tones, strength and timing of contractions, and resting uterine tone at least every 15 minutes or more often if indicated. Continuous observation of patient required. (4) Monitor oral fluid intake and observe for signs of fluid retention. Water intoxication has caused maternal death. (5) Oxytocins must be administered by only one route at a time. For instance, do not combine oral and IV routes. (6) Severe hypertension can result in the presence of local anesthesia, regional anesthesia (caudal or spinal), and with dopamine (Intropin), ephedrine, epinephrine, methoxamine (Vasoxyl), and other vasopressors. Chlorpromazine (Thorazine) IV will reduce this hypertension. (7) Refrigerate to store for long periods. (8) May be found in breast milk; consider postponing nursing for 24 hours after discontinued. (9) Oxytocin challenge test is an antepartum test of uteroplacental insufficiency in high-risk pregnancy. Infuse properly diluted oxytocin (10 mU/ml) at an initial rate of 0.5 mU/min. Gradually increase rate until contractions are every 3 to 4 minutes. Monitor fetal heart rate concurrently. Observe signs of fetal distress with contractions. Distress indicates inadequate placental reserve. Stop infusion. Test done only by a qualified physician.

Contraindications: Abruptio placentae, cephalopelvic disproportion, cesarean section (previous) or uterine surgery, dead fetus, fetal distress, fetal malpresentation, hypersensitivity, hypertonic uterine contractions, lack of satisfactory progress with adequate uterine activity, prolonged use in uterine inertia, serious medical or obstetrical conditions (past or present), toximia (severe), vaginal delivery contraindicated (e.g., active herpes genitalis, cord presentation or prolapse, invasive cervical carcinoma, total placenta previa and vasa previa.

Incompatible with: Levarterenol (Levophed), prochlorperazine (Compazine), warfarin (Coumadin).

Side effects: *Maternal:* Anaphylaxis; cardiac dysrhythmias; fatal afibinogenemia; fluid retention leading to water intoxication and coma, convulsion, and death; hypertension; increased blood loss; nausea; pelvic hematoma; PVCs; postpartum hemorrhage; severe uterine hypertonicity, spasm or contraction; subarachnoid hemorrhage; uterine rupture; vomitng.

Fetal: Bradycardia, brain damage, CNS damage, death, low Apgar scores, neonatal jaundice, retinal hemorrhage.

Antidote: Nausea and vomiting are tolerable and can be treated symptomatically. Immediately call the physician's attention to any side effect noted or suspected; many can be fatal. Discontinue the drug immediately for any signs of fetal distress, uterine hyperactivity, tetanic contractions, uterine resting tone exceeding 15 to 20 mm H_20 or water intoxication. Use of a Y-connection or three-way stopcock, allowing the oxytocin drip to be discontinued while the vein is kept open, is required. Turn mother on side (prevent fetal anoxia) and administer oxygen. Restriction of fluids, diuresis, hypertonic saline solutions IV, correction of electrolyte balance, control of convulsions with cautious use of barbiturates, or the use of magnesium sulfate may be required. These side effects can occur during labor and delivery and into the postpartum period. Treat nausea and vomiting symptomatically. Careful evaluation and selection of patients eliminate many hazards, but the nurse must be prepared for an emergency.

PANCURONIUM BROMIDE pH 4.0

(Pavulon)

Usual dose: Must be individualized, depending on previous drugs administered and degree and length of muscle relaxation required. 0.04 to 0.1 mg/kg of body weight initially. 0.01 mg/kg in increments as required to maintain muscle relaxation.
Endotracheal intubation: 0.06 to 0.1 mg/kg.

Neonatal dose: Extreme sensitivity to pancuronium exists during the first month of life. Begin with a test dose of 0.02 mg/kg and assess responsiveness.

Dilution: May be given undiluted.

Rate of administration: A single dose over 60 to 90 seconds.

Actions: A skeletal muscle relaxant five times as potent as tubocurarine chloride (curare). Causes paralysis by interfering with neural transmission at the myoneural junction. Onset of action is dose dependent. May occur in 30 seconds and lasts about 25 minutes. It may take another 30 minutes or up to several hours before complete recovery occurs. Excreted in the urine.

Indications and uses: (1) Adjunctive to general anesthesia; (2) facilitate endotracheal intubation; (3) management of patients undergoing mechanical ventilation; (4) paralytic agent when no other drug has controlled severe agitation, inhibiting specific treatments in intensive care units.

Precautions: (1) Best if stored in refrigerator. Will maintain potency at room temperature for up to 6 months. (2) Administered only by or under the direct observation of the anesthesiologist. (3) This drug produces apnea. Controlled artificial ventilation with oxygen must be continuous and under direct observation at all times. Maintain a patent airway. (4) Use a peripheral nerve stimulator to monitor response to pancuronium and avoid overdose. (5) Repeated doses may produce a cumulative effect. (6) Impaired pulmonary function or respiratory deficiencies can cause critical reactions. Use caution in impaired liver or kidney function. (7) Myasthenia gravis increases sensitivity to drug. (8) Potentiated by hypokalemia, some carcinomas, inhalant anesthetics (e.g., ether), neuromuscular blocking antibiotics (e.g., clindamycin [Cleocin], kanamycin [Kantrex], gentamicin [Garamycin]), calcium salts, CO_2, diuretics, diazepam (Valium) and other muscle relaxants, digitalis, magnesium sulfate, MAO inhibitors, quinidine, morphine, lidocaine, meperidine, propranalol (Inderal), succinylcholine, and others. Markedly reduced dose of pancuronium must be used with caution. (9) Antagonized by acetylcholine, anticholinesterases, aminophylline, azathioprine, carbamazepine, and potassium. Hyperkalemia may cause cardiac dysrhythmias and increased paralysis. (10) Succinylcholine must show signs of wearing off before pancuronium is given. Use caution. (11) Patient may be conscious and completely unable to communicate by any means. Pancuronium has no analgesic properties. Respiratory depression with morphine may be preferred in some patients requiring mechanical ventilation. (12) Action is altered by dehydration, electrolyte imbalance, body temperatures, and acid-base imbalance.

Contraindications: Known hypersensitivity to pancuronium or bromides.

Incompatible with: Specific information not available. Note Precautions.

Side effects: Prolonged action resulting in respiratory insufficiency or apnea. Airway closure caused by relaxation of epiglottis, pharynx, and tongue muscles. Hypersensitivity reactions are possible. Anaphylaxis, histamine release, hypotension, and shock may occur.

Antidote: All side effects are medical emergencies. Treat symptomatically. Controlled artificial ventilation must be continuous. Pyridostigmine (Mestinon) or neostigmine (Prostigmin) given with atropine will probably reverse the muscle relaxation. Not effective in all situations; may aggravate severe overdose. Resuscitate as necessary.

PAPAVERINE HYDROCHLORIDE

pH 3.0 to 4.5

Usual dose: 1 to 4 ml (30 to 120 mg) every 3 to 6 hours if indicated. Second dose may be given in 10 minutes only when treating extrasystoles.

Pediatric dose: 1.5 mg/kg of body weight every 6 hours.

Dilution: May be given undiluted or may be diluted in an equal amount of sterile water for injection. Usually not added to IV solutions. May be given through Y-tube or three-way stopcock of infusion set.

Rate of administration: 1 ml (30 mg) or fraction thereof over 2 minutes.

Actions: A nonnarcotic opium alkaloid, it is a direct smooth muscle relaxant and antispasmodic. More effective on muscle in spasm, it has an affinity for the smooth muscle of blood vessels. Affects cardiac muscle to depress conduction and increase refractory period. Improved circulation and muscle relaxation decrease pain. Metabolized in the liver and excreted in the urine.

Indications and uses: (1) Vascular spasm associated with an acute myocardial infarction; (2) peripheral or pulmonary embolism; (3) peripheral vascular disease and cerebral angiospastic states; (4) visceral spasm of ureteral, biliary, or GI colic; (5) angina pectoris.

Precautions: (1) Rarely used; active therapeutic value is questioned. (2) May be used with narcotics if the relaxant effect is not adequate to relieve discomfort. Narcotic dosage should be reduced. (3) Rapid IV injection may cause death. (4) IM injection is preferred. (5) Use with caution in glaucoma and impaired liver function. (6) Antagonizes effects of levodopa. (7) Potentiates diazoxide IV; severe hypotension may occur. Do not administer within 6 hours of each other. (8) Safety for use in pregnancy and lactation and in children not established.

Contraindications: Complete AV heart block.

Incompatible with: Alkaline solutions, aminophylline, bromides, iodides, lactated Ringer's injection.

Side effects: *Minor:* Blurred or double vision, diaphoresis, discomfort (generalized), flushing, hypertension (slight), hypotension, respiratory depth increase, scleral jaundice, sedation, tachycardia.

Major: Respiratory depression, seizures, ventricular ectopic rhythms, sudden death.

Antidote: Notify the physician of any minor side effects. If minor symptoms progress or any major side effect appears, discontinue the drug immediately and notify the physician. Treatment of toxicity will be symptomatic and supportive. Consider diazepam (Valium) or phenytoin (Dilantin) for convulsions. Anesthesia with thiopental and paralysis with a neuromuscular blocking agent (e.g., tubocurarine [curare]) may be required. Use dopamine (Intropin) for hypotension. Calcium gluconate may reduce toxic cardiovascular effects. Monitor ECG. Resuscitate as necessary.

PARALDEHYDE

Usual dose: 3 to 5 ml or 0.2 to 0.4 ml/kg of body weight. May repeat in 6 to 8 hours with extreme caution.

Dilution: Each 1 ml should be diluted with at least 20 ml of sodium chloride for injection.

Rate of administration: Each 21 ml or fraction thereof of diluted medication over at least 3 to 5 minutes.

Actions: A potent CNS depressant. Used as a sedative and a hypnotic. Effective within 30 minutes, lasts 6 to 8 hours. Metabolized in the liver and partly excreted in the lungs.

Indications and uses: (1) Delirium tremens; (2) tetanus; (3) eclampsia; (4) status epilepticus; (5) poisoning from convulsant drugs.

Precautions: (1) A lethal and addictive drug. Rarely used because of severity of side effects. (2) Use a glass syringe, reacts rapidly with plastics. (3) Use IV route only in an emergency. Oral or rectal route as efficient with fewer side effects. (4) Use only fresh, clear solutions. (5) Air exposure converts paraldehyde to toxic acetic acid; discard unused medication carefully. Corrosive to tissues. (6) Avoid extravasation; thrombophlebitis is frequent. (7) Position patient on side to prevent aspiration of increased bronchial secretions. (8) Breath will have a distinctive odor. (9) Do not use concurrently with sulfonamides or disulfiram (Antabuse). (10) Additive effects with anesthetics, MAO inhibitors (e.g., isocarboxazid [Marplan]), and tricyclic antidepressants (e.g., amitriptyline [Elavil]). (11) Produces excitement or delirium in presence of pain.

Contraindications: Severe hepatic insufficiency, respiratory disease, gastroenteritis with ulceration.

Incompatible with: Plastics, chlorpromazine (Thorazine), prochlorperazine (Compazine); do not mix in syringe or solution with any other drug.

Side effects: Acidosis, circulatory collapse, cough, cyanosis, dilation of right side of heart, hypotension, liver damage, pulmonary edema, pulmonary hemorrhage, rapid labored respiration, renal damage, death.

Antidote: Discontinue the drug and notify the physician of any side effects. Symptomatic and supportive treatment is most important in overdose. Mechanical respiration may be essential in respiratory depression. Doxapram (Dopram) may be useful.

PENICILLIN G AQUEOUS — pH 6.0 to 7.0

(Penicillin G Potassium, Penicillin G Sodium, Pfizerpen)

Usual dose: 1 to 20 million units/24 hr equally distributed over 24 hours as a continuous infusion. Doses up to 80 million units/24 hr have been given in life-threatening infections. (400,000 units equals approximately 250 mg.)

Pediatric dose: 50,000 to 300,000 units/kg of body weight/24 hr in equally divided doses every 4 to 6 hours. Dosage can vary greatly and must be adjusted according to the severity of the infection.

Neonatal dose: *Under 2,000 Gm; age up to 7 days:* 50,000 units/kg body weight/24 hr in equally divided doses every 12 hours (meningitis, 100,000 units); *Over 7 days:* 75,000 units/kg/24 hr in equally divided doses every 8 hours (meningitis, 150,000 units).

Over 2,000 Gm; age up to 7 days: 50,000 units/kg/24 hr in equally divided doses every 8 hours (meningitis, 150,000 units); *Over 7 days:* 100,000 units/kg/24 hr in equally divided doses every 6 hours (meningitis, 200,000 units).

Dilution: Initial dilution must be with sterile water for injection. Direct flow of water against sides of the vial while gently rotating vial. Shake vigorously. Directions on vial should be followed to provide desired number of units per milliliter. Available with 200,000 and 500,000 units and 1, 5, 10, and 20 million units per vial. May be added to 0.9% sodium chloride or dextrose solutions for infusion.

Rate of administration: Penicillin is not given by direct IV route. Administer as ordered as continuous IV drip; for example, 5 million units in 1,000 ml of 5% dextrose in water over 12 hours. Is sometimes given by intermittent infusion (a single dose in 100 ml every 2, 4, or 6 hours). Dosage level must be maintained to provide therapeutic serum levels. Too rapid administration or excessive doses may cause electrolyte imbalance and/or seizures. Stable at room temperature for at least 24 hours.

Actions: Bactericidal against penicillin-sensitive microorganisms during the stage of active multiplication. Appears in most body fluids. Absorption into spinal fluid minimal unless inflammation is present. Crosses the placental barrier. Excreted in the urine. Secreted in breast milk. Available in a potassium or sodium salt containing 1.7 mEq of the salt in 1 million units (39 to 46 mg).

Indications and uses: (1) Severe infections caused by penicillin G–sensitive gram-positive, gram-negative, and anaerobic microorganisms (e.g., streptococcal, pneumococcal, Vincent's gingivitis, spirochetal infections, meningitis, endocarditis); (2) prophylaxis against bacterial endocarditis in specific situations.

Precautions: (1) Sensitivity studies necessary to determine susceptibility of the causative organism to penicillin. (2) Adjust dosage down for individuals with impaired kidney function. Elimination rate markedly reduced in neonates. (3) Allergic reactions are most likely to occur in patients with a history of sensitivity to multiple allergens. (4) Periodic evaluation of renal and hematopoietic systems is recommended in prolonged therapy. (5) Electrolyte imbalance from potassium or sodium content is very possible. (6) Avoid prolonged use of drug; superinfection caused by overgrowth of nonsusceptible organisms may result. (7) Penicillins interact with many drugs; some of these, such as antibiotics (chloramphenicol, erythromycin, tetracyclines), will inactivate the bactericidal activity of penicillins. Inactivated by acids, alkalies, oxidizing agents, and carbohydrate solutions with an alkaline pH. (8) Optimum pH range 6.0 to 7.0. (9) Observe for thrombophlebitis. (10) Potassium penicillin most frequently used. (11) Concomitant use with β-adrenergic blockers (e.g., propranolol [Inderal]) may increase risk of anaphylaxis and inhibit treatment. (12) Risk of bleeding with anticoagulants (e.g., heparin) is increased. (13) Inactivates aminoglycosides (e.g., gentamicin [Garamycin]); administer in separate infusions. (14) Oral probenecid will achieve higher and more prolonged blood levels. May be desirable or may cause toxicity. (15) May decrease effectiveness of oral contraceptives; breakthrough bleeding or pregnancy could result.

Contraindications: Known sensitivity to any penicillin.

Incompatible with: To preserve bactericidal action, do not mix other agents with penicillin in the infusion solution. Acid media, alcohol 5% in dextrose, alkaline media, amikacin (Amikin), aminophylline, amphotericin B (Fungizone), ascorbic acid, cephalothin (Keflin), chlorpromazine (Thorazine), dextran, dopamine (Intropin), heparin, hydroxyzine (Vistaril), lincomycin (Lincocin), metaraminol (Aramine), metoclopramide (Reglan), pentobarbital (Nembutal), phenytoin (Dilantin), prochlorperazine (Compazine), promazine (Sparine), promethazine (Phenergan), sodium bicarbonate, tetracycline, thiopental (Pentothal), trifluoperazine (Stelazine), vancomycin (Vancocin), vitamin B complex with C.

Side effects: *Minor:* Arthralgia, chills, edema, fever, prostration, skin rash, urticaria.

Major: Acute interstitial nephritis, anaphylaxis, convulsions, hemolytic anemia, hyperreflexia, neurotoxicity, potassium poisoning with coma, sodium-induced congestive heart failure.

Antidote: For all side effects, discontinue the drug, treat the allergic reaction or resuscitate as necessary, and notify the physician. Treat minor side effects symptomatically according to physician's order.

PENTAMIDINE ISETHIONATE pH 4.09 to 5.4

(Pentam 300)

Usual dose: 4 mg/kg of body weight once daily for 14 days. Reduce dose in renal failure.

Dilution: Initially dilute each 300 mg or fraction thereof in 3 to 5 ml sterile water or 5% dextrose in water for injection. A single dose must be further diluted in 50 to 250 ml of 5% dextrose in water and given as an infusion.

Rate of administration: A single dose should be evenly distributed over 60 minutes.

Actions: An antiprotozoal agent. Specifically active against *Pneumocystis carinii.* It is thought to interfere with nuclear metabolism and inhibit the synthesis of DNA, RNA, phospholipids, and proteins. Excreted in urine. Accumulates in renal failure.

Indications and uses: Treatment of *Pneumocystis carinii* pneumonia.

Investigational use: Treatment of trypanosomiasis and visceral leishmaniasis.

Precautions: (1) Specific use only; establish correct diagnosis. (2) Trimethoprim/sulfamethoxazole is the drug of choice for treatment of *Pneumocystis* pneumonia. Pentamidine causes numerous and serious side effects and is indicated only if the patient does not respond to or tolerate TMP/SMX. (3) Has caused fatalities resulting from severe hypotension, hypoglycemia, and cardiac dysrhythmias even with the administration of the first dose. Keep patient supine, observe continuously for any sign of adverse reaction, and monitor blood pressure continuously during infusion and afterward until stable. (4) Emergency equipment for resuscitation must be immediately available. (5) Monitor blood glucose levels daily during therapy and several times after therapy is complete. Pancreatic necrosis and very high plasma insulin levels have occurred. May also cause hyperglycemia and diabetes mellitus. (6) Before, during, and after therapy obtain a BUN (daily), CBC, platelet count, alkaline phosphatase, bilirubin, SGOT, SGPT, serum calcium, and ECG. (7) Use extreme caution in patients with hypertension, hypotension, hypoglycemia, hyperglycemia, hypocalcemia, leukopenia, thrombocytopenia, anemia, hepatic or renal dysfunction, ventricular tachycardia, pancreatitis, and Stevens-Johnson syndrome. (8) Use only when clearly needed during pregnancy and lactation. Hazards to fetus or infant are unknown. (9) Stable at room temperature for 48 hours. Discard unused portion.

Contraindications: None if the diagnosis of *Pneumocystis carinii* pneumonia is confirmed.

Incompatible with: Specific information not available. Consider incompatible in syringe or solution because of specific use and frequent side effects.

Side effects: Occur in more than 50% of patients and may be life threatening. Some side effects occur after the course of treatment is completed. Acute renal failure, anemia, anorexia, bad taste in mouth, cardiac dysrhythmias including ventricular tachycardia, confusion, dizziness, elevated serum creatinine and liver function tests, fever, hallucinations, hyperglycemia, hyperkalemia, hypocalcemia, hypoglycemia, hypotension, leukopenia, nausea, neuralgia, phlebitis, rash, thrombocytopenia.

Antidote: Discontinue the drug and resuscitate as necessary for any life-threatening side effects. Notify physician of all side effects. Symptomatic treatment is indicated.

PENTAZOCINE LACTATE pH 4.0 to 5.0

(Talwin)

Usual dose: 5 to 30 mg. May repeat every 3 to 4 hours or decrease to 5 to 15 mg and repeat every 2 hours. 360 mg equals maximum dose in 24 hours.

Dilution: May be given undiluted. It is preferable to dilute each 5 mg with at least 1 ml of sterile water for injection.

Rate of administration: Each 5 mg or fraction thereof over 1 minute.

Actions: A synthetic narcotic agonist-antagonist with a potent analgesic action, pentazocine is somewhat less effective than morphine and meperidine in equivalent doses. Onset of action is prompt, 2 to 3 minutes, and lasts about 2 hours. Metabolized in the liver. Excreted in urine. Crosses the placental barrier. Secreted in breast milk.

Indications and uses: (1) Relief of moderate to severe pain; (2) preoperative medication; (3) support of anesthesia; (4) obstetrical analgesia.

Precautions: (1) Oxygen and controlled respiratory equipment must always be available. (2) Observe patient continuously during injection and frequently thereafter. Monitor vital signs. (3) Low addictive element. (4) Use with caution in bronchial asthma, relief of biliary pain, history of drug abuse, myocardial infarction (especially if nausea and vomiting are present; increases cardiac workload), decreased renal or hepatic function, respiratory depression from any cause, a history of seizures and during delivery of premature infants. (5) Mild narcotic antagonist. May precipitate withdrawal symptoms in patients accustomed to narcotics. (6) May have less effective analgesia in heavy smokers. (7) Use caution with CNS depressants such as narcotic analgesics, general anesthetics, alcohol, anticholinergics, antihistamines, barbiturates, hypnotics, sedatives, psychotropic agents, MAO inhibitors, and neuromuscular blocking agents (e.g., tubocurarine). Reduced doses of both drugs may be indicated.

Contraindications: Children under 12 years, head injury, hypersensitivity to pentazocine, pathological brain conditions, increased intracranial pressure.

Incompatible with: All barbiturates, aminophylline, glycopyrrolate (Robinul), sodium bicarbonate.

Side effects: Allergic reactions, apprehension, blurred vision, circulatory depression, confusion, constipation, cramps, depression, diarrhea, disorientation, double vision, dreams, drug dependence, dry mouth, dyspnea, facial edema, floating feeling, flushing, hallucinations, headache, hypertension, insomnia, muscle tremor, neonatal apnea, nervousness, nystagmus, paresthesias, perspiration, pruritus, respiratory depression, sedation, seizures, shock, tachycardia, taste alteration, urinary retention, uterine contraction depression.

Antidote: For any side effect, discontinue the drug and notify the physician. Treat side effects symptomatically. For overdose or respiratory depression, naloxone hydrochloride (Narcan) is the antidote of choice. If naloxone is not available, methylphenidate (Ritalin) may be of value in respiratory depression (only available in oral form).

PENTOBARBITAL SODIUM — pH 9.0 to 10.5

(Nembutal Sodium)

Usual dose: 100 mg initially. Wait 1 full minute between each dose to determine drug effect. Additional doses in increments of 25 to 50 mg may be given as indicated. Maximum dosage ranges from 200 to 500 mg.

Pediatric dose: Initial dose is 50 mg.

Dilution: May be given undiluted or, preferably, may be further diluted in sterile water, sodium chloride for injection, or Ringer's injection. Any desired amount of diluent may be used. 9 ml of diluent with 1 ml of pentobarbital (50 mg) equals 5 mg/ml.

Rate of administration: 50 mg or fraction thereof over 1 minute. Titrate slowly to desired effect.

Actions: A sedative, hypnotic barbiturate of short duration with anticonvulsant effects. Pentobarbital is a CNS depressant. Onset of action is prompt by the IV route and lasts about 3 to 4 hours. Will effectively depress the motor cortex if adequate doses are administered. Pain perception is unimpaired. Detoxified in the liver and excreted fairly quickly in the urine in changed form. Crosses the placental barrier. Secreted in breast milk.

Indications and uses: (1) Preanesthetic sedation; (2) dental and minor surgical sedation; (3) control of convulsions caused by disease and drug poisoning; (4) sedation in psychotic states.

Precautions: (1) Use only absolutely clear solutions. (2) Rapid injection rate may cause symptoms of overdose. (3) Record blood pressure, pulse, and respiration every 3 to 5 minutes. Keep patient under constant observation. (4) Maintain a patent airway. (5) Treat the cause of a convulsion. (6) May be habit forming. Status epilepticus can occur from too rapid withdrawal. (7) Use caution in status asthmaticus, shock, severe liver diseases, uremia, and depressive state after a convulsion. (8) Determine absolute patency of vein; use of large veins preferred to prevent thrombosis. Avoid extravasation. Intraarterial injection will cause gangrene. (9) Use extreme caution if any other CNS depressants have been given, such as alcohol, narcotic analgesics, anesthetics, antidepressants, antihistamines, hypnotics, MAO inhibitors, phenothiazines, sedatives, aminoglycoside antibiotics, or tranquilizers; potentiation with respiratory depression may occur. (10) Inhibits effectiveness of propranolol (Inderal), corticosteroids, doxycycline (Vibramycin), oral anticoagulants, oral contraceptives, quinidine, and theophylline. Capable of innumerable interactions with many drugs. (11) May increase orthostatic hypotension with furosemide (Lasix). (12) Monitor phenytoin and barbiturate levels when both drugs are used concurrently. (13) Will cause birth defects. (14) May cause paradoxical excitement in children or the elderly.

Contraindications: Delivery (when maximum drug effect would be at the time of delivery), history of porphyria, known hypersensitivity to barbiturates, impaired liver function, pregnancy, premature delivery, severe respiratory depression.

Incompatible with: Atropine, benzquinamide (Emete-Con), brompheniramine (DimetaneTen), butorphanol (Stadol), cefazolin (Kefzol), cephalothin (Keflin), chlordiazepoxide (Librium), chlorpheniramine (Chlor-Trimeton), chlorpromazine (Thorazine), cimetidine (Tagamet), clindamycin (Cleocin), codeine, dimenhydrinate (Dramamine), diphenhydramine (Benadryl), droperidol (Inapsine), ephedrine, erythromycin (Ilotycin), fentanyl, fructose solutions, glycopyrrolate (Robinul), hydrocortisone sodium succinate (Solu-Cortef), hydroxyzine (Vistaril), insulin (aqueous), kanamycin (Kantrex), levarterenol (Levophed), levorphanol (Levo-Dromoran), meperidine (Demerol), methadone, midazolam (Versed), morphine, nalbuphine (Nubain), opium alkaloids, penicillins, pentazocine (Talwin), phenytoin (Dilantin), prochlorperazine (Compazine), promazine (Sparine), promethazine (Phenergan), ranitidine (Zantac), sodium bicarbonate, streptomycin, succinylcholine (Anectine), tetracycline, triflupromazine (Vesprin), vancomycin (Vancocin).

Side effects: *Average dose:* Asthma, bronchospasm, depression, dermatitis, facial edema, fever, hypotension, neonatal apnea, pain at or below injection site, respiratory depression (slight), thrombocytopenic purpura.

Overdose: Apnea, coma, cough reflex depression, flat EEG (reversible unless hypoxic damage has occurred), hypotension, laryngospasm, lowered body temperature, pulmonary edema, renal shutdown, respiratory depression, sluggish or absent reflexes.

Antidote: Discontinue drug immediately for pain at or below injection site. Notify the physician of any side effects. Symptomatic and supportive treatment are most important in overdose. Maintain an adequate airway with artificial ventilation if indicated. Keep the patient warm. IV volume expanders (dextran) and IV fluids will help maintain adequate circulation. Diuretics or hemodialysis will promote the elimination of the drug. Vasopressors (dopamine [Intropin]) will maintain blood pressure.

PERPHENAZINE pH 4.2 to 5.6

(Trilafon)

Usual dose: 1 mg, repeat as necessary, allowing 2 to 3 minutes between doses, only until symptoms are controlled. Do not exceed 5 mg.

Dilution: Each 5 mg (1 ml) must be diluted with 9 ml of normal saline for injection. Shake well. 1 ml will equal 0.5 mg. May be further diluted and given as an infusion under observation of anesthesiologist (use an infusion pump or a microdrip, 60 gtt/ml).

Rate of administration: 0.5 mg or fraction thereof over 1 minute.

Actions: A phenothiazine derivative said to be six times more potent than chlorpromazine (Thorazine) with effects on the central, autonomic, and peripheral nervous systems. Decreases anxiety and tension, relaxes muscle, produces sedation, and tranquilizes. A potent antiemetic. Onset of action is prompt and lasting. Excretion is slow through the kidneys.

Indications and uses: Control of severe vomiting, intractable hiccups, or acute symptoms such as violent retching during surgery.

Precautions: (1) Use IV only when absolutely necessary. (2) Check label on ampoule. Only single-dose, 5 mg ampoules may be given IV. (3) Handle carefully; may cause contact dermatitis. Sensitive to light. Slightly yellow color does not affect potency. Discard if markedly discolored. (4) Keep patient in supine position and monitor blood pressure and pulse between doses. (5) May mask diagnosis of brain tumor, drug intoxication, and intestinal obstruction. (6) Use caution in coronary disease, severe hypertension or hypotension, and epilepsy. (7) Temperature without etiology indicates drug intolerance. (8) Potentiates CNS depressants such as narcotics, barbiturates, alcohol, anesthetics, MAO inhibitors (e.g., pargyline [Eutonyl]), oral antidiabetics, insulin, anticholinergics, antihistamines, antihypertensives, hypnotics, muscle relaxants, and Rauwolfia alkaloids. Reduce dosage of any medication potentiated by phenothiazines by one fourth to one half; has less potentiating effect than other phenothiazines. (9) Contraindicated with quinidine, epinephrine, and thiazide diuretics. (10) Capable of innumerable other interactions. (11) Not recommended for use in children under 12 years. (12) May cause pardoxical excitation in children and the elderly.

Contraindications: Comatose or severely depressed states, hypersensitivity to phenothiazines.

Incompatible with: Aminophylline, cefoperazone (Cefobid), midazolam (Versed), opium alkaloids, oxytocin, pentobarbital (Nembutal), secobarbital (Seconal), thiopental (Pentothal), vitamin B complex.

Side effects: Usually transient if drug is discontinued, but may require treatment if severe: anaphylaxis, blurring of vision, cardiac arrest, dermatitis, dizziness, dryness of mouth, dysphagia, extrapyramidal symptoms (e.g., abnormal positioning, extreme restlessness, pseudoparkinsonism, weakness of extremities), elevated blood pressure, excitement, hypersensitivity reactions, hypotension, slurred speech, spastic movements (especially about the face), tachycardia, temperature without etiology, tightness of the throat, tongue discol oration, tongue protrusion, and many others. Overdose can cause convulsions, hallucinations, and death.

Antidote: Discontinue the drug at onset of any side effect and notify the physician. Counteract hypotension with IV fluids, dopamine (Intropin), or levarterenol (Levophed) and extrapyramidal symptoms with benztropine mesylate (Cogentin) or diphenhydramine (Benadryl). Epinephrine is contraindicated for hypotension; further hypotension will occur. Use diazepam (Valium) or phenobarbital for convulsions or hyperactivity. Phenytoin may be helpful in ventricular dysrhythmias. In treating respiratory depression and unconsciousness, avoid analeptics such as doxapram (Dopram); they may cause convulsions. Resuscitate as necessary.

PHENOBARBITAL SODIUM pH 8.5 to 10.5

(Luminal Sodium)

Usual dose: 100 to 300 mg. May be repeated in 6 hours. Do not exceed 600 mg/24 hr.

Pediatric dose: *Anticonvulsant:* 20 mg/kg of body weight, then 6 mg/kg every 20 minutes as needed. Maximum dose 40 mg/kg/24 hr.

Dilution: Sterile powder must be slowly diluted with sterile water for injection. Use a minimum of 10 ml of diluent regardless of dose desired. Also available in a sterile solution. Further dilute solution up to 10 ml with sterile water for injection.

Rate of administration: 65 mg (gr 1) or fraction thereof over 1 minute. Titrate slowly to desired effect.

Actions: A sedative, hypnotic barbiturate of long duration with potent anticonvulsant effects. Phenobarbital is a CNS depressant. Onset of action is prompt by the IV route and becomes rapidly more intense. Effects last from 6 to 10 hours. Will effectively depress the motor cortex with small doses. Pain perception is unimpaired. Rapidly absorbed by all body tissues and excreted in changed form in the urine. Excreted more readily in alkaline urine. Crosses the placental barrier. Secreted in breast milk.

Indications and uses: (1) Prolonged sedation (medical and psychiatric); (2) anticonvulsant.

Precautions: (1) Solutions from powder form must be freshly prepared. Use only absolutely clear solutions. Discard powder or solution exposed to air for 30 minutes. (2) Use only enough medication to achieve the desired effect. May take up to 15 minutes to reach peak levels in the brain; guard against overdose and excessive respiratory depression. Rapid injection rate may cause symptoms of overdose. (3) IV route used only if oral or IM route not feasible. (4) Keep patient under constant observation. Record vital signs every hour, or more often if indicated. (5) Maintain a patent airway. (6) Treat the cause of a convulsion. (7) Keep equipment for artificial ventilation available. (8) Determine absolute patency of vein; use of large veins preferred to prevent thrombosis. Avoid extravasation. Intraarterial injection will cause gangrene. (9) May be habit forming. Status epilepticus can occur from too rapid withdrawal. (10) Use caution in elderly and debilitated patients and those with asthma, pulmonary disease, shock, and uremia. (11) Use extreme caution if any other CNS depressants have been given, such as alcohol, narcotic analgesics, anesthetics, antidepressants, antihistamines, hypnotics, MAO inhibitors, phenothiazines, sedatives, aminoglycoside antibiotics, and tranquilizers. Potentiation with respiratory depression may occur. (12) Inhibits effectiveness of propranolol (Inderal), corticosteroids, doxycycline (Vibramycin), oral anticoagulants, oral contraceptives, quinidine, and theophylline. Capable of innumerable interactions with many drugs. (13) May increase orthostatic hypotension with furosemide (Lasix). (14) Monitor phenytoin and barbiturate levels when both drugs are used concurrently. (15) Will cause birth defects. (16) May cause paradoxical excitement in children or the elderly.

Contraindications: History of porphyria, impaired renal function, known hypersensitivity to barbiturates, previous addiction, severe respiratory depression including dyspnea, obstruction, or cor pulmonale.

Incompatible with: Acidic solutions, alcohol 5% in dextrose, aminophylline, benzquinamide (Emete-Con), calcium chloride, cephalothin (Keflin), chlorpromazine (Thorazine), cimetidine (Tagamet), clindamycin (Cleocin), codeine, diphenhydramine (Benadryl), droperidol (Inapsine), ephedrine, erythromycin (Ilotycin), hydralazine (Apresoline), hydrocortisone sodium succinate (Solu-Cortef), hydroxyzine (Vistaril), insulin (aqueous), kanamycin (Kantrex), levarterenol (Levophed), levorphanol (Levo-Dromoran), meperidine (Demerol), magnesium sulfate, methadone, morphine, pancuronium bromide (Pavulon), parabens, penicillin G potassium, pentazocine (Talwin), phenytoin (Dilantin), phytonadione (Aquamephyton), procaine (Novocain), prochlorperazine (Compazine), promazine (Sparine), promethazine (Phenergan), propiomazine (Largon), ranitidine (Zantac), sodium bicarbonate, streptomycin, succinylcholine (Anectine), tetracycline, thiamine, trifluoperazine (Stelazine), tripelennamine (Pyribenzamine), vancomycin (Vancocin), warfarin (Coumadin).

Side effects: Rarely occur with slow injection of average doses.

Average dose: Asthma, bronchospasm, depression, dermatitis, facial edema, fever, headache, hypotension, nausea, neonatal apnea, respiratory depression (slight), thrombocytopenic purpura, vertigo.

Overdose: Apnea, coma, cough reflex depression, delirium, flat EEG (reversible unless hypoxic damage has occurred), hypotension, laryngospasm, lowered body temperature, pulmonary edema, renal shutdown, respiratory depression, sluggish or absent reflexes, stupor.

Antidote: Notify the physician of any side effects. Symptomatic and supportive treatment is most important in overdose. Maintain an adequate airway with artificial ventilation if indicated. Keep the patient warm. IV volume expanders (dextran) and other IV fluids will help maintain adequate circulation. Diuretics or hemodialysis will promote the elimination of the drug. Vasopressors (e.g., dopamine [Intropin]) will maintain blood pressure.

PHENOLSULFONPHTHALEIN INJECTION (P.S.P.)

Usual dose: 1 ml (6 mg) as a single dose.

Dilution: May be given undiluted.

Rate of administration: 1 ml over 1 minute.

Actions: A dye used to determine the excretory function of the kidneys. In the normal kidney the dye appears in the urine within 3 to 5 minutes.

Indications and uses: Kidney function test.

Precautions: (1) Accurate results are not obtained if there is residual urine in the bladder, if there is circulatory inadequacy, if the patient is taking probenecid (Benemid), or if dehydration is present. (2) Have patient empty bladder completely before giving dye. (3) Collect voided specimens of at least 40 ml at exactly 1 hour and 2 hours after injection. (4) Urine will have a reddish orange color.

Contraindications: Known sensitivity to phenolsulfonphthalein.

Incompatible with: Any other drug in syringe.

Side effects: Almost nonexistent, but hypersensitivity reactions including anaphylaxis are possible.

Antidote: For hypersensitivity reactions, discontinue the drug, treat as necessary with antihistamines and/or epinephrine, and notify the physician. Resuscitate as necessary.

PHENTOLAMINE MESYLATE pH 4.5 to 6.5

(Regitine)

Usual dose: Preoperatively, 5 mg 1 to 2 hours before surgery. May be repeated. During surgery the same doses are used as indicated to control epinephrine intoxication. To prevent necrosis caused by levarterenol, add 10 mg of phentolamine to each 1,000 ml of IV solution containing levarterenol (norepinephrine).

Test dose for diagnosis of pheochromocytoma: 2.5 to 5 mg.

Pediatric dose: 1 mg, 0.1 mg/kg of body weight, or 3 mg/M^2.

Dilution: Each 5 mg should be diluted with 1 ml of sterile water for injection. May be further diluted with 5 to 10 ml of sterile water for injection.

Rate of administration: Each 5 mg or fraction thereof over 1 minute. Inject test dose rapidly after pressor response to venipuncture has subsided.

Actions: An α-blocking agent that actually inhibits hypertension resulting from elevated levels of epinephrine and norepinephrine. A vasodilator, it causes some GI stimulation.

Indications and uses: (1) Prevention and treatment of hypertensive episodes of pheochromocytoma preoperatively and during surgery; (2) prevention and treatment of necrosis and sloughing occurring with dopamine (Intropin) and norepinephrine (Levophed); (3) definitive diagnosis of pheochromocytoma.

Investigational uses: Hypertensive crisis due to MAO inhibitor/sympathomimetic amine interactions and rebound hypertension after discontinuation of clonidine, propranolol, or other hypertensive agents.

Precautions: (1) Use only freshly prepared solutions. (2) For diagnosis of pheochromocytoma, urinary tests such as vanillylmandelic acid (VMA) are safer. Phentolamine is used only when absolutely necessary. Specific procedure must be followed. Consult with physician and pharmacist. (3) Use care in the presence of any dysrhythmia. It is preferable to have a normal sinus rhythm. (4) Monitor vital signs every 2 minutes. (5) May be used concomitantly with propranolol (Inderal). (6) Antagonizes effects of epinephrine and ephedrine. (7) Safety for use during pregnancy and lactation not established. Use with extreme caution, only when clearly indicated. (8) Use caution in gastritis or peptic ulcer disease.

Contraindications: Coronary artery disease, coronary insufficiency, hypersensitivity to phentolamine, myocardial infarction (previous or present).

Incompatible with: Iron salts.

Side effects: *Minor:* Abdominal pain, diarrhea, dizziness, hypotension, nasal stuffiness, nausea, tachycardia, tingling of skin, weakness, vomiting.

Major: Cardiac dysrhythmias, cerebrovascular occlusion, cerebrovascular spasm, hypotension (severe), myocardial infarction, shock, tachycardia, vomiting under anesthesia.

Antidote: For minor side effects, notify the physician. If symptoms progress or any major side effect occurs, discontinue drug and notify the physician immediately. Administer dopamine (Intropin) for shock caused by hypotension. Do not use epinephrine. Maintain the patient as indicated. If tachycardia or cardiac dysrhythmias occur, defer use of digitalis derivatives if possible until rhythm returns to normal.

PHENYLEPHRINE HYDROCHLORIDE

pH 3.0 to 6.5

(Neo-Synephrine)

Usual dose: 0.2 mg. From 0.1 to 0.5 mg may be used initially. May be repeated every 10 to 15 minutes. Never exceed 0.5 mg in a single dose. Highly individualized.

Dilution: *Direct IV:* Dilute each 1 mg with 9 ml of sterile water for injection (0.1 mg equals 1 ml).

Infusion: Dilute 10 mg in 500 ml of dextrose or sodium chloride for injection to provide a 1:50,000 solution.

Rate of administration: *Direct IV:* Single dose over 20 to 30 seconds to treat paroxysmal supraventricular tachycardia; over 1 minute in other situations.

Infusion: Regulate drip rate to provide and maintain individual's low normal blood pressure. Use an infusion pump or microdrip (60 gtt/ml) to administer.

Actions: A sympathomimetic, similar to epinephrine. A potent long-lasting vasoconstrictor. Unique in that it slows the heart rate, increases stroke volume, and does not induce any change in rhythm of the pulse. Renal vessel constriction will occur. Repeated injections produce comparable results. Effective within seconds and lasts about 15 minutes.

Indications and uses: (1) To maintain adequate blood pressure in inhalation and spinal anesthesia, shocklike states, drug-induced hypotension, and hypersensitivity reactions; (2) to treat paroxysmal supraventricular tachycardia; (3) to prolong anesthesia; (4) specific antidote for hypotension produced by chlorpromazine hydrochloride (Thorazine).

Precautions: (1) Check blood pressure every 2 minutes until stabilized at the desired level. (2) Start with a small dose, giving only as much of the drug as required to alleviate undesirable symptoms. (3) Blood volume depletion should be corrected. May be administered concurrently with blood volume replacement. (4) Hypotension of powerful peripheral adrenergic blocking agents, chlorpromazine, or pheochromocytomectomy may require carefully calculated increased dosage therapy. (5) Discontinue IV administration if vein infiltrates or is thrombosed; can cause tissue necrosis and sloughing. (6) Use extreme caution in the elderly, hyperthyroidism, bradycardia, partial heart block, myocardial disease, or severe arteriosclerosis. (7) May cause severe hypertension with ergonovine or oxytocin. (8) Potentiated by halothane anesthetics, tricyclic antidepressants (e.g., desipramine [Norpramin]), guanethidine, MAO inhibitors (e.g., isocarboxazid [Marplan]), other vasopressors (epinephrine [Adrenalin]); hypertensive crisis and death can result. (9) Use caution with digitalis; dysrhythmias may occur. (10) Will cause bradycardia and hypotension with hydantoins (e.g., phenytoin [Dilantin]).

Contraindications: Anesthesia with inhalant anesthetics (e.g., halothane), hypertension, myocardial infarction, ventricular tachycardia.

Incompatible with: Alkaline solutions, iron salts, phenytoin (Dilantin).

Side effects: Bradycardia, fullness of head, headache, hypertension, tingling of extremities, tremulousness, ventricular extrasystoles, ventricular tachycardia (short paroxysms), vertigo.

Antidote: To prevent sloughing and necrosis in areas where extravasation has occurred, with a fine hypodermic needle inject 5 to 10 mg of phentolamine (Regitine) diluted in 10 to 15 ml of normal saline liberally throughout the tissue in the extravasated area. Treatment should be started as soon as extravasation is recognized. Notify the physician of all side effects. IM injection may be preferable. Treat hypertension with phentolamine (Regitine). Treat cardiac dysrhythmias as indicated and resuscitate as necessary.

PHENYTOIN SODIUM pH 12.0

(Dilantin, Dilantin Sodium)

Usual dose: *Anticonvulsant:* (1) 100 to 250 mg initially. 100 to 150 mg may be repeated in 30 minutes if indicated. Higher doses may be required. Initial dose may be repeated every 4 hours. (2) A loading dose of 600 to 1,000 mg in divided doses over 8 to 12 hours is an alternate dosing schedule. Do not exceed a total dose of 20 mg/kg of body weight.

Status epilepticus: IV diazepam is the drug of choice for initial treatment. Concurrent administration of phenytoin in the above doses is recommended by some specialists to maintain control.

Antiarrhythmic: 50 to 100 mg every 10 to 15 minutes. Do not exceed a total dose of 15 mg/kg of body weight.

Pediatric dose: *Anticonvulsant:* 250 mg/M^2 or 10 to 15 mg/kg of body weight/day in divided doses of 5 to 10 mg/kg.

Neonatal dose: *Anticonvulsant:* 15 to 20 mg/kg of body weight/day in divided doses of 5 to 10 mg/kg.

Dilution: Special solvent provided; add 2.2 ml to 100 mg vial and 5.2 ml to 250 mg vial. 1 ml equals 50 mg. Shake to dissolve. Immerse vial in warm water to dissolve phenytoin powder. Do not add to IV solutions. May be injected through Y-tube or three-way stopcock of infusion set. Recent studies have utilized infusion solutions (normal saline or lactated Ringer's injection) prepared immediately before use in suitable concentrations (from 100 mg in 25 to 50 ml diluent up to 1 Gm in 1 L) to facilitate required rate and fluid limitations or requirements. An in-line filter is required. Method not recommended by manufacturer or established in common use as yet (see incompatibilities).

Rate of administration: *Anticonvulsant:* 50 mg or fraction thereof over 1 minute.

Antiarrhythmic: 25 mg or fraction thereof over 1 minute.

Infusion: Concentrated dilutions should be given within 1 hour. Dilute solutions (1 Gm in 1 L) may be given over 4 to 8 hours.

Actions: A synthetic anticonvulsant, chemically related to barbiturates. Selectively stabilizes seizure threshold and depresses seizure activity in the motor cortex. Effective control in emergency treatment of seizures may take 15 to 20 minutes because of rate of injection required. Also exerts a depressant effect on the myocardium by selectively elevating the excitability threshold of the cell, reducing the cell's response to stimuli. Readily absorbed, phenytoin is metabolized in the liver and excreted in changed form in the urine. Crosses placental barrier. Secreted in breast milk.

Indications and uses: (1) Control of grand mal and psychomotor seizures; (2) control of seizures in neurosurgery; (3) treatment of status epilepticus (grand mal seizures); (4) treatment of supraventricular and ventricular dysrhythmias including those caused by digitalis intoxication. Especially useful for patients who are unable to tolerate quinidine or procainamide (not FDA approved, but in common usage).

Precautions: (1) Use solution only when completely dissolved and clear; discard if hazy or if a precipitate forms. May be light yellow in color. (2) Determine absolute patency of vein. Avoid extravasation. Very alkaline; follow each injection with sterile normal saline to reduce local venous irritation. (3) May cause convulsions in hypoglycemia caused by pancreatic tumor. (4) Use caution, lower dosage, and slower rate of administration in the seriously ill, elderly, and those with impaired liver or renal function. (5) Narrow margin of error between therapeutic and toxic dose. Plasma levels above 10 mcg/ml usually control seizure activity. The acceptable range is 5 to 20 mcg/ml. Toxicity begins with nystagmus at levels exceeding 20 mcg/ml. Lethal dose estimated at 2 to 5 Gm. (6) Capable of innumerable catastrophic drug interactions; nursing observation of patient symptoms and effectiveness of medications is imperative. Potentiated by amphetamines, analeptics, anticoagulants, antidepressants, antihistamines, benzodiazepines (e.g., diazepam [Valium]), chloramphenicol, cimetidine (Tagamet), disulfiram (Antabuse), estrogens, myocardial depressants, phenothiazines, sulfonamides, valproic acid, and others. Toxicity and fatality may result. (7) Inhibited by alcohol, antineoplastics, antituberculosis drugs, barbiturates, carbamazepine (Tegretol), folic acid, theophylline, and others. (8) Potentiates CNS depressants, folic acid antagonists, and muscle relaxants. (9) Inhibits corticosteroids, digitalis, diuretics, levodopa, quinidine, and others. (10) Alters some clinical laboratory tests. (11) Severe hypotension and bradycardia result with concomitant administration with dopamine (Intropin) and all other sympathomimetic antihypertensive drugs. (12) Status epilepticus can occur from abrupt withdrawal of hydantoins. (13) Not effective for petit mal seizures; combined therapy required if both conditions present. (14) May cause birth defects (see literature).

Contraindications: Bradycardia; sinoatrial, second-, or third-degree heart block; Stokes-Adams syndrome; known sensitivity to hydantoin derivatives.

Incompatible with: Any other drug in syringe or solution. Will precipitate if pH is altered. Clear tubing with normal saline if possible before and after administration through Y-tube or three-way stopcock.

Side effects: *Minor:* Ataxia, confusion, dizziness, drowsiness, fever, hyperplasia of gums, nervousness, nystagmus, skin eruptions, tremors, visual disturbances.

Major: Bradycardia, cardiac arrest, heart block, hypotension, respiratory arrest, tonic seizures, ventricular fibrillation.

Antidote: Notify the physician of any side effects. If minor symptoms progress or any major side effect occurs, discontinue the drug and notify the physician. Maintain a patent airway and resuscitate as necessary. Symptoms of heart block or bradycardia may be reversed with IV atropine. Epinephrine may also be useful. Hemodialysis may be required in overdose.

PHOSPHATE pH 5.0 to 7.8

(Potassium Phosphate, Sodium Phosphate)

Usual dose: Dependent on individual needs of the patient. In total parenteral nutrition (TPN), 10 to 15 mM of phosphorus/L of TPN solution should maintain normal serum phosphate. Larger amounts may be required.

Pediatric dose: *Infants receiving TPN:* 1.5 to 2 m M/kg of body weight/day.

Dilution: Must be diluted in a larger volume of suitable IV solution and given as an infusion. Soluble in all commonly used IV solutions except protein hydrolysate. Mix thoroughly.

Rate of administration: Dependent on individual needs of the patient. Consider sodium/potassium content. Infuse slowly.

Actions: Helps to maintain calcium levels, has a buffering effect on acid-base equlibrium, and influences renal excretion of the hydrogen ion. Normal levels in adults, 3.0 to 4.5 mg/dl of serum; in children, 4.0 to 7.0 mg/dl.

Indications and uses: To prevent or correct hypophosphatemia in patients with restricted or no oral intake.

Precautions: (1) Rapid infusion may cause phosphate or potassium intoxication. Serum calcium may be reduced rapidly causing hypocalcemic tetany. (2) Monitor serum calcium, potassium, phosphate, chlorides, and sodium. Discontinue when serum phosphate exceeds 2 mg/dl. (3) Use sodium phosphate with caution in renal impairment, cirrhosis, cardiac failure, or any edematous, sodium-retaining state. (4) Use potassium phosphate with caution in cardiac disease, renal disease, and digitalized patients. May cause hyperkalemia with potassium-sparing diuretics (e.g., amiloride) or angiotensin-converting enzyme inhibitors (e.g., enalapril [Vasotec]). (5) Safety for use in pregnancy not established.

Contraindications: Any disease with high phosphate or low calcium levels, hyperkalemia, (potassium phosphate), hypernatremia (sodium phosphate).

Incompatible with: Calcium salts, dextrose in Ringer's, dobutamine (Dobutrex), Ionosol solutions (specific), magnesium, Ringer's lactate. Mix thoroughly after each addition of supposedly compatible drugs or solutions.

Side effects: Elevated phosphates; reduced calcium levels and hypocalcemic tetany; elevated potasssium levels causing cardiac dysrhythmias; flaccid paralysis; heaviness of the legs; hypotension; listlessness; mental confusion; paresthesia of the extremities.

Antidote: For any side effect, discontinue the drug and notify the physician. Restore serum calcium with calcium gluconate or chloride. Shift potassium from serum to cells with 150 ml of ⅙ molar sodium lactate or 10% to 20% dextrose with 10 units regular insulin for each 20 Gm dextrose at 300 to 500 ml/hr. Correct acidosis with sodium bicarbonate. Reduce sodium by restriction, diuretics, or hemodialysis. Resuscitate as necessary.

PHYSOSTIGMINE SALICYLATE pH 3.5 to 5.0

(Antilirium)

Usual dose: 0.5 to 2 mg initially. 1 to 4 mg may be repeated as necessary as life-threatening signs recur (dysrhythmias, convulsions, deep coma).

Postanesthesia: 0.5 to 1 mg initially. Repeat at 10- to 30-minute intervals until desired results obtained.

Pediatric dose: *To be used in life-threatening situations only.* 0.5 mg initially. May be repeated at 5- to 10-minute intervals only if toxic effects persist and there is no sign of cholinergic effects. Maximum total dose is 2 mg.

Dilution: May be given undiluted. Do not add to IV solutions. May be given through Y-tube or three-way stopcock of infusion set.

Rate of administration: 1 mg or fraction thereof over 1 to 3 minutes.

Pediatric dose: 0.5 mg or fraction thereof over at least 1 minute.

Actions: An extract of *Physostigma venenosum* seeds. It inhibits the destructive action of cholinesterase and prolongs and exaggerates the effects of acetylcholine.

Stimulates parasympathetic nerve stimulation (pupil contraction, increased intestinal musculature tonus, bronchial constriction, salivary and sweat gland stimulation). Does enter the CNS. Onset of action occurs in 5 minutes and lasts about 1 hour.

Indications and uses: To reverse CNS toxic effects caused by drugs capable of producing anticholinergic poisoning including atropine, glycopyrrolate, and other anticholinergics; antispasmodics (e.g., diazepam [Valium]); and tricyclic antidepressants.

Precautions: (1) Rapid IV administration may cause bradycardia, hypersalivation, respiratory distress, and convulsions. (2) Atropine must always be available. (3) Potentiates narcotic analgesics (e.g., morphine, codeine, meperidine) and succinylcholine (Anectine). (4) Antagonizes ganglionic blocking agents (e.g., trimethaphan [Arfonad]), and aminoglycoside antibiotics (e.g., kanamycin [Kantrex]). (5) Potentiated by colistimethate (Coly-Mycin M); neuromuscular block may be accentuated.

Contraindications: Asthma, cardiovascular disease, diabetes, gangrene, mechanical obstruction of the intestines or urogenital tract, vagotonic states, patients receiving choline esters or depolarizing neuromuscular blocking agents (succinylcholine).

Incompatible with: No specific information available. Because of potential toxicity, should not be mixed with any other drug.

Side effects: Anxiety, bradycardia, cholinergic crisis (overdose), coma, defecation, delirium, disorientation, emesis, hallucinations, hyperactivity, hypersensitivity, nausea, salivation, seizures, sweating, urination.

Antidote: Keep physician informed of side effects. For excessive nausea or sweating, reduce dose. Discontinue drug for excessive defecation, emesis, salivation, or urination. Treat cholinergic crisis or hypersensitivity with the specific antagonist atropine sulfate in doses of 0.6 mg IV. May be repeated every 3 to 10 minutes. Endotracheal intubation or tracheostomy are considered prophylactic in anesthesia or crisis. Artificial ventilation, oxygen therapy, cardiac monitoring, adequate suctioning, and treatment of shock or convulsions must be instituted and maintained as necessary.

PHYTONADIONE pH 3.5 to 7.0

(Aquamephyton, Vitamin K_1)

Usual dose: 2.5 to 25 mg. Up to 50 mg in rare instances. A single dose is preferred, but it may be repeated if clinically indicated.

Newborn dose: 0.5 to 1.0 mg IM or SC only.

Dilution: May be diluted only with normal saline for injection or 5% dextrose in saline. Dilution with at least 10 ml of diluent is recommended to facilitate prescribed rate of administration.

Rate of administration: Each 1 mg or fraction thereof over 1 minute or longer.

Actions: Vitamin K, a fat-soluble vitamin, is essential for the production of prothrombin by the liver. Hemorrhage will occur in its absence. Fastest-acting vitamin K_1 preparation. Results should be detectable in 1 to 2 hours. Usually controls hemorrhage in 3 to 6 hours, and normal prothrombin levels should be obtained in 12 to 14 hours. Metabolized completely by the body. Excreted as metabolites in the urine.

Indications and uses: (1) Anticoagulant-induced prothrombin deficiency (warfarin or dicumarol); (2) hemorrhagic disease of the newborn; (3) hypoprothrombinemia resulting from antibacterial therapy and salicylates; (4) hypoprothrombinemia resulting from obstructive jaundice, biliary fistula, sprue, ulcerative colitis, celiac disease, intestinal resection, cystic fibrosis of the pancreas, and regional enteritis—these diseases limit the absorption and synthesis of vitamin K.

Precautions: (1) Discontinue drugs adversely affecting the coagulation mechanism if possible (e.g., salicylates, antibiotics). (2) Dosage and effect determined by prothrombin times. Keep the physician informed. (3) Use the smallest dose that achieves effective results to prevent clotting hazards. (4) Supplement with whole blood transfusion if indicated. (5) Photosensitive; protect from light in all dilutions. (6) Discard after single use. (7) IV is not route of choice; used only when IM or SC route cannot be used. (8) May cause temporary resistance to prothrombin-depressing oral anticoagulants by increasing amount of phytonadione in the liver and blood. Anticoagulation will require larger doses of same or use of heparin sodium. (9) Pain and swelling at injection site can occur. (10) Use extreme caution in premature infants and neonates. Excessive doses may cause increased bilirubinemia. Severe hemolytic anemia, hemoglobinuria, kernicterus, brain damage, and death may occur.

Contraindications: Liver disease if the response to an initial dose is not satisfactory; hypersensitivity to components.

Incompatible with: Acid pH barbiturates, ascorbic acid, cyanocobalamin (vitamin B_{12}), dextran, pentobarbital (Nembutal), phenobarbital (Luminal), phenytoin (Dilantin), vancomycin (Vancocin), warfarin (Coumadin).

Side effects: Cyanosis, diaphoresis, dizziness, dyspnea, hypotension, peculiar taste sensations, tachycardia, transient flushing sensation. Anaphylaxis, shock, and death have occurred with IV injection.

Antidote: Should not be necessary if dosage is accurately calculated before administration. Action can be reversed by warfarin or heparin if indicated. Discontinue the drug and notify the physician of any side effects. For most side effects the physician will probably choose to continue the drug at a decreased rate of administration. Treat allergic reactions as necessary.

PIPERACILLIN SODIUM pH 5.5 to 7.5

(Pipracil)

Usual dose: 3 to 4 Gm (200 to 300 mg/kg of body weight/24 hr) in equally divided doses every 4, 6, 8, or 12 hours. Maximum dose usually 24 Gm/24 hr.

Perioperative prophylaxis: 2 to 4 Gm 30 minutes to 1 hour before incision. Repeat every 4 to 6 hours for up to 24 hours if indicated. Specific doses for specific procedures (see literature).

Dilution: Each 1 Gm or fraction thereof should be diluted with at least 5 ml of sterile water or 0.9% sodium chloride for injection. Shake vigorously to dissolve.

May be further diluted to desired volume (50 to 100 ml) with 5% dextrose in water, 0.9% normal saline, or other compatible infusion solutions (see literature) and given as an intermittent infusion.

Rate of administration: *Direct IV:* A single dose over 3 to 5 minutes.

Intermittent infusion: A single dose properly diluted over 30 minutes. Discontinue primary IV infusion during administration.

Actions: An extended spectrum penicillin. Bactericidal against a variety of gram-negative and gram-positive bacteria including aerobic and anaerobic strains. Especially effective against *Klebsiella* and *Pseudomonas.* Well distributed in all body fluids, tissue, and bone and through inflamed meninges. Onset of action is prompt. Excreted in bile and urine. Crosses the placental barrier. Secreted in breast milk.

Indications and uses: (1) Treatment of serious lower respiratory tract, intraabdominal, urinary tract, gynecologic, skin and skin structure, bone and joint, and gonococcal infections and septicemia caused by susceptible organisms. May be used in either liver or renal impairment since excretion occurs in bile and urine. Frequently used to initiate therapy in serious infections because of broad spectrum. (2) Perioperative prophylaxis.

Precautions: (1) Stable at room temperature for 24 hours. (2) Frequently used concurrently with aminoglycosides (e.g., kanamycin [Kantrex]), but must be administered in separate infusions; inactivates aminoglycosides. (3) Sensitivity studies indicated to determine susceptibility of the causative organism to piperacillin. (4) Oral probenecid will achieve higher and more prolonged blood levels. May be desirable or may cause toxicity. (5) Watch for early symptoms of allergic reaction. (6) Avoid prolonged use of drug; superinfection caused by overgrowth of nonsusceptible organisms may result. (7) Periodic evaluation of renal, hepatic, and hematopoietic systems and serum potassium is recommended in prolonged therapy. (8) Electrolyte imbalance and cardiac irregularities resulting from high sodium content are very possible. Contains 1.98 mEq sodium/Gm. (9) Confirm patency of vein, avoid extravasation or intraarterial injection. Slow infusion rate for pain along venipuncture site. (10) Usual duration of therapy is 7 to 10 days. Continue at least 2 days after symptoms of infection disappear. (11) Reduce dose only in severe renal impairment with creatinine clearance temporarily below 40 ml/min. May be given to patients undergoing hemodialysis and peritoneal dialysis (see literature for dose). (12) Concomitant use with β-adrenergic blockers (e.g., propranolol [Inderal]) may increase risk of anaphylaxis and inhibit treatment. (13) Risk of bleeding with anticoagulants (e.g., heparin) is increased. (14) Inactivated by chloramphenicol, erythromycin, and tetracyclines. Bactericidal action is actually negated by these drugs. (15) May inhibit effectiveness of oral contraceptives; could result in breakthrough bleeding or pregnancy. (16) Use only if absolutely necessary in pregnancy and lactation. Safety for use in children under 12 years not established. (17) Neuromuscular excitability or convulsions may be caused by higher than normal doses.

Contraindications: History of allergic reaction to any penicillin or cephalosporin, neonates.

Incompatible with: Aminoglycosides (e.g., amikacin, colistimethate, gentamicin, kanamycin, streptomycin, tobramycin), amphotericin B (Fungizone), chloramphenicol, lincomycin, polymyxin B, promethazine (Phenergan), tetracycline (Achromycin), vitamin B with C.

Side effects: Anaphylaxis, convulsions, diarrhea, dizziness, fatigue, headache, increased creatinine or BUN, leukopenia, muscle relaxation (prolonged), nausea, neutropenia, pruritus, thrombocytopenia, thrombophlebitis, skin rash, vomiting.

Antidote: Notify the physician immediately of any adverse symptoms. For severe symptoms, discontinue the drug, treat allergic reaction (antihistamines, epinephrine, corticosteroids), and resuscitate as necessary. Hemodialysis is effective in overdose.

PLASMA PROTEIN FRACTION pH 6.7 to 7.3

(Plasmanate, Plasma-Plex, Plasmatein, Protenate)

Usual dose: Variable, depending on indication for use, condition of patient, and response to therapy. Range is from 250 to 1,500 ml/24 hr. Suggested initial doses are as follows:

Shock: 250 to 500 ml.

Burns: 500 to 1,000 ml.

Hypoproteinemia: 1,000 to 1,500 ml/24 hr. Each 500 ml bottle yields 25 Gm of plasma protein. Do not exceed 250 Gm in 48 hours. Whole blood or plasma probably indicated.

Pediatric dose: 20 to 30 ml/kg of body weight to treat acute shock.

Dilution: Available as a 5% solution buffered with saline in 250 and 500 ml bottles with injection sets. Plasmanate also available in a 50 ml size. No further dilution is required.

Rate of administration: Variable, depending on indication, present blood volume, and patient response. Averages are:

Normal blood volume: 1 ml/min.

Treatment of shock and burns in the adult: 5 to 8 ml/min. Higher rates may be tolerated if necessary. Rapid infusion (over 10 ml/min) may cause hypotension. Decrease flow rate as patient improves.

Treatment of shock in infants and children: 5 to 10 ml/min. Do not exceed 10 ml/min in children.

Treatment of hypoproteinemia: Single 500 ml dose over 1 hour. For larger amounts the maximum rate is 100 ml/hr.

Actions: A sterile natural plasma protein substance containing 88% albumin, 7% alpha globulin, and 5% beta globulin. Contains 130 to 160 mEq sodium/L. It expands intravascular volume, maintains colloid osmotic pressure, prevents marked hemoconcentration, and maintains appropriate electrolyte balance in burns.

Indications and uses: (1) Emergency treatment of shock caused by burns, infections, surgery, or trauma; (2) temporary treatment of hemorrhage when whole blood unavailable; (3) hypoproteinemia until cause determined and corrected.

Precautions: (1) Use immediately after opening and discard any unused portion. Contains no preservatives. (2) Do not use if solution turbid or a sediment visible. (3) May be given without regard to blood group or type. (4) Adjust or slow rate according to clinical response and rising blood pressure. (5) Monitor vital signs (including central venous pressure if possible) and urine output every 5 to 15 minutes for 1 hour and hourly thereafter depending on condition. (6) Observe carefully for increased bleeding resulting from higher than normal blood pressure, circulatory embarrassment, pulmonary edema, or hypervolemia. (7) Whole blood may be indicated for considerable red blood cell loss or anemia caused by large amounts of plasma protein. (8) Additional fluids are required for dehydrated patients. Tissue dehydration caused by osmotic action of plasma proteins can be acute. (9) Hemoglobin, hematocrit, electrolyte, and serum protein evaluations are necessary during therapy. May cause an elevated alkaline phosphatase level. (10) Not effective for coagulation mechanism defects. (11) Added protein load requires caution in hepatic or renal impairment. (12) If continuous protein loss occurs or edema is present, normal serum albumin (25%) may be the preferred product.

Contraindications: Cardiac failure, cardiopulmonary bypass, history of allergic reactions to albumin, normal or increased intravascular volume, severe anemia.

Incompatible with: Alcohol, norepinephrine (Levophed).

Side effects: Allergic and/or pyrogenic reactions can occur. Incidence of toxicity is low when administered with appropriate caution. Slight nausea does occur. Hypotension can be sudden if administered too rapidly.

Antidote: Notify the physician of all symptoms and side effects. Discontinue infusion for sudden hypotension. Decrease flow rate if indicated and treat symptomatically. Resuscitate as necessary.

PLICAMYCIN pH 7.0

(Mithracin, Mithramycin)

Usual dose: *Testicular tumors:* 25 to 30 mcg/kg of body weight/24 hr. Repeat daily for 8 to 10 days unless significant side effects or toxicity occur. Repeat at monthly intervals if indicated.

Hypercalcemia and hypercalciuria: 25 mcg/kg of body weight/24 hr for 3 or 4 days. Repeat weekly as required to maintain normal calcium levels.

Dilution: *Specific techniques required, see Precautions.* Each 2.5 mg vial must be initially diluted with 4.9 ml of sterile water for injection (1 ml equals 500 mcg). A single daily dose must be further diluted in 1,000 ml of 5% dextrose in water and given as an infusion. Do not use a filter smaller than 5 microns. Loss of potency will occur.

Rate of administration: A single dose every 24 hours over 4 to 6 hours.

Actions: A potent antibiotic, antineoplastic agent. Interferes with cell division by binding with DNA to inhibit and slow production of RNA. Exact mechanism unknown. Cytotoxic to HeLa cell tissue culture and some animal tumors. Will produce hypocalcemia in patients with cancer.

Indications and uses: (1) Testicular tumors not treatable with surgery and/or radiation; (2) hypercalcemia and hypercalciuria associated with many advanced neoplasms.

Precautions: (1) Follow guidelines for handling cytotoxic agents. See Appendix, p. 677. (2) Administered by or under the direction of the physician specialist. (3) Determine absolute patency of vein; cellulitis and tissue necrosis may result from extravasation. Discontinue injection, use another vein. Elevate extremity and apply warm moist heat to the extravasated area. (4) Store in refrigerator before dilution. Prepare fresh daily and discard any unused portion. (5) Dosage based on average weight in presence of edema or ascites. (6) Severe sudden onset of hemorrhage and even death can result from use. (7) Maintain hydration and correct electrolyte imbalance before treatment. (8) Use extreme caution in impaired renal or hepatic function. (9) Monitor platelet count, PT, and bleeding time during and after therapy. (10) Safety for use in pregnancy and lactation and in men and women capable of conception not documented. (11) Many drug interactions possible; observe patient closely. (12) Do not administer vaccines or chloroquine to patients receiving antineoplastic drugs. (13) Observe closely for all signs of infection. (14) Prophylactic antiemetics may reduce nausea and vomiting and increase patient comfort.

Contraindications: Thrombocytopenia, thrombocytopathy, coagulation disorders or any susceptibility to bleeding, impairment of bone marrow function, lack of hospital and laboratory facilities.

Incompatible with: Specific information not available. Should be considered incompatible with any other drug because of toxicity and specific use.

Side effects: *Minor:* Anorexia, depression, diarrhea, drowsiness, fever, flushing, headache, nausea, skin rash, stomatitis, vomiting.

Major: Abnormal clot retraction, abnormal liver function tests, abnormal renal function tests, elevation of bleeding and clotting time, epistaxis (severe), hematemesis, hemoglobin depression, leukopenia (unusual), platelet count depression, prothrombin content depression, serum calcium, phosphorus, and potassium depression.

Antidote: Minor side effects will be treated symptomatically. Discontinue the drug and notify the physician immediately of any major side effects. Platelet-rich plasma may help to elevate platelet count. Provide immediate treatment or supportive therapy as indicated; bleeding episodes can be fatal. If extravasation has occurred, long-acting dexamethasone injected into the indurated area with a fine hypodermic needle may be helpful. Apply moderate heat.

POLYMYXIN B SULFATE pH 5.0 to 7.5

(Aerosporin)

Usual dose: 15,000 to 25,000 units/kg of body weight/24 hr. Give one half of total 24-hour dose every 12 hours. Normal renal function is necessary for this dose. In impaired renal function, decrease dose from 15,000 units/kg/24 hr downward.

Infant dose: With normal kidney function, up to 40,000 units/kg of body weight/ 24 hr.

Dilution: Each 500,000 units of powder must be initially diluted with 5 ml of sterile water or normal saline for injection (100,000 units/ml). Each single dose must be further diluted in 300 to 500 ml of 5% dextrose in water and given as a continuous infusion.

Rate of administration: Each single dose properly diluted over a minimum of 60 to 90 minutes.

Actions: A polypeptide antibiotic with neuromuscular blocking action. Bactericidal against many gram-negative organisms. Poorly absorbed into serum and tissue. Does not pass the blood-brain barrier. Slowly excreted in the urine. Development of resistant strains seldom occurs.

Indications and uses: Treatment of acute infections caused by susceptible gram-negative organisms, especially *Pseudomonas aeruginosa*.

Precautions: (1) Refrigerate unused medication after initial dilution and discard after 72 hours. (2) Sensitivity studies necessary to determine susceptibility of the causative organism to polymyxin B. (3) Watch for decrease in urine output, rising BUN and serum creatinine, and declining creatinine clearance levels. Drug may need to be discontinued. Routine serum levels and renal function evaluation are necessary. (4) Potentiated by anesthetics, other neuromuscular blocking antibiotics (e.g., kanamycin, streptomycin), anticholinesterases (e.g., edrophonium, [Tensilon]), antineoplastics (e.g., nitrogen mustard), barbiturates, muscle relaxants (e.g., tubocurarine), phenothiazines (e.g., promethazine [Phenergan]), procainamide, quinidine, and sodium citrate. *Apnea can occur.* Concurrent use not recommended. (5) Superinfection may occur from overgrowth of nonsusceptible organisms. (6) Maintain good hydration.

Contraindications: Known polymyxin sensitivity, pregnancy.

Incompatible with: Strong acids or alkalies; cobaltous, ferrous, magnesium, or manganous ions; amphotericin B; ampicillin (Omnipen); cefazolin (Kefzol); cephalothin (Keflin); chloramphenicol (Chloromycetin); chlorothiazide (Diuril); heparin; magnesium sulfate; prednisolone (Hydeltrasol); tetracycline (Achromycin).

Side effects: Albuminuria; apnea; ataxia; azotemia; cylindruria; dizziness; fever; flushing; increasing blood levels without increased dose; increased BUN, nonprotein nitrogen, creatinine; oliguria; peripheral paresthesias; rash; thrombophlebitis.

Antidote: Discontinue the drug and notify the physician of all side effects. Depending on diagnosis, dosage may be reduced or an alternate drug indicated. Nephrotoxicity is reversible. Most treatment will be symptomatic. Maintain an adequate airway and artificial ventilation as indicated. Treat allergic reactions and resuscitate as necessary.

POTASSIUM CHLORIDE AND POTASSIUM ACETATE

pH 4.0 to 8.0

Usual dose: 20 to 60 mEq/24 hr. Up to 400 mEq/24 hr has been given in selected situations with extreme caution.

Pediatric dose: 3 mEq/kg of body weight. Do not exceed 40 mEq/day.

Dilution: Each individual dose must be diluted in a larger volume of suitable IV solution and given as an infusion. Soluble in all commonly used IV solutions. Avoid layering of potassium by thoroughly agitating the prepared IV solution. Do not add potassium to an IV bottle in the hanging position. In severe hypokalemia, solutions without dextrose are preferred (dextrose might decrease serum potassium level).

Rate of administration: A maximum of 10 mEq/hr of potassium chloride in any given amount of infusion fluid should not be exceeded. With serious potassium depletion (under 2.5 mEq/L serum), 40 mEq/hr has been given with extreme caution.

Actions: Helps to maintain osmotic pressure and ion balance. Flow of potassium into the cell (serum deficiency) increases membrane resting potential and decreases membrane permeability. Flow of potassium out of the cell (serum excess) decreases resting membrane potential and increases membrane permeability. Essential for intracellular tonicity; nerve impulse transmission; cardiac, skeletal, and smooth muscle contraction; normal renal function; metabolism of carbohydrates and proteins; and enzyme reactions. Excreted in urine.

Indications and uses: Prophylaxis or treatment of potassium deficiency (e.g., hypokalemia due to diuretic therapy, digitalis intoxication, low dietary potassium intake, vomiting and diarrhea, diabetic acidosis, metabolic alkalosis, corticosteroid therapy, increased renal excretion resulting from acidosis, hemodialysis).

Precautions: (1) Use only clear solutions. (2) Normal kidney function of utmost importance. (3) Routine serum potassium, calcium, and sodium levels; pH; ECGs; adequate hydration; and evaluation of adequate urine output are mandatory. (4) Continuous cardiac monitoring is preferable for infusion of over 10 mEq of potassium in 1 hour. (5) Confirm absolute patency of vein. Extravasation will cause necrosis. (6) Potentiated by angiotensin-converting enzyme inhibitors (e.g., spironolactone [Aldactone]). (7) Digitalis intoxication may occur with hypokalemia. Use with extreme caution in patients taking digitalis. (8) Potassium-sparing diuretics (e.g., amiloride) may cause hypokalemia. (9) Potassium phosphate is preferred for specific intracellular deficiency not caused by alkalosis, since phosphate is the usual ion attached to potassium in the body. Not used in the presence of kidney failure. (10) Potassium acetate preferred for potassium deficiency patients with renal tubular acidosis. Metabolic acidosis and hyperchloremia are most likely present. (11) Use caution in pregnancy and lactation.

Contraindications: Adrenal cortex insufficiency, hyperkalemia, impaired renal function, patients on digitalis with severe or complete heart block, postoperative oliguria (not absolute), shock with hemolytic reactions and/or dehydration.

Incompatible with: Amikacin (Amikin), amphotericin B (Fungizone), dobutamine (Dobutrex), fat emulsion 10%, mannitol, penicillin G sodium.

Side effects: Bradycardia, cardiac arrest, confusion, diarrhea, dysphagia, ECG changes (including increased amplitude of T wave, decreased amplitude of R wave, below baseline depression of S wave, disappearing P wave, PR prolongation), hyperkalemia, respiratory distress, weakness, ventricular fibrillation, voluntary muscle paralysis, death.

Antidote: For any side effect, discontinue the drug and notify the physician. For severe hyperkalemia (over 8 mEq/L plasma), use IV dextrose, 10% to 20%, with 10 units of regular insulin for each 50 Gm of dextrose (give 300 to 500 ml/hr) or 150 ml of ⅙ molar sodium lactate. Use IV sodium bicarbonate to correct acidosis. Eliminate potassium-containing foods and medicines. Monitor ECG continuously. If P waves are absent, give calcium gluconate or chloride (do not use if patient receiving digitalis). All of these measures cause a shift of potassium into the cells and may be used simultaneously. Sodium polystyrene sulfonate (Kayexalate) orally or as retention enemas is used to actually remove potassium from the body. Hemodialysis or peritoneal dialysis may be useful. Use caution in the digitalized patient; too rapid removal of potassium may cause digitalis toxicity. Resuscitate as necessary. For extravasation, inject area with 1% procaine and hyaluronidase (Wydase). Use a 27- or 25-gauge needle. Apply warm moist compresses.

PRALIDOXIME CHLORIDE pH 3.5 to 4.5

(Protopam chloride)

Usual dose: *Poisoning:* 1 Gm initially. Repeat in 1 hour if indicated. Double dose for overwhelming toxicity. If symptoms continue, additional doses can be given with extreme caution. Atropine must be given before pralidoxime but after adequate ventilation has been established.

Cholinergic crisis due to overdose of carbamate anticholinesterase drugs (e.g., neostigmine, pyridostigmine): 1 to 2 Gm followed by 250 mg every 5 minutes.

Pediatric dose: 20 to 40 mg/kg of body weight as initial dose in poisoning.

Dilution: Each 1 Gm of sterile powder is diluted with 20 ml of sterile water for injection. Should be further diluted in 100 ml of normal saline and given as an IV infusion.

Rate of administration: Each 1 Gm or fraction thereof over 5 minutes.

Infusion: given over 15 to 30 minutes.

Actions: An anticholinesterase antagonist that reactivates cholinesterase inhibited by phosphate esters. A chemical reaction with anticholinesterases and depolarization at the neuromuscular junction also takes place. Rapidly absorbed and well dispersed throughout body fluids. Most of a single dose is excreted within 6 hours in the urine.

Indications and uses: (1) Antidote for anticholinesterase drug or chemical overdose or poisoning. Primarily useful for many phosphate ester insecticide poisons with anticholinesterase activity (e.g., parathion). (2) Control of overdose of anticholinesterase drugs used to treat myasthenia gravis. Confirm diagnosis with edrophonium (Tensilon).

Precautions: *In all indications including poisoning:* (1) Establish and maintain an adequate airway and controlled respiration as indicated. (2) Give atropine, 2 to 4 mg IV, after cyanosis disappears. Repeat every 10 minutes until atropine toxicity (pulse 140 beats/min). Ventricular fibrillation can occur if oxygenation is inadequate. Maintain atropinization for up to 48 hours. (3) Monitor vital signs and ECG continuously. (4) Morphine, theophylline (aminophylline), succinylcholine, reserpine compounds, and phenothiazines are contraindicated. May defeat effectiveness. Potentiates barbiturates.

In poisoning: (5) Wear rubber gloves to protect hands. (6) Remove contaminated clothing and cleanse contaminated skin surfaces with water, baking soda solution, and alcohol. (7) Thiopental sodium may be required to stop convulsions. Use with extreme caution. May cause additional respiratory depression. (8) Maintain adequate urine output. (9) Use caution in myasthenia gravis; may cause a myasthenic crisis. (10) Toxicity may recur as poison is absorbed from bowel. (11) Reduce dose in renal impairment.

Contraindications: None when indicated. Increases toxicity of Sevin (carbamate insecticide).

Incompatible with: Any other drug in syringe or solution because of specific use.

Side effects: Usually minor and transient: blurred vision, diplopia, dizziness, headache, impaired accommodation, laryngospasm, muscle rigidity, nausea, pharyngeal pain, tachycardia.

Antidote: Has not been needed. Patient should be observed for atropine intoxication. Maintain vital signs by any means necessary.

PREDNISOLONE SODIUM PHOSPHATE

pH 7.0 to 8.0

(Hydeltrasol, Key-Pred SP, Predicort-RP, Prednisolone Phosphate)

Usual dose: 4 to 60 mg/24 hr initially. 10 to 20 mg every 3 to 4 hours may be given. Total dose usually does not exceed 400 mg every 24 hours. Dosage individualized according to the severity of the disease and the response of the patient.

Pediatric dose: Smaller dosage is usually required.

Dilution: May be given without mixing or dilution. Always use a separate syringe for Hydeltrasol. May be added to sodium chloride injection or dextrose injection and given by IV infusion. Use solution within 24 hours of dilution.

Rate of administration: 10 mg or fraction thereof over 1 minute. Decrease rate of injection if any complaints of burning or tingling along injection site.

Actions: Rapidly absorbed synthetic adrenocortical steroid with potent metabolic and antiinflammatory actions. May be used in conjunction with other forms of therapy, such as epinephrine for acute allergic reactions or antibiotics in acute infections. It is three to four times more potent than hydrocortisone. It is absorbed primarily into the lymph stream and probably excreted in the urine. Crosses the placental barrier. Secreted in breast milk.

Indications and uses: (1) Supplementary therapy for severe allergic reactions (use epinephrine first); (2) adrenocortical insufficiency: total, relative, and operative; (3) shock unresponsive to conventional therapy; (4) acute exacerbations of disease for patients on steroid therapy; (5) acute life-threatening infections with massive antibiotic therapy; (6) to induce remission of some malignancies; (7) viral hepatitis; (8) thyroid crisis; (9) diagnostic aid to distinguish between adrenocortical hyperplasia and adrenocortical tumor.

Precautions: (1) Give a single daily dose by 9 AM to reduce suppression of individual's own adrenocortical activity. (2) Sensitive to heat. (3) May cause elevated blood pressure and salt and water retention. (4) Salt restriction and potassium replacement necessary. (5) May mask signs of infection. (6) To avoid adrenocortical insufficiency, do not stop therapy abruptly; taper off. Patient is observed carefully, especially under stress, for up to 2 years. (7) Maintain on ulcer regimen and antacid prophylactically. (8) May increase insulin needs in diabetes. (9) Caution when used with cyclophosphamide (Cytoxan). Dosage adjustments may be required. (10) Inhibits anticoagulants, isoniazid, and salicylates. (11) Inhibited by some antihistamines, barbiturates, hydantoins, rifampin, and troleandomycin. (12) Potentiates theophyllines and cyclosporine. (13) Monitor serum potassium levels; may cause hypokalemia with digitalis products, amphotericin B, or potassium-depleting diuretics. (14) Do not vaccinate with attenuated-virus vaccines (e.g., smallpox) during therapy. (15) Altered protein-binding capacity will impact effectiveness of this drug.

Contraindications: *Absolute contraindications, except in life-threatening situations:* Hypersensitivity to any product component including sulfites; systemic fungal infections.

Relative contraindications: Active or latent peptic ulcer, active or healed tuberculosis, acute psychoses, chickenpox, diabetes mellitus, diverticulitis, fresh intestinal anastomoses, hypertension, myasthenia gravis, ocular herpes simplex, osteoporosis, pregnancy, psychotic tendencies, renal insufficiency, thromboembolic tendencies, vaccinia.

Incompatible with: Calcium gluceptate, calcium gluconate, dimenhydrinate (Dramamine), metaraminol (Aramine), methotrexate, polymyxin B (Aerosporin), prochlorperazine (Compazine), promazine (Sparine), promethazine (Phenergan). Not generally mixed with any other drug in a solution.

Side effects: Do occur, but are usually reversible: anaphylaxis, Cushing's syndrome (moon face, fat pads, etc.), decrease in spermatozoa, euphoria, fat emboli, fluid and electrolyte imbalance with edema, increased intracranial pressure, menstrual irregularities, peptic ulcer with perforation and hemorrhage, protein catabolism with negative nitrogen balance, relative adrenocortical insufficiency, spontaneous fractures, suppression of growth, transitory burning or tingling, and many others.

Antidote: Notify the physician of any side effect. Will probably treat the side effect. Resuscitate as necessary for anaphylaxis and notify the physician. Keep epinephrine immediately available.

PROCAINAMIDE HYDROCHLORIDE pH 4.0 to 6.0

(Pronestyl)

Usual dose: 0.2 to 1 Gm (100 mg/ml). 100 mg every 5 minutes (600 mg over 30 minutes) may be given as an infusion until dysrhythmia suppressed or maximum initial dose (1 Gm) is reached. An initial loading dose of 12 mg/kg of body weight (total dose) may also be given by the above method as an alternate dosage regimen. Follow either choice of initial dosage with an infusion of 1 to 6 mg/min. Titrate to control dysrhythmias (0.02 to 0.08 mg/kg/min is an alternate dosing regimen for maintenance). Maintain with oral procainamide as soon as possible but at least 4 hours after last IV dose.

Pediatric dose: 2 to 5 mg/kg of body weight. Do not exceed 100 mg. Repeat as indicated every 10 to 30 minutes. Maximum dose in 24 hours is 30 mg/kg. An alternate dose regimen is 3 to 6 mg given over 5 minutes; follow with a maintenance infusion of 0.02 to 0.08 mg/kg/min to control dysrhythmias.

Dilution: *Direct IV:* Dilute each 100 mg with 10 ml of 5% dextrose in water or sterile water for injection.

Infusion: Add 1 Gm of procainamide to 250 to 500 ml of 5% dextrose in water. Solution gives 4 or 2 mg procainamide for each milliliter.

Rate of administration: 20 mg or fraction thereof over 1 minute. Use an infusion pump or a microdrip (60 gtt/ml) for infusion. Up to 50 mg may be given direct IV over 1 minute with extreme caution. After initial dosage follow with a maintenance infusion at 1 to 6 mg/min.

Actions: A procaine derivative. Exerts a depressing antiarrhythmic action on the heart, slowing the rate, slowing conduction, reducing myocardial irritability, and prolonging the refractory period. Decreases membrane permeability of the cell and prevents loss of sodium and potassium ions. Onset of action should occur in 2 to 3 minutes. Crosses the placental barrier. Plasma levels decrease slowly; it is excreted in the urine.

Indications and uses: (1) Ventricular and supraventricular dysrhythmias such as extrasystoles and tachycardia; (2)

atrial fibrillation; (3) paroxysmal atrial tachycardia; (4) dysrhythmias caused by anesthesia; (5) prevent recurrence of ventricular tachycardia after conversion to sinus rhythm by other drugs or methods.

Precautions: (1) Photosensitive; protect from light. Store in refrigerator. (2) Solution should be clear, may be light yellow. Discard if darker than light amber. (3) Monitor the patient's ECG and blood pressure continuously. Keep patient in a supine position. (4) Oral or IM administration is the route of choice; IV route for emergencies only. (5) Discontinue IV use when the cardiac dysrhythmia is interrupted or when the ventricular rate slows without regular atrioventricular conduction. (6) Small emboli may be dislodged when atrial fibrillation is corrected. (7) Use extreme caution in first or second degree blocks, ventricular tachycardia after a myocardial infarction, digitalis intoxication, and impaired liver and kidney function. (8) Potentiates or is potentiated by neuromuscular blocking antibiotics (e.g., kanamycin [Kantrex]), anticholinergics (e.g., atropine), thiazide diuretics, antihypertensive agents, muscle relaxants, succinylcholine (Anectine), cimetidine (Tagamet), and others. (9) Use care with digitalis, lidocaine (Xylocaine), and quinidine. Lower doses of both drugs may be required. (10) Antagonizes anticholinesterases (e.g., neostigmine). (11) Alcohol may increase hepatic metabolism. (12) May elevate SGOT levels. (13) Safety for use in pregnancy and lactation and in children not established.

Contraindications: Complete atrioventricular heart block, second and third degree AV block unless an electrical pacemaker is operative, torsade de pointes, known sensitivity to procainamide or any other local anesthetic of the amide type, myasthenia gravis, systemic lupus erythematosus.

Incompatible with: Phenytoin (Dilantin). Physically compatible with many drugs. However, combination is not practical because of individualized rate adjustments necessary to achieve desired effects.

Side effects: *Minor:* Anorexia, bleeding, bruising, chills, fever, flushing, hallucinations, giddiness, joint swelling or pain, mental confusion, nausea, skin rash, vomiting, weakness.

Major: Agranulocytosis, hypotension with a blood pressure drop over 15 mm Hg, lupus erythematosus-like symptoms, PR interval prolongation, QRS complex widening, QT interval prolongation, ventricular asystole, ventricular fibrillation, ventricular tachycardia.

Antidote: Notify the physician of any side effect. If minor symptoms progress or any major side effect appears, discontinue the drug immediately and notify the physician. Use dopamine (Intropin) or phenylephrine hydrochloride (Neo-Synephrine) to correct hypotension. Treatment of toxicity is symptomatic and supportive. Infusion of ⅙ molar sodium lactate injection may reduce cardiotoxic effects. Hemodialysis may be indicated or urinary acidifiers may increase renal clearance. Resuscitate as necessary. Depending on dysrhythmia, quinidine or lidocaine is an effective alternate. Consider insertion of a ventricular pacing electrode as a precautionary measure in case serious AV block develops.

PROCHLORPERAZINE EDISYLATE pH 4.2 to 6.2

(Compazine, ✱ Stemetil)

Usual dose: 5 to 10 mg, may be repeated one time in 1 to 2 hours if indicated. 40 mg/24 hr is the maximum parenteral dose.

Management of emetic-inducing chemotherapy: 20 mg 30 minutes before and 3 hours after treatment.

Dilution: Each 5 mg (1 ml) should be diluted with 9 ml of normal saline for injection. 1 ml will equal 0.5 mg. Add 10 to 20 mg to 1 liter of isotonic IV solution and give as an infusion. Prochlorperazine may cause the solution to turn a light yellow color.

Rate of administration: *Direct IV:* Each 5 mg or fraction thereof over 1 minute.

Intermittent IV: A single dose over 20 minutes in management of emetic-inducing chemotherapy.

Infusion: May be given at ordered rate, or rate may be increased or decreased as symptoms indicate. Use an infusion pump or a microdrip (60 gtt/ml) for infusion.

Actions: A phenothiazine derivative said to be four times more potent than chlorpromazine (Thorazine), with effects on the central, autonomic, and peripheral nervous systems. Decreases anxiety and tension, relaxes muscle, produces sedation, and tranquilizes. A potent antiemetic. Onset of action is prompt and lasting. Excretion is slow through the kidneys.

Indications and uses: (1) Control of nausea, vomiting, retching, and hyperexcitability before, during, and after surgery; (2) treatment of withdrawal symptoms from alcohol, barbiturates, or narcotics; (3) antipsychotic drug.

Precautions: (1) Use IV only when absolutely necessary. IV not recommended for children. (2) Sensitive to light. Slightly yellow color does not affect potency. Discard if markedly discolored. (3) Handle carefully; may cause contact dermatitis. (4) Keep patient in supine position and monitor blood pressure and pulse before administration and between doses. (5) May mask diagnosis of brain tumor, drug intoxication, and intestinal obstruction. (6) Use caution in coronary disease, severe hypertension or hypotension, and epilepsy. (7) Potentiates CNS depressant effects of narcotics, barbiturates, alcohol, anesthetics. Additive effects with MAO inhibitors (e.g., pargyline [Eutonyl]), oral antidiabetics, insulin, anticholinergics, antihistamines, antihypertensives, hypnotics, muscle relaxants, phenytoin (Dilantin), propranolol (Inderal), and Rauwolfia alkaloids. Reduce dosage of any medication potentiated by phenothiazines by one fourth to one half. (8) Contraindicated with quinidine, epinephrine, and thiazide diuretics. (9) Capable of innumerable other interactions. (10) Greater extrapyramidal and antiemetic effects than other phenothiazines with less sedative and hypotensive reactions. (11) May discolor urine pink to reddish brown. (12) Photosensitivity of skin is possible. (13) May cause paradoxical excitation in children and the elderly.

Contraindications: Bone marrow depression, children under 2 years or 10 kg (22 lb), comatose or severely depressed states, hypersensitivity to phenothiazines, lactation, and pregnancy, except labor and delivery; do not use in pediatric surgery.

Incompatible with: Aminophylline, amobarbital (Amytal), amphotericin B, ampicillin, calcium gluceptate, calcium gluconate, cephalothin (Keflin), chloramphenicol (Chloromycetin), chlorothiazide (Diuril), dexamethasone (Decadron), dimenhydrinate (Dramamine), epinephrine (Adrenalin), erythromycin (Ilotycin), heparin, hydrocortisone sodium succinate (Solu-Cortef), hydromorphone (Dilaudid), kanamycin (Kantrex), levallorphan (Lorfan), methicillin (Staphcillin), methohexital (Brevital), midazolam (Versed) oxytocin, paraldehyde, penicillin G potassium and sodium, pentobarbital (Nembutal), phenobarbital (Luminal), phenytoin (Dilantin), prednisolone (Hydeltrasol), secobarbital (Seconal), tetracycline, thiopental (Pentothal), vancomycin (Vancocin), vitamin B complex with C. *Should be considered incompatible in syringe with any other drug.*

Side effects: Usually transient if drug discontinued but may require treatment if severe: anaphylaxis, blurring of vision, cardiac arrest, dermatitis, dizziness, dryness of mouth, dysphagia, elevated blood pressure, extrapyramidal symptoms (e.g., abnormal positioning, extreme restlessness, pseudoparkinsonism, weakness of extremities), excitement, hypersensitivity reactions, hypotension, slurred speech, spastic movements (especially about the face), tachycardia, temperature without etiology, tightness of the throat, tongue discoloration, tongue protrusion, and many others. Overdose can cause convulsions, hallucinations, and death.

Antidote: Discontinue the drug at onset of any side effect and notify the physician. Counteract hypotension with IV fluids and dopamine (Intropin) and extrapyramidal symptoms with benztropine mesylate (Cogentin) or diphenhydramine (Benadryl). Epinephrine is contraindicated for hypotension. Further hypotension will occur. Use diazepam (Valium) or phenobarbital for convulsions or hyperactivity. Phenytoin may be helpful in ventricular dysrhythmias. In treating respiratory depression and unconsciousness, avoid analeptics such as doxapram (Dopram); they may cause convulsions. Resuscitate as necessary.

PROMAZINE HYDROCHLORIDE pH 4.0 to 5.5

(Norazine, Prozine, Sparine)

Usual dose: 25 to 50 mg. May repeat as indicated by symptoms. If necessary to repeat within 1 hour, use caution.

Dilution: May be given undiluted, but never exceed a concentration of 25 mg/ml. Each 25 to 50 mg (1 ml, depending on initial dilution) should be further diluted with 9 ml of normal saline for injection. 1 ml of diluted solution will equal 2.5 to 5 mg of promazine.

Rate of administration: 25 mg or fraction thereof over 1 minute.

Actions: A phenothiazine derivative, primarily an antianxiety agent, with effects on the central, autonomic, and peripheral nervous systems. Decreases anxiety and tension, relaxes muscle, produces sedation, and tranquilizes. A potent antiemetic. Onset of action is prompt and lasting. Excretion is slow through the kidneys.

Indications and uses: (1) Control of nausea, vomiting, retching, hiccups, and hyperexcitability before, during, and after surgery; (2) treatment of withdrawal symptoms from alcohol, barbiturates, or narcotics; (3) antipsychotic drug.

Precautions: (1) Use IV only when absolutely necessary. Establish unquestionable patency of vein. Avoid extravasation. (2) Intraarterial injection will cause gangrene. (3) Handle carefully; may cause contact dermatitis. (4) Monitor blood pressure and pulse before administration and between doses. Keep patient in supine position. (5) Use with caution in the presence of cerebral arteriosclerosis, coronary heart disease, severe hypertension or hypotension, epilepsy, heat exhaustion, liver disease, and respiratory problems. (6) May mask diagnosis of brain tumor, drug intoxication, and intestinal obstruction. (7) Potentiates CNS depressant effects of narcotics, barbiturates, alcohol, anesthetics, polypeptide antibiotics (e.g., bacitracin), and procarbazine. Additive effects with MAO inhibitors (e.g., pargyline [Eutonyl]), oral antidiabetics, insulin, anticholinergics, antihistamines, antihypertensives, hypnotics, muscle relaxants, phenytoin (Dilantin), propranolol

(Inderal), Rauwolfia alkaloids, and tricyclic antidepressants. Reduce dosage of any medication potentiated by phenothiazines by one fourth to one half. (8) Contraindicated with quinidine, epinephrine, and thiazide diuretics. (9) Capable of innumerable other interactions. (10) In large doses, extrapyramidal, antiemetic, and sedative effects are moderate. Hypotensive effects are very prominent. (11) May discolor urine pink to reddish brown. (12) Photosensitivity of skin is possible.

Contraindications: Bone marrow depression, children under 12 years, comatose or severely depressed states, hypersensitivity to phenothiazines, lactation, and pregnancy, except labor and delivery.

Incompatible with: Aminophylline, amobarbital (Amytal), ampicillin (Polycillin), atropine, chloramphenicol (Chloromycetin), chlorothiazide (Diuril), dimenhydrinate (Dramamine), epinephrine (Adrenalin), heparin, hydrocortisone phosphate, hydrocortisone sodium succinate (Solu-Cortef), methicillin (Staphcillin), methohexital (Brevital), nafcillin (Unipen), normal saline, penicillin G potassium and sodium, pentobarbital (Nembutal), phenobarbital (Luminal), phenytoin (Dilantin), prednisolone (Hydeltrasol), sodium bicarbonate, thiopental (Pentothal), vitamin B with C, warfarin (Coumadin).

Side effects: Usually transient if drug is discontinued but may require treatment if severe; considered less toxic than prochlorperazine. Anaphylaxis, blurring of vision, cardiac arrest, cerebral edema, convulsions, dermatitis, dizziness, dryness of mouth, dysphagia, extrapyramidal symptoms (e.g., abnormal positioning, extreme restlessness, pseudoparkinsonism, weakness of extremities), elevated blood pressure, excitement, hypersensitivity reactions, hypotension, slurred speech, spastic movements (especially about the face), tachycardia, temperature without etiology, tightness of the throat, tongue discoloration, tongue protrusion, and many others.

Antidote: Discontinue the drug at onset of any side effect and notify the physician. Counteract hypotension with dopamine (Intropin) and IV fluids; extrapyramidal symptoms with benztropine mesylate (Cogentin) or diphenhydramine (Benadryl). Epinephrine is contraindicated for hypotension. Further hypotension will occur. Use diazepam (Valium) or phenobarbital for convulsions or hyperactivity. Phenytoin may be helpful in ventricular dysrhythmias. In treating respiratory depression and unconsciousness, avoid analeptics such as doxapram (Dopram); they may cause convulsions. Resuscitate as necessary.

PROMETHAZINE HYDROCHLORIDE

pH 4.0 to 5.5

(Anergan 25, Phenazine 25, Phenergan, Prometh-25, Prorex, Prothazine, V-Gan 25)

Usual dose: 12.5 to 25 mg. May be repeated in 4 to 6 hours if indicated. Maintain with IM or oral medication as soon as feasible. Ampoule must state "for IV use."

Pediatric dose: 1 mg/kg of body weight every 4 to 6 hours. IV rarely used. Do not exceed one half of adult dose.

Dilution: Never exceed a concentration of 25 mg/ml. Each 25 to 50 mg (1 ml), depending on initial dilution, should be diluted with 9 ml of normal saline for injection. 1 ml of diluted solution will equal 2.5 to 5 mg of promethazine.

Rate of administration: Each 25 mg or fraction thereof over 2 minutes.

Actions: A phenothiazine derivative with effects on the central, autonomic, and peripheral nervous systems. It has potent antihistaminic, antiemetic, and amnesic actions. Potentiates the analgesic and sedative effects of narcotics and other CNS depressants. Promethazine relaxes smooth muscle. Onset of action is prompt and lasts 4 to 6 hours. Readily absorbed, primarily metabolized in the liver and excreted in the urine.

Indications and uses: (1) Prophylaxis or treatment of minor transfusion reactions; (2) treatment of hypersensitivity reactions; (3) treatment of acute nausea, vomiting, and motion sickness; (4) adjunct to narcotic analgesics in control of postoperative pain; (5) sedation to meet surgical and obstetrical needs.

Precautions: (1) Multiple-dose vials or diluted solutions should be refrigerated. (2) Sensitive to light. Slightly yellow color does not alter potency. Discard if greatly discolored. (3) Handle carefully; may cause contact dermatitis. (4) Determine absolute patency of vein; extravasation will cause necrosis. (5) Keep patient in supine position. Monitor blood pressure and pulse before administration and between doses. (6) Potentiates CNS depressant effects of narcotics, alcohol, anesthetics, and barbiturates. Additive effects with MAO inhibitors (e.g., pargyline [Eutonyl]), oral antidiabetics, anticholinergics, antihistamines, antihypertensives, hypnotics, insulin, muscle relaxants, phenytoin (Dilantin), propranolol (Inderal), Rauwolfia alkaloids, and sulfonamides. Reduce dosage of any medication potentiated by phenothiazines by one fourth to one half. (7) May produce apnea with neuromuscular blocking antibiotics (e.g., gentamicin). (8) Contraindicated with quinidine, epinephrine, and thiazide diuretics. (9) Capable of innumerable other interactions. (10) Sedative effect may require ambulation to be monitored. (11) Use with extreme caution in children and the elderly. (12) May cause paradoxical excitation in children and the elderly. (13) Use phenothiazines with extreme caution in children with a history of sleep apnea, a family history of sudden infant death syndrome, or in the presence of Reye's syndrome. (14) May lower seizure threshold; use extreme caution in patients with known seizure disorders and with narcotics or local anesthetics that also lower seizure threshold.

Contraindications: Bone marrow depression, comatose or severely depressed states, hypersensitivity to phenothiazines, jaundice, lactation, pregnancy. Never inject into an artery.

Incompatible with: Aminophylline, calcium gluconate, carbenicillin (Geopen), chloramphenicol (Chloromycetin), chlordiazepoxide (Librium), chlorothiazide (Diuril), codeine, dextran, diatrizoate sodium and meglumine, dimenhydrinate (Dramamine), heparin, hydrocortisone sodium succinate (Solu-Cortef), iodipamide sodium and meglumine, methicillin (Staphcillin), methohexital (Brevital), methylprednisolone (Solu-Medrol), morphine, penicillin G potassium and sodium, pentobarbital (Nembutal), phenobarbital (Luminal), phenytoin (Dilantin), secobarbital (Seconal), thiopental (Pentothal), vitamin B with C.

Side effects: *Average dose:* Blurring of vision, dizziness, dryness of mouth, hyperexcitability, hypersensitivity reactions, hypertension (rare), hypotension (mild), nightmares, spastic movements of upper extremities.

Overdose: Anaphylaxis, cardiac arrest, coma, convulsions, deep sedation, respiratory depression. All side effects of phenothiazines are possible, but rarely occur. See prochlorperazine (Compazine).

Antidote: Discontinue the drug at onset of any side effect and notify the physician. Counteract hypotension with dopamine (Intropin) and IV fluids; extrapyramidal symptoms with benztropine mesylate (Cogentin) or diphenhydramine (Benadryl). Epinephrine is contraindicated for hypotension. Further hypotension will occur. Use diazepam (Valium) or phenobarbital for convulsions or hyperactivity. Phenytoin may be helpful in ventricular dysrhythmias. In treating respiratory depression and unconsciousness, avoid analeptics such as doxapram (Dopram); they may cause convulsions. Resuscitate as necessary.

PROPIOMAZINE HYDROCHLORIDE

pH 4.7 to 5.3

(Largon)

Usual dose: 10 to 40 mg (20 mg average) given alone or in conjunction with one-fourth to one-half the usual dose of narcotics. May be repeated in 3 to 4 hours as indicated.

Pediatric dose: 0.5 (average dose) to 1 mg/kg of body weight, but do not exceed adult dose.

Dilution: Each 20 mg (1 ml) should be diluted with 9 ml of normal saline for injection. 1 ml will equal 2 mg.

Rate of administration: Each 10 mg or fraction thereof over 1 minute. A slower rate of injection may be indicated by the accompanying narcotic.

Actions: A phenothiazine derivative that potentiates the analgesic and sedative effects of narcotics. Used alone it produces sedation and reduces anxiety. Has some antihistaminic effect and a mild antiemetic effect. Prompt onset of action with a short duration of effect is a desirable action. Slowly excreted through the kidneys.

Indications and uses: Sedation and relief of restlessness preoperatively, during surgery, and during labor and delivery.

Precautions: (1) Solution must be clear. Discard if cloudy or if a precipitate is present. (2) Establish unquestionable patency of vein. Avoid extravasation; severe cellulitis and tissue necrosis will result. Intraarterial injection will cause gangrene. (3) Monitor blood pressure and pulse before administration and between doses. Keep patient in supine position. (4) Use with caution in cerebral arteriosclerosis, coronary heart disease, severe hypertension, epilepsy, heat exhaustion, liver disease, pregnancy, and respiratory problems. (5) May mask diagnosis of brain tumor, drug intoxication, and intestinal obstruction. (6) Potentiates CNS depressant effects of narcotics, barbiturates, alcohol, and anesthetics. Additive with MAO inhibitors (e.g., pargyline [Eutonyl]), oral antidiabetics, insulin, anticholinergics, antihistamines, antihypertensives, hypnotics, muscle relaxants, phenytoin (Dilantin), propranolol (Inderal), and Rauwolfia alkaloids. Reduce dosage of any medication potentiated by phenothiazines by one fourth to one half. (7) Contraindicated with quinidine, epinephrine, and thiazide diuretics. (8) Capable of innumerable other interactions.

Contraindications: Bone marrow depression, comatose or severely depressed states, first trimester of pregnancy, hypersensitivity to phenothiazines, lactation.

Incompatible with: Alkaline solutions, barbiturates. Sufficient information not available, but refer to other phenothiazines such as promazine (Sparine).

Side effects: Dryness of mouth, hypertension (moderate), hypotension, tachycardia, thrombophlebitis. All side effects of phenothiazines could occur, but rarely do.

For additional possible side effects see prochlorperazine (Compazine).

Antidote: Dryness of mouth, moderate hypertension, and tachycardia are usually tolerable. Notify physician if excessive. For all other side effects discontinue drug at onset and notify the physician. Counteract hypotension with dopamine (Intropin) and extrapyramidal symptoms with benztropine mesylate (Cogentin) or diphenhydramine (Benadryl). Epinephrine is contraindicated for hypotension. Further hypotension will occur. Resuscitate as necessary.

PROPRANOLOL HYDROCHLORIDE pH 2.8 to 3.5
(Inderal)

Usual dose: 0.5 to 3 mg given 1 mg at a time. If there is no change in rhythm for at least 2 minutes after the initial dose, cycle may be repeated one time. *No further propranolol may be given by any route for at least 4 hours.*

Dilution: Each 1 mg can be diluted in 10 ml of 5% dextrose in water for injection or may be given undiluted. May be diluted in 50 ml of normal saline for infusion.

Rate of administration: Each 1 mg or fraction thereof must be given over 1 minute. Give 1 mg as an infusion over 10 to 15 minutes. Allow adequate time for circulation. Observe monitor and discontinue propranolol as soon as rhythm change occurs.

Actions: Propranolol is a β-adrenergic blocker with antiarrhythmic effects. Cardiac response to sympathetic nerve stimulation is inhibited, slowing the heart rate (especially ventricular rate) by inhibiting atrioventricular conduction, decreasing the force of cardiac contractility, and decreasing arterial pressure and cardiac output. Propranolol also decreases the plasma level of free fatty acid and blood glucose. Well distributed throughout the body, the onset of action occurs within 1 to 2 minutes and lasts about 4 hours. Metabolized in the liver. Some excreted in the urine.

Indications and uses: (1) Management of life-threatening cardiac dysrhythmias such as paroxysmal atrial tachycardia, sinus tachycardia, atrial or ventricular extrasystoles, and atrial flutter and fibrillation; tachyarrhythmia caused by digitalis intoxication, anesthesia (other than chloroform and ether, etc.), thyrotoxicosis, and catecholamines (epinephrine, norepinephrine); (2) ventricular tachycardia and dysrhythmias caused by tumor manipulation during excision of pheochromocytoma after treatment with an α-adrenergic blocking agent; (3) reduce blood pressure in systolic hypertension caused by hyperdynamic β-adrenergic circulatory state that occurs in younger persons.

Precautions: (1) Continuous ECG and blood pressure monitoring is mandatory during administration of IV propranolol. Monitoring of pulmonary wedge pressure or central venous pressure is recommended. Discontinue the drug when a rhythm change is noted and wait to note full effect before giving additional medication if indicated. (2) Oral administration is preferred. Use IV administration only when necessary. (3) Not considered the drug of choice for dysrhythmias in myocardial infarction. (4) Antagonizes antihistamines, antiinflammatory agents, isoproterenol (Isuprel), ritodrine, and others. (5) Potentiated by general anesthetics, cimetidine (Tagamet), furosemide, phenothiazines (e.g., promethazine [Phenergan]), phenytoin (Dilantin), and urethane. Death can occur. (6) Potentiates antidiabetics, barbiturates, catecholamine-depleting drugs (e.g., reserpine), insulin, lidocaine, narcotics, muscle relaxants, theophyllines, and thyroid agents; dosage adjustment may be required. Increased CNS depression may cause death. (7) Used concurrently with digitalis or α-adrenergic blockers as indicated. May cause life-threatening hypotension and bradycardia with haloperidol (Haldol). (8) Use with extreme caution in asthmatics, diabetics, or patients with a history of hypoglycemia. May cause hypoglycemia and mask the symptoms. (9) Epinephrine concurrently is contraindicated. (10) Use with clonidine may precipitate acute hypertension. (11) Use with verapamil may potentiate both drugs and lead to severe depression of myocardium and AV conduction. (12) BUN may be elevated in patients with impaired renal function. (13) Should be discontinued 48 hours before major surgery (β-blockade interferes with cardiac response to reflex stimuli). (14) May cause severe bradycardia in patients with Wolff-Parkinson-White syndrome. (15) Reduce dose gradually to avoid rebound angina, myocardial infarction, or ventricular dysrhythmias. (16) May aggravate rebound hypertension if clonidine stopped abruptly. (17) Safety for use in pregnancy and lactation and in children not established. Use only when clearly indicated.

Contraindications: Allergic rhinitis, bronchial asthma, bronchospasm, cardiogenic shock, complete heart block, congestive heart failure (unless caused by tachycardia), chronic obstructive pulmonary disease, hypersensitivity to β-adrenergic blocking agents, myocardial-depressing anesthetics (e.g., chloroform, ether), right ventricular failure caused by pulmonary hypertension, second-degree heart block, sinus bradycardia; contraindicated concurrently with all antihypertensive drugs including diuretics, and may not be given to patients receiving antidepressants or MAO inhibitors (e.g., pargyline [Eutonyl]), until after a 2-week withdrawal period.

Incompatible with: Any other drug in a syringe or solution because of toxicity. Note Precautions and Contraindications.

Side effects: Bradycardia, cardiac failure, cardiac standstill, erythematous rash, hallucination, hypotension, laryngospasm, paresthesia of the hands, respiratory distress, syncopal attacks, vertigo, visual disturbances.

Antidote: For any side effect, discontinue the drug and notify the physician immediately. Effects can be reversed by dopamine, isoproterenol, or levarterenol, but protracted severe hypotension may result. Use atropine for bradycardia, digitalis and diuretics for cardiac failure, epinephrine for hypotension, aminophylline and isoproterenol (with extreme care) for bronchospasm, and glucagon for hypoglycemia. Treat other side effects symptomatically and resuscitate as necessary.

PROTAMINE SULFATE pH 6.0 to 7.0

Usual dose: 1 mg for every 100 USP units of heparin. May be repeated if needed in 10 to 15 minutes. Never exceed 50 mg in any 10-minute period. The dose of protamine required decreases rapidly with the time elapsed after heparin injection. (30 minutes after IV heparin, 0.5 mg of protamine will neutralize 100 USP units of heparin.)

Dilution: Each 50 mg of powder is diluted with 5 ml sterile bacteriostatic water for injection. Shake vigorously. May be further diluted with at least an equal volume of normal saline or 5% dextrose in water. May be given as an infusion by diluting in a given amount of the same infusion solutions.

Rate of administration: 20 mg (2 ml) or fraction thereof over 1 to 3 minutes. Do not exceed 50 mg in 10 minutes. As an infusion, may be given over 2 to 3 hours with dosage titrated according to coagulation studies. Use infusion pump or microdrip (60 gtt/ml) to administer.

Actions: An anticoagulant if administered alone. In the presence of heparin, protamine forms a stable salt, neutralizing the anticoagulant effect of both drugs. Each 1 mg of protamine can neutralize 100 USP units of heparin. It is effective for about 2 hours.

Indications and uses: (1) To neutralize the anticoagulant activity of heparin in severe heparin overdosage; (2) post–coronary artery bypass graft neutralization of heparin.

Precautions: (1) Refrigerate before dilution. Use immediately after dilution. Discard remaining medication. (2) Prompt administration of protamine sulfate may decrease dosage requirements. (3) Dosage adjusted as indicated by coagulation studies. (4) Facilities to treat shock must be available. (5) After cardiac surgery, even with adequate neutralization, further bleeding may occur any time within 24 hours (heparin "rebound"). Observe the patient continuously. Additional protamine sulfate may be indicated. (6) Safety for use in children, pregnancy, or lactation not established. (7)

Potential for hypersensitivity increased in patients with allergies to fish.

Contraindications: None when used as indicated.

Incompatible with: Cephalosporins, penicillins. Should be considered incompatible in syringe or solution with any other drug because of individualized rate adjustment necessary to produce desired effects.

Side effects: Occur more frequently with too rapid injection; anaphylaxis, bradycardia, dyspnea, feeling of warmth, flushing, severe hypertension or hypotension.

Antidote: Discontinue the drug and notify the physician, who may recommend a decrease in rate of administration or, if side effects are severe, symptomatic treatment such as administration of whole blood, vasopressors (e.g., dopamine [Intropin]) for hypotension, atropine for bradycardia, and oxygen for dyspnea. Resuscitate as necessary.

PROTEIN (AMINO ACID) PRODUCTS

pH 5.0 to 7.0

(Aminess 5.2%; Aminosyn 3.5%, 3.5% M, 5%, 7%, 8.5%, and 10%; Aminosyn 7% and 8.5% with Electrolytes; Aminosyn (pH 6) 8.5%, and 10%; Aminosyn HBC 7%; Aminosyn II 3.5%, 3.5% M, 5%, 7%, 8.5%, and 10%; Aminosyn II 7%, 8.5%, and 10% with Electrolytes; Aminosyn II 3.5% in 5% or 25% Dextrose; Aminosyn II 5% in 25% Dextrose; Aminosyn II 3.5% M in 5% Dextrose; Aminosyn II 4.25% in 10%, 20%, and 25% Dextrose; Aminosyn II 4.25% M in 10% Dextrose; Aminosyn PF 7% and 10%; Aminosyn RF 5.2%; crystalline amino acid infusions; 4% Branch Amin; FreAmine HBC 6.9%; FreAmine III 8.5%, 10%, and 3% and 8.5% with Electrolytes; HepaAmine; hyperalimentation; Nephramine 5.4%; Novamine; Novamine 15%; ProcalAmine; protein hydrolysates, RenAmin, total parenteral nutrition; Travasol 5.5%, 8.5%, and 10% without Electrolytes; Travasol 3.5% M, 5.5% and 8.5% with Electrolytes; TrophaAmine 6% and 10%).

Usual dose: Based on protein requirements, physical condition, and weight (actual grams of available protein vary with various brands). Consider total body fluid needs. Average adult will require 2 L/24 hr providing 1 to 2 Gm protein/kg of body weight. Glucose supplies nonprotein calories. Protein amino acid products are available in general, renal failure, hepatic failure/encephalopathy, and metabolic stress formulations.

Pediatric and infant dose: Sufficient milliliters to provide 2 to 3 Gm protein/kg of body weight/24 hr to meet average needs. Infants and children require different percentages of all components.

Dilution: If required, dilute under strict aseptic techniques according to manufacturer's specific instructions. Various brands supply additional calories with alcohol, fructose, or glucose. These additional calories permit available protein to be used for repair of tissue in addition to meeting basic caloric needs.

Rate of administration: Start with 1 L/24 hr and gradually increase by 1 L/24 hr to desired amount. Begin infusion at a rate of approximately 1 ml/kg of body weight/hr. Gradually increase to 2 ml/kg/hr. *Total daily dose should be evenly distributed over the 24-hour period. Maintain a constant drip rate.* Never exceed 4 ml/kg/hr. Use of infusion pump and microfilter recommended.

Actions: Supplies essential and nonessential amino acids and calories with the intent of promoting protein production (anabolism) and preventing protein breakdown (catabolism), promotes wound healing, and acts as a buffer in intracellular and extracellular body fluids.

Indications and uses: Maintenance of positive nitrogen balance in severe illness when oral alimentation is not practical for prolonged periods or normal GI absorption is impaired.

Precautions: (1) Use promptly after mixing; laminar flow hood preferred; refrigerate briefly if necessary, and discard any unused portion. (2) Use only clear solutions; observe against adequate light for particulate matter or evidence of container damage. (3) Catheter insertion for administration of central parenteral nutrition is a sterile surgical procedure (must be a large vein [subclavian or superior vena cava preferred]; 50% glucose is a sclerosing solution). (4) Peripheral veins are suitable for specific products (peripheral parenteral nutrition), when amino acid products are diluted with 2.5%, 5%, or 10% dextrose. (5) Follow a strict, regular aseptic routine to care for insertion site. (6) Single-port central venous catheters to be used only for the nutritional regimen. Do not draw blood, samples, transfuse blood, or administer other medications. Pseudoagglutination and thrombosis can occur, risk of contamination is great, and validity of results are compromised. Multiple-port central venous catheters may be used for these additional procedures. Observe specific protocols. (7) Specific baseline studies are required before administration: CBC, platelet count, PT, BUN SMA-6, SMA-12, magnesium, phosphorus, weight, body length and head circumference (in infants), and immunocompetence.

During stabilization (3 to 5 days), measure urine glucose and ketones every shift, SMA-6, phosphorus, intake and output, weight, and plasma and urine osmolarity. Arterial blood gases and pH, blood glucose levels, cholesterol, serum proteins, magnesium, phosphate, PT, and electrolytes also need to be monitored during therapy. (8) Monitor BUN frequently. Discontinue infusion if BUN exceeds normal postprandial limits and continues to rise. Blood ammonia levels important especially in infants. (9) After stabilization, measure urine glucose and ketones at least every 8 hours; record intake and output and daily weight. (10) Check frequently for any signs of extravasation. (11) Observe for any signs of infection. (12) Additional insulin coverage may be required, especially when dosage is increased too rapidly or with maximum doses. (13) To prevent rebound hypoglycemia, decrease rate gradually over at least 24 hours to discontinue administration. Follow with use of fluids containing 5% or 10% dextrose for several days. (14) RDA vitamins, trace metals, potassium, magnesium, phosphates, sodium, calcium, and chlorides needed. Usually added as prescribed with aseptic technique. Heparin has been added. (15) Amino acids given without carbohydrates may cause ketone accumulation. (16) Frequently used in conjunction with IV fat emulsion as a nonprotein calorie source. Use a separate port; never mixed together in a container. (17) Tetracycline may reduce protein-sparing effects. (18) Discard any single bottle after 24 hours. Replace administration set every 24 to 48 hours. (19) Use hypertonic dextrose with extreme caution in low-birth-weight or septic infants. May cause severe hyperglycemia. (20) Fatty infiltration of the liver, acute respiratory failure, and difficulty in weaning hypermetabolic patients from the respirator may be caused by excessive carbohydrate calories.

Contraindications: Hypersensitivity to any component, acidosis, anuria, azotemia, decreased circulating blood volume, severe liver disease, metabolic disorders with impaired amino acid metabolization.

Incompatible with: Amobarbital (Amytal), chlorothiazide (Diuril), penicillins, sodium bicarbonate, thiopental (Pentothal), many other drugs, and whole blood. Most incompatibilities relate to the preparation (chloride as opposed to phosphate), amount of medication added, other additives present, and thoroughness of mixing. Consult with the pharmacist before mixing any drugs in protein (amino acid) products. Only required nutritional products should be added.

Side effects: Abdominal pains, anaphylaxis, bone demineralization, changes in levels of consciousness, convulsions, dehydration, edema at the site of injection, electrolyte imbalances, glycosuria, hyperammonemia, hyperglycemia, hyperpyrexia, hypertension, metabolic acidosis and/or alkalosis, osmotic dehydration, phlebitis and thrombosis, pulmonary edema, rebound hypoglycemia, septicemia, vasodilation, vomiting, weakness.

Antidote: Notify the physician of all side effects. An alternate brand may cause fewer problems, or amounts of glucose or additives may be adjusted to correct the problem. Many of the side effects listed will respond to a reduced rate. Some will require catheter insertion at a new site. Treat symptomatically and resuscitate as necessary.

PROTIRELIN

(Relefact TRH, Thypinone)

Usual dose: 200 to 500 mcg. 500 mcg is optimum dose. Specific procedure required (see Precautions).

Pediatric dose: *Ages 6 to 16 years:* 7 mcg/kg of body weight up to 500 mcg. Experience is limited in infants and children under 6 years of age, but the same dose has been used.

Dilution: May be given undiluted.

Rate of administration: A single dose over 15 to 30 seconds.

Actions: This synthetic hormone is similiar to natural thyrotropin-releasing hormone produced by the hypothalamus. It increases release of thyroid-stimulating hormone (TSH) from the anterior pituitary. Effective within 5 minutes, peaks in 20 to 30 minutes, and is completely excreted in about 3 hours.

Indications and uses: As an adjunct in (1) the diagnostic assessment of thyroid function; (2) other diagnostic procedures in pituitary or hypothalamic dysfunction; (3) evaluation of the effectiveness of thyrotropin suppression with T_4 in patients with nodular or diffuse goiter; (4) primary hypothyroidism to facilitate adjustment of thyroid hormone dosage.

Precautions: (1) Patient should remain supine throughout the test. Moderate transient hypertension is frequent; monitor blood pressure frequently until it returns to pretreatment baseline. (2) Draw one blood sample for TSH assay just before injection, and another 30 minutes after injection. (3) Assay methods and thus results vary with each laboratory performing this test. (4) Discontinue liothyronine (T_3) 7 days before test and medications containing levothyroxine (T_4) 14 days before test except when testing effectiveness of thyroid suppression with T_4 or for adjustment of thyroid dosage. (5) Adrenocortical drugs used in maintenance therapy of hypopituitarism may be continued. Only large doses will reduce the TSH response. (6) Response may be inhibited by aspirin and levodopa. (7) Should not be repeated for at least 7 days or TSH response will be reduced. (8) Will not differentiate primary hypothyroidism from normal. (9) Safety for use during pregnancy not established.

Contraindications: None stated in literature.

Incompatible with: Specific information not available. Consider specific use.

Side effects: Occur frequently; are usually minor and subside quickly. Abdominal discomfort, bad taste, breast enlargement and leakage in lactating women, dry mouth, flushed sensation, headache, hypertension, hypotension, lightheadedness, nausea, urge to urinate. Anxiety, convulsions in patients with epilepsy or brain damage, drowsiness, pressure in the chest, sweating, tightness in the throat, tingling sensation, and transient amaurosis in patients with pituitary tumors may occur.

Antidote: Notify physician and manage side effects as indicated by severity. Treat allergic reactions and resuscitate as necessary.

PYRIDOSTIGMINE BROMIDE pH 5.0

(Mestinon, Regonol)

Usual dose: *Myasthenia gravis:* One thirtieth of the oral dose, or about 2 mg. Highly individualized. Observe for cholinergic crisis.

Muscle relaxant antagonist: 0.1 to 0.25 mg/kg of body weight (usually 10 to 20 mg) as a single dose. Give atropine first (see Precautions) and maintain ventilation.

Dilution: May be given undiluted. Do not add to IV solutions. May be given through Y-tube or three-way stopcock of infusion set.

Rate of administration: *Myasthenia gravis:* Each 0.5 mg or fraction thereof over 1 minute.

Muscle relaxant antagonist: Each 5 mg or fraction thereof over 1 minute.

Actions: An anticholinesterase muscle stimulant and antagonist of skeletal muscle relaxants. Inhibits the enzyme cholinesterase, allowing acetylcholine to accumulate at the myoneural junction. Restores normal transmission of nerve impulses and makes muscle contraction stronger and more prolonged. Has fewer side effects and longer duration of action than neostigmine (Prostigmin).

Indications and uses: (1) Treatment of myasthenia gravis during physically stressful situations when oral dosage is not practical (labor, postpartum, surgery); (2) antagonist to nondepolarizing muscle relaxants (e.g., gallamine [Flaxedil], tubocurarine [curare]).

Precautions: (1) A physician should be present when this drug is used. IM route preferred. (2) Used as a curariform antagonist; administer atropine sulfate, 0.6 to 1.2 mg IV, immediately before pyridostigmine. *Caution:* atropine may mask symptoms of pyridostigmine overdose. Cholinergic crisis may result. Maintain a patent airway and use artificial ventilation as indicated. (3) Edrophonium (Tensilon) can differentiate between increased symptoms of myasthenia and cholinergic crisis. (4) Epinephrine and atropine should always be available. (5) Use caution in bronchial asthma, cardiac dysrhythmias, and patients receiving anticholinesterase drugs. (6) Potentiates narcotic analgesics (e.g., morphine, codeine, meperidine) and succinylcholine (Anectine). (7) Antagonizes anesthetics (ether), ganglionic blocking agents (e.g., trimethaphan [Arfonad]), and aminoglycoside antibiotics (e.g., kanamycin [Kantrex]); neuromuscular block may be accentuated. (8) May be inhibited by corticosteroids and magnesium. (9) A peripheral nerve stimulator device can monitor effectiveness. (10) May induce premature labor in pregnancy near term. Transient muscular weakness in swallowing, sucking, and breathing has been observed in neonates of myasthenic mothers. Confirm distinction between cholinergic and myasthenic crisis in neonate with edrophonium test. Treat neonate with IM pyridostigmine 0.05 to 0.15 mg/kg if indicated.

Contraindications: Known sensitivity to anticholinesterase agents or bromides, mechanical intestinal or urinary obstruction, urinary tract infections, patients taking mecamylamine.

Incompatible with: Limited information available. Because of potential toxicity, pyridostigmine should not be mixed with any other drug. Unstable in alkaline solutions.

Side effects: *Usually caused by overdose:* Abdominal cramps, anorexia, anxiety, bradycardia, cardiac dysrhythmias and arrest, cholinergic crisis, cold moist skin, convulsions, diaphoresis, diarrhea, hypotension, increased bronchial secretions, increased lacrimation, increased salivation, miosis, muscle cramps, muscle weakness, nausea, pulmonary edema, respiratory paralysis with apnea, skin rash (bromide), thrombophlebitis, vomiting.

Antidote: *Atropine sulfate.* If side effects occur, discontinue the drug and notify the physician. Atropine sulfate in doses of 0.6 mg IV will counteract most side effects and may be repeated every 3 to 10 minutes. Endotracheal intubation or tracheostomy is considered prophylactic in anesthesia or crisis. Artificial ventilation, oxygen therapy, cardiac monitoring, adequate suctioning, and treatment of shock or convulsions must be instituted and maintained as necessary. Treat allergic reactions with epinephrine. Pralidoxime chloride 1 to 2

Gm IV followed by 250 mg every 5 minutes may be required to reactivate cholinesterase and reverse paralysis.

PYRIDOXINE HYDROCHLORIDE pH 2.0 to 3.8

(Beesix, Hexa-Betalin, Vitamin B_6)

Usual dose: 10 to 100 mg/24 hr. Up to 4 Gm may be given in severe isoniazid poisoning (over 10 Gm). Follow with 1 Gm IM every 30 minutes. Total dose to equal dose of isoniazid.

Dilution: May be given by direct IV administration undiluted or added to most IV solutions and given as an infusion.

Rate of administration: 50 mg or fraction thereof over 1 minute if given undiluted.

Actions: Vitamin B_6 is water soluble. It is a coenzyme, necessary for the metabolism of amino acids and fatty acids. It also aids in the conversion of tryptophan to nicotinamide and energy transformation in brain and nerve cells. Easily absorbed and utilized, metabolized by the liver, and excreted in the urine.

Indications and uses: Adjunctive therapy in treatment of alcoholism, hyperemesis gravidarum, irradiation sickness, vitamin B_6 deficiency, pellagra, and isoniazid poisoning.

Investigational use: Hydrazine poisoning.

Precautions: (1) Deteriorates in excessive heat; may be refrigerated. (2) Large doses in utero can cause pyridoxine-dependency syndrome in the newborn. (3) May inhibit lactation. (4) Used IV only when oral dosage not acceptable. (5) An antagonist to levodopa. (6) Isoniazid is a vitamin B_6 antagonist and will cause deficiency disease. Cycloserine, penicillamine, hydralazine, and oral contraceptives may increase pyridoxine requirements. (7) Deficiency can cause an abnormal EEG. (8) Excessive doses may elevate SGOT. (9) Protect from heat and light. (10) Safety for use in children not established. (11) Need for pyridoxine increases with the amount of protein in the diet. (12) Inhibits phenobarbital and phenytoin (Dilantin).

Contraindications: Known sensitivity to pyridoxine.

Incompatible with: Sufficient information not available; alkaline solutions, iron salts, oxidizing solutions.

Side effects: Almost nonexistent; some slight flushing or feeling of warmth may occur. With larger doses, ataxia, low folic acid levels, paresthesias, somnolence, and withdrawal seizures in infants with high maternal doses may occur.

Antidote: No antidote is known or has been needed. Symptomatic treatment of side effects may be indicated.

QUINIDINE GLUCONATE INJECTION

pH 5.5 to 7.0

Usual dose: 200 mg. May be repeated as indicated to effect control of the dysrhythmia. 330 mg or less effective in most patients. Up to 1 Gm has been required. Highly individualized. Maintain with oral quinidine sulfate. Do not exceed 5 Gm total dose in 24 hours.

Dilution: 800 mg (10 ml) must be diluted in at least 40 ml of 5% dextrose for injection. 1 ml of properly diluted solution equals 16 mg quinidine.

Rate of administration: 1 ml (16 mg) or fraction thereof of properly diluted solution over 1 minute. Use an infusion pump or microdrip (60 gtt/ml).

Actions: A dextro-isomer of quinine. Exerts a depressing antiarrhythmic action on the heart, slowing the rate, slowing conduction, reducing myocardial contractility, and prolonging the refractory period. Increases potassium levels within the cells while it decreases sodium levels. Can have a vasodilating effect. Onset of action occurs when an effective blood concentration has been reached (15 to 30 minutes usually), and lasts 4 to 6 hours. Metabolized in the liver, most of the drug is excreted in the urine.

Indications and uses: (1) Cardiac dysrhythmias, including atrial fibrillation, atrial flutter, premature asystoles, supraventricular tachycardia, ventricular tachycardia, and paroxysmal rhythms; (2) treatment of chloroquine-resistant *Plasmodium falciparum* infections if quinine dihydrochloride is unavailable.

Precautions: (1) Monitor patient's ECG and blood pressure continuously. Too rapid administration may cause a marked decrease in arterial pressure. (2) Keep patient in supine position. (3) Oral or IM administration is route of choice. (4) Discontinue IV use when the normal sinus rhythm returns, the heart rate falls to 120 beats/min, or any signs of cardiac toxicity occur (increased PR and QT intervals, over a 50% prolongation of QRS complex, or P waves disappear). (5) Use extreme caution in first or second degree blocks, extensive myocardial damage, digitalis intoxication, and impaired liver or kidney function. (6) Use caution in atrial flutter or fibrillation; may require pretreatment with digitalis to prevent progressive reduction of AV block and an extremely rapid ventricular rate. (7) A test dose of 200 mg IM for idiosyncrasy is desired if time permits. (8) Lidocaine or procainamide are generally used in preference to quinidine. (9) Monitor serum levels if quinidine is used over 48 hours. (10) Potentiates or is potentiated by neuromuscular blocking antibiotics (e.g., kanamycin [Kantrex]), anticholinergics (e.g., atropine), thiazide diuretics, antihypertensive agents, cimetidine (Tagamet), muscle relaxants, anticoagulants, phenothiazines, (e.g., prochlorperazine [Compazine]), reserpine, succinylcholine (Anectine), urinary alkalinizers, and others. Cardiac dysrhythmias and other serious side effects may occur. (11) Use caution with digitalis, procainamide, and propranolol. Lower doses of both drugs may be required. (12) May cause increased urine catecholamines, an increased PT, and a positive Coombs' test. (13) Inhibited by phenobarbital, phenytoin (Dilantin), nifedipine, and rifampin; adjust dosage. (14) May cause severe hypotension with verapamil, especially in patents with hypertrophic cardiomyopathy. (15) Use only clear, colorless solutions.

Contraindications: Partial AV or complete heart block,

any severe intraventricular conduction defects, aberrant impulses and abnormal rhythms because of escape mechanism, known hypersensitivity to quinidine or cinchona, lactation, myasthenia gravis, history of thrombocytopenic purpura with quinidine administration.

Incompatible with: Alkalies and iodides. Most other drugs in syringe or solution. Combination impractical because of possible side effects and need to determine effectiveness. Has been shown to be compatible with bretylium, cimetidine, and verapamil through Y-tube connection.

Side effects: *Minor:* Apprehension, cramps, diaphoresis, fever, headache, nausea, rash, tinnitus, urge to defecate, urge to void, vertigo, visual disturbances, vomiting.

Major: Atrioventricular heart block; cardiac standstill; hypotension (acute); prolonged PR or QT intervals, or 50% widening of QRS complex; tachycardia; thrombocytopenia purpura; urticaria; ventricular fibrillation.

Antidote: Notify the physician of any side effects. If minor symptoms progress or any major side effect appears, discontinue the drug immediately and notify the physician. Use dopamine (Intropin), metaraminol (Aramine), or angiotensin (Hypertensin) to correct hypotension, and ⅙ molar sodium lactate to block effects of quinidine on the myocardium. Treatment of toxicity is symptomatic and supportive. Hemodialysis may be indicated. Do not administer any CNS depressants in overdose. Resuscitate as necessary. Depending on dysrhythmia, procainamide or lidocaine is effective alternate.

RANITIDINE pH 6.7 to 7.3

(Zantac)

Usual dose: *Direct IV or intermittent infusion:* 50 mg (2 ml) every 6 to 8 hours. Increase frequency, not amount, if necessary for pain relief. Do not exceed 400 mg/day.

Continuous infusion: 150 mg may be given as a continuous infusion equally distributed over 24 hours.

To maintain intergastric acid secretion at 10 mEq/hr or less, dose range may be higher in patients with pathological hypersecretory (Zollinger-Ellison) syndrome. Literature suggests an initial dose of 1.0 mg/kg/hr. Measure gastric acid output in 4 hours; if above 10 mEq/hr or symptoms recur, adjust dose upwards in 0.5 mg/kg/hr increments. Up to 2.5 mg/kg/hr has been used. Increase intervals between injections to achieve pain relief with least frequent dosage in impaired renal function.

Prevention of pulmonary aspiration during anesthesia: 50 mg 60 to 90 minutes before anesthesia.

Dilution: *Direct IV:* Each 50 mg must be diluted with 20 ml of normal saline or other compatible infusion solution for injection (5% or 10% dextrose in water, lactated Ringer's solution, 5% sodium bicarbonate). Do not dilute beyond this 2.5 mg/ml solution.

Intermittent infusion: Each 50 mg may be diluted in 50 ml (1 mg/ml) to 100 ml (0.5 mg/ml) of 5% dextrose in water or other compatible infusion solution and given piggyback. Do not dilute beyond a 0.5 mg/ml solution. Discontinue primary IV during intermittent infusion. Do not use premixed plastic containers in series connections; may cause air embolism.

Continuous infusion: Total daily dose may be diluted in 250 ml of 5% dextrose in water or other compatible infusion solution. For Zollinger-Ellison patients, do not dilute beyond a 2.5 mg/ml solution.

In all situations, avoid any contact with aluminum during administration (e.g., needles).

Rate of administration: *Direct IV:* Each 50 mg or fraction thereof at a rate not to exceed 4 ml/min diluted solution (20 ml over 5 minutes).

Intermittent infusion: Each 50 mg dose over 15 to 20 minutes. Should not exceed a rate of 5 to 7 ml/min.

Continuous infusion: Total daily dose equally distributed over 24 hours. Should not exceed a rate of 6.25 mg/hr (10.7 ml/hr if 150 mg [6 ml ranitidine] is diluted in 250 ml). Use of infusion pump preferred to avoid complications of overdose or too rapid administation.

Actions: A histamine H_2 antagonist, it inhibits both daytime and nocturnal basal gastric acid secretion. It also inhibits gastric acid secretion stimulated by food, histamine, bentazole, and pentagastrin. Not an anticholinergic agent. Does not lower calcium levels in hypercalcemia. Onset of action is prompt and effective for 6 to 8 hours. Metabolized in the liver. Excreted in the urine. Crosses placental barrier. Secreted in breast milk.

Indications and uses: (1) Short-term treatment of intractable duodenal ulcers and pathological hypersecretory conditions in the hospitalized patient; (2) treatment of active benign gastric ulcers in those patients unable to take oral medication.

Investigational use: Preoperatively to prevent pulmonary aspiration of acid during anesthesia.

Precautions: (1) Too rapid administration has precipitated rare instances of bradycardia, tachycardia, and PVCs. (2) Use antacids concomitantly to relieve pain. (3) May potentiate warfarin-type anticoagulants; monitor prothrombin times. (4) Gastric malignancy may be present even though patient is asymptomatic. (5) Use caution in patients with impaired hepatic function. Monitor SGPT if therapy exceeds 400 mg for over 5 days. (6) Inspect for color and clarity. Slight darkening of solution does not affect potency. Stable at room temperature for 48 hours after dilution. (7) Gastric pain and ulceration may recur after medication stopped. (8) Effects maintained with oral dosage. Total treatment usually discontinued after 6 weeks. (9) Potentiates effects of procainamide (Pronestyl), sulfonylureas (Glipizide). (10) May potentiate theophyllines (e.g., aminophylline). (11) Use during pregnancy or lactation only when clearly needed. (12) Safety for use in children not established. (13) Has been added to specific total parenteral nutrition fluids; consult with pharmacist.

Contraindications: Known hypersensitivity to ranitidine or its components.

Incompatible with: Amphotericin B (Fungizone), chlorpromazine (Thorazine), clindamycin (Cleocin), diazepam (Valium), hydroxyzine (Vistaril), midazolam (Versed), opium alkaloids, pentobarbital (Nembutal), phenobarbital (Luminal). Do not add any other drugs to premixed ranitidine in plastic containers.

Side effects: Abdominal discomfort, burning and itching at IV site, constipation, diarrhea, headache (severe), and nausea and vomiting are the most common side effects. Allergic reactions (bronchospasm, fever, rash, eosinophilia) can occur. Agitation, arthralgias, bradycardia, confusion, depression, dizziness, elevated SGPT, hallucinations, hepatitis (reversible), impotence, insomnia, malaise, muscular pain, PVCs, somnolence, tachycardia, and vertigo occur rarely.

Antidote: Notify physician of all side effects. May be treated symptomatically or may respond to decrease in frequency of dosage. Resuscitate as necessary for overdose. Hemodialysis or peritoneal dialysis may be indicated in overdose.

RIFAMPIN — pH 7.8 to 8.8

Rifadin

Usual dose: *Tuberculosis:* 600 mg daily as a single dose. Prescribed concurrently with at least one other antituberculin drug (e.g., ethambutol [Myambutol], izoniazid, pyrazinamide, or streptomycin).

Meningococcal carriers: 600 mg daily as a single dose for 4 days or 600 mg every 12 hours for 2 days.

In all situations use oral dose form as soon as practical.

Pediatric dose: *Tuberculosis and meningococcal carriers:* 10 to 20 mg/kg of body weight daily as a single dose. Do not exceed 600 mg. See information in adult dose.

Neonatal dose: *Meningococcal carriers:* Under 1 month of age: 5 mg/kg every 12 hr for 2 days.

Over 1 month of age: 10 mg/kg every 12 hr for 2 days.

Reduced dose: Required in impaired hepatic function. No dose adjustment is necessary in impaired renal function; serum concentrations do not change.

Dilution: Each 600 mg vial must be initially diluted in 10 ml of sterile water for injection (60mg/ml). Swirl gently to dissolve. Withdraw desired dose and further dilute in 500 ml (preferred) or 100 ml of 5% dextrose in water. If dextrose is contraindicated, normal saline may be used but will slightly decrease the stability of the solution. 100 ml dilution used only in selected situations. Stable for 24 hours at room temperature after reconstitution. Protect from light prior to dilution.

Rate of administration: A single dose equally distributed as an infusion over 3 hours. In selected situations a single dose diluted in 100 ml may be administered over 30 minutes.

Actions: A semisynthetic antituberculosis antibiotic. Has a bactericidal or bacteriostatic action that is effective in susceptible cells during cell division or at the resting stage. Onset of peak plasma levels is prompt, and average levels are maintained for 8 to 12 hours based on dose. Rapidly absorbed throughout the body and present in many organs and body fluids including CSF. Metabolized in the liver and excreted in bile. Crosses the placental barrier. Secreted in breast milk.

Indications and uses: (1) Treatment or retreatment of tuberculosis when the drug cannot be taken by mouth; (2) treatment of asymptomatic carriers of *Neisseria* meningitis. Not indicated for treatment of meningococcal infection because of rapid emergence of resistant meningococci.

Precautions: (1) For IV use only. Do not administer IM or SC. (2) Obtain a complete blood count, bilirubin level, and transaminase level prior to initiating rifampin. Draw a blood sample for baseline chemistries. (3) Monitor SGPT and SGOT or AST and ALT prior to therapy and every 2 to 3 weeks during therapy. (4) Risk of liver damage is markedly increased if impaired liver function is present. Hepatotoxicity, hepatic encephalopathy, and death associated with jaundice have occurred in patients with liver disease and when rifampin is given with other hepatotoxic agents (e.g., isoniazid, halothane). Discontinue one or both drugs for signs of hepatocellular damage. Notify physician immediately if flulike symptoms develop. (5) Thrombocytopenia has occurred. Reversible if rifampin is discontinued as soon as purpura occurs. Cerebral hemorrhage has occurred when rifampin has been continued or resumed after the appearance of purpura. Contact physician immediately if purpura occurs. (6) Susceptibility tests required before use as treatment for asymptomatic carriers of neisseria meningitis and if positive cultures persist after use. (7) Confirm patency of IV; avoid extravasation. Restart IV at a new site for any signs of inflammation or irritation. (8) Inhibits activity and decreases plasma levels of acetaminophen (Tylenol), analgesics (e.g., narcotics), barbiturates (e.g., phenobarbital), benzodiazepines (e.g., diazepam [Valium]), beta blockers (e.g., propranolol [Inderal]), chloramphenicol, clofibrate (Atromid-S), corticosteroids (e.g., prednisone), cyclosporine (Sandimmune), dapsone, digoxin and digitoxin, disopyramide (Norpace), estrogens, hydantoins (phentoin [Dilantin]), methadone, mexiletine (Mexitil), oral antidiabetics (tolbutamide), oral anticoagulants (warfarin [Coumadin]), oral contraceptives, quinidine, theophyllines (e.g., aminophylline, tocainide (Tonocard), and verapamil (Isoptin). Increased doses of these drugs may be required. Monitor carefully; obtain prothrombin daily when used with oral anticoagulants (e.g., warfarin); use of nonhormonal contraceptives recommended during rifampin therapy; and diabetes may be more difficult to control. (9) Treatment failure of ketoconazole (Nizoral) or rifampin may occur when given concomitantly. (10) Inhibited by clofazimine (Lamprene). Decreases rate of absorption and delays peak plasma levels of rifampin. (11) Potentiated by probenecid. (12) May cause hypertension with enalapril (Vasotec). (13) Para-aminosalicylic acid (PAS) will decrease serum lelvels of rifampin. Drugs should be taken at least 8 hours apart. (14) May cause an early rise in bilirubin during initial days of treatment; should subside. Throughout treatment transient abnormalities in liver function tests will occur. Reduced biliary excretion of contrast media for gallbladder studies may occur. Do all lab tests and affeted radiology studies before daily dose of medication. (15) Therapeutic levels inhibit assays of serum folate and vitamin B_{12}. (16)

May exacerbate porphyria. (17) Urine, feces, saliva, sputum, sweat, and tears may be colored red-orange. Soft contact lenses may be permanently stained. CSF may be light yellow. (18) Has teratogenic potential. Safety for use during pregnancy not established. Benefit must outweigh risk. Administration during the last few weeks of pregnancy may cause postnatal hemorrhages in mother and infant; treatment with vitamin K may be required. Closely monitor neonates of rifampin-treated mothers for adverse effects. (19) Discontinue breast feeding if mother requires treatment.

Contraindications: Hypersensitivity to any rifamycins; individuals with liver disease are at higher risk for complications.

Incompatible with: Media containing sodium lactate.

Side effects: *Average dose:* Anaphylaxis may occur even with repeat doses. Abnormal liver function tests, anorexia, ataxia, behavioral changes, conjunctivitis (exudative), cramps, diarrhea, edema of face and extremities, epigastric distress, dizziness, eosinophilia, fatigue, flushing, flulike symptoms (e.g., chills, fever, headache, malaise, muscle and bone pain), gas, heartburn, hematuria, hemolytic anemia, hepatic reactions, hepatitis, hypotension, leukopenia, menstrual disturbances, mental confusion myopathy (rare), muscle weakness, nausea, numbness (generalized), pain in extremities, purpura, pruritis, rash, renal failure (acute), shortness of breath, sore mouth and tongue, thrombocytopenia, urticaria, visual disturbances, vomiting, wheezing.

Overdose: Bilirubin levels increase rapidly; Brown-red discoloration of feces, skin, sweat, tears, and urine is proportional to amount of overdose; lethargy, nausea, and vomiting are immediate; liver enlargement and tenderness; unconsciousness.

Antidote: With increasing severity of any side effect, alterations in liver function tests, flulike symptoms, purpura, thrombocytopenia, or symptoms of overdose, discontinue the drug and notify the physician immediately. Forced diuresis will promote excretion. Bile drainage may be indicated in the presence of seriously impaired hepatic function lasting more than 24 to 48 hours. Hemodialysis may be useful. Treat anaphylaxis and resuscitate as necessary.

RITODRINE HYDROCHLORIDE pH 4.8 to 5.5

(Yutopar)

Usual dose: 0.1 mg/min (0.33 ml/min or 20 gtt/min) initially. Gradually increase by 0.05 mg/min (0.17 ml/min or 10 gtt/min) every 10 minutes until desired result obtained. Continue infusion until 12 hours after contractions cease, then begin oral ritodrine (approximately 30% of IV potency) immediately. Administer first oral dose 30 minutes before IV is discontinued.

Dilution: Each 150 mg (three 50 mg ampoules) must be diluted in 500 ml of 5% dextrose in water for infusion. Use normal saline, Ringer's solution, or Hartmann's solution only when dextrose is not appropriate (e.g., diabetes mellitus). Concentration will be 0.33 mg/ml.

Rate of administration: Specific instructions included under Usual dose. Usually effective between 0.15 and 0.35 mg/min (0.50 to 1.17 ml/min or 30 to 70 gtt/min). Use of a microdrip chamber (60 gtt/ml) required; infusion pump preferred. Estimates based on suggested dilution. Adjust if more or less diluent is used. Highly individualized based on patient's response and side effects.

Actions: A β-adrenergic stimulator that acts to inhibit contractility of uterine smooth muscle. Increases pulse rate and widens pulse pressure moderately. Onset of action is prompt and lasts about 2 hours. Crosses the placental barrier. Primary excretion in the urine.

Indications and uses: (1) To arrest preterm labor; (2) temporarily prevent labor during preparation for operative delivery; (3) prevent fetal distress during transportation to a hospital.

Precautions: (1) Most effective if begun as soon as diagnosis of preterm labor established. (2) Do not use if solution discolored or contains particulate matter or precipitate. (3) Discard solution after 48 hours. (4) Obtain maternal baseline ECG to rule out heart disease. Monitor uterine contractions, maternal pulse rate, blood pressure, and fetal heart rate every 5 minutes until stable, every 15 to 30 minutes thereafter until infusion discontinued. (5) Maintain adequate hydration, but avoid fluid overload and observe for signs of pulmonary edema (may unmask unknown cardiac disease). Respiratory rate above 20 or pulse rate sustained at 140 or above may indicate onset of pulmonary edema. (6) Maintain patient in left lateral position during infusion to minimize hypotension. (7) Use extreme caution if indicated in maternal mild to moderate preeclampsia, hypertension, or diabetes. (8) Evaluate fetal maturity (sonography). (9) Maternal hyperglycemia must be monitored and treated if indicated. May precipitate reactive hypoglycemia in the infant. Monitor insulin, glucose, and electrolyte levels in selected patients or long-term therapy. Normal levels will be altered. (10) Corticosteroids concomitantly may precipitate pulmonary edema. (11) Inhibited by β-adrenergic blockers (e.g., propranolol [Inderal]). (12) Potentiated by other sympathomimetic amines (e.g., epinephrine [Adrenalin], dopamine [Intropin]). Effects may be additive. Do not administer concurrently; allow adequate time intervals before initiating therapy with any sympathomimetic drug. (13) Cardiovascular effects (cardiac dysrhythmias, hypotension) potentiated by diazoxide (Hyperstat IV), magnesium sulfate, meperidine (Demerol), and general anesthetics. (14) Increased hypertension may occur with atropine. (15) Concomitant use with sulfites may cause severe allergic reaction.

Contraindications: Before the twentieth week of pregnancy; conditions during pregnancy that are hazardous to the mother or infant, that is, antepartum hemorrhage, cardiac disease (maternal), chorioamnionitis, diabetes mellitus (uncontrolled), eclampsia (or severe preeclampsia), hypersensitivity to ritodrine or its components, hyperthyroidism (maternal), intrauterine fetal death, pulmonary hypertension, preexisting maternal medical conditions adversely affected by β-mimetic drugs (bronchial asthma treated with β-mimetics or steroids, cardiac dysrhythmias with tachycardia or digitalis intoxication), hypovolemia, hypertension (uncontrolled), and pheochromocytoma.

Incompatible with: Should be considered incompatible in solution with any other drug because of specific use, accurate rate calculation, and potential for additive toxicity.

Side effects: Anaphylaxis, anxiety, cardiac dysrhythmias, chest pain, constipation, decreased diastolic pressure, diarrhea, epigastric distress, elevated systolic pressure, erythema, glycosuria, headache, hemolytic icterus, hyperventilation, ileus, jitteriness, lactic acidosis, malaise, nausea, nervousness, palpitations, pulmonary edema, pulse pressure widened, restlessness, tachycardia, tightness of the chest, tremor, vomiting.

Antidote: Keep physician informed of all side effects. Most side effects are expected and will be tolerated or treated symptomatically (note drug interactions). Marked hypotension, tachycardia, cardiac dysrhythmias, and other signs of β-adrenergic stimulation will require discontinuation of the drug. Uterine relaxation may persist for several hours, and oral therapy may be considered. A β-blocker (propranolol [Inderal]) may be required. Discontinue drug and treat anaphylaxis as indicated. At first signs of fluid overload or pulmonary edema, notify physician immediately and treat as indicated.

SARGRAMOSTIM pH 7.1 to 7.7

(GM-CSF, human granulocyte-macrophage colony stimulating factor, Leukine, Prokine)

Usual dose: 250 mcg/M^2 as an infusion daily for 21 days. Range may be from 60 to 1,000 mcg/M^2/day. Initial infusion must begin 2 to 4 hours after the autologous bone marrow infusion and not less than 24 hours after the last dose of chemotherapy and 12 hours after the last dose of radiation. May require dose reduction in impaired renal or hepatic function. Based on individual patient response.

Dilution: Each 250 or 500 mcg vial must be diluted with 1 ml sterile water for injection without preservative. Confirm expiration date to ensure valid product. Direct diluent to the side of the vial and swirl gently. Avoid foaming or vigorous agitation. Do not shake. Must be further diluted in normal saline for infusion. If the final concentration of sargramostim will be below 10 mcg/

ml, albumin (human) must be added to the normal saline before addition of the sargramostim (1 ml of 5% albumin to each 50 ml normal saline). This will prevent absorption of the drug into the components of the IV delivery system. Contains no preservatives. Use sterile technique; enter vial only to dilute and to withdraw a single dose. Discard any unused portion. Should be clear and colorless. Should be used promptly, but the reconstituted or the diluted solution can be refrigerated temporarily at 2° to 8° C (36° to 46° F). Must be completely administered within 6 hours.

Rate of administration: Each single dose must be evenly distributed over 2 hours. Reduce rate or temporarily discontinue for onset of any side effects that cause concern (e.g., allergic reaction).

Actions: Colony-stimulating factors are glycoproteins that bind to specific hematopoietic cell surface receptors and stimulate proliferation, differentiation commitment, and some end-cell functional activation. Utilizing recombinant DNA technology, sargramostim is produced in a yeast (*S. cerevisiae*). It differs slightly from endogenous GM CSF. It induces partially committed progenitor cells to divide and differentiate in the granulocyte-macrophage pathways. Can also activate mature granulocytes and macrophages. It is a multilineage factor and has dose-dependent effects. It increases the cytotoxicity of monocytes toward certain neoplastic cell lines and activates polymorphonuclear neutrophils to inhibit the growth of tumor cells. It significantly improves the time to neutrophil recovery (engraftment), decreases length of hospitalization, shortens the duration of infectious episodes, and decreases antibiotic usage. Detected in the serum in 5 minutes; peak levels are reached 2 hours after injection and last at least 6 hours.

Indications and uses: Acceleration of hematopoietic recovery (engraftment) in patients undergoing autologous bone marrow transplantation (AuBMT) because of lymphoid malignancies (ALL [acute lymphoblastic leukemia], NHL [non-Hodgkin's lymphoma], and HD [Hodgkin's disease]).

Investigational use: Acceleration of myeloid recovery following peripheral blood stem cell transplantation.

Precautions: (1) Should be administered under the direction of a physician knowledgeable about appropriate use. (2) Obtain a complete blood count with differential before administration and twice weekly thereafter to monitor for excessive leukocytosis (WBC greater than 50,000 cells/mm^3) or an absolute neutrophil count (ANC) greater than 20,000 cells/mm^3. (3) Myeloproliferative effects may be potentiated by lithium or corticosteroids; use with caution. (4) Observe for fluid retention, may cause peripheral edema, pleural effusion, and/or pericardial effusion. May occur more frequently in individuals with preexisting lung disease or cardiac disease, including a history of dysrhythmias. Use with caution. (5) Use caution in patients with preexisting renal or hepatic dysfunction, an increased serum creatinine or increased bilirubin and hepatic enzymes may occur. Reversible if drug discontinued. Monitor renal and hepatic function biweekly. (6) Use caution if considered for use in any malignancy with myeloid characteristics. Can act as a growth factor for any tumor type, particularly myeloid malignancies. (7) Can be effective in patients receiving purged bone marrow if the purging process preserves a sufficient number of progenitors. (8) Effects may be limited in patients previously exposed to intensive chemotherapy or radiation therapy. (9) Neutralizing antibodies may form after receiving sargramostim and may inhibit therapeutic effect. (10) Has been used in more than 100 children from 4 months of age to 18 years with similar experience to the adult population, even though literature says safety not established. (11) Safety for use in pregnancy and lactation not established; use only if clearly needed. (12) Must be refrigerated in all forms; do not freeze or shake.

Contraindications: Hypersensitivity to any of the components of sargramostim; patients with leukemic myeloid blasts in the bone marrow or peripheral blood equal to 10% or more.

Incompatible with: Specific information not available. Manufacturer recommends that no medication other than albumin be added to the infusion solution.

Side effects: Asthenia, diarrhea, malaise, rash are most common. Allergic reactions, including anaphylaxis, are possible; dyspnea, hypoxia, local injection site reactions, pericardial effusion, peripheral edema, pleural effusion, and supraventricular dysrhythmias have been reported.

Antidote: For anaphylaxis, accidental overdose: if blast cells appear or there is progression of underlying disease, discontinue sargramostim. For an ANC above 20,000 cells/mm^3 or a platelet count above 500,000/mm^3, reduce dose by one half or temporarily discontinue. Blood count should return to baseline level in 3 to 7 days. For any side effect that causes concern, reduce dose or temporarily discontinue. Keep physician informed. Treat anaphylaxis and resuscitate as necessary.

SECOBARBITAL SODIUM pH 9.7 to 10.5

(Seconal Sodium)

Usual dose (for adults and children): *Moderate sedation:* 1 to 1.5 mg/kg of body weight.

Hypnotic: 2 mg/kg.

Convulsions due to tetanus: 5.5 mg/kg. Any dose may be repeated in 3 to 4 hours as indicated. 250 mg is usual maximum single dose, but 500 mg is never exceeded.

Dilution: Dilute with sterile water for injection. Any desired amount of dilutent may be used. 9 ml of diluent with 1 ml of secobarbital (50 mg) equals 5 mg/ml. Dilute secobarbital in powder form to a 5 solution (add 5 ml to 250 mg). Rotate ampoule gently while introducing diluent. Further dilute if desired.

Rate of administration: 50 mg or fraction thereof over 1 minute. Never exceed a rate of 50 mg or fraction thereof over 15 seconds. Titrate slowly to desired effect.

Actions: A sedative, hypnotic barbiturate of short duration with anticonvulsant effects. Secobarbital is a CNS depressant. Onset of action is prompt by IV route and lasts about 3 or 4 hours. Will effectively depress motor cortex if adequate doses are administered. Pain perception is unimpaired. Rapidly absorbed by all body tissues and excreted fairly quickly in the urine in changed form. Crosses placental barrier. Secreted in breast milk.

Indications and uses: (1) Preanesthetic sedation; (2) dental and minor surgical sedation; (3) sedation during labor; (4) control of convulsions caused by tetanus; (5) sedation in psychotic states.

Precautions: (1) Store in refrigerator. (2) Hydrolyzes in dry or solution form when exposed to air. Use only absolutely clear solutions and discard powder or solution that has been exposed to air for 30 minutes. (3) Use only enough medication to achieve desired effect. Rapid injection rate may cause symptoms of overdose. (4) Record blood pressure, pulse, and respiration every 3 to 5 minutes. Keep patient under constant observation. (5) Maintain a patent airway. Keep equipment for artificial ventilation available. (6) Treat the cause of a convulsion. (7) May be habit forming. Status epilepticus can occur from too rapid withdrawal. (8) Determine absolute patency of vein; use of large veins preferred to prevent thrombosis. Avoid extravasation. Intraarterial injection will cause gangrene. (9) Use caution in asthma, pulmonary and cardiovascular diseases, toxemia of pregnancy, history of bleeding, impaired renal function, shock, uremia, and depressive states after a convulsion. (10) Use extreme caution if any other CNS depressants have been given such as alcohol, narcotic analgesics, anesthetics, antidepressants, antihistamines, hypnotics, MAO inhibitors, phenothiazines, sedatives, neuromuscular blocking antibiotics, or tranquilizers. Potentiation with respiratory depression may occur. (11) Inhibits effectiveness of propranolol (Inderal), corticosteroids, doxycycline (Vibramycin), oral anticoagulants, oral contraceptives, quinidine, and theophylline. Capable of innumerable interactions with many drugs. (12) May increase orthostatic hypotension with furosemide (Lasix). (13) Monitor phenytoin and barbiturate levels when both drugs are used concurrently. (14) May not drive, etc., if given on an outpatient basis. (15) May cause paradoxical excitement in children or the elderly.

Contraindications: Delivery (when maximum drug effect would be achieved at the time of delivery), history of porphyria, impaired liver function, known hypersensitivity to barbiturates, premature delivery, severe respiratory depression.

Incompatible with: Atracurium (Tracrium), benzquinamide (Emete-Con), chlordiazepoxide (Librium), chlorpromazine (Thorazine), cimetidine (Tagamet), clindamycin (Cleocin), codeine, diphenhydramine (Benadryl), droperidol (Inapsine), ephedrine, erythromycin (Ilotycin), glycopyrrolate (Robinul), hydrocortisone sodium succinate (Solu-Cortef), insulin (aqueous), isoproterenol (Isuprel), levarterenol (Levophed), levorphanol (Levo-Dromoran), meperidine (Demerol), metaraminol (Aramine), methadone, methyldopate (Aldomet), pancuronium bromide (Pavulon), penicillin G potassium, pentazocine (Talwin), phenytoin (Dilantin), phytonadione (Aquamephyton), procaine (Novocain), prochlorperazine (Compazine), promethazine (Phenergan), propiomazine (Largon), sodium bicarbonate, streptomycin, succinycholine (Anectine), tetracycline, vancomycin (Vancocin).

Side effects: *Average dose:* Asthma, bronchospasm, depression, dermatitis, facial edema, fever, hypotension, neonatal apnea, respiratory depression (slight), thrombocytopenic purpura.

Overdose: Apnea, coma, cough reflex depression, flat EEG (reversible unless hypoxic damage has occurred), hypotension, laryngospasm, lowered body temperature, pulmonary edema, sluggish or absent reflexes, renal shutdown, respiratory depression.

Antidote: Notify the physician of any side effects. Symptomatic and supportive treatment is most important in overdose. Maintain an adequate airway with artificial ventilation if indicated. Keep the patient warm. IV volume expanders (dextran) and IV fluids will help maintain adequate circulation. Diuretics or hemodialysis will promote the elimination of the drug. Vasopressors (e.g., dopamine [Intropin]) will maintain blood pressure.

SECRETIN

(Secretin-Boots, Secretin-Ferring)

Usual dose: Skin test before injection of clinical dose.

Pancreatic function testing: 1 unit/kg of body weight as a single dose.

Diagnosis of gastrinoma (Zollinger-Ellison syndrome): 2 units/kg as a single dose.

Dilution: Each vial containing 100 (75) units must be diluted with 10 (7.5) ml of normal saline for injection. 10 units/ml.

Rate of administration: A single dose evenly distributed over 1 minute.

Actions: A polypeptide composed of many amino acids. It acts to increase the secretory function of pancreatic exocrine glands. Measuring and analyzing duodenal fluid aids in the determination of pancreatic function. Peak output occurs in 30 minutes and may continue for 2 hours. Degraded in the liver. IV secretin has a serum half-life of 18 minutes.

Indications and uses: (1) Diagnosis of chronic pancreatic dysfunction; (2) diagnosis of gastrinoma (Zollinger-Ellison syndrome); (3) may aid in the diagnosis of some hepatobiliary diseases by providing cells for cytopathologic examination.

Precautions: (1) Must be refrigerated at 2° to 7° C (36° to 45° F); check expiration date. (2) Use diluted solution immediately and discard unused portion. (3) Skin testing recommended with 0.1 ml of properly diluted solution. Use a control skin test with 0.1 ml of plain normal saline (without preservatives) for injection. If the secretin causes a greater reddened area than the control area, do not give IV. (4) Pancreatic dysfunction diagnosis is accomplished by inserting a specific double-lumen gastric tube after a 12-hour fast. Correct positioning under fluoroscopic guidance is required. Aspirate gastric contents continuously to prevent passage into the duodenum. Collect duodenal contents for 10 to 20 minutes until a clear, bile-stained, uncontaminated fluid with a pH of 6.0 is obtained. Administer secretin (usually done by physician). Collect four duodenal samples in separate sterile specimen containers (one sample at 10 minutes, one at 20 minutes, one at 40 minutes, and the last at 1 hour after administration of secretin). Sometimes the samples are collected at four 20-minute intervals. (5) Gastrinoma diagnosis begins with a 12-hour fast. Draw two blood samples for fasting serum gastrin levels. Administer secretin. Collect blood samples at 1, 2, 5, 10, and 30 minutes for serum gastrin concentrations. (6) Use with extreme caution in acute pancreatitis; defer use in pregnancy if possible. (7) Safety for use in children not established. (8) Inhibited by carbonic anhydrase inhibitors (e.g., acetazolamide [Diamox]) and anticholinergics (e.g., atropine).

Contraindications: History of asthma or allergy, positive skin test to secretin, known hypersensitivity to secretin, acute pancreatitis until attack subsided.

Incompatible with: Specific information not available. Should be considered incompatible with any drug in the syringe because of specific use.

Side effects: Allergic reactions from impure preparations and/or repeat injections do occur. Thrombophlebitis can occur.

Antidote: Discontinue the drug immediately for any signs of allergic reaction. Treat anaphylaxis with epinephrine, antihistamines (e.g., diphenhydramine [Benadryl]), vasopressors (e.g., dopamine [Intropin]), aminophylline, and corticosteroids as indicated. Maintain a patent airway and resuscitate as necessary.

SERMORELIN ACETATE pH 5.5

(Geref)

Usual dose: 1.0 mcg/kg of body weight as a single test dose. Schedule in the morning following an overnight fast. Specific procedure required. Draw venous blood samples for growth hormone determinations 15 minutes before, immediately prior to administration, and every 15 minutes times four after administration. Use a

3 ml normal saline flush immediately after injection of sermorelin.

Dilution: Each 50 mcg ampule must be diluted with a minimum of 0.5 ml of the 2 ml normal saline provided. Solution must be clear and used immediately after reconstitution. Do not use if cloudy or discolored. Discard any unused material.

Rate of administration: A single dose as a bolus injection followed by a 3 ml normal saline flush.

Actions: A sterile lyophilized white powder, this synthetic hormone is identical in amino acid composition to endogenous natural growth hormone–releasing factor (GHRF; GRF). Increases plasma growth hormone concentrations by direct stimulation of the somatotroph cells of the anterior pituitary gland to release growth hormone. Does not have stimulatory effects on the secretion of other pituitary hormones (e.g., prolactin, TSH, FSH, LH, or ACTH). An increase in peak levels begins within 5 minutes, and maximum levels occur 30 to 60 minutes after injection. Plasma half-life is 6 to 8 minutes. Rapidly distributed and then degraded to an inactive fragment.

Indications and uses: Evaluation of the ability of the somatotroph of the pituitary gland to secrete growth hormone (GH).

Precautions: (1) A normal plasma GH response (28 ± 15 ng/ml within 30 minutes) to sermorelin acetate demonstrates that the somototroph is intact. 50% of patients who do not respond to standard testing will show a normal response to sermorelin. GH deficiency may still be the result of hypothalamic dysfunction in the presence of an intact somatotroph. (2) Test is most easily interpreted when there is a subnormal response to conventional provocative testing and a normal response to sermorelin. The site of dysfunction cannot be determined if both conventional and sermorelin testing result in subnormal GH responses. (3) Not useful in the diagnosis of acromegaly. (4) Discontinue exogenous growth hormone therapy at least 1 week before testing. (5) Do not test in the presence of drugs that directly affect the pituitary secretion of somatotropin (e.g., insulin, glucocorticoids [e.g., dexamethasone, cortisone, prednisone], cyclooxygenase inhibitors [e.g., aspirin or indomethacin]. (6) Transiently elevated somatotropin levels can occur with clonidine, levodopa, and insulin-induced hypoglycemia. (7) Response inhibited by muscarinic antagonists (e.g., atropine), antithyroids (e.g., propylthiouracil), and in hypothyroid patients. Response may be inhibited by obesity, hyperglycemia, and elevated plasma fatty acids. (8) Safety for use in pregnancy and lactation not established. Has been shown to produce minor variations in fetuses of rats and rabbits. Use during pregnancy or lactation only if benefits outweigh risk. (9) Dry powder stable for 1 year from date of manufacture if stored in refrigerator.

Contraindications: Hypersensitivity to sermorelin acetate or any of its components (e.g., mannitol, albumin).

Incompatible with: Specific information not available. Consider incompatible in syringe or solution due to specific use.

Side effects: *Average dose:* Allergic reactions (e.g., redness, swelling, and urticaria at the injection site [25% of patients develop antibodies]); flushing of the face; headache; nausea; pain at the injection site; paleness; strange taste in mouth; tightness in the chest; transient warmth; vomiting.

Overdose: Blood pressure and heart rate changes have been reported with doses over 10 mcg/kg. Cardiovascular collapse is conceivable but has not happened.

Antidote: Notify physician of all side effects; may be transient or may require symptomatic treatment. Treat allergic reactions with diphenhydramine (Benadryl) or epinephrine. Resuscitate as necessary.

SINCALIDE pH 5.5 to 6.5

(Kinevac)

Usual dose: *Contraction of the gallbladder:* 0.02 mcg/kg of body weight (1.4 mcg/70 kg [154 lb]). May repeat in 15 minutes if satisfactory contraction of the gallbladder does not occur. After the injection, take x-rays at 5-minute intervals to visualize the gallbladder and 1-minute intervals during the first 5 minutes to visualize the cystic duct.

Secretin-sincalide test of pancreatic function: Skin testing required, refer to Secretin. Initiate an infusion of secretin 0.25 units/kg. Follow in 30 minutes through a separate IV site with an infusion of sincalide 0.02 mcg/kg.

Dilution: Each 5 mcg vial must be initially diluted with 5 ml of sterile water for injection.

Contraction of the gallbladder: May be given without additional dilution.

Secretin-sincalide test of pancreatic function: Further dilute the calculated dose (1.4 mcg/70 kg [1.4 ml]) in 30 ml normal saline for injection. Further dilute the calculated dose of secretin in 60 ml normal saline for injection.

Rate of administration: *Contraction of the gallbladder:* A single dose evenly distributed over 30 to 60 seconds.

Secretin-sincalide test of pancreatic function: Evenly distribute secretin over 60 minutes (approximately 1 ml/min). Evenly distribute sincalide over 30 minutes (approximately 1 ml/min).

Actions: Causes the gallbladder to contract and evacuate bile in a manner similar to endogenous cholecystokinin. Maximum effect is achieved in 5 to 15 minutes. Causes delayed gastric emptying and increased intestinal motility. When given in conjunction with secretin, both the volume of pancreatic secretion and the output of bicarbonate and protein enzymes are increased. By analyzing and measuring the duodenal aspirate, pancreatic function (volume of the secretion, bicarbonate concentration, amylase content) can be assessed.

Indications and uses: (1) To provide a sample of gallbladder bile for analysis of its composition (aspirated from the duodenum). (2) To stimulate pancreatic secretion for analysis of its composition and examination of cytology. Used in conjunction with secretin. Specimen aspirated from the duodenum. (3) Postevacuation cholecystography when indicated and intake of a fatty meal is not desired.

Precautions: (1) Store at room temperature before and after dilution. Use diluted solution immediately and discard unused portion. (2) Small gallbladder stones may be evacuated from the gallbladder. They could lodge in the cystic duct or common bile duct. Not highly probable because contraction of the gallbladder is not complete. (3) Safety for use during pregnancy not established; use only when benefits outweigh risk to fetus. Safety for use in children not established.

Contraindications: Known hypersensitivity to sincalide.

Incompatible with: Specific information not available. Should be considered incompatible with any drug in the syringe or solution because of specific use.

Side effects: Abdominal discomfort, abdominal pain, and urge to defecate usually occur because of delayed gastric emptying and increased intestinal motility. Dizziness, flushing, and nausea may occur.

Antidote: Keep physician informed of side effects. Assist patient with comfort measures. Resuscitate as necessary.

SODIUM ACETATE — pH 6.0 to 7.0

Usual dose: Determined by nutritional needs, evaluation of electrolytes, and degree of hyponatremia. Each gram contains 7.3 mEq of sodium and acetate.

Dilution: Must be added to larger volumes of IV infusion solutions including total parenteral nutrition.

Rate of administration: Administer at prescribed rate for infusion solutions.

Actions: An alkalizing agent and sodium salt. Sodium is

the predominant cation of extracellular fluid. It controls water distribution throughout the body. Hypothalamus osmoreceptors, sensitive to osmolarity changes in the blood, control serum sodium concentration (142 mEq/L). Body fluid is lost when sodium content decreases and retained when sodium content increases. The acetate ion fully metabolizes outside the liver to bicarbonate.

Indications and uses: (1) To prevent or correct hyponatremia in patients with restricted intake, especially in individualized IV formulations when basic needs are not met by standard solutions; (2) treatment of mild to moderate acidotic states; (3) source of sodium ions in hemodialysis and peritoneal dialysis.

Precautions: (1) Evaluate electrolytes frequently during treatment. Evaluate fluid balance. (2) Use with caution in impaired renal function, congestive heart failure, hypertension, peripheral or pulmonary edema, any condition resulting in salt retention, and in patients receiving corticosteroids. (3) Rapid or excessive administration may produce alkalosis or hypokalemia. Cardiac dysrhythmias may result from an intracellular shift of potassium. Many other complications may arise from electrolyte imbalance. (4) Temporary therapy in acidosis. Treatment of primary condition must be instituted. (5) Sodium bicarbonate is the drug of choice for use in severe acidosis that requires immediate correction. (6) Store at room temperature.

Contraindications: Metabolic alkalosis, respiratory alkalosis.

Incompatible with: None when used as indicated.

Side effects: Hypernatremia, sodium level over 147 mEq/L, is most common (congestive heart failure, delirium, dizziness, edema, fever, flushing, headache, hypotension, oliguria, pulmonary edema, reduced salivation and lacrimation, respiratory arrest, restlessness, swollen tongue, tachycardia, thirst, weakness). Alkalosis and fluid or solute overload can occur.

Antidote: Notify the physician of any side effect. Reduce rate and notify physician at first sign of congestion or fluid overload. May be treated by sodium restriction and/or use of diuretics (e.g., furosemide [Lasix]) or dialysis. Resuscitate as necessary.

SODIUM BICARBONATE pH 7.0 to 8.5

Usual dose: Adjusted according to pH, $Paco_2$, calculated base deficit, clinical response, and fluid limitations of the patient. In the presence of a low CO_2 content, adjust gradually to avoid unrecognized alkalosis. Correction to a CO_2 of 20 mEq/L within 24 hours will most likely result in a normal pH if the cause of acidosis is controlled and normal kidney function is present.

Cardiac arrest: 0.5 to 1 mEq/kg body weight, only when appropriate. Repeat half dose in 10 minutes if indicated by blood pH and $Paco_2$. Available as:

4.2% sodium bicarbonate solution: 5 mEq/10 ml (0.5 mEq/ml).

5% sodium bicarbonate solution: 297.5 mEq/500 ml (0.595 mEq/ml).

7.5% sodium bicarbonate solution : 44.6 mEq/50 ml or 8.9 mEq/10 ml (0.892 mEq/ml).

8.4% sodium bicarbonate solution: 50 mEq/50 ml or 10 mEq/10 ml (1.0 mEq/ml).

neut (4% sodium bicarbonate solution): 2.4 mEq/5 ml (0.48 mEq/ml).

Dilution: May be given in prepared solutions. 7.5% and 8.4% solutions should be diluted with equal amount of water for injection, or dilute with compatible IV solutions, depending on desired dosage and desired rate of administration. 4.2% solution is preferred for infants and children.

Rate of administration: Usual rate of administration of any solution is 2 to 5 mEq/kg over 4 to 8 hours. Do not exceed 50 mEq/hr. Decrease rate for children. For neonates and children up to 2 years of age do not exceed a rate of 8 mEq/kg/24 hr.

Cardiac arrest: Up to 1 mEq/kg of body weight properly diluted over 1 to 3 minutes.

Actions: An alkalizing agent and sodium salt. Helps to maintain osmotic pressure and ion balance. It is the buffering agent in blood. Bicarbonate ion elevates blood pH promptly. 99% reabsorbed with normal kidney function. Only 1% is excreted in the urine.

Indications and uses: (1) Metabolic acidosis (blood pH

below 7.25) caused by circulatory insufficiency resulting from shock or severe dehydration, extracorporeal circulation of blood, severe renal disease, severe dehydration, cardiac arrest, salicylate intoxication, uncontrolled diabetes with ketoacidosis, and primary lactic acidosis; (2) hyperkalemia; (3) hyponatremia (administer with 5% sodium chloride, usually 1 part sodium bicarbonate to 3 parts sodium chloride); (4) relieve bronchospasm in status asthmaticus; (5) barbiturate or salicylate intoxication; (6) buffering solution to raise pH of IV fluids and medications.

Precautions: (1) Confirm absolute patency of vein. Extravasation may cause chemical cellulitis, necrosis, ulceration, or sloughing. (2) Flush IV line thoroughly before and after administration; many incompatabilities. Use only clear solutions. (3) Determine blood pH, Po_2, Pco_2, and electrolytes several times daily during intensive treatment and daily in most other situations. Determine base excess or deficit in infants and children (dose = 0.3 × kg × base deficit). Notify physician of all results. (4) Temporary therapy in metabolic acidosis. Treatment of primary condition must be instituted. (5) Use with caution in cardiac, liver, or renal disease resulting from salt retention; and in patients receiving corticosteroids. (6) Rapid or excessive administration may produce alkalosis, hypokalemia, and hypocalcemia. Cardiac dysrhythmias may result from an intracellular shift of potassium. Many other complications may arise from electrolyte imbalance. (7) Doses in excess of 8 mEq/kg/24 hr and/or given too rapidly (10 ml/min) may cause intracranial hemorrhage, hypernatremia, and decrease in cerebrospinal fluid pressure in neonates and children under 2 years. (8) Use only 50 ml ampoules in cardiac arrest to prevent accidental overdose. Recent practice indicates smaller doses (0.5 mEq/kg) may be appropriate when indicated in cardiac arrest and may prevent secondary alkalosis. Adequate alveolar ventilation is imperative. Evaluate patient response and blood gases. (9) Inhibits tetracyclines, chlorpropamide, lithium carbonate, and salicylates. (10) Potentiates amphetamines, ephedrine, flecainide, mecamylamine, and quinidine.

Contraindications: Edema, hypertension, hypocalcemia,

hypochloremia (from vomiting, GI suction, or diuretics), impaired renal function, metabolic alkalosis, respiratory alkalosis or acidosis.

Incompatible with: 5% alcohol with 5% dextrose, amino acids, ascorbic acid, atropine, calcium chloride, calcium gluconate, carmustine (BiCNU), cefotaxime (Claforan), chlorpromazine (Thorazine), cisplatin (Platinol), codeine, corticotropin (ACTH), dobutamine (Dobutrex), dopamine (Intropin), epinephrine (Adrenalin), glycopyrrolate (Robinul), hydromorphone (Dilaudid), insulin (aqueous), Ionosol solutions, isoproterenol (Isuprel), labetalol (Normodyne), lactated Ringer's injection, levarterenol (Levophed), levorphanol (Levo-Dromoran), lincomycin (Lincocin), magnesium sulfate, meperidine (Demerol), methadone, methicillin (Staphcillin), metoclopramide (Reglan), morphine, penicillin G potassium, pentobarbital (Nembutal), pentazocine (Talwin), phenobarbital (Luminal), procaine (Novocain), promazine (Sparine), Ringer's injection, secobarbital (Seconal), sodium lactate injection (1/6 molar), streptomycin, succinylcholine (Anectine), tetracycline, thiopental (Pentothal), tubocurarine (Curare), vancomycin (Vancocin), vitamin B complex with C.

Side effects: Rare when used with caution: alkalosis, hyperexcitability, hypokalemia, irritability, restlessness, tetany.

Antidote: Discontinue the drug and notify the physician of any side effect. Hypokalemia usually occurs with alkalosis. Sodium and potassium chloride must be supplemented as indicated for correction. Treatment of alkalosis often results in more alkalosis. Rebreathing expired air from a paper bag may help to control beginning symptoms of alkalosis; calcium gluconate may help in severe alkalosis. Administration of a balanced hypotonic electrolyte solution (Isolyte H, Normosol-M, Plasma-lyte 56) with sodium and potassium chloride added may help to excrete the bicarbonate ion in the urine. Ammonium chloride may be indicated. Treat tetany as indicated (calcium gluconate). Treat extravasation with injection of lidocaine or hyaluronidase (Wydase). Use a 27- or 25-gauge needle. Elevate the extremity and apply warm moist compresses. Resuscitate as necessary.

SODIUM CHLORIDE pH 5.5

Usual dose: Highly individualized and related to specific condition, concentration of salts in the plasma, and/or loss of body fluids.

Isotonic: (0.9%, 9 Gm of sodium chloride/L or 154 mEq of sodium and 154 mEq of chloride), 1.5 to 3 L/24 hr.

Hypotonic: (0.45%, 4.5 Gm of sodium chloride/L or 77 mEq of sodium and 77 mEq of chloride), 2 to 4 L/24 hr.

Hypertonic: Calculate sodium deficit. (5%, 50 Gm of sodium chloride/L or 850 mEq of sodium and 850 mEq of chloride; or 3%, 30 Gm of sodium chloride/L or 510 mEq of sodium and 510 mEq of chloride), 200 to 400 ml/24 hr. Continue until sodium is 130 mEq/L or neurological symptoms improve. Occasionally may have to be repeated within the 24-hour period. See Precautions.

Dilution: Available as *isotonic* (10 ml, 20 ml, 30 ml, 50 ml, 100 ml, 150 ml, 250 ml, 500 ml, 1 liter); *hypotonic* (500 ml, 1 liter); or *hypertonic* (500 ml) solution in vials and/or bottles for injection or infusion and ready for use. Isotonic and hypotonic sodium chloride are frequently combined with dextrose 5% or 10%.

Rate of administration: *Isotonic and hypotonic:* A single daily dose equally distributed over 24 hours. Rate is dependent on age, weight, and clinical condition of the patient.

Hypertonic: One-half the calculated dose over at least 8 hours. Do not exceed 100 ml over 1 hour.

Actions: Sodium is the predominant cation of extracellular fluid. It controls water distribution throughout the body. Hypothalamus osmoreceptors, sensitive to osmolarity changes in the blood, control serum sodium concentration (142 mEq/L). Body fluid is lost when sodium content decreases and retained when sodium content increases. Readily absorbed in kidney tubules. Frequently exchanged for hydrogen and potassium ions. Excess excreted in urine.

Indications and uses: (1) To replace lost sodium and chloride ions in the body (e.g., hyponatremia or low salt syndrome); to maintain electrolyte balance.

Isotonic: To replace sodium and chloride lost from vomiting because of obstructions and/or aspiration of GI fluids; treatment of metabolic alkalosis with fluid loss and sodium depletion.

Hypotonic: Water replacement without increase of osmotic pressure or serum sodium levels; treatment of hyperosmolar diabetes requiring considerable fluid without excess sodium.

Hypertonic: Used only when high sodium and/or chloride content without large amounts of fluid is required. Also used in addisonian crisis and diabetic coma.

(2) Diluent in parenteral preparations.
(3) To initiate and terminate blood transfusions without hemolyzing red blood cells.
(4) Maintain patency and perform routine irrigations of many types of intravascular devices (e.g., catheters, implanted ports.)
(5) Priming solution in hemodialysis procedures.

Precautions: (1) Use caution in circulatory insufficiency, congestive heart failure, edema with sodium retention, kidney dysfunction, hepatic disease, hypoproteinemia, in elderly or debilitated individuals, and in patients receiving corticosteroids. (2) Maintain accurate intake and output. (3) Monitor vital signs as indicated. (4) More than 1 liter of normal saline may cause hypernatremia, which can result in loss of bicarbonate ions and acidosis. (5) Normal saline can cause sodium retention during or immediately after surgery. (6) Excessive administration of potassium-free solutions may cause hypokalemia. (7) Before and during use of hypertonic sodium chloride, determine osmolar concentrations and chloride and bicarbonate content of the serum. Observe patient continuously to prevent pulmonary edema. (8) Store below 40° C (104° F). Do not freeze. Change IV tubing at least every 24 to 48 hours. (9) Benzyl alcohol preservative in bacteriostatic sodium chloride has caused toxicity in newborns. Do not use.

Contraindications: Hypernatremia; fluid retention; situations where sodium or chloride could be detrimental. 3% and 5% sodium chloride solutions are contraindicated with elevated, normal, or slightly decreased serum sodium and chloride levels.

Incompatible with: Amphotericin B (Fungizone), levarterenol (Levophed), mannitol.

Side effects: Due to sodium excess: aggravation of existing acidosis, anorexia, cellular dehydration, deep respiration, disorientation, distention, edema, hydrogen loss, hyperchloremic acidosis, hypertension, increased BUN, nausea, oliguria, potassium loss, pulmonary edema, water retention, weakness.

Antidote: Discontinue or decrease the rate of infusion and notify the physician of side effects. Sodium excess can be treated by sodium restriction and/or use of diuretics or hemodialysis to remove excessive amounts. Observe the patient carefully and treat symptomatically. Save balance of fluid for examination.

SODIUM LACTATE

pH 6.0 to 7.3

(1/6 Molar sodium lactate)

Usual dose: Determined by severity of acidosis based on evaluation of pH, Pa_{CO_2}, age, weight, clinical response, and fluid limitations of the patient. Dose in ml of 1/6 molar sodium lactate = (60 − plasma CO_2) × (0.8 × body weight in pounds). Oxidative processes must be intact. Available as:

1/6 Molar sodium lactate: (167 mEq each of sodium and lactate ions in 150, 250, 500, and 1,000 ml.

Sodium lactate : (50 mEq in 10 ml vial [5 mEq/ml each of sodium and lactate ions]).

Also a component in lactated Ringer's injection.

Dilution: May be given in prepared solutions. 1/6 Molar sodium lactate is usually given as an IV infusion; sodium lactate (5 mEq/ml) must be added to larger volumes of IV infusion solutions including total parenteral nutrition.

Rate of administration: Usual rate of administration of any solution is 2 to 5 mEq/kg over 4 to 8 hours. Do not exceed 300 ml/hr of 1/6 molar sodium lactate in adults. Decrease rate for children. For neonates and children up to 2 years of age do not exceed a rate of 8 mEq/kg/24 hr.

Actions: An alkalizing agent and sodium salt. A sterile solution of lactic acid in water. Its activity depends on conversion to bicarbonate. Oxidized in the liver to bicarbonate and glycogen. Slowly metabolized to CO_2 and H_2O. The bicarbonate ion elevates blood pH, but the process takes 1 to 2 hours.

Indications and uses: Treatment of mild to moderate metabolic acidosis in patients with restricted oral intake with liver function adequate to oxidize sodium lactate to bicarbonate and glycogen.

Precautions: (1) Sodium bicarbonate is the drug of choice for use in severe acidosis that requires immediate correction. Sodium lactate has a 1- to 2-hour delay in correcting acidosis. (2) Determine blood glucose, pH, Po_2, Pco_2, and electrolytes daily during treatment. Evaluate fluid balance. (3) Temporary therapy in metabolic acidosis. Treatment of primary condition must be instituted. (4) Use with caution in anuria, oliguria, congestive heart failure, edema, any condition resulting in salt retention, and in patients receiving corticosteroids. (5) Conversion to bicarbonate and glycogen is delayed in tissue anoxia, impaired liver function, metabolic acidosis associated with circulatory insufficiency, extracorporeal circulation, hypothermia, glycogen storage disease, shock, cardiac decompensation, beriberi, and other disorders resulting in reduced perfusion of body tissues. Use sodium bicarbonate. (6) Rapid or excessive administration may produce alkalosis or hypokalemia. Cardiac dysrhythmias may result from an intracellular shift of potassium. Many other complications may arise from electrolyte imbalance. (7) Safety for use in pregnancy not established; use only if clearly needed. (8) Store at room temperature.

Contraindications: Severe acidosis, lactic acidosis (sodium lactate may be harmful), metabolic alkalosis, respiratory alkalosis.

Incompatible with: Sodium bicarbonate.

Side effects: Alkalosis, congestive conditions (e.g., pulmonary edema), electrolyte dilution, fluid or solute overload, hypernatremia with or without edema, hypokalemia, phlebitis, thrombosis.

Antidote: Discontinue the drug and notify the physician of any side effect. Reduce rate and notify physician at first sign of congestion or fluid overload. Hypokalemia usully occurs with alkalosis. Sodium and potassium chloride must be supplemented as indicated for correction. Treatment of alkalosis often results in more alkalosis. Rebreathing expired air from a paper bag may help to control beginning symptoms of alkalosis. Resuscitate as necessary.

SODIUM NITRITE AND SODIUM THIOSULFATE

pH 7.0 to 9.0
pH 6.0 to 9.5

Usual dose: *Cyanide poisoning:* Following administration of amyl nitrite inhaler, give 300 mg (10 ml) sodium nitrite IV followed by sodium thiosulfate 12.5 Gm (125 ml) IV. One half of the initial dose of both drugs may be given in the same order if indicated.

Arsenic poisoning: (Sodium thiosulfate only) 100 mg (1 ml) on the first day. Increase dose by 100 mg each day until 500 mg dose is reached. Thereafter, give 500 mg every other day as needed.

Pediatric dose: *Cyanide poisoning:* Following administration of amyl nitrite inhaler, give 180 to 240 mg (6 to 8 ml) of sodium nitrite/M^2 followed by sodium thiosulfate 7 Gm/M^2. Do not exceed adult doses.

Dilution: May both be given undiluted.

Rate of administration: *Cyanide poisoning:* Sodium nitrite at 2.5 ml/min; sodium thiosulfate, a single dose equally distributed over 10 minutes or longer.

Arsenic poisoning: A single dose equally distributed over at least 2 minutes.

Actions: Sodium nitrite produces methemoglobinemia that combines with the cyanide ion to make cyanmethemoglobin. It dissociates to make free cyanide, which is then converted to thiocyanate by sodium thiosulfate. The end product is excreted in urine.

Indications and uses: A cyanide antidote kit to facilitate the removal of cyanide in intoxication. Sodium thiosulfate is also used as an injection into tissue infiltrated by extravasation of mechlorethamine.

Precautions: (1) Monitor the patient very carefully, maintain a patent airway, and provide oxygen. Control shock with IV fluids, blood, and vasopressors, and correct acidosis if indicated. (2) Read instructions supplied in kit thoroughly. (3) Ampoule must be airtight for storage. (4) Dimercaprol (BAL) IM is more commonly used as an antidote for arsenic poisoning.

Contraindications: None when used for specific indication.

Incompatible with: Acids, oxidizing agents, salts of heavy metals.

Side effects: Abdominal pain, angina, apprehension, dizziness, headache (severe), hypotension, involuntary passing of urine and feces, nausea and vomiting, paradoxical bradycardia, restlessness, tachycardia, weakness, vertigo.

Antidote: Keep physician informed of all side effects; will be treated symptomatically. A decrease in rate of administration may be necessary. Resuscitate as indicated.

SODIUM PHOSPHATE P 32 — pH 5.0 to 6.0

Usual dose: Measured by appropriate radioactivity calibration system immediately before administration by the radiation oncologist. See literature for specific calibrations.

Polycythemia vera: Leukocyte count should be 5,000/mm^3 or more, and platelet count should be above 150,000/mm^3. 1 to 8 mCi depending on stage of disease and patient size. Must be individualized.

Chronic myelocytic leukemia: Leukocyte count should be 20,000/mm^3 or more. 6 to 15 mCi.

Chronic lymphocytic leukemia: 6 to 15 mCi.

Skeletal metastases: Leukocyte count should be $5,000/mm^3$ or more, and platelet count should be above $100,000\ mm^3$.

Dilution: May be given undiluted. May be given direct IV or through Y-tube or three-way stopcock of a free-flowing IV infusion. May be further diluted in 50 to 100 ml of normal saline or 5% dextrose in water or saline and given as an infusion.

Rate of administration: *Direct IV:* Total desired dose over 2 to 3 minutes.

IV infusion: Total dose over 30 minutes.

Actions: Phosphorus is required in the metabolic and proliferative activity of cells. Radioactive phosphorus concentrates in rapidly proliferating tissue (e.g., bone marrow, spleen, liver). Beneficial only when in direct contact with malignancy or absorbed into bone. Halflife is 14.3 days. Decays by β-emission.

Indications and uses: (1) Trcatment of polycythemia vera, chronic myelocytic leukemia, and chronic lymphocytic leukemia; (2) palliative treatment of selected patients with multiple areas of skeletal metastases.

Precautions: (1) Rarely used. Follow specific guidelines for handling radioactive agents to ensure minimum radiation exposure to patients and occupational workers consistent with appropriate patient management. Contact radiation safety officer. (2) Radiopharmaceuticals usually administered in the hospital by or under the direction of the physician specialist whose experience and training have been approved by the appropriate government agency. (3) Monitor blood and bone marrow at regular intervals. (4) Prepare IV set-up and prime IV tubing in advance. Ensure there will be no dripping or spills of radioactive material. (5) Stored at room temperature in special containers in specific areas. (6) Oral administration in a fasting patient may be as effective as IV administration. (7) Not usually effective in retinoblastomas. (8) Use radiopharmaceuticals when indicated within 10 days of onset of menses in women of childbearing age. (9) Safety for use in pregnancy not established. Use only when clearly indicated and benefits exceed hazards to fetus. Discontinue breast feeding. (10) Safety for use in children not established. (11) Maintain adequate hydration.

Contraindications: Sequential treatment with a chemotherapeutic agent. See Usual dose for specific limitations based on leukocyte and platelet counts.

Incompatible with: Specific information not available. Consider incompatible with any other drug in syringe or solution because of radioactivity and specific use.

Side effects: None when used as indicated with appropriate precautions.

Antidote: Keep physician informed of patient status and results of blood and bone marrow studies.

STREPTOKINASE — pH 6.0 to 8.0

(Kabikinase, Streptase)

Usual dose: *Coronary artery thrombi:* 1.5 million IU direct IV within 6 hours of onset of symptoms of acute transmural myocardial infarction or as an alternative, 750,000 IU direct IV within 3 hours of onset of symptoms of acute transmural myocardial infarction. Follow 750,000 IU dose with 250,000 IU in 30 to 60 minutes. Another alternative is 20,000 IU given directly into coronary artery within 6 hours of onset of symptoms of acute transmural myocardial infarction. Follow with 2,000 IU/min for 1 hour.

Deep vein thrombosis, pulmonary or arterial embolism, arterial thrombosis: Loading dose: 250,000 IU. *Maintenance dose:* 100,000 IU/hr for 24 to 72 hours depending on diagnosis. May be increased based on PT evaluations.

Arteriovenous cannula occlusion: 250,000 IU into each occluded limb of cannula.

Dilution: *All uses except cannula occlusion and direct IV:* Each vial (250,000, 600,000, or 750,000 IU) must be diluted with 5 ml of normal saline for injection (preferred) or 5% dextrose for injection. Add diluent slowly, direct to sides of vial, roll and tilt gently. Do not shake. Further slowly dilute each vial to a total volume of 45 ml (preferred). May be diluted to a maximum of 500 ml in 45 ml increments (preferred). Discard solution with large amounts of flocculation or any solution remaining after 24 hours. Should be infused through a 0.22 or 0.45 micron filter.

Direct IV: Dilute each vial of a single dose with 5 ml normal saline. Further dilute 750,000 IU dose in 50 ml normal saline or 5% dextrose in water. Further dilute 1.5 million IU dose in 100 ml or more of normal saline or 5% dextrose in water. Use care in dilution as above in both situations.

Arteriovenous cannula occlusion: Each vial (250,000 IU) must be diluted with 2 ml sodium chloride for injection. Use care in dilution as above.

Rate of administration: Volumetric or syringe infusion pump required except for direct IV use. Reconstituted streptokinase will alter drop-size and impact correct dosage with drop-size mechanisms.

Direct IV use for coronary artery thrombi: 1.5 million IU dose evenly distributed over 60 minutes. 750,000 IU dose evenly distributed over 5 to 10 minutes.

Coronary artery thrombi: Bolus dose over 15 to 30 seconds via coronary catheter placed by Judkins or Sones technique directly to thrombosed site verified by selective coronary angiography. Follow with 2,000 IU/min for 60 minutes.

Deep vein thrombosis, pulmonary arterial embolism, arterial thrombi: Loading dose: a single dose equally distributed over 25 to 30 minutes.

Maintenance dose: 100,000 IU or more as ordered equally distributed every hour for 24 to 72 hours. Dissolution of arterial thrombi may occur in 24 hours or less, deep vein thrombi may take up to 72 hours.

Arteriovenous cannula occlusion: A single dose slowly (do not force) into each occluded limb of cannula. Clamp for 2 hours, then aspirate contents, flush with saline, and reconnect.

Actions: An enzyme prepared from filtrates of β-hemolytic streptococci. It combines with plasminogen and converts it to plasmin, which degrades fibrin clots, fibrinogen, and other plasma proteins. This activation takes place within a thrombus as well as on the surface. Onset of action is prompt and may last up to 12 to 24 hours. End products of this activity possess an anticoagulant effect. Bleeding may be very difficult to control.

Indications and uses: (1) Lysis of coronary artery thrombi; (2) lysis of acute massive pulmonary emboli if one or more lobes are involved or if hemodynamics are unstable; (3) lysis of an equivalent amount of thrombi in other vessels (deep veins); (4) lysis of acute arterial thrombi and arterial emboli; (5) clearing of occluded arteriovenous cannulae as an alternative to surgical revision.

Precautions: (1) Administered only in the hospital under the direction of a physician knowledgeable in its use and with appropriate diagnostic and laboratory facilities available. Observe patient continuously. Monitor hematocrit, platelet count, activated PTT, thrombin time, and PT before therapy. In 4 hours and during therapy thrombin time or PT changes are monitored and will reflect effectiveness of treatment. Keep physician continuously informed. Request specific parameters for notifying physician after initial supervised injection. (2) Before direct IV use, obtain CPK in addition to above baseline blood tests. Give diphenhydramine (Benadryl) 50 mg IV prophylactically. Monitor ECG and record strips with greatest ST segment elevation initially and every 15 minutes for at least 4 hours. When thrombin time is less than twice the normal control value, initiate heparin infusion to keep PTT at 60 seconds. Prompt, easy treatment a distinct advantage over catheter procedure. (3) For coronary catheter procedure, diagnosis of acute myocardial infarction must be confirmed and the site of the coronary thrombosis confirmed with selective angiography. Concurrent heparin therapy may be required in this situation. (4) Diagnosis of pulmonary or other emboli should be confirmed. Best results obtained if started within 7 days of onset of emboli. Discontinue streptokinase if PT or other lysis parameters are not above 1½ times normal in 4 hours. Excessive resistance may be present. (5) A greater alteration of hemostatic status than with heparin; use care in handling patient, avoid arterial puncture, venipuncture, and IM injection. Use extreme precautionary methods (use of radial artery, not femoral; extended pressure application of up to 30 minutes) if above procedures absolutely necessary. Minor bleeding occurs often at streptokinase insertion sites. Do not reduce or stop streptokinase as lytic activity will be increased and cause more bleeding. (6) Use extreme caution in presence of atrial fibrillation or mitral stenosis with atrial fibrillation; very high risk of stroke from dislodged emboli. (7) Monitor for dysrhythmias during therapy; atrial and ventricular dysrhythmias can occur. (8) Simultaneous use of anticoagulants not recommended except for coronary artery thrombi. Do not use either drug until the effects of the previous drug are diminished. (9) Avoid use of drugs that may alter platelet function (e.g., aspirin, indomethacin, phenylbutazone). (10) Intensive follow-up therapy with continuous infusion of heparin (without a loading dose) is indicated in all situations to prevent recurrent thrombosis. Begin in about 3 to 4 hours of completion of streptokinase, when the PT is reduced to less than twice the normal control value. (11) Do not take blood pressure in lower extremities; thrombi may be dislodged. (12) Prior sensitization to streptokinase increases risk of allergic reaction in subsequent courses of treatment. (13) Attempt to clear arteriovenous cannulae occlusions with good syringe technique and heparinized saline before using streptokinase. Allow effect of heparin to diminish. Instruct patient to exhale and hold his breath any time the catheter is not connected to thc IV tubing or a syringe to prevent air from entering the open catheter and thus the circulatory system. (14) Use extreme caution in the following situations: any surgical procedure, biopsy, lumbar puncture, thoracentesis, paracentesis, multiple cutdowns, or intraarterial diagnostic procedures within 10 days; ulcerative wounds; recent trauma with possible internal injury; visceral malignancy; pregnancy and first 10 days postpartum; any lesion of GI or GU tract with a potential for bleeding (e.g., diverticulitis, ulcerative colitis); severe hypertension; acute or chronic hepatic or renal insufficiency; uncontrolled hypocoagulable state; chronic lung disease with cavitation; rheumatic valvular disease; and any condition where bleeding might be hazardous or difficult to manage because of location. (15) Refrigerate after initial dilution.

Contraindications: Active internal bleeding, cerebral vascular accident within 2 months, intracranial or intraspinal surgery, intracranial neoplasm, hypersensitivity to streptokinase, subacute bacterial endocarditis.

Incompatible with: Specific information not available. Should be considered incompatible in solution because of specific use and hazards of use.

Side effects: Allergic reactions including anaphylaxis are not uncommon with streptokinase. Fever increase of 1° to 2° F is common. Bleeding can be life threatening.

Antidote: Notify physician of all side effects. Note even the minutest bleeding tendency. Therapy may have to be discontinued with serious blood loss and bleeding not controlled by local pressure. Whole blood, packed red blood cells, cryoprecipitate, fresh frozen plasma, and aminocaproic acid may all be indicated. Do not use Dextran. Treat minor allergic reactions symptomatically. Discontinue drug and treat anaphylaxis as indicated; resuscitate as necessary.

STREPTOZOCIN — pH 3.5 to 4.5

(Zanosar)

Usual dose: 500 mg/M^2 for 5 consecutive days. Repeat every 6 weeks until maximum benefit or treatment-limiting toxicity observed. May also give 1,000 mg/M^2 weekly for 2 doses. May then increase up to 1,500 mg/M^2 to achieve therapeutic response if significant toxicity not observed. Overall cumulative dose to onset of response is 2,000 mg/M^2. Maximum response is usually achieved with 4,000 mg/M^2 total cumulative dose.

Reduced dose may be required in impaired renal function; note Precautions.

Dilution: Specific techniques required; see Precautions. Each 1 Gm vial must be diluted with 9.5 ml 0.9% sodium chloride or dextrose for injection (100 mg/ml). May be further diluted in larger amounts (50 to 250 ml) of the same solutions if desired.

Rate of administration: A single dose in minimum diluent may be given over 5 to 15 minutes. Increase injection time if additional diluent used or if indicated for patient comfort.

Actions: An alkylating agent of the nitrogen mustard group with antitumor activity, cell cycle phase nonspecific. Disappears from the blood serum rapidly. Concentrates in the liver and kidneys. 20% excreted in the urine.

Indications and uses: Suppress or retard neoplastic growth in metastatic pancreatic islet cell carcinoma. Use limited by renal toxicity to those with symptomatic or progressive metastatic disease.

Precautions: (1) Follow guidelines for handling cytotoxic agents recommended. See Appendix, p. 677. (2) Administered by or under the direction of the physician specialist. (3) Renal toxicity is dose related, cumulative, and can be fatal. Monitor renal function before, weekly, and for 4 weeks after each course of therapy (serial urinalysis, BUN, plasma creatinine, serum electrolytes, creatinine clearance). Reduce dose or discontinue drug if mild proteinuria occurs. Further deterioration of renal function will occur. (4) Determine absolute patency and quality of vein and adequate circulation of extremity. Severe cellulitis may result from extravasation. (5) Store in refrigerator before and after dilution. Discard within 12 hours of dilution. Contains no preservatives. Protect from light. (6) This drug used to induce hypoinsulinemia diabetes mellitus in experimental animals. (7) Monitor CBCs and liver function tests weekly. (8) Can be used with other antineoplastic drugs in reduced doses to achieve tumor remission. (9) Will produce teratogenic effects on the fetus. Has mutagenic potential. Discontinue breast feeding. (10) Nausea and vomiting have occurred in all patients and can be severe. Prophylactic administration of antiemetics recommended. (11) Do not administer vaccine or chloroquine to patients receiving antineoplastic drugs.

(12) Avoid contact of streptozocin solution with the skin. Severe carcinogenic hazard. (13) Potentiates or is potentiated by hepatotoxic or nephrotoxic medications and radiation therapy. May be fatal. (14) Observe for any signs of infection. (15) Maintain hydration.

Contraindications: Hypersensitivity to streptozocin. Severely impaired liver or renal function may be a contraindication.

Incompatible with: Consider incompatible in syringe or solution because of toxicity and specific use.

Side effects: Anemia, decreased platelet count (precipitous), diarrhea, elevated SGOT and LDH, hepatic toxicity (usually reversible), hypoalbuminemia, hypoglycemia, insulin shock, leukopenia (precipitous), nausea and vomiting (severe), proteinuria, thrombocytopenia.

Antidote: Notify physician of all side effects. Nausea and vomiting, hematological changes, and renal toxicity (proteinuria) may require dose reduction or discontinuation of the drug. There is no specific antidote. Supportive therapy as indicated will help sustain the patient in toxicity. For extravasation, elevate extremity, consider injection of long-acting dexamethasone (Decadron LA) or hyaluronidase (Wydase) throughout extravasated tissue. Use a 27- or 25-gauge needle. Apply warm moist compresses.

SUCCINYLCHOLINE CHLORIDE pH 3.0 to 4.5

(Anectine, Quelicin, Sucostrin, Sux-cert)

Usual dose: 0.3 to 1.1 mg/kg of body weight initially for short-term muscle relaxation (average is 0.6 mg/kg). If muscle relaxation must be sustained over a long period of time, maintain with 0.04 to 0.07 mg/kg at appropriate intervals. Highly individualized, depending on response and degree of relaxation required. 1 mg/kg of body weight is sufficient to cause respiratory paralysis. Never exceed 150 mg total dose. A test dose of 0.1 mg is sometimes used to test patient sensitivity and recovery time.

Pediatric dose: *Infants and small children:* 2 mg/kg.

Older children and adolescents: 1 mg/kg.

Dilution: May be given undiluted if short-term muscle relaxation is desired. For intermittent or continuous infusion during anesthesia add 1 Gm of succinylcholine to 1 liter of 5% dextrose solution or isotonic saline solution. 1 ml of diluted solution delivers 1 mg of succinylcholine. For all other uses, 100 mg in 1 liter delivers 0.1 mg succinylcholine.

Rate of administration: *Direct IV:* Single initial dose over 30 seconds.

Intermittent or continuous infusion: Variable, depending on individual response and muscle relaxation required. Use an infusion pump or microdrip (60 gtt/ml) for accuracy. Never exceed 10 mg/min.

Actions: An ultra-short-acting skeletal muscle relaxant. Causes paralysis by interfering with neural transmission at the myoneural junction. Onset of action is within 1 or 2 minutes and lasts about 5 minutes. Complete recovery from a single dose occurs in about 10 minutes. Metabolized to succinic acid and choline. Only a small amount is excreted in the kidneys. Crosses placental barrier.

Indications and uses: (1) Skeletal muscle relaxation during operative and manipulative procedures; (2) facilitate management of patients undergoing mechanical ventilation; (3) termination or prevention of convulsive episodes resulting from drug toxicity or electroshock therapy.

Precautions: (1) Primarily used by or under the direct observation of the anesthesiologist. (2) This drug produces apnea. Controlled artificial ventilation must be continuous and under direct observation at all times. (3) Use only freshly prepared solutions. Store in refrigerator. Multidose vials stable at room temperature for up to 14 days. Powder for infusion may be stored at room temperature before preparation. (4) Should be administered after unconsciousness induced to reduce patient discomfort. Small doses of nondepolarizing muscle relaxants (e.g., tubocurarine) will reduce severity of muscle fasciculations and incidence of myoglobinuria (occurs more frequently in children) but may cause a prolonged mixed block. (5) Use caution in extensive tissue trauma, fractures, severe burns, nerve damage, and paralysis. Hyperkalemia may cause cardiac dysrhythmias. (6) Observe for early signs of malignant hyperthermic crisis (jaw muscle spasm, lack of laryngeal relaxation, rigidity, unresponsive tachycardia). (7) Use caution in anemia; cardiovascular, hepatic, pulmonary, metabolic, and renal disorders; or malnutrition. Decreased plasma cholinesterase activity potentiates this drug. May increase intraocular pressure. (8) Use extreme caution in pregnancy. There is greater potential for prolonged apnea. May also affect the fetus. (9) Potentiated by neuromuscular blocking antibiotics (e.g., streptomycin, kanamycin, neomycin), β-adrenergic blocking agents (e.g., propranolol [Inderal]), furosemide (Lasix), procainamide (Pronestyl), organic phosphate compounds (insecticides), anticholinesterase drugs (e.g., neostigmine, edrophonium), cimetidine (Tagamet), cyclophosphamide (Cytoxan), lidocaine, quinine, quinidine, and magnesium salts. Capable of innumerable other drug interactions. (10) Inhibited by previous administration of diazepam (Valium). (11) May cause cardiac dysrhythmias in digitalized patients resulting from loss of potassium from muscle cells.

Contraindications: Hypersensitivity to succinylcholine, family history of malignant hyperthermia, genetic disorders of plasma pseudocholinesterase, myopathies associated with elevated CPK values, acute narrow-angle glaucoma, penetrating eye injuries.

Incompatible with: Alkaline solutions, barbiturates (e.g., amobarbital [Amytal], methohexital [Brevital], pentobarbital [Nembutal], phenobarbital, secobarbital [Seconal], thiopental [Pentothal]), chlorpromazine (Thorazine), nafcillin (Unipen).

Side effects: *Minor:* Bradycardia, muscular twitching, respiratory depression.

Major: Cardiac dysrhythmias, hyperthermia, malignant hyperthermic crisis, prolonged apnea with progression to a phase II block (usually results from repeated or prolonged administration).

Antidote: Discontinue drug with onset of any major side effect. An anesthesiologist should be present. Controlled artificial ventilation must be continuous. Endotracheal intubation or tracheostomy is considered prophylactic if necessary for adequate respiratory exchange. Confirm diagnosis of phase II block by using a peripheral nerve stimulator; presence of muscle twitch must also have returned for at least 20 minutes. Both of these are necessary before reversal with anticholinesterase drugs (e.g., neostigmine) is attempted. Whole blood transfusion may restore absent cholinesterase activity and stimulate voluntary respiration in unresponsive cases. Atropine should help to control bradycardia. Treat malignant hyperthermic crisis symptomatically with cooling measures, restoration of electrolyte balance, IV fluids, and maintenance of urinary output. Sodium bicarbonate may be indicated. Dantrolene may be indicated. Resuscitate as necessary.

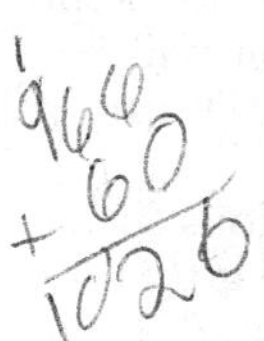

TERBUTALINE SULFATE pH 3.0 to 5.0

(Brethine, Bricanyl)

Usual dose: *All IV doses are investigational.* Literature recommends hydrating the patient with IV fluids (5% dextrose in lactated Ringers or 0.45% saline) for 30 minutes. If no adverse effects, try oral terbutaline 2.5 mg. If contractions remain strong and regular after 30 minutes, begin IV dosing at 10 mcg/min initially (120 gtt/min if 60 gtt = 1 ml, 30 gtt/min if 15 gtt = 1 ml). Gradually increase by 5 mcg/min at 10 to 20 minute intervals until desired result obtained or a maximum dose of 25 mcg/min is reached (some literature states 80 mcg/min). Continue infusion for 30 to 60 minutes after contractions cease. Reduce infusion by 5 mcg/min at 30 minute intervals, until the lowest effective maintenance dose is reached. Maintain this dose for at least 8 hours after uterine contractions have ceased. Immediately follow with SC therapy at 250 mcg every 6 hr for 3 days followed by oral terbutaline 5 mg 3 times daily (some follow immediately with oral dosing eliminating SC).

Dilution: Each 5 mg (five 1 mg ampoules) must be diluted in 1,000 ml of 5% dextrose in water for infusion. Use normal saline only when dextrose is not appropriate (e.g., diabetes mellitus). Concentration will be 5 mcg/ml. Use only clear, colorless solutions. Discard solution after 48 hours.

Rate of administration: Specific instructions included under usual dose. Use of a microdrip (60 gtt/ml) required; infusion pump preferred. Estimates based on suggested dilution. Adjust if more or less diluent is used. Highly individualized based on patient's response and side effects.

Actions: A beta-adrenergic stimulator. Primary actions are bronchodilation and inhibition of uterine smooth muscle contractility. Increases pulse rate and widens pulse pressure moderately. Onset of action is prompt and lasts about 2 hours. Metabolized in the liver. Crosses the placental barrier. Primary excretion in the urine. Secreted in breast milk.

Indications and uses: *All IV uses are investigational.* (1)

To arrest preterm labor; (2) temporarily prevent labor during preparation for operative delivery; (3) prevent fetal distress during transportation to a hospital.

Precautions: (1) *Not FDA approved for IV use. Both manufacturers state their product is for SC use only and state "not for IV use."* Is being used IV throughout the United States and in other countries. Considered by many to be as effective as ritodrine (Yutopar), to have fewer serious side effects, and to be more economical. (2) Generally used in patients with preterm labor with regular uterine contractions at less than 10 minute intervals. A complete evaluation of the mother must be made (e.g., history, physical, prenatal record, reports from previous ultrasound, routine lab including urine culture and sensitivity). *This is an experimental drug. Although it has been used for this purpose for many years, your hospital may require a documented informed consent.* (3) Most effective if begun as soon as diagnosis of preterm labor established. (4) Obtain maternal baseline ECG to rule out heart disease. Monitor frequency and duration of uterine contractions, maternal pulse rate, blood pressure, and fetal heart rate every 5 minutes until stable, every 15 minutes thereafter until infusion discontinued. (5) Maintain adequate hydration, but avoid fluid overload and observe for signs of pulmonary edema. Respiratory rate above 20 or pulse rate sustained at 150 or above may indicate onset of pulmonary edema. Infusion time exceeding 24 hours, sodium-containing solution, and multiple pregnancy may precipitate pulmonary edema. (6) Use extreme caution if indicated in maternal mild to moderate preeclampsia, hypertension, or diabetes. (7) Evaluate fetal maturity (sonography). (8) Maternal hyperglycemia must be monitored and treated if indicated. May precipitate reactive hypoglycemia in the infant. Monitor insulin, glucose, and electrolyte levels in selected patients or long-term therapy. Normal levels will be altered. (9) Inhibited by beta-adrenergic blockers (e.g., propranolol [Inderal]). (10) Potentiated by other sympathomimetic amines (e.g., epinephrine [Adrenalin], dopamine [Intropin]). Effects, including cardiovascular effects, may be additive. Do not administer concurrently; allow adequate time intervals before initiating therapy with any sympathomimetic drug. (11) MAO inhibitors (e.g., pargyline [Eutonyl]) will potentiate effects on the vascular system. (12) Ampoules are stored at room temperature protected from light.

Contraindications: Before the twentieth week of pregnancy; conditions during pregnancy that are hazardous to the mother or infant (e.g., antepartum hemorrhage, cardiac disease [maternal], chorioamnionitis, diabetes mellitus [uncontrolled], eclampsia [or severe preeclampsia], hypersensitivity to terbutaine or its components, hyperthyroidism [maternal], intrauterine fetal death, pulmonary hypertension, preexisting maternal medical conditions adversely affected by beta-mimetic drugs [bronchial asthma treated with beta-mimetics or steroids], cardiac arrhythmias with tachycardia or digitalis intoxication); hypovolemia; hypertension (uncontrolled); and pheochromocytoma. *Probable contraindications* may include infection; placenta abruptio; placenta previa; premature rupture of the membranes; severe Rh disease, including erythroblastosis fetalis.

Incompatible with: Bleomycin (Blenoxane). Should be considered incompatible in solution with any other drug because of specific use, accurate rate calculation, and potential for additive toxicity.

Side effects: *Maternal:* Allergic reactions including anaphylaxis; cardiac dysrhythmias; chest pain; chest discomfort or burning sensation; decreased diastolic pressure; diaphoresis; dizziness; drowsiness; dyspnea; elevated systolic pressure; flushing; headache; hyperglycemia; hyperinsulinemia; hypokalemia; hyperlactacidemia; hypocalcemic nausea; myocardial ischemia; nervousness; pain at injection site; palpitations; pulmonary edema; pulse pressure widening; sweating; tachycardia; tremors; vomiting; weakness.

Fetal: Tachycardia, neonatal hypoglycemia.

Antidote: Keep physician informed of all side effects. Notify immediately if contractions persist (terbutaline ineffective) or if any signs of maternal or fetal stress occur. Some side effects are expected and will be tolerated or treated symptomatically (note drug interactions). Marked hypotension, tachycardia, cardiac arrhythmias, and other signs of beta-adrenergic stimulation will require discontinuation of the drug. Uterine relaxation may persist for several hours, and SC and oral therapy instead of IV may be considered. Discontinue drug and treat anaphylaxis as indicated. At first signs of fluid overload or pulmonary edema, notify physician immediately and treat as indicated. Additional reasons for discontinuing terbutaline are: evidence of overt amnionitis; fetal distress; fetal heart rate above 200/min, maternal heart rate above 150/min, or respiratory rate less than 10/min; persistent maternal dysrhythmia; progressive cervical dilatation to greater than 7cm.

TERIPARATIDE ACETATE

(Parathar)

Usual dose: 200 units. Specific procedure required (see Precautions and manufacturer's literature).

Pediatric dose: *Children over 3 years of age:* 3 units/kg of body weight. Do not exceed 200 units.

Dilution: Diluent provided; 10 ml equals 200 units. Must be used within 4 hours.

Rate of administration: A single dose equally distributed over 10 minutes.

Actions: A synthetic polypeptide hormone containing a specific fragment of human parathyroid hormone. One effect of this hormone is to stimulate the release of cyclic adenosine monophosphate (cAMP) in the urine. This effect makes it useful as a diagnostic agent.

Indications and uses: To distinguish between hypoparathyroidism and pseudohypoparathyroidism in patients with clinical laboratory evidence of hypocalcemia, which may be caused by either condition.

Precautions: (1) To differentiate between hypoparathyroidisms (modified Ellsworth-Howard test) the patient must drink 200 ml of water/hr beginning 2 hours before the study begins and every hour until it is complete. This ensures adequate urine output. Collect a baseline urine specimen for 60 minutes immediately before administration of teriparatide. Collect urine specimens from 0 to 30 minutes, 30 to 60 minutes, and 60 to 120 minutes. All specimens must be in separate containers and labeled appropriately. Change in urinary cAMP excretion in the 0- to 30-minute period is the most sensitive indicator for separation of hypoparathyroidisms. Measurement of urinary cAMP and phosphate must be corrected for creatinine excretion. (2) Discard any unused reconstituted solution. (3) Use caution in borderline hypercalcemic patients (10.5 mg/dl); a single dose can cause hypercalcemia. (4) Not intended for recurrent or chronic use. (5) Allergic reactions may be caused by peptide content. Have epinephrine available. (6) Safety for use in pregnancy and lactation not established; use only when clearly indicated. (7) Limited data available on children over 3 years of age.

Contraindications: Hypersensitivity to teriparatide or any component of this preparation.

Incompatible with: Specific information not available. Consider specific use.

Side effects: Allergic reactions including anaphylaxis; cramps, diarrhea, hypercalcemia, hypocalcemia, metallic taste, nausea, pain at injection site, tingling of extremities. Hypertensive crisis occurred in one patient with a history of hypertension.

Antidote: Notify physician and manage side effects as indicated by severity. Treat allergic reactions with epinephrine. If hypercalcemia occurs, discontinue drug immediately and ensure adequate hydration. Treat hypocalcemia with calcium if indicated. Resuscitate as necessary.

TETANUS ANTITOXIN

Usual dose: 50,000 to 100,000 units. Give part of the dose IV and the remainder IM. Used only when tetanus immune globulin IM is not available. Testing for sensitivity to horse serum required before use (see Precautions).

Dilution: May be given undiluted.

Rate of administration: To be given very slowly. Titrate carefully to patient reaction.

Actions: A sterile solution of purified antitoxic substances prepared from the blood serum of horses immunized against tetanus toxin. Neutralizes the toxins produced by *Clostridium tetani*.

Indications and uses: Treatment of patients with clinical symptoms of tetanus. Given IM for all other indications.

Precautions: (1) Read drug literature supplied with antitoxin completely before use. Essential to evaluate symptoms and individual status of each patient. (2) Determine patient response to any previous injections of serum of any type and history of any allergic-type reactions. (3) Hospitalize patient if possible. (4) Test every patient for sensitivity to horse serum without exception (1 ml vial of 1:10 dilution horse serum supplied). Conjunctival test and skin test recommended for maximum safety. Always begin with the conjunctival test.

Conjunctival test: Instill 1 drop 1:10 horse serum into conjunctival sac for adults (1 drop 1:100 dilution for children). Itching, redness, burning, and/or lacrimation within 30 minutes is a positive reaction. A drop of normal saline in the opposite eye is used as a control and should be asymptomatic. Reverse adverse effects of positive reaction with 1 drop epinephrine ophthalmic solution.

Scratch test: Make a ¼ inch skin scratch through a drop of 1:100 dilution in normal saline. Make a similar scratch through a drop of normal saline on a comparable skin site as a control. Compare sites in 20 minutes. An urticarial wheal surrounded by a zone of erythema is a positive reaction.

Skin test: Inject 0.02 to 0.1 ml of 1:100 horse serum intradermally. In patients with a history of allergies use a 1:1,000 solution. A like injection of normal saline can be used as a control. An urticarial wheal surrounded by a zone of erythema is a positive reaction. Compare in 20 minutes.

Other testing methods may be used. Use at least two. Concomitant use of antihistamines may interfere with sensitivity tests. (5) Initiate active tetanus immunization with tetanus toxoid concomitantly. (6) Use of a different syringe and a different IM site for tetanus toxoid and tetanus antitoxin is recommended. (7) Store at 2° to 8° C (35° to 46° F).

Contraindications: Hypersensitivity to horse serum unless only treatment available for a life-threatening situation. Several techniques, including preload of antihistamines and/or desensitization, may be considered (see literature).

Incompatible with: Specific information not available. Do not mix with any other drug in syringe or solution because of specific use.

Side effects: Acute anaphylaxis with urticaria, respiratory distress, vascular collapse. Serum sickness may occur. Usually appears in 7 to 12 days. Local pain, local erythema, and urticaria without systemic reaction can occur.

Antidote: Discontinue the drug and notify the physician of all side effects. Treat anaphylaxis immediately. Epinephrine (Adrenalin) and diphenhydramine (Benadryl), oxygen, vasopressors (dopamine), corticosteroids, and ventilation equipment must always be available. Resuscitate as necessary.

TETRACYCLINE HYDROCHLORIDE

pH 2.0 to 3.0

(Achromycin, Achromycin IV)

Usual dose: 250 to 500 mg every 12 hours. Maximum dose in 24 hours is 500 mg every 6 hours. Normal renal function required.

Pediatric dose: *Over 8 years of age:* 12 mg/kg of body weight/24 hr in 2 equal doses. May vary from 10 to 20 mg/kg/24 hr.

Dilution: Each 250 mg or fraction thereof is diluted with 5 ml of sterile water for injection. Must be further diluted with a minimum of 100 ml of 5% dextrose in water or isotonic saline for infusion, or preferably added to larger volumes of standard infusion solutions such as normal saline, dextrose in water or saline, or Ringer's solution.

Rate of administration: Each 100 mg or fraction thereof over a minimum of 5 minutes. Never exceed this rate. Must be completed within 12 hours of dilution.

Actions: A broad-spectrum antibiotic that is bacteriostatic against many gram-positive and gram-negative organisms. Thought to interfere with protein synthesis of microorganisms. Well distributed in most body tissues and often bound to plasma protein, tetracyclines are concentrated in the liver and excreted through the bile to urine and feces in a biologically active state. Crosses the placental barrier. Secreted in breast milk.

Indications and uses: (1) Infections caused by susceptible strains or organisms such as rickettsiae, spirochetal agents, viruses, and many other gram-negative and gram-positive bacteria; (2) to substitute for contraindicated penicillin or sulfonamide therapy; (3) adjunct to amebicides in acute intestinal amebiasis.

Precautions: (1) Initiate oral therapy as soon as possible. (2) Must be stored away from heat and light. (3) Check expiration date; outdated ampoules may cause nephrotoxicity. (4) Stable at room temperature no longer than 12 hours after dilution. (5) Buffered with ascorbic acid. (6) Sensitivity studies necessary to determine susceptibility of the causative organism to tetracycline. (7) Avoid prolonged use of drug. Superinfection caused by overgrowth of nonsusceptible organisms may result. (8) Use caution in impaired liver or renal function. Tetracycline serum concentrations and liver and kidney function tests are indicated. (9) May cause skeletal retardation in the fetus and infants, and permanent tooth discoloration in children under 8 years, including in utero or through mother's milk. Do not use during pregnancy; discontinue breast feeding. (10) Inhibits oral contraceptives; may result in pregnancy or breakthrough bleeding. (11) Monitor blood glucose; may reduce insulin requirements. (12) May alter lithium levels. (13) Inhibits bactericidal action of penicillins (e.g., penicillin G sodium, ampicillin, oxacillin, methicillin). May be toxic with sulfonamides. (14) May potentiate digoxin and anticoagulants. Reduced doses of these drugs may be necessary. (15) Potentiated by alcohol, cimetidine (Tagamet), methoxyflurane (Penthrane), and other hepatotoxic drugs; severe liver damage may result. (16) Inhibited by alkalinizing agents; calcium, iron, and magnesium salts; riboflavin; sodium bicarbonate; and others. (17) Alert patient to photosensitive skin reaction. (18) Determine absolute patency of vein and avoid extravasation; thrombophlebitis is not infrequent. (19) Organisms resisitant to one tetracycline are usually resistant to others. (20) If syphilis is suspected, perform a dark-field examination before initiating tetracyclines.

Contraindications: Children under 8 years of age, known hypersensitivity to tetracyclines, pregnancy, lactation.

Incompatible with: Amikacin (Amikin), aminophylline, amobarbital (Amytal), amphotericin B (Fungizone), calcium salts and solution, carbenicillin (Geopen), cefazolin (Kefzol), cephalothin (Keflin), cephapirin (Cefadyl), chloramphenicol (Chloromycetin), chlorothiazide (Diuril), dimenhydrinate (Dramamine), erythromycin (Ilotycin, Erythrocin), fat emulsion 10% IV, heparin, hyaluronidase (e.g., Wydase), hydrocortisone sodium succinate (Solu-Cortef), methicillin (Staphcillin), methohexital (Brevital), methyldopate (Aldomet), methylprednisolone (Solu-Medrol), metoclopramide (Reglan), oxacillin (Prostaphlin), penicillins, pentobarbital (Nembutal), phenobarbital (Luminal), phenytoin (Dilantin), polymyxin B (Aerosporin), prochlorperazine (Compazine), riboflavin, secobarbital (Seconal), sodium bicarbonate, thiopental (Pentothal), vitamin B complex, warfarin (Coumadin).

Side effects: Relatively nontoxic in average doses. More toxic in large doses or if given too rapidly.

Minor: Anogenital lesions, anorexia, blood dyscrasias, diarrhea, dysphagia, enterocolitis, nausea, skin rashes, vomiting.

Major: Hypersensitivity reactions, including anaphylaxis; blurred vision and headache (benign intracranial hypertension); bulging fontanels in infants; liver damage; photosensitivity; systemic candidiasis; thrombophlebitis.

Antidote: Notify the physician of all side effects. If minor side effects are progressive or any major side effect occurs, discontinue the drug, treat allergic reaction, or resuscitate as necessary.

THEOPHYLLINE AND DEXTROSE pH 4.2 to 4.7

(Theophylline and 5% Dextrose [100% Theophylline])

Usual dose: Initial loading dose of 4.7 mg/kg of lean body weight (theophylline does not distribute into fatty tissue). Follow with a continuous infusion from 0.5 to 0.7 mg/kg/hr for first 12 hours and 0.1 to 0.5 mg/kg/hr thereafter, depending on condition and response. Reduce initial dose and maintenance doses in individuals who are presently taking theophylline medications. Measurement of actual serum concentration is preferred.

Pediatric dose: 4.7 mg/kg of body weight is maximum IV loading dose. Follow with a continuous infusion from 1.0 to 1.2 mg/kg/hr for first 12 hours and 0.8 to 1.0 mg/kg/hr thereafter, depending on age, condition, and response. Reduce initial and maintenance dose as for adults.

Dilution: Available in Viaflex plastic containers as a prediluted solution (200 mg in 50 ml [4 mg/ml] or 100 ml [2 mg/ml]; 400 mg in 100 ml [4 mg/ml], 250 ml [1.6 mg/ml], 500 ml [0.8 mg/ml], or 1 liter [0.4 mg/ml]; 800 mg in 250 ml [3.2 mg/ml], 500 ml [1.6 mg/ml] or 1 liter [0.8 mg/ml]).

Rate of administration: A single dose over a minimum of 20 to 30 minutes. Do not exceed a rate of 20 mg/min. Discontinue primary infusion if theophylline administered by piggyback or additive tubing and a possible incompatibility problem exists. Rapid administration will cause ventricular fibrillation or cardiac arrest.

Actions: An alkaloid xanthine derivative, it relaxes smooth muscle and the bronchial tubes. Cardiac output, urinary output, and sodium excretion are increased. Skeletal and cardiac muscles are stimulated, as is the CNS to a lesser degree. There is peripheral vasodilation. It decreases pulmonary artery pressure and lowers the threshold of the respiratory center to CO_2. Well distributed throughout the body and excreted in a changed form in the urine. Crosses the placental barrier. Secreted in breast milk.

Indications and uses: (1) Bronchial asthma; (2) reversible bronchospasm of chronic bronchitis or emphysema.

Precautions: (1) Verify actual milligrams of theophylline content. Theophylline and dextrose is 100% theophylline; aminophylline (theophylline ethylenediamine) is 79% theophylline. (2) Check solution carefully; must state for IV use; warm to room temperature. Change IV tubing every 24 hours. (3) Monitor serum levels to achieve maximum benefit with minimum risk. Each 0.5 mg/kg will increase serum theophylline by 1 mcg/ml. 10 to 20 mcg/ml is considered therapeutic. Peak serum levels best measured 15 to 20 minutes after initial loading dose. (4) Long-term use in any form has a cumulative effect or may render the drug ineffective. (5) Use with caution in cardiac disease, congestive heart failure, coronary occlusion, cor pulmonale, peptic ulcer disease, renal and hepatic disease, severe hypertension, severe hypoxemia, severe myocardial damage, hyperthyroidism, glaucoma, and in the elderly. (6) Do not use one xanthine derivative concurrently with another xanthine derivative, ephedrine or other sympathomimetic drugs. (7) Use with extreme caution in children. Has caused fatal reactions. (8) Use in pregnancy and during lactation only if clearly indicated. (9) Elimination of drug is prolonged in premature infants, neonates, and children up to 1 year. (10) Xanthines antagonize or potentiate or are themselves antagonized or potentiated by many drug groups. Examples are: inhibited (serum level decreased) by aminoglutenide, barbiturates, β-adrenergic blockers (e.g., propranolol [Inderal]), carbamazipine, hydantoins (e.g., phenytoin [Dilantin]), primidone, rifampin; potentiated (serum level increased) by alcohol, cimetidine (Tagamet), clindamycin (Cleocin), erythromycin, halothane or ketamine anesthesia, quinolone antibiotics (e.g., ciprofloxacin [Cipro]), troleandomycin (TAO); potentiates erythromycin; inhibits nondepolarizing muscle relaxants (e.g., tubocurarine [curare]). Review of patient drug profile by pharmacist imperative. (11) May cause tachycardia with reserpine. (12) Smokers may require higher dose range. (13) Oral therapy may be initiated 4 to 6 hours after the last IV dose or as soon as symptoms are adequately improved. Serum levels may be measured.

Contraindications: Known sensitivity to theophylline, infants under 6 months of age except for apnea and bradycardia of prematurity.

Incompatible with: Ampicillin (Ampicin), cimetidine (Tagamet), clindamycin (Cleocin), hetastarch (Hespan). According to the manufacturer, cefazolin (Kefzol), erythromycin lactobionate, and gentamicin (Garamycin) are compatible in some dilutions. Consult pharmacist.

Side effects: Toxicity resulting in death may occur suddenly, especially with serum levels above 20 mcg/ml. Anxiety, cardiac arrest, convulsions, delirium, dizziness, headache, hyperpyrexia, nausea, peripheral vascular collapse, restlessness, temporary hypotension, ventricular fibrillation, vomiting.

Antidote: With onset of any side effect, discontinue the drug and notify the physician. For mild symptoms the physician may choose to continue the drug at a decreased rate of administration. All side effects will be treated symptomatically. Maintain adequate ventilation and adequate hydration. Grand mal seizures may not respond to anticonvulsants. Diazepam (Valium) may be most effective. Treat atrial dysrhythmias with verapamil, ventricular dysrhythmias with lidocaine or procainamide. Use dopamine (Intropin) for hypotension. Do not use stimulants. Consider charcoal hemoperfusion dialysis for serum levels above 40 mcg/ml. Resuscitate as necessary.

THEOPHYLLINE ETHYLENEDIAMINE

pH 8.6 to 9.0

(Aminophylline [79% Theophylline])

Usual dose: Initial loading dose of 6 mg/kg of lean body weight (theophylline does not distribute into fatty tissue). Follow with a continuous infusion from 0.5 to 0.7 mg/kg/hr for first 12 hours and 0.1 to 0.5 mg/kg/hr thereafter, depending on condition and response. Reduce initial dose and maintenance doses in individuals who are presently taking theophylline medications. Measurement of actual serum concentration is preferred.

Pediatric dose: 6 mg/kg of body weight is maximum IV loading dose. Follow with a continuous infusion from 1.0 to 1.2 mg/kg/hr for first 12 hours and 0.8 to 1.0 mg/kg/hr thereafter, depending on age, condition, and response. Reduce initial and maintenance dose as for adults.

Neonatal dose: *Apnea and bradycardia of prematurity:* 1 mg/kg for each 2 mcg/ml serum theophylline concentration desired. Maintain with *(preterm [less than 40 weeks postconception])* 1 mg/kg lean body weight every 12 hours; *(term [40 weeks postconception] and up to 4 weeks postnatal)* 1 to 2 mg/kg every 12 hours; *(4 to 8 weeks)* 1 to 2 mg/kg every 8 hours; *(over 8 weeks)* 1 to 3 mg/kg every 6 hours.

Dilution: Only the 25 mg/ml solution may be given by direct IV undiluted, or it can be further diluted in at least 100 to 200 ml of 5% dextrose in water and given as an infusion.

Rate of administration: A single dose over a minimum of 20 to 30 minutes. Do not exceed an average rate of 1 ml or 20 mg/min when giving direct IV or as an infusion. Rapid administration will cause ventricular fibrillation or cardiac arrest. Discontinue primary infusion if theophylline administered by piggyback or additive tubing and a possible incompatibility problem exists.

Actions: An alkaloid xanthine derivative, it relaxes smooth muscle and the bronchial tubes. Cardiac output, urinary output, and sodium excretion are increased. Skeletal and cardiac muscles are stimulated, as is the CNS to a lesser degree. There is peripheral vasodilation. It decreases pulmonary artery pressure and lowers the threshold of the respiratory center to CO_2. Well distributed throughout the body and excreted in a changed form in the urine. Crosses the placental barrier. Secreted in breast milk.

Indications and uses: (1) Bronchial asthma; (2) reversible bronchospasm of chronic bronchitis or emphysema.

Investigational use: Apnea and bradycardia of prematurity.

Precautions: (1) Check vial carefully; must state for IV use. Minimum dilution must be 25 mg/ml; warm to room temperature. Verify actual milligrams of theophylline content. (2) Monitor serum levels to achieve maximum benefit with minimum risk. Each 0.6 mg/kg will increase serum theophylline by 1 mcg/ml. 10 to 20 mcg/ml is considered therapeutic. Peak serum level is best measured 15 to 20 minutes after initial loading dose. (3) Long-term use in any form has a cumulative effect or may render the drug ineffective. (4) Use with caution in cardiac disease, congestive heart failure, coronary occlusion, cor pulmonale, peptic ulcer disease, renal and hepatic disease, severe hypertension, severe hypoxemia, severe myocardial damage, hyperthyroidism, glaucoma, and in the elderly. (5) Do not use one xanthine derivative concurrently with another xanthine derivative, ephedrine, or other sympathomimetic drugs. (6) Use with extreme caution in children. Has caused fatal reactions. (7) Use in pregnancy and during lactation only if clearly indicated. (8) Elimination of drug is prolonged in premature infants, neonates, and children up to 1 year. (9) Xanthines antagonize or potentiate or are themselves antagonized or potentiated by many drug groups. Examples are: inhibited (serum level decreased) by β-adrenergic blockers (e.g., propranolol [Inderal]), hydantoins (e.g., phenytoin [Dilantin]); potentiated (serum level increased) by alcohol, cimetidine (Tagamet), clindamycin (Cleocin), halothane or ketamine anesthesia, quinolone antibiotics (e.g., ciprofloxacin [Cipro]), troleandomycin (TAO); potentiates erythromycin; inhibits nondepolarizing muscle relaxants (e.g., tubocurarine [curare]). Review of patient drug profile by pharmacist imperative. (10) May cause tachycardia with reserpine. (11) Crystals will form if solution pH falls below 8.0. (12) Smokers may require higher dose range. (13) Initiate oral therapy as soon as symptoms are adequately improved. Wait 4 to 6 hours after last IV dose or measure serum levels.

Contraindications: Known sensitivity to theophylline or ethylenediamine, infants under 6 months of age except for apnea and bradycardia of prematurity.

Incompatible with: Acid solutions, amikacin (Amikin), ascorbic acid, bleomycin (Blenoxane), cephalothin (Keflin), cephapirin (Cefadyl), chloramphenicol, chlorpromazine (Thorazine), cimetidine (Tagamet), clindamycin (Cleocin), codeine, corticotropin (Acthar), dimenhydrinate (Dramamine), dobutamine (Dobutrex), doxapram (Dopram), doxorubicin (Adriamycin), doxycycline (Vibramycin), epinephrine (Adrenalin), erythromycin (Ilotycin), fructose solution, heparin, hydralazine, hydroxyzine (Vistaril), insulin, invert sugar solutions, isoproterenol (Isuprel), levarterenol (Levophed), levorphanol (Levo-Dromoran), meperidine (Demerol), methadone, methicillin (Staphcillin), methylprednisolone (SoluMedrol), morphine, nafcillin, papaverine, penicillin G sodium and potassium, pentazocine (Talwin), phenobarbital (Luminal), phenytoin (Dilantin), procaine, prochlorperazine (Compazine), promazine (Sparine), promethazine (Phenergan), succinylcholine (Anectine), tetracycline (Achromycin), vancomycin (Vancocin), vitamin B complex, vitamin B with C.

Side effects: Toxicity resulting in death may occur suddenly, especially with serum levels above 20 mcg/ml. Anxiety, cardiac arrest, convulsions, delirium, dizziness, flushing, headache, hyperpyrexia, nausea, peripheral vascular collapse, restlessness, temporary hypotension, ventricular fibrillation, vomiting.

Antidote: With onset of any side effect, discontinue the drug and notify the physician. For mild symptoms the physician may choose to continue the drug at a decreased rate of administration. All side effects will be treated symptomatically. Maintain adequate ventilation and adequate hydration. Grand mal seizures may not respond to anticonvulsants. Diazepam (Valium) may be most effective. Treat atrial dysrhythmias with verapamil, ventricular dysrhythmias with lidocaine or procainamide. Use dopamine (Intropin) for hypotension. Do not use stimulants. Consider charcoal hemoperfusion dialysis for serum levels above 40 mcg/ml. Resuscitate as necessary.

THIAMINE HYDROCHLORIDE pH 2.5 to 4.5

(Betalin S, Vitamin B_1)

Usual dose: Up to 30 mg 3 times daily.

Pediatric dose: 10 to 25 mg/24 hr.

Dilution: May be given by direct IV administration or added to most IV solutions and given as an infusion.

Rate of administration: 100 mg or fraction thereof over 5 minutes.

Actions: A water-soluble vitamin, thiamine is necessary to most metabolic processes in humans, especially carbohydrate metabolism. Many cells require its presence both for growth and maturation and for accomplishing group formations and transfers. Found in all body tissues, stored in the liver, and excreted in urine.

Indications and uses: (1) Wet beriberi with myocardial failure; (2) neuritis and polyneuritis of any etiology; (3) vitamin B_1 deficiency resulting from supply or absorption (e.g. alcoholism).

Precautions: (1) Not commonly administered IV; IM is preferred. (2) Rarely used alone, it is more often administered as a multiple B vitamin. (3) Intradermal test dose recommended in suspected sensitivity. (4) Can be refrigerated; protect from freezing and from light. (5) In thiamine deficiency, administer thiamine before giving any glucose load to prevent the sudden onset of Wernicke's encephalopathy.

Contraindications: Known hypersensitivity to thiamine hydrochloride.

Incompatible with: Amobarbital (Amytal), phenobarbital (Luminal), solutions with neutral or alkaline pH such as carbonates, citrates, barbiturates, acetates, sulfites.

Side effects: Anaphylaxis and death caused by sensitivity reaction can occur with IV administration.

Antidote: Discontinue the drug, treat allergic reaction or resuscitate as necessary, and notify the physician.

THIOPENTAL SODIUM pH 10.0 to 11.0

(Pentothal Sodium)

Usual dose: *Convulsions:* 75 to 125 mg. Up to 250 mg may be required.

Dilution: Each 500 mg ampoule of sterile thiopental powder is diluted with 20 ml of sterile water for injection (supplied) to make a 2.5% solution. Prepared solutions also available. Each 1 ml equals 25 mg. Soluble only in isotonic saline or 5% glucose in water for infusion.

Rate of administration: Each 25 mg or fraction thereof over 1 minute. Titrate slowly to desired effect. Rapid injection rate may cause symptoms of overdose.

Actions: An ultra-short-acting barbiturate and CNS depressant that produces hypnosis and anesthesia without analgesia. Has potent anticonvulsant effects. Onset of action is prompt and lasts about 15 to 30 minutes. Rapidly absorbed by all body tissues. Some is retained in fatty tissue, causing sustained or delayed effect. Excreted in changed form in the urine. Crosses the placental barrier. Secreted in breast milk.

Indications and uses: Control of convulsive states. Administration for any other indication is limited to the anesthesiologist.

Precautions: (1) Usually administered by or under direct observation of a physician. (2) Use only freshly prepared clear solutions. (3) Determine absolute patency of vein. Extravasation will cause necrosis and sloughing; intraarterial injection can cause gangrene. (4) Use only enough medication to achieve desired effect. (5) Record vital signs every 3 to 5 minutes. Keep patient under constant observation. (6) Treat the cause of the convulsion. (7) Maintain a patent airway and have equipment for artificial ventilation available. (8) Reduce dosage and use caution in cardiovascular disease, hypotension, shock, medication potentiation, impaired renal or liver function, Addison's disease, myxedema, elevated blood urea, elevated intracranial pressure, asthma, and myasthenia gravis. (9) May be habit forming. Status epilepticus can occur from too rapid withdrawal. (10) Use with extreme caution if any other CNS depressants have been given, such as alcohol, narcotic analgesics, anesthetics, antidepressants, antihistamines, hypnotics, MAO inhibitors, phenothiazines, sedatives, neuromuscular blocking antibiotics, or tranquilizers. Potentiation with respiratory depression may occur. (11) Inhibits effectiveness of propranolol (Inderal), corticosteroids, doxycycline (Vibramycin), oral anticoagulants, oral contraceptives, quinidine, and theophylline. Capable of innumerable interactions with many drugs. (12) May increase orthostatic hypotension with furosemide (Lasix). (13) Monitor phenytoin and barbiturate levels when both drugs are used concurrently. (14) May cause paradoxical excitement in children or the elderly.

Contraindications: History of porphyria, known hypersensitivity to barbiturates, status asthmaticus, suitable veins not available.

Incompatible with: Acid solutions, amikacin (Amikin), aminophylline, arginine, atracurium (Tracrium), benzquinamide (Emete-Con), calcium salts, cephalothin (Keflin), cephapirin (Cefadyl), cimetidine (Tagamet), clindamycin (Cleocin), chlorpromazine (Thorazine), codeine, dimenhydrinate (Dramamine), diphenhydramine (Benadryl), doxapram (Dopram), droperidol (Inapsine), ephedrine, glycopyrrolate (Robinul), hydromorphone (Dilaudid), insulin (aqueous), levarterenol (Levophed), levorphanol (Levo-Dromoran), magnesium sulfate, meperidine (Demerol), metaraminol (Aramine), methadone, methylprednisolone (Solu-Medrol), morphine, para-aminobenzoic acid (PABA), penicillins, procaine (Novocain), prochlorperazine (Compazine), promazine (Sparine), promethazine (Phenergan), Ringer's solutions, sodium bicarbonate, solutions with more than 5% sugar, succinylcholine (Anectine), tetracycline, tubocurarine (Curare).

Side effects: *Average dose:* Asthma, bronchospasm, depression, dermatitis, facial edema, fever, hypotension, neonatal apnea, respiratory depression (slight), thrombocytopenic purpura.

Overdose: Apnea, cardiac dysrhythmias, coma, cough reflex depression, flat EEG (reversible unless hypoxic damage has occurred), hypotension, hypothermia, laryngospasm, pulmonary edema, renal shutdown, respiratory depression, sluggish or absent reflexes.

Antidote: Call any side effect to the physician's attention. Symptomatic and supportive treatment is most important in overdosage. Keep the patient warm. IV volume expanders (dextran) and IV fluids will help maintain adequate circulation. Diuretics or hemodialysis will promote the elimination of the drug. Vasopressors (e.g., dopamine [Intropin]) will maintain blood pressure. For extravasation, local injection of 1% procaine will relieve pain and promote vasodilation. Local heat application may be helpful.

TICARCILLIN AND CLAVULANATE

pH 5.5 to 7.5

(Timentin)

Usual dose: *Over 60 kg (132 lb):* 3.1 Gm every 4 to 6 hours.

Under 60 kg: 200 to 300 mg/kg of body weight/24 hr in equally divided doses every 4 to 6 hours.

Normal renal function required. Dosages vary depending on the severity of the infection, susceptibility of the organism, and condition of the patient. Treatment usually continued for 10 to 14 days, may be extended if required. Continue for at least 2 days after signs and symptoms of infection have disappeared.

Dilution: Each 3.1 Gm or fraction thereof is diluted with 13 ml of sterile water or normal saline for injection (200 mg/ml). Shake well. A single dose must be further diluted in 50 to 100 ml or more of 5% dextrose in water, 0.9% sodium chloride, or lactated Ringer's injection and given as an intermittent infusion.

Rate of administration: *Intermittent infusion:* A single dose over 30 minutes. May be given through Y-tube or three-way stopcock of infusion set. Discontinue primary IV during administration. Too rapid injection may cause seizures.

Actions: An extended spectrum penicillin. Bactericidal for many gram-negative, gram-positive, and anaerobic organisms. This specific formulation extends activity by protecting ticarcillin from degradation by β-lactamase enzymes. Large doses with high blood levels are well tolerated. Widely absorbed in all body fluids and tissues. Appears in cerebrospinal fluid only if inflammation is present. Crosses the placental barrier. Excreted in the urine. Secreted in breast milk.

Indications and uses: Bacterial septicemia, acute and chronic infections of the respiratory tract, skin and skin structure, bone and joint, endometrium, and urinary tract caused by β-lactamase–producing organisms. Useful in infections complicated by impaired renal functions or in patients receiving immunosuppressive or oncolytic drugs.

Precautions: (1) Stable at room temperature for at least 6 hours or for 72 hours under refrigeration. Stability extended after further dilution (see literature). (2) Specific process sensitivity studies indicated to determine susceptibility of the causative organism to ticarcillin and clavulanate. (3) Oral probenecid will achieve higher and more prolonged blood levels of ticarcillin, will not affect clavulanate levels. May be desirable or may cause toxicity. (4) Reduce total daily dose if renal function impaired. Calculated according to degree of impairment (see literature). (5) Periodic evaluation of renal, hepatic, and hematopoietic systems is recommended in prolonged therapy. (6) Superinfection caused by overgrowth of nonsusceptible organisms can occur. (7) Electrolyte imbalance and cardiac irregularities from sodium content are possible. Contains 4.75 mEq sodium/Gm. Observe for hypokalemia. (8) Slow infusion rate for pain along venipuncture site. (9) Aminoglycosides (e.g., gentamicin, tobramycin) used concurrently in severe infection but must be administered in separate infusions; inactivates aminoglycosides. (10) Use only when clearly indicated in pregnancy. (11) Inactivated by chloramphenicol, erythromycin, and tetracyclines. Bactericidal action is actually negated by these drugs. (12) Concomitant use with β-adrenergic blockers (e.g., propranolol [Inderal]) may increase risk of anaphylaxis and inhibit treatment. (13) Risk of bleeding is increased. Monitoring of coagulation tests may be indicated. Use caution with anticoagulants (e.g., heparin). (14) May inhibit effectiveness of oral contraceptives; breakthrough bleeding or pregnancy could result. (15) Neuromuscular excitability or convulsions may be caused by higher than normal doses. (16) Safety for use in infants and children under 12 not established. (17) May produce pseudoproteinuria. (18) Clavulanic acid may cause a false positive Coombs' test.

Contraindications: Known penicillin or cephalosporin sensitivity.

Incompatible with: All aminoglycosides (e.g., gentamicin [Garamycin], kanamycin [Kantrex], tobramycin [Nebcin]), amikacin (Amikin), colistimethate (Coly-Mycin), sodium bicarbonate.

Side effects: Anaphylaxis; anemia; arthralgia; chest discomfort; chills; convulsions; diarrhea; disturbances of taste and smell; elevated alkaline phosphatase, BUN, LDH, serum bilirubin, SGOT, and SGPT; eosinophilia; fever; flatulence; epigastric pain; headache; hypernatremia; hypokalemia; leukopenia; myalgia; nausea; neutropenia; phlebitis; prolonged clotting time or PT; pruritus; skin rash; stomatitis; thrombocytopenia; urticaria; vomiting.

Antidote: Notify the physician immediately of any adverse symptoms. For severe symptoms, discontinue the drug, treat allergic reaction (epinephrine, antihistamines, corticosteroids), and resuscitate as necessary. Hemodialysis may be indicated in overdose.

TICARCILLIN DISODIUM — pH 6.0 to 8.0

(Ticar)

Usual dose: 150 to 300 mg/kg of body weight/24 hr in divided doses every 3, 4, or 6 hours. All dosages vary depending on the severity of the infection. Maximum dose is 24 Gm/24 hr.

Pediatric dose: *Under 40 kg (88 lb):* 50 to 300 mg/kg of body weight/24 hr in divided doses every 4, 6, or 8 hours. Do not exceed adult dose.

Neonatal dose: *Under 2,000 Gm; age up to 7 days:* 75 mg/kg of body weight every 12 hours. *Over 7 days of age:* 75 mg/kg every 8 hours.

Over 2,000 Gm; age up to 7 days: 75 mg/kg every 8 hours. *Over 7 days of age:* 100 mg/kg every 8 hours.

Dilution: Each 1 Gm or fraction thereof is diluted with 4 ml of sterile water for injection. Further dilution of each gram with an additional 10 to 20 ml or more of sterile water for injection, 5% dextrose, or normal saline is required for direct IV administration or intermittent piggyback infusion. May be added to larger volumes or standard IV fluids and given as a continuous infusion.

Rate of administration: Too rapid injection may cause seizures.

Direct IV: 1 Gm or fraction thereof over 5 minutes or more to reduce vein irritation.

Intermittent infusion: A single dose over 30 minutes to 2 hours. In neonate give over 10 to 20 minutes.

Continuous infusion: At specified rate not to exceed rate and concentration of intermittent infusion.

Actions: An extended spectrum penicillin. Bactericidal for many gram-negative, gram-positive, and anaerobic organisms. Large doses with high blood levels are well tolerated. Appears in cerebrospinal fluid only if inflammation is present. Crosses the placental barrier. Excreted in the urine. Secreted in breast milk.

Indications and uses: Bacterial septicemia, acute and chronic infections of the respiratory tract, skin and soft tissue, intraabdominal area, female pelvis, genital tract, and urinary tract. Useful in infections complicated by impaired renal functions or in patients receiving immunosuppressive or oncolytic drugs.

Precautions: (1) Stable at room temperature for at least 48 hours. (2) Sensitivity studies indicated to determine susceptibility of the causative organism to ticarcillin. (3) Oral probenecid will achieve higher and more prolonged blood levels. May be desirable or may cause toxicity. (4) Reduce daily dose commensurate with amount of renal impairment. Intervals between injections should also be increased. (5) Periodic evaluation of renal, hepatic, and hematopoietic systems is recommended in prolonged therapy. (6) Superinfection caused by overgrowth of nonsusceptible organisms can occur. (7) Electrolyte imbalance and cardiac irregularities from high sodium content are possible. (8) Slow infusion rate for pain along venipuncture site. (9) Gentamicin and tobramycin used concurrently in severe infection but must be administered in separate infusions; inactivate aminoglycosides. (10) Use caution in pregnancy. (11) Inactivated by chloramphenicol, erythromycin, and tetracyclines. Bactericidal action is actually negated by these drugs. (12) Concomitant use with β-adrenergic blockers (e.g., propranolol [Inderal]) may increase risk of anaphylaxis and inhibit treatment. (13) Risk of bleeding with anticoagulants (e.g., heparin) is increased. (14) May inhibit effectiveness of oral contraceptives; breakthrough bleeding or pregnancy could result. (15) Neuromuscular excitability or convulsions may be caused by higher than normal doses. (16) Elimination rate markedly reduced in neonates.

Contraindications: Known penicillin or cephalosporin sensitivity.

Incompatible with: All aminoglycosides (e.g., Amikacin [Amikin], gentamicin [Garamycin], kanamycin [Kantrex], netilmicin [Neutromycin], tobramycin [Nebcin]) colistimethate (Coly-Mycin).

Side effects: Abnormal clotting time or PT, anaphylaxis, anemia, convulsions, elevated SGOT and SGPT, eosinophilia, fever, leukopenia, nausea, neutropenia, phlebitis, pruritus, skin rash, thrombocytopenia, urticaria, vomiting.

Antidote: Notify the physician immediately of any adverse symptoms. For severe symptoms, discontinue the drug, treat allergic reaction (epinephrine, antihistamines, corticosteroids), and resuscitate as necessary. Hemodialysis is effective in overdose.

TOBRAMYCIN SULFATE pH 6.0 to 8.0

(Nebcin)

Usual dose: 3 mg/kg of body weight/24 hr equally divided into 3 or 4 doses. Up to 5 mg/kg may be given if indicated. Reduce to usual dose as soon as feasible. Normal renal function necessary. Dosage based on lean body weight plus 40% for obese patients.

Pediatric dose: 6 to 7.5 mg/kg of body weight/24 hr in 3 or 4 equally divided doses every 6 or 8 hours.

Newborn dose: *1 week of age or less:* 4 mg/kg of body weight/24 hr in 2 equal doses every 12 hours. Lower doses may be safer because of immature kidney function. 2.5 mg/kg every 18 hours or 3 mg/kg every 24 hours may provide acceptable peak and trough levels in neonates weighing less than 2,000 Gm.

Dilution: Prepared solutions equal 10 or 40 mg/ml. Further dilute each single dose in 50 to 100 ml of IV normal saline or 5% dextrose in water and administer through an additive tubing. Reduce volume of diluent proportionately for children.

Rate of administration: Each single dose, properly diluted, over a minimum of 20 and a maximum of 60 minutes.

Actions: An aminoglycoside antibiotic with potential neuromuscular blocking action. Inhibits protein synthesis in bacterial cells. Bactercidal against specific gram-negative and gram-positive bacilli, including *Escherichia coli, Klebsiella, Proteus,* and *Pseudomonas.* Well distributed through all body fluids. Usual half-life is 2 to 2.5 hours. Half-life is prolonged in infants, postpartum females, fever, liver disease and ascites, spinal cord injury, cystic fibrosis, and the elderly; shorter in severe burns. Crosses the placental barrier. Excreted in the kidneys.

Indications and uses: (1) Short-term treatment of serious infections caused by susceptible organisms, (e.g., septicemia, meningitis, peritonitis); (2) primarily used when penicillin and other less toxic antibiotics ineffective or contraindicated; (3) concurrent therapy with a penicillin or cephalosporin sometimes indicated.

Precautions: (1) Use extreme caution if therapy is required over 7 to 10 days. (2) Sensitivity studies necessary to determine susceptibility of causative organism to tobramycin. (3) Reduce daily dose commensurate with amount of renal impairment. Intervals between injections should also be increased. (4) Watch for decrease in urine output, rising BUN and serum creatinine, and declining creatinine clearance levels. Dosage may require decreasing. Routine evaluation of hearing is recommended. (5) Narrow range between toxic and therapeutic levels. Monitor peak and trough concentrations to avoid peak serum concentrations above 12 mcg/ml and trough concentrations above 2 mcg/ml. Therapeutic levels are between 4 and 8 mcg/ml. (6) Use caution in infants, children, and the elderly. (7) Potentiated by anesthetics, other neuromuscular blocking antibiotics (e.g., kanamycin, streptomycin), anticholinesterases (e.g., edrophonioum [Tensilon]), antineoplastics (e.g., nitrogen mustard, cisplatin), barbiturates, cephalosporins, muscle relaxants (e.g., tubocurarine), phenothiazines (e.g., promethazine [Phenergan]), procainamide, quinidine, and sodium citrate (citrate-anticoagulated blood). *Apnea can occur.* (8) Ototoxicity may be potentiated by loop diuretics (e.g., ethacrynic acid [Edecrin], furosemide [Lasix]). An elevated serum level of tobramycin may occur, increasing nephrotoxicity and neurotoxicity. (9) Inactivated in solution with carbenicillin and other penicillins. Synergistic when used in combination with penicillins and cephalosporins. Dose adjustment and appropriate spacing required because of physical incompatibilities and interactions. (10) Superinfection may occur from overgrowth of nonsusceptible organisms. (11) Maintain good hydration. (12) Use during pregnancy and lactation only when absolutely necessary.

Contraindications: Known tobramycin or aminoglycoside sensitivity.

Incompatible with: Cefamandole (Mandol), clindamycin (Cleocin), heparin. Any other drug in syringe or solution. Administer separately. Note precautions.

Side effects: Occur more frequently with impaired renal function, higher doses, or prolonged administration.

Minor: Dizziness; fever; headache; increased SGOT, SGPT, and serum bilirubin; itching; lethargy; rash; roaring in the ears; urticaria; vomiting.

Major: Apnea; blood dyscrasias; cylindruria; elevated BUN, nonprotein nitrogen, and creatinine; hearing loss; neuromuscular blockade; oliguria; proteinuria; seizures (large doses); tinnitus; vertigo.

Antidote: Notify the physician of all side effects. If minor side effects persist or any major symptom appears, discontinue the drug and notify the physician. Treatment is symptomatic or a reduction in dose may be required. In overdose, hemodialysis may be indicated. Complexation with ticarcillin or carbenicillin may be as effective as hemodialysis. Consider exchange transfusion in the newborn. Calcium salts or neostigmine may reverse neuromuscular blockade. Resuscitate as necessary.

TOLAZOLINE HYDROCHLORIDE pH 3.0 to 4.0

(Priscoline)

Neonatal dose: 1 to 2 mg/kg of body weight via scalp vein as an initial dose. Follow with an infusion of 1 to 2 mg/kg/hr. Usually discontinued within 48 hours.

Dilution: May be given undiluted. May be further diluted to be given as an infusion. Compatible with many commonly used solutions (e.g., Dextran 6% in dextrose or saline, dextrose in water or saline, fructose in water or saline, invert sugar in water or saline, Ionosol products, lactated Ringer's injection, normal or half-normal saline, Protein hydrolysate 5%, Ringer's injection, sodium lactate ⅙ molar). Amount of diluent based on total dose and fluid needs of infant. May be given through Y-tube or three-way stopcock of infusion set.

Rate of administration: Each 10 mg or fraction thereof over 1 minute directly into scalp vein. Rate of infusion should deliver desired dose over each hour.

Actions: An adrenergic blocking agent. Decreases peripheral resistance and increases venous capacitance. Usually reduces pulmonary arterial pressure and vascular resistance. Onset of action is within 30 minutes; half-life in neonates is from 3 to 10 hours. Excreted in the urine.

Indications and uses: Treatment of persistent pulmonary hypertension of the newborn (systemic arterial oxygenation cannot be adequately sustained by usual supportive care of oxygen and mechanical ventilation).

Precautions: (1) For use only in a highly supervised setting such as an intensive care nursery. Vital signs, oxygenation, acid-base status, and fluid and electrolyte balance must be monitored and maintained. (2) Stimulates gastric secretion and may activate stress ulcers. Pretreat infants with antacids to prevent GI bleeding. (3) Observe for signs of systemic hypotension. Treat promptly. (4) Use with caution in patients with known or suspected mitral stenosis. Priscoline may produce a rise or fall in pulmonary artery pressure and total pulmonary resistance. (5) Effectiveness may be pH dependent. Acidosis may decrease effectiveness. (6) Use caution with epinephrine; severe hypotension with exaggerated rebound will occur.

Contraindications: Hypersensitivity to tolazoline.

Incompatible with: Ethacrynic acid (Edecrin), hydrocortisone sodium succinate (Solu-Cortef), methylprednisolone sodium succinate (Solu-Medrol).

Side effects: *Average dose:* Cardiac dysrhythmias, diarrhea, edema, flushing, GI hemorrhage, hematuria, hepatitis, hypertension, hypotension, increased pilomotor activity with tingling or chilliness, leukopenia, nausea, oliguria, pulmonary hemorrhage, rash, tachycardia, thrombocytopenia, tingling, vomiting.

Overdose: Hypotension and shock in addition to flushing, increased pilomotor activity, and peripheral vasodilation.

Antidote: Notify the physician of all side effects. If minor symptoms progress or major side effects appear, discontinue the drug immediately and notify the physician. Treat hypotension with IV fluids, a head-low position, and ephedrine if necessary. Epinephrine and levarterenol (Levophed) are contraindicated for hypotension. Further hypotension will occur. Treat all other side effects symptomatically and resuscitate as necessary.

TOLBUTAMIDE SODIUM pH 8.0 to 9.8

(Orinase Diagnostic)

Usual dose: 1 Gm. Specific procedure required (see Precautions and manufacturer's literature).

Dilution: Diluent provided, 20 ml for 1 Gm. Prepare immediately before use.

Rate of administration: A single dose equally distributed over 2 to 3 minutes.

Actions: Will cause a rapid fall in blood sugar for 30 to 45 minutes followed by a return to normal limits in 90 to 180 minutes in normal individuals. Results in patients with functioning insulinomas or pancreatic islet cell adenomas are distinctively different.

Indications and uses: Adjunct in the diagnosis of (1) islet cell adenoma to prevent surgical intervention when it is not indicated; (2) insulinomas.

Precautions: (1) Results vary with laboratory methods. Use only a true glucose procedure (Somogyi-Nelson, Modified Folin-Wu, AutoAnalyzer, or glucose oxidase). (2) A high-carbohydrate diet (150 to 300 Gm/day) must be eaten for 3 days before the test. (3) To test for islet cell adenoma, draw a fasting blood glucose the morning of the test, administer tolbutamide, draw venous blood glucose samples 20, 30, 45, 60, 90, 120, 150, and 180 minutes after midpoint of tolbutamide administration. (4) To test for insulinomas, draw venous blood samples for serum insulin levels before and 10, 20, and 30 minutes after midpoint of tolbutamide administration. (5) Terminate the test with breakfast, oral glucose, or 50% glucose IV (followed by 10% dextrose in water as an infusion) depending on patient condition. Nondiabetics and individuals with atherosclerosis may develop a severe hypoglycemic reaction. If this occurs, terminate test after the 30-minute blood sample or sooner if indicated. (6) Physician will refer to manufacturer's literature for interpretation of results. (7) False positive results can occur in patients with liver disease, alcohol hypoglycemia, idiopathic hypoglycemia of infancy, severe undernutrition, azotemia, sarcoma, or other extrapancreatic insulin-producing tumors. (8) May cause severe and prolonged hypoglycemia with impaired renal or hepatic function. (9) Not recommended for use during pregnancy; teratogenic in rats and prolonged severe hypoglycemia has occurred in newborns of mothers taking sulfonylureas. Discontinue breast feeding. (10) Potentiated by β-adrenergic blocking agents (e.g., propranolol [Inderal]), chloramphenicol, dicumarol, MAO inhibitors, phenylbutazone, probenecid, salicylates, and sulfonamides. Hypoglycemia may be severe and test results will not be accurate. (11) Must be completely dissolved and solution must be clear. Use within 1 hour of reconstitution.

Contraindications: Children, hypersensitivity to tolbutamide or related sulfonylureas.

Incompatible with: Specific information not available. Consider specific use.

Side effects: Allergic reactions including anaphylaxis, burning sensation at injection site (too rapid injection), thrombophlebitis. Hypoglycemia, mild (fatigue, hunger, nausea, nervousness, sweating, trembling, weakness) or severe (confusion, coma, lethargy, loss of consciousness, stupor), will occur.

Antidote: Notify physician and manage side effects as indicated by severity. Treat mild hypoglycemia with oral glucose. For severe hypoglycemia with loss of consciousness, treat with 50% glucose IV and hospitalize. Follow with 10% dextrose in water as an IV infusion and maintain blood glucose above 100 mg/dl. Monitor for at least 48 hours; hypoglycemia may recur. Treat allergic reactions and resuscitate as necessary.

TRACE METALS

(M.T.E.-4, 5, 6, & 7, M.T.E.-4, 5, & 6 Concentrated, Chromium, Conte-Pak-4, Copper, Iodine, Manganese, Molybdenum, Multi-Pak-4, Multiple Trace Element, Multiple Trace Element Concentrated, Selenium, T.E.C., Trace-4, Trace Metals Additive in 0.9% NaCl, Zinc.) Neotrace-4, Ped-Pak-4, Pedtrace-4, Pediatric Multiple Trace Element, P.T.E.-4 & 5, Tracelyte, Tracelyte with Double Electrolytes, Tracelyte II, Tracelyte II with Double Electrolytes.

Usual dose: *Available as single elements, selected combined elements in various strengths, and in combination with electrolytes.* Selection of correct product based on minimum daily requirement and individual needs.

Zinc: 2.5 to 4 mg/day; add 2 mg in acute catabolic states. Increase to 12.2 mg/L of total parenteral nutrition (TPN) if there is fluid loss from the small bowel.

Copper: 0.5 to 1.5 mg/day.

Manganese: 0.15 to 0.8 mg/day.

Molybdenum: 20 to 120 mcg/day. Increase to 163 mcg/day for 21 days in deficiency states resulting from prolonged TPN.

Chromium: 10 to 15 mcg/day. Increase to 20 mcg/day with intestinal fluid loss.

Selenium: 20 to 50 mcg/day. Increase to 100 mcg/day for 31 days in deficiency states resulting from prolonged TPN.

Iodine: 1 to 2 mcg/kg of body weight/day. Increase to 2 to 3 mcg/kg/day in growing children, pregnant and lactating women.

Pediatric dose: *Zinc:* 100 mcg/kg/day for full-term infants and children up to 5 years of age. 300 mcg/kg/day for premature infants with birth weights from 1,500 Gm to 3 kg.

Copper: 20 mcg/kg/day.

Manganese: 2 to 10 mcg/kg/day.

Molybdenum: Dosage must be calculated by extrapolation; consult pharmacist.
Chromium: 0.14 to 0.2 mcg/kg/day.
Selenium: 3 mcg/kg/day.

Dilution: Must be added to daily volume of IV infusion fluids including TPN.

Rate of administration: Administer properly diluted at rate prescribed for IV infusion fluids or TPN.

Actions: All are basic elements present in the human body. Specific amounts required to initiate, facilitate, or maintain appropriate body systems.

Indications and uses: Nutritional supplement to IV solutions given for total parenteral or central nutrition.

Precautions: (1) Monitor serum trace metal concentration to avoid accumulation. Results will also determine use of a single element or a combined product. (2) Reduce or omit dose in impaired renal function or GI malfunction. (3) Use in pregnancy only if clearly indicated. (4) Selenium enhances vitamin E and decreases the toxicity of mercury, cadmium, and arsenic. (5) Use manganese with caution in the nursing mother.

Contraindications: Do not give direct IV; hypersensitivity to any component. Manganese contraindicated in presence of high manganese levels. Molybdenum without copper supplementation contraindicated in copper-deficient patients.

Incompatible with: None when used as directed.

Side effects: Toxicity is rare at recommended doses. Iodine may cause anaphylaxis.

Antidote: Dosage will be adjusted based on serum levels. Keep physician informed. Resuscitate as necessary.

TRANEXAMIC ACID pH 6.5 to 7.5

(✤ Cyclokapron, Cyklokapron)

Usual dose: *Dental extraction in patients with hemophilia:* 10 mg/kg of body weight immediately before surgery. Follow with 25 mg/kg orally after surgery and for 2 to 8 days. 10 mg/kg IV may be given 3 to 4 times daily the day before surgery, followed by the above regimen. In patients unable to take oral medicine, use 10 mg/kg IV 3 to 4 times daily for 2 to 8 days. Normal renal function required.

Dilution: 100 mg equals 1 ml of prepared solution. Further dilute a single dose with at least 50 ml compatible infusion solutions (e.g., normal saline, dextrose in saline or distilled water, Ringer's solution, amino acids, dextran). Heparin may be added to solution if indicated.

Rate of administration: 100 mg or fraction thereof over at least 1 minute. Too rapid infusion may cause hypotension.

Actions: A synthetic amino acid with the specific action of inhibiting plasminogen activator substances; to a lesser degree inhibits plasmin activity. Increases fibrinogen activity in clot formation by inhibiting the enzyme required for destruction of formed fibrin. More potent than aminocaproic acid. Onset of action is prompt. Half-life approximately 2 hours. Readily excreted in the urine. Crosses the placental barrier. Secreted in breast milk.

Indications and uses: Reduce or prevent hemorrhage and reduce the need for replacement therapy in hemophilia patients during and following tooth extraction.

Precautions: (1) For short-term use only (2 to 8 days). (2) Prepare solution immediately before use; discard any unused solution. (3) Reduce dose in impaired renal function; specific calculation required (see literature). (4) In repeated treatment or if treatment will last more than several (2 to 3) days, a complete ophthalmological examination (visual acuity, color vision, eyeground, visual fields) should be done before and at regular intervals during treatment. Discontinue use if changes are found. (5) Use extreme caution; retinal changes, leukemia, hyperplasia of the biliary tract, cholangioma, and adenocarcinoma of the intrahepatic biliary system have been found in laboratory animal studies. (6) Use caution and only if clearly needed in pregnancy and lactation. (7) Use only in conjunction with general and specific tests to determine the amount of fibrinolysis present. (8) Rapid administration in any form may cause hypotension. (9) Whole blood transfusions may be given if necessary but must be given through a second infusion site.

Contraindications: Acquired defective color vision, subarachnoid hemorrhage.

Incompatible with: Blood, penicillins.

Side effects: Diarrhea, giddiness, hypotension, nausea and vomiting.

Antidote: All side effects may subside with reduced dosage or rate of administration. Discontinue use of drug if any changes are found during follow-up ophthalmological examinations. Resuscitate as necessary.

TRIETHYLENETHIOPHOSPHORAMIDE pH 7.6

(Tespa, Thiotepa, TSPA)

Usual dose: 0.3 to 0.4 mg/kg of body weight as initial dose. Maintenance dose and frequency adjusted according to blood cell counts before and after treatment. Usually given at 1-to 4-week intervals. Dosage based on average weight in presence of ascites or edema.

Dilution: *Specific techniques required, see Precautions.* Each 15 mg of drug is diluted with 1.5 ml of sterile water for injection. Shake solution gently and allow to stand until clear. May be given through Y-tube or three-way stopcock of a free-flowing IV infusion. May be added to selected IV solutions (see literature).

Rate of administration: 60 mg or fraction thereof over 1 minute direct IV.

Actions: An alkylating agent of the nitrogen mustard group with antitumor activity. Cell cycle phase nonspecific. Thought to have a radiomimetic action, which releases ethylenimine radicals to destroy actively dividing cells. Well absorbed and distributed, it is excreted unchanged in the urine.

Indications and uses: To suppress or retard neoplastic growth. Used infrequently, but good response has been experienced in Hodgkin's disease, non-Hodgkin's lymphomas, retinoblastoma, and adenocarcinomas of the breast and ovary.

Investigational use: Prevention of pterygium recurrences following surgery.

Precautions: (1) Follow guidelines for handling cytotoxic agents. See Appendix, p. 677. (2) Administered by or under the direction of the physician specialist. (3) Must be refrigerated before and after dilution. Potency maintained for 5 days after dilution. (4) Do not use if a precipitate is present. (5) Daily blood cell counts are necessary during initial treatment and weekly thereafter until 3 weeks after therapy is discontinued. Very toxic to hematopoietic system. (6) Use caution in leukopenia, thrombocytopenia, recent radiation therapy, and infection. (7) May cause irreversible bone marrow damage with other neoplastic drugs or any drugs that cause bone marrow depression. Allow complete recovery verified by white blood cell count before using a second agent. (8) Will produce teratogenic effects on the fetus. Has a mutagenic potential and must be given with caution to men and women capable of conception. (9) Potentiates anticoagulants (e.g., heparin) and nondepolarizing muscle relaxants (e.g., pancuronium [Pavulon], tubocurarine [Curare]). (10) Be alert for signs of bone marrow depression or infection. (11) Do not administer any vaccines or chloroquine to patients receiving antineoplastic drugs. (12) Local anesthetic at injection site may reduce pain during administration. (13) Used in combination with urokinase to treat bladder cancer. (14) Allopurinol may prevent formation of uric acid crystals. (15) Prophylactic antiemetics may increase patient comfort. (16) Has been given directly into tumor mass in different doses. Toxicity still occurs from systemic absorption.

Contraindications: Hepatic, renal, or bone marrow damage unless need is greater than the risk; known hypersensitivity to triethylenethiophosphoramide.

Incompatible with: Sufficient information not available. Consider incompatible in syringe or solution with any other drug.

Side effects: *Minor:* Amenorrhea, anorexia, dizziness, fever, headache, hives, hyperuricemia, nausea, pain at injection site, skin rash, throat tightness, vomiting.

Major: Anaphylaxis, bone marrow depression, hemorrhage, intestinal perforation, leukopenia, septicemia, thrombocytopenia.

Antidote: Minor side effects will be treated symptomatically if necessary. Discontinue the drug and notify the physician of major side effects. If platelet count below 150,000/mm^3 or white blood cells below 3,000/mm^3, discontinue use and notify physician. Administration of whole blood, platelets, or leukocytes may be required. Treat allergic reaction as indicated.

TRIMETHAPHAN CAMSYLATE — pH 4.9 to 5.6

(Arfonad)

Usual dose: 1 to 4 mg/min. Up to 6 mg/min has been used.

Pediatric dose: 50 to 150 mcg/kg of body weight/min.

Dilution: Each 500 mg (10 ml) or fraction thereof must be diluted in at least 500 ml of 5% dextrose in water and given as an IV infusion. 1 mg equals 1 ml.

Rate of administration: Correct dose/min of properly diluted solution as indicated to maintain blood pressure at the desired level. Use of an infusion pump or microdrip (60 gtt/ml) is indicated.

Actions: A ganglionic blocking agent and a potent vasodilator. Does not alter membrane potential. Liberates histamine. Will lower blood pressure in normotensive as well as hypertensive individuals. It has an extremely short duration of action. Blood pressure may return to normal within 5 to 10 minutes after trimethaphan is discontinued. Excreted by the kidneys.

Indications and uses: (1) Induce and maintain controlled hypotensive state in neurosurgery and vascular surgery; (2) hypertensive crises; (3) pulmonary edema secondary to hypertension; (4) cardiogenic shock; (5) dissecting aortic aneurysm.

Precautions: (1) Most often administered by or under the direction of the anesthesiologist. (2) Must be refrigerated. Prepare solution just prior to use, and discard any remaining portion after 24 hours. (3) Keep patient in supine or reverse Trendelenburg position to prevent cerebral anoxia. (4) Check blood pressure every 2 minutes until stabilized at desired level. Check every 5 minutes thereafter until the drug is discontinued. (5) Adequate oxygenation and ventilation must be maintained continuously. Use artificial means if necessary. (6) Use extreme caution in Addison's disease, allergic individuals, arteriosclerosis, cardiac disease, children, debilitated individuals, degenerative CNS disease, diabetes, hepatic or renal disease, the elderly, in the immediate postoperative period, and in patients taking steroids. (7) Potentiated by antihypertensives, anesthetics (local or regional), alcohol, and thiazide diuretics. Reduced dosage of both drugs may be required to prevent additive hypotensive effect. (8) Potentiates succinylcholine (Anectine) and nondepolarizing muscle relaxants (e.g., tubocurarine [Curare]); prolonged *apnea may result.* (9) Pupillary dilation may occur with trimethaphan; other observations must be used to evaluate anoxia or depth of anesthesia.

Contraindications: Anemia, blood replacement not practical, coronary or cerebrovascular insufficiency, hypovolemia, IV fluids not immediately available, MAO inhibitors in drug regimen within previous 3 weeks, pregnancy, respiratory insufficiency, shock.

Incompatible with: Any other drug in syringe, solution, or infusion tubing. Alkaline solutions, bromides, iodides, gallamine triethiodide (Flaxedil), thiopental (Pentothal), tubocurarine (Curare).

Side effects: Blurring of vision, cerebral ischemia, dryness of mouth, ileus, lowering of central venous pressure, postural hypotension, respiratory depression or arrest, severe hypotension, tachycardia, urinary retention.

Antidote: Notify the physician of all side effects and discontinue the drug if indicated. Reduced central venous pressure may be a desirable effect, as in left ventricular failure. Vasopressors (e.g., phenylephrine [NeoSynephrine]) may be used to treat overdose. If ineffective, use dopamine (Intropin). Resuscitate as necessary.

TRIMETHOPRIM-SULFAMETHOXAZOLE pH 10.0

(Bactrim, Co-Trimoxazole, Septra, Sulfamethoprim, TMP-SMZ)

Usual dose: *Severe urinary tract infections and shigellosis:* 8 to 10 mg/kg of body weight in equally divided doses every 6, 8, or 12 hours for 14 days (urinary tract infections) or 5 days (shigellosis).

Pneumocystis carinii pneumonitis: 15 to 20 mg/kg in equally divided doses every 6 or 8 hours for up to 14 days.

Prophylaxis in neutropenic patients: 800 mg sulfamethoxazole with 160 mg trimethoprim (10 ml before appropriate dilution) every 12 hours.

Normal renal function required for usual dose.

Dilution: Each 5 ml ampoule must be diluted in 125 ml 5% dextrose in water and given as an infusion. Reduce diluent to 75 ml for each ampoule only if fluid restriction required. Standard dilution must be used within 6 hours; fluid restriction dilution must be used within 2 hours. Discard if cloudiness or crystallization is present.

Rate of administration: A single dose must be infused over 60 to 90 minutes. When administered by an infusion device, thoroughly flush all lines used to remove any residual trimethoprim-sulfamethoxazole.

Actions: A broad-spectrum antibacterial and antiprotozoal combination agent with bacteriostatic action effective against gram-positive and gram-negative organisms. Prevents formation of folic acid and reduction of folates essential to organism growth. Combination contains 400 mg sulfamethoxazole and 80 mg trimethoprim per each 5 ml. Effective ratio of sulfamethoxazole to trimethoprim is 20 to 1. Widely distributed in all body fluids and tissues, including cerebrospinal fluid, sputum, and bile. Crosses placental barrier. Onset of action is prompt and serum levels are maintained up to 10 hours. Metabolized in the liver and up to 60% is excreted in urine in 24 hours. Secreted in breast milk.

Indications and uses: (1) Severe urinary tract infections; (2) *Pneumocystis carinii* pneumonitis; (3) shigellosis; (4) prophylaxis in neutropenic patients.

Investigational use: Treatment of cholera and *Salmonella*-type infections.

Precautions: (1) Avoid rapid infusion or bolus injection. (2) Sensitivity studies indicated to determine susceptibility of the causative organism to trimethoprim-sulfamethoxazole. (3) Stable at room temperature; do not refrigerate. (4) Maintain adequate hydration to prevent crystalluria and stone formation. (5) CBC required before and during therapy. Discontinue for any significant reduction in a blood-forming element. Urinalysis and renal function tests also indicated. (6) Reduce dose by one-half for creatinine clearance between 15 and 30 ml/min. (7) If extravasation occurs, discontinue and restart at a new site. May cause phlebitis. (8) Not for IM use. (9) Use caution in impaired liver or renal function, possible folate deficiency, allergic individuals, bronchial asthma, porphyria, and glucose 6-phosphate dehydrogenase (G-6PD) deficiency, and in the elderly. (10) A sulfonamide drug, allergic reactions can occur. Use caution in patients hypersensitive to furosemide (Lasix), thiazide diuretics (e.g., chlorothiazide), sulfonylureas (e.g., tolbutamide), or carbonic anhydrase inhibitors (e.g., acetazolamide). (11) Potentiated by probenecid; sulfinpyrazone toxicity may result. (12) Will inhibit bactericidal action of penicillins and renal excretion of methotrexate. (13) Concurrent use with methenamines (e.g., Urised) may increase incidence of crystalluria and is not recommended. (14) Inhibits cyclosporine (Sandimmune) and increases nephrotoxicity. (15) May potentiate warfarin (Coumadin), phenytoin (Dilantin), oral hypoglycemics, and phenylbutazone (Butazolidin). (16) Inhibited by aminobenzoic acid

(PABA), alkalinizing agents, and thiopental (Pentothal). (17) Incidence of side effects markedly increased in AIDS patients. May not tolerate or respond to this drug.

Contraindications: Infants less than 2 months of age (may cause kernicterus), creatinine clearance below 15 ml/min, hypersensitivity to trimethoprim or sulfonamides, megaloblastic anemia resulting from folate deficiency, pregnancy and lactation, streptococcal pharyngitis.

Incompatible with: Do not mix in syringe or solution with any other drug (manufacturer's directive).

Side effects: All side effects of sulfonamides including allergic reaction are possible. Nausea, vomiting, and rash occur most frequently. Ataxia, convulsions, tremors, and respiratory depression are symptoms of major toxicity. With high doses or administration over an extended period of time, bone marrow depression (leukopenia, megaloblastic anemia, thrombocytopenia) may occur.

Antidote: Notify the physician of any side effect. Discontinue the drug at any sign of major toxicity or bone marrow depression. Treat bone marrow depression with leucovorin 3 to 6 mg IM daily for 3 days or until normal hematopoiesis occurs. Peritoneal dialysis is not effective in toxicity; hemodialysis may be moderately effective in reducing serum levels. Acidification of urine may increase excretion. Treat anaphylaxis with epinephrine, corticosteroids, antihistamines, and vasopressors as indicated.

TROMETHAMINE

pH 10.0 to 11.5

(Tham, Tham-E)

Usual dose: Limit dose to amount needed to increase blood pH to normal limits (7.35 to 7.45) and to correct acid-base derangements. Tham-E contains electrolytes.

Acidosis: Required dose (ml of 0.3 molar solution) = to body weight in kilograms × base deficit in mEq/L × 1.1.

Acidosis in cardiac bypass surgery: 9 ml/kg of body weight. 500 ml is an average adult dose. Up to 1,000 ml has been used.

Acidity of ACD priming blood: Average of 60 ml to each 500 ml of stored blood adequate. Varies from 15 to 77 ml to correct pH of 6.80 to 6.22.

Acidosis in cardiac arrest: Use only if indicated. Initial dose of 3.5 to 6.0 ml/kg. Additional doses should be based on evaluation of base deficit. If the chest is not open, use a large peripheral vein. Do not inject into cardiac muscle.

Dilution: May be given undiluted as an infusion or added to pump oxygenator blood, other priming fluid, or ACD blood.

Rate of administration: Slow IV infusion recommended. 5 ml or less/min would deliver up to 300 ml in 1 hour. Rate dictated by patient's condition and intended use (see Precautions).

Actions: Acts as a proton acceptor and actively binds hydrogen ions in metabolic acids and carbonic acid. Releases bicarbonate anions. Rapidly excreted in the urine, it has an osmotic diuretic effect, increases urine output, urine pH, and excretion of fixed acids, CO_2, and electrolytes. Also capable of neutralizing acidic ions of the intracellular fluid.

Indications and uses: Prevention and correction of systemic acidosis, particularly that associated with cardiac bypass surgery.

Precautions: (1) Determine blood pH, P_{CO_2}, bicarbonate, glucose, and electrolytes before, during, and after administration. (2) Avoid overdose (total drug or too rapid rate). Severe alkalosis and/or prolonged hypoglycemia may result. (3) Use a large peripheral vein. Determine absolute patency of vein; necrosis may result from extravasation. (4) Reduced rate may control venospasm. (5) May severely depress respiration; oxygen and controlled ventilation equipment must always be available. (6) Use extreme caution in impaired renal function or decreased urine output. ECG monitoring and frequent serum potassium measurements are required. (7) Intended for short-term use only (1 day). (8) Severe hypoglycemia or severe hemorrhagic liver necrosis may occur in premature or full-term infants. (9) Sodium bicarbonate or sodium lactate is effective in most acidotic situations and has fewer side effects. (10) Potentiates amphetamines, ephedrine, and quinidine. (11) Inhibits lithium, methotrexate, and salicylates.

Contraindications: Hypersensitivity to tromethamine, anuria, and uremia. Pregnancy is a probable contraindication.

Incompatible with: Sufficient information not available. Should be administered alone because of specific use and potential side effects.

Side effects: Hyperkalemia, hypoglycemia, phlebitis, respiratory depression, thrombosis.

Antidote: Notify physician of all side effects. Reduced rate of infusion may prevent hypoglycemia. Use glucose if indicated. Discontinue drug immediately for hyperkalemia or extravasation. Local infiltration with 1% procaine with hyaluronidase or phentolamine may reduce tissue necrosis. Use a no. 25 needle. Symptomatic treatment is indicated. Alternate drugs are indicated (sodium bicarbonate, sodium lactate).

TUBOCURARINE CHLORIDE — pH 2.5 to 5.0

(Curare, ✤ Tubarine)

Usual dose: *Aid to controlled ventilation:* 16.5 mcg (0.0165 mg)/kg of body weight. Adjust as needed.

Muscle contraction or convulsions: 0.15 mg (1 unit)/kg minus 3 mg (20 units). May repeat as necessary.

Diagnosis of myasthenia gravis: 4 to 33 mcg (0.004 to 0.033 mg)/kg.

Dilution: May be given undiluted in 3 mg/ml concentration.

Myasthenia testing: Dilute single dose to 4 ml with sterile normal saline for injection.

Rate of administration: A single dose over 60 to 90 seconds. Too rapid injection will cause symptoms of overdose and histamine release resulting in severe bronchospasm and profound hypotension.

Myasthenia testing: 0.5 ml diluted medication over 2 minutes.

Actions: A short-acting skeletal muscle relaxant. Causes paralysis by interfering with neural transmission at the myoneural junction. Onset of action is within 2 or 3 minutes and may last up to 60 minutes. Complete recovery from a single dose may take several hours. Metabolized in the liver and excreted in the urine. Crosses the placental barrier.

Indications and uses: (1) Muscle relaxation in severe muscle contraction or convulsion caused by disease, drugs, or electrical stimulation; (2) diagnosis of myasthenia gravis if other tests inconclusive; (3) facilitate management of patients undergoing mechanical ventilation; (4) adjunctive to general anesthesia.

Precautions: (1) Administered by or under the direction of the anesthesiologist. (2) This drug produces apnea. Controlled artificial ventilation with oxygen must be continuous and under direct observation at all times. Maintain a patent airway. (3) Repeated doses may produce cumulative effect. (4) Impaired pulmonary function or respiratory deficiencies can cause critical reactions. Use caution in impaired liver or kidney function. (5) Use extreme caution in pregnancy; has caused fetal malformation. Use caution in lactation; safety not established. (6) Myasthenia gravis increases sensitivity to drug. Terminate testing process within 2 to 3 minutes with 1.5 mg of neostigmine to avoid prolonged respiratory paralysis. (7) Use only clear solutions. Faint discoloration is acceptable. (8) Potentiated by inhalant anesthetics (e.g., ether), neuromuscular blocking antibiotics (e.g., kanamycin [Kantrex]), calcium and magnesium salts, CO_2, digitalis, diuretics, muscle relaxants, (e.g., diazepam [Valium]), lidocaine, MAO inhibitors, propranolol (Inderal), quinidine, tetracyclines, succinylcholine, verapamil, and others. Markedly reduced dose of tubocurarine must be used with caution. (9) Antagonized by acetylcholines, anticholinesterases, carbamazepine, and potassium. (10) Hyperkalemia may cause cardiac dysrhythmias and increased paralysis. Body temperature, some carcinomas, dehydration, and renal disease will adversely affect the action of this drug. (11) Confirm adequate potassium levels before use. Consider witholding diuretics for at least 4 days before elective surgery. (12) Patient may be conscious and completely unable to communicate by any means. Tubocurarine has no analgesic properties. (13) Use of a peripheral nerve stimulator is recommended to monitor effectiveness of this drug.

Contraindications: Known sensitivity, patients in whom histamine release is definite hazard.

Incompatible with: All barbiturates. Consider incompatible in a syringe with any other drug. Evaluation of predictable results imperative.

Side effects: Airway closure caused by relaxation of epiglottis, pharynx, and tongue muscles. Allergic reactions including anaphylaxis, histamine release, profound hypotension, respiratory deficiency, respiratory failure, severe bronchospasm, and shock may occur.

Antidote: All side effects are medical emergencies. Treat symptomatically. Controlled artificial ventilation must be continuous. Edrophonium or neostigmine methylsulfate with atropine may help to reverse muscle relaxation. Not effective in all situations; may aggravate severe overdose. Treat allergic reactions and resuscitate as necessary.

UREA-STERILE USP — pH 5.5 to 7.5

(Ureaphil)

Usual dose: 0.5 to 1.5 Gm/kg of body weight. Highly individualized according to clinical condition of the patient. Do not exceed total dose of 120 Gm/24 hr. A 30% in 1 liter equals approximately 5,250 mOsm/L.

Pediatric dose: 0.5 Gm/kg of body weight.

Infant dose: *Under 2 years:* 0.1 Gm/kg of body weight may be sufficient.

Dilution: Must be diluted to a 30% solution (30 Gm/dl diluent) with 5% or 10% dextrose for infusion or 10% invert sugar in water. Diluent provided by some manufacturers.

30% solution: Add 105 ml recommended diluent to 40 Gm of urea. Total volume equals 135 ml (300 mg/ml).

Rate of administration: 100 ml of a 30% solution is usually given over 1 or 2 hours. Do not exceed infusion rate of 1,200 mg/min (60 gtt or 4 ml of a 30% solution).

Actions: Normal degradation product of amino acids. Hypertonic urea increases blood tonicity. A greater urea concentration in the blood absorbs fluid from extravascular tissue, brain, and intraocular and cerebrospinal fluid into the blood. Effective within 15 minutes, peaks in 1 to 2 hours, lasts 3 to 10 hours. Rebound may occur within 12 hours. Increased urea in the glomerular filtrate inhibits reabsorption of water.

Indications and uses: Reduction of intracranial pressure, cerebrospinal fluid pressure, and intraocular pressure.

Precautions: (1) Mannitol is usually the preferred drug when an osmotic diuretic is desired. (2) Use only freshly prepared solutions; discard unused portion. (3) Determine absolute patency of vein; extravasation may cause necrosis. (4) Observe infusion site; chemical phlebitis and thrombosis do occur. (5) Frequent electrolyte panels and kidney function tests necessary. Observe for early signs of hypokalemia and hyponatremia. (6) Observe urine output continuously; insert Foley catheter if necessary. (7) Use caution in pregnancy, lactation, childbearing years, and liver impairment. (8) Do not administer through same infusion set with blood. (9) Observe for reactivation of intracranial bleeding. (10) May mask symptoms of excessive blood loss. Blood replacement should be adequate. (11) Concomitant use of hypothermia increases risk of venous thrombosis and hemoglobinuria. (12) Will increase renal excretion of lithium.

Contraindications: Impaired renal function (severe), active intracranial bleeding, marked dehydration, liver failure, edema of cardiac failure, lower extremity infusion in the elderly.

Incompatible with: Alkaline solutions, whole blood. Additional information not available. Consider specific indication for administration.

Side effects: Congestive heart failure, disorientation, headache, hemolysis, hypokalemia, hyponatremia, nausea, pulmonary edema, syncope, thrombophlebitis, vomiting.

Antidote: Notify the physician of all side effects. Treatment will probably be symptomatic. Resuscitate as necessary.

UROKINASE

pH 6.0 to 7.5

(Abbokinase, Abbokinase Open-Cath)

Usual dose: *Pulmonary embolism:* 4,400 IU/kg of body weight is given as an initial priming dose over 10 minutes. Follow with a continuous infusion of 4,400 IU/kg/hr for 12 hours. Total volume of infusion must not exceed 200 ml. To be sure entire dose is administered, follow entire procedure with a flush of normal saline or 5% dextrose for infusion. Use a volume equal to the volume of the catheter. Keep line open with this solution at 15 ml/hr.

Coronary artery thrombi: Initially give a bolus dose of heparin 2,500 to 10,000 units directly into the coronary artery. Consider any heparin administered in the previous 4 to 6 hours when calculating this dose. Follow with prepared solution of urokinase directly into the coronary artery at 4 ml/min (6,000 IU/min) for up to 2 hours. Continue until artery is maximally opened, usually 15 or 30 minutes after the initial breakthrough. Average required total dosage is 500,000 IU. Obtain coagulation parameters. Continue heparin therapy.

IV catheter clearance: 5,000 IU (1 ml specifically diluted solution). More or less can be used. Amount should be equal to the volume of the catheter.

Dilution: Each vial (250,000 IU) must be diluted with 5.2 ml of sterile water for injection without preservatives. Add diluent slowly, direct to sides of vial, roll and tilt gently. Do not shake. Terminally filter through a 0.45 micron or smaller cellulose membrane filter.

For IV infusion in pulmonary embolism: Each dose must be further diluted with sufficient normal saline to administer a total infusion of 195 ml.

For lysis of coronary artery thrombi: Dilute three 250,000 IU vials as described. Add the contents of these three vials to 500 ml of 5% dextrose in water for infusion (1,500 IU/ml).

For IV catheter clearance: Add 1 ml of the initially reconstituted drug to 9 ml of sterile water for injection without preservatives (1 ml equals 5,000 IU). Prepare immediately before using and discard any solution remaining in vial after dose removed.

Rate of administration: *Pulmonary embolism:* Initial priming dose is delivered equally distributed over 10 minutes. Follow with continuous infusion of calculated total dose over 12 hours. Use of an infusion pump capable of administering the total volume (195 ml) over 12 hours is required. Keep vein open (see Usual dose).

Lysis of coronary artery thrombi: 4 ml/min (6,000 IU).

IV catheter clearance: Confirm occlusion by gently attempting to aspirate blood with a 10 ml syringe. Slowly and gently inject specifically diluted and premeasured amount of urokinase into the catheter (usually 1 ml in a tuberculin syringe). Connect a 5 ml syringe to the catheter and wait 5 minutes. Gently aspirate to remove clot. Repeat aspiration every 5 minutes until clot clears or for 30 minutes. If unsuccessful, cap catheter for 30 to 60 minutes and attempt to aspirate again. If still unsuccessful, a second dose of urokinase may be required. Maintain absolute sterility of IV system in all situations. When successful aspirate 5 ml of blood to ensure removal of clots and medication. Gently irrigate the catheter with 10 ml of normal saline. Reconnect to IV tubing.

Actions: An enzyme obtained from human kidney cells by tissue-culturing techniques. It converts plasminogen to plasmin, which degrades fibrin clots, fibrinogen, and other plasma proteins. This activation takes place both within a thrombus and on the surface. Onset of action is prompt and may last up to 12 to 24 hours. End products of this activity possess an anticoagulant effect. Bleeding may be very difficult to control.

Indications and uses: (1) Lysis of acute massive pulmonary emboli if one or more lobes are involved or if hemodynamics are unstable; (2) lysis of coronary artery thrombi, (3) restore patency of IV catheters occluded by clotted blood or fibrin (includes central venous catheters). Rarely used except for catheter clearance. tPA or streptokinase generally preferred for other uses.

Precautions: (1) Administered only in the hospital under the direction of a physician knowledgeable in its use and with appropriate diagnostic and laboratory facilities available. Observe patient continuously. Monitor hematocrit, platelet count, thrombin time, and activated PTT or PT before therapy. Thrombin time or activated PTT should be less than twice the normal control value before thrombolytic therapy is started. In 4 hours and during therapy, thrombin time or PT changes are monitored and will reflect effectiveness of treatment. Keep physician informed. Request specific parameters for notifying physician after initial supervised injection. (2) Diagnosis of pulmonary or other emboli should be confirmed. (3) Best results obtained if started within 7 days of onset of emboli. (4) For coronary catheter procedure, diagnosis of acute myocardial infarction must be confirmed and the site of the coronary thrombosis confirmed with selective angiography. Best results obtained within 4 to 6 hours of infarct. (5) A greater alteration of hemostatic status than with heparin; use care in handling patient, avoid arterial puncture, venipuncture, and IM injection. Use extreme precautionary methods (use of radial artery, not femoral; extended pressure application of up to 30 minutes) if above procedures absolutely necessary. (6) Use caution in presence of atrial fibrillation. (7) Monitor for dysrhythmias during therapy; atrial and ventricular dysrhythmias can occur. (8) Simultaneous use of anticoagulants not recommended except in lysis of coronary artery. Do not use either drug until the effects of the previous drug are diminished. Intensive follow-up therapy with heparin is indicated. Do not use a loading dose with continuous heparin therapy. Thrombin time should be reduced to less than twice the normal control value before heparin therapy begins. Usually occurs in 3 to 4 hours. (9) Avoid use of drugs that may alter platelet function (e.g., aspirin, indomethacin, phenylbutazone). (10) Do not take blood pressure in lower extremities; thrombi may be dislodged. (11) Urokinase has less potential for allergic reaction than streptokinase and is indicated if repeated therapy necessary. (12) Avoid force while attempting to clear catheters; may rupture catheter or dislodge clot into the circulation. Instruct the patient to exhale and hold his breath any time the catheter is not connected to the IV tubing or a syringe to prevent air from entering the open catheter and the circulatory system. (13) Will not dissolve drug precipitate or anything other than blood products. Use caution so as not to dislodge foreign bodies into the circulatory system. (14) Use extreme caution in the following situations: any surgical procedure, biopsy, lumbar puncture, thoracentesis, paracentesis, multiple cutdowns, or intraarterial diagnostic procedures within 10 days; ulcerative wounds; recent trauma with possible internal injury; visceral or intracranial malignancy; pregnancy and first 10 days postpartum; any lesion of GI or GU tract with a potential for bleeding (e.g., diverticulitis, ulcerative colitis); severe hypertension; acute or chronic hepatic or renal insufficiency; uncontrolled hypocoagulable state; chronic lung disease with cavitation; rheumatic valvular disease; recent cerebral embolism; and any condition where bleeding might be hazardous or difficult to manage because of location. (15) Contains no preservatives; reconstitute immediately before use. Visually inspect; should be a clear, colorless solution. Do not use highly colored solutions. Discard unused portions.

Contraindications: Active internal bleeding, cerebrovascular accident within 2 months, intracranial or intraspinal surgery, intracranial neoplasm, hypersensitivity to urokinase, liver disease, subacute bacterial endocarditis, visceral malignancy.

Incompatible with: Specific information not available. Should be considered incompatible in syringe or solution because of specific use and hazards of use.

Side effects: Mild allergic reactions (bronchospasm, skin rash); bleeding can be life threatening.

Antidote: Notify physician of all side effects. Note even the minutest bleeding tendency. Therapy may have to be discontinued with blood loss and/or serious bleeding not controlled by local pressure. Whole blood, packed red blood cells, cryoprecipitate, fresh frozen plasma, and aminocaproic acid may all be indicated. Do not use dextran. Treat minor allergic reactions symptomatically. Discontinue drug and treat anaphylaxis as indicated, resuscitate as necessary.

VANCOMYCIN HYDROCHLORIDE pH 2.4 to 4.5

(Lyphocin, Vancocin, Vancoled, Vancor)

Usual dose: 500 mg every 6 hours or 1 Gm every 12 hours. Maximum dosage of 3 to 4 Gm/24 hr used only in extreme situations. Normal renal function required.

Prevention of bacterial endocarditis in penicillin-allergic patients having dental procedures or upper respiratory tract surgery or instrumentation: Adults and children: Over 27 kg (59½ lb), 1 Gm IV 1 hour before the procedure; under 27 kg, 20 mg/kg of body weight 1 hour before before the procedure. Repeat dose in 8 to 12 hours for high-risk patients.

Prevention of bacterial endocarditis in penicillin-allergic patients having GI or GU surgery or instrumentation: Adults and children: Over 27 kg (59½ lb), 1 Gm IV 1 hour before the procedure (gentamicin 1.5 mg/kg given concurrently); under 27 kg, 20 mg/kg 1 hour before the procedure (gentamicin 2 mg/kg given concurrently). Repeat dose in 8 to 12 hours for high-risk patients.

Pediatric dose: 40 mg/kg of body weight/24 hr divided into 4 equal doses. Do not exceed 2 Gm in 24 hours. *See Usual dose for specific uses.*

Infant and neonatal dose: 15 mg/kg as an initial dose. Follow with 10 mg/kg every 12 hours for infants up to 1 month of age and every 8 hours for infants over 1 month of age.

Dilution: Each 500 mg is initially diluted with 10 ml of sterile water for injection. Each 500 mg must be further diluted with 100 ml of normal saline or 5% dextrose in water and given as an intermittent infusion. If absolutely necessary, 1 to 2 Gm may be further diluted in sufficient amounts of the same infusion fluids and given over 24 hours. Not recommended.

Rate of administration: A single dose properly diluted over 60 minutes. Preferred route of administration because of high incidence of thrombophlebitis.

Actions: A very potent tricyclic glycopeptide antibiotic, it is bacterial against gram-positive cocci. Use limited because of ototoxic and nephrotoxic side effects. Well distributed in all body tissues and fluids including spinal fluid if the meninges are inflamed. Vancomycin is excreted in biologically active form in the urine.

Indications and uses: (1) Life-threatening gram-positive infections that do not respond or are resistant to other less toxic antibiotics, such as penicillins or cephalosporins; (2) to substitute for contraindicated penicillin therapy if absolutely necessary; (3) treatment of endocarditis caused by *Streptococcus viridans* or *S. bovis* concurrently with an aminoglycoside antibiotic; (4) prophylaxis against bacterial endocarditis in high-risk (rheumatic or congenital heart disease) patients undergoing dental, upper respiratory, GI, or GU surgery or instrumentation.

Precautions: (1) Store in refrigerator after initial dilution. Maintains potency for 2 weeks. Solutions prepared from ADD-vantage vials stable at room temperature for 24 hours. (2) Sensitivity studies necessary to determine susceptibility of the causative organism to vancomycin. (3) Prolonged use of drug may result in superinfection caused by overgrowth of nonsusceptible organisms. (4) Ototoxic and nephrotoxic. Use extreme caution in impaired hearing, impaired renal function, pregnancy, lactation, neonates, and the elderly. Reduce total daily dose if renal function impaired. Neonates have immature renal function; blood levels may be excessive. (5) Blood levels of vancomycin, auditory testing, and renal function tests are necessary when this drug is used. (6) Determine absolute patency of vein. Necrosis and sloughing will result from extravasation. Rotate injection sites every 2 to 3 days. (7) Use caution with dimenhydrinate (Dramamine), which can mask ototoxicity. Neuromuscular blocking antibiotics (e.g., kanamycin [Kantrex]) and other nephrotoxic or ototoxic drugs (e.g., cisplatin, ethacrynic acid [Edecrin]) may potentiate vancomycin. (8) Observe for furry tongue, diarrhea, and foul-smelling stools. (9) Severe hypotension, with or without red blotching of the face, neck, chest, and extremities, and cardiac arrest can occur with too rapid injection. Monitor blood pressure continuously during infusion to prevent a precipitous drop.

Contraindications: Known hypersensitivity to vancomycin.

Incompatible with: Aminophylline, amobarbital (Amytal), chloramphenicol (Chloromycetin), chlorothiazide (Diuril), dexamethasone (Decadron), heparin, hydrocortisone sodium succinate (Solu-Cortef), methicillin (Staphcillin), penicillins, pentobarbital (Nembutal), phenobarbital (Luminal), phenytoin (Dilantin), prochlorperazine (Compazine), secobarbital (Seconal), sodium bicarbonate, vitamin B complex with C, warfarin (Coumadin).

Side effects: *Minor:* Chills, fever, macular rashes, nausea, pain at injection site, tinnitus, urticaria.

Major: Anaphylaxis, cardiac arrest, eosinophilia, hearing loss, hypotension, redneck or redman syndrome, thrombophlebitis.

Antidote: Notify the physician of all side effects. Hearing loss may progress even if drug is discontinued. If minor side effects are progressive or any major side effect occurs, discontinue the drug, treat allergic reaction, or resuscitate as necessary. Prevent severe hypotension by slowing infusion rate to 2 hours. Fluids, antihistamines, corticosteroids, and vasopressors (e.g., dopamine [Intropin]) may be required. Hemodialysis or CAPD will not decrease blood levels in toxicity.

VECURONIUM BROMIDE pH 4.0

(Norcuron)

Usual dose: Must be individualized, depending on previous drugs administered and degree and length of muscle relaxation required. 0.08 to 0.1 mg/kg of body weight initially as an IV bolus. Patient should be unconscious before administration. Reduce dose by 15% if administered more than 5 minutes after inhalation general anesthetics. Reduce dose to 0.04 to 0.06 mg/kg if following succinylcholine administration. Determine need for maintenance dose based on beginning symptoms of neuromuscular blockade reversal determined by a peripheral nerve stimulator. 0.010 to 0.015 mg/kg will be required in approximately 25 to 40 minutes and every 12 to 20 minutes thereafter to maintain muscle relaxation. Higher doses (0.15 to 0.28 mg/kg) at longer intervals have been given with proper ventilation without causing adverse cardiac effects.

Pediatric dose: *7 weeks to 10 years of age:* May require high end of initial adult dose, and maintenance dose may be required on a more frequent basis.

Dilution: Each 10 mg must be diluted with 5 ml sterile water for injection (supplied). May be given direct IV or may be further diluted in normal saline, 5% dextrose in water or normal saline, or lactated Ringer's and given as an infusion titrated to symptoms of neuromuscular blockade reversal.

Rate of administration: A single dose as an IV bolus over 30 to 60 seconds. If maintenance dose is given as an infusion, adjust rate to specific dose desired.

Actions: A nondepolarizing skeletal muscle relaxant about one-third more potent than pancuronium with a shorter duration of neuromuscular blockade. Causes paralysis by interfering with neural transmission at the myoneural junction. Onset of action is dose dependent. Onset of action is within 30 seconds, produces maximum neuromuscular blockade within 3 to 5 minutes, and lasts about 25 minutes. It may take up to 60 minutes or more before complete recovery occurs. Up to three times the therapeutic dose has been given without significant changes of hemodynamic parameters. Excreted as metabolites in bile and urine. Crosses the placental barrier.

Indications and uses: (1) Adjunctive to general anesthesia; (2) facilitate endotracheal intubation; (3) management of patients undergoing mechanical ventilation.

Precautions: (1) For IV use only. (2) Administered only by or under the direct observation of the anesthesiologist. (3) This drug produces apnea. Controlled artificial ventilation with oxygen must be continuous and under direct observation at all times. Maintain a patent airway. (4) Use a peripheral nerve stimulator to monitor response to vecuronium and avoid overdose. (5) Repeated doses have no cumulative effect if recovery is allowed to begin before administration. (6) Use extreme caution in patients with cirrhosis, cholestasis, obesity, or circulatory insufficiency. Reduced dose may be required in renal failure. (7) Myasthenia gravis and other neuromuscular diseases increase sensitivity to drug. Can cause critical reactions. (8) Potentiated by hypokalemia, some carcinomas, general anesthetics (e.g., enflurane, isoflurane, halothane), neuromuscular blocking antibiotics (e.g., clindamycin [Cleocin], kanamycin [Kantrex], gentamicin [Garamycin]), polypeptide antibiotics (e.g., bacitracin, colistimethate), tetracyclines, diuretics, diazepam (Valium) and other muscle relaxants, magnesium sulfate, quinidine, morphine, meperidine, succinylcholine, verapamil, and others. Reduced dose of vecuronium must be used with caution. (9) Antagonized by acetylcholine, anticholinesterases, azathioprine, carbamazepine, phenytoin, and theophylline. (10) Succinylcholine must show signs of wearing off before vecuronium is given. Use caution. (11) Patient may be conscious and completely unable to communicate by any means. Has no analgesic properties. Respiratory depression with morphine may be preferred in some patients requiring mechanical ventilation. (12) Action is altered by dehydration, electrolyte imbalance, body temperatures, and acid-base imbalance. (13) Use in pregnancy only if use justifies potential risk to fetus. Has been used during cesarean section; monitor infant carefully. Use caution during lactation. (14) Safety for use in infants under 7 weeks of age not established. (15) Store under refrigeration. Discard after 24 hours.

Contraindications: None known.

Incompatible with: Specific information not available.

Side effects: No side effects have occurred except with overdose: prolonged action resulting in respiratory insufficiency or apnea, airway closure caused by relaxation of epiglottis, pharynx, and tongue muscles. Hypersensitivity reactions including anaphylaxis are possible.

Antidote: All side effects are medical emergencies. Treat symptomatically. Controlled artificial ventilation must be continuous until full muscle control returns. Pyridostigmine (Mestinon) or neostigmine (Prostigmin) given with atropine will probably reverse the muscle relaxation but should not be required because of short time of effectiveness. Not effective in all situations; may aggravate severe overdose. Resuscitate as necessary.

VERAPAMIL HYDROCHLORIDE pH 4.1 to 6.0

(Isoptin)

Usual dose: 5 to 10 mg initially (0.075 to 0.15 mg/kg of body weight). 10 mg (0.15 mg/kg) may be repeated in 30 minutes if needed to achieve appropriate response.

Pediatric dose: *Infants up to 1 year of age:* 0.1 to 0.2 mg/kg of body weight (usually 0.75 to 2 mg). Repeat in 30 minutes if indicated.

1 to 15 years of age: 0.1 to 0.3 mg/kg (usually 2 to 5 mg). Repeat in 30 minutes if indicated.

Do not exceed 5 mg.

Dilution: May be given undiluted through Y-tube or threeway stopcock of tubing containing dextrose 5%, sodium chloride 0.9%, or Ringer's solution for infusion.

Rate of administration: A single dose over 2 minutes for adults and children. Extend to 3 minutes in the elderly.

Actions: A calcium (and possibly sodium) ion inhibitor through slow channels. Slows conduction through SA and AV nodes, prolongs effective refractory period in the AV node, and reduces ventricular rates. Prevents reentry phenomena through the atrioventricular node. Reduces myocardial contractility, afterload, arterial pressure, vascular tone, and oxygen demand. Effective within 1 to 5 minutes. Hemodynamic effects last about 20 minutes, but antiarrhythymic èffects last up to 6 hours. Does not alter total serum calcium levels. Metabolized in the liver. Crosses the placental barrier. Excreted in urine and feces. Secreted in breast milk.

Indications and uses: Treatment of supraventricular tachyarrhythmias including conversion to normal sinus rhythm of paroxysmal supraventricular tachycardia (includes Wolff-Parkinson-White and Lown-Ganong-Levine syndromes) and temporary control of rapid ventricular rate in atrial flutter or atrial fibrillation.

Precautions: (1) ECG monitoring during administration mandatory for infants and children, recommended for all others. Monitor blood pressure very closely. (2) Protect from light. Do not use if discolored or particulate matter present. (3) Valsalva maneuver recommended before use of verapamil in all paroxysmal supraventricular tachycardias if clinically appropriate. (4) Emergency resuscitation drugs and equipment must always be available. (5) Treat heart failure with digitalis and diuretics before using verapamil. (6) Pulmonary wedge pressure above 20 mm Hg and/or ejection fraction below 20% indicates acute heart failure. (7) Monitor for side effects (AV block) and digoxin levels when used concurrently with digitalis. Potentiates digoxin; lower dose may be appropriate. (8) Do not give concomitantly (within a few hours) with oral or IV β-adrenergic blocking drugs (e.g., propranolol [Inderal]) (see Contraindications). Both drugs depress myocardial contractility and AV node conduction. (9) Do not administer disopyramide (Norpace) within 48 hours before or 24 hours after verapamil. (10) Potentiates cyclosporine and carbamazepine. Potentiates nondepolarizing muscle relaxants (e.g., tubocurarine); use lower doses of muscle relaxant and extreme caution. (11) Caution required in hepatic and renal disease, especially if repeated dosage is required. Use extreme caution in patients with hypertrophic cardiomyopathy. (12) May precipitate respiratory muscle failure in patients with muscular dystrophy or increase intracranial pressure during anesthesia induction in patients with supratentorial tumors. Use caution. (13) Safety for use in pregnancy not yet established; use only when clearly indicated. Discontinue breast feeding. (14) May cause excessive hypotension with other antihypertensive drugs (vasodilators and diuretics) and quinidine. (15) May inhibit other highly protein-bound drugs (e.g., oral hypoglycemics, warfarin). Use caution. (16) Abrupt withdrawal can precipitate rebound angina. Gradually decrease dose. (17) Children under 6 months of age may not respond to treatment with verapamil. (18) Discard unused solution.

Contraindications: Atrial fibrillation or flutter when associated with an accessory bypass tract (e.g., Wolff-Parkinson-White or Lown-Ganong-Levine syndromes), cardiogenic shock, congestive heart failure (severe) unless secondary to supraventricular tachyarrhythmia treatable with verapramil, known sensitivity to verapamil, second or third degree AV block, severe hypotension, sick sinus syndrome (unless functioning artificial pacemaker in place), patients receiving IV β-adrenergic blocking drugs (e.g., propranolol [Inderal]) within 2 to 4 hours, ventricular tachycardia.

Incompatible with: Albumin, amphotericin B (Fungizone), ampicillin (Polycillin-N), dobutamine (Dobutrex), hydralazine (Apresoline), mezlocillin (Mezlin), nafcillin sodium, oxacillin (Prostaphlin), sodium bicarbonate, trimethoprim-sulfamethoxazole.

Side effects: Abdominal discomfort, allergic reactions including anaphylaxis, asystole, bradycardia, dizziness, headache, heart failure, hypotension (symptomatic), increased ventricular response in atrial flutter, fibrillation (Wolff-Parkinson-White and Lown-Ganong-Levine syndromes), nausea, PVCs, tachycardia.

Antidote: Notify physician promptly of all side effects. Treatment will depend on clinical situation. Calcium chloride may reverse effects of verapamil and can be used in toxicity. Rapid ventricular response in atrial flutter/fibrillation should respond to cardioversion, procainamide, and/or lidocaine. Treat bradycardia, AV block, and asystole with standard AHA protocol (atropine, isoproterenol, pacing). Levarterenol or dopamine will reverse hypotension. Treat allergic reactions or resuscitate as necessary.

VIDARABINE pH 5.0 to 6.2

(ARA-A, Adenine Arabinoside, Vira-A)

Usual dose: *Herpes simplex virus encephalitis:* 15 mg/kg of body weight/day for 10 days.
Herpes zoster: 10 mg/kg/day for 5 days.
Reduce dose in impaired renal function, may be necessary in impaired hepatic function.

Pediatric dose: *Neonatal herpes simplex virus infections:* 15 mg/kg of body weight/day. Reduce dose as noted in Usual dose.

Dilution: Each 1 mg of vidarabine requires 2.22 ml of infusion solution to dissolve. (450 mg requires a minimum of 1 liter of fluid). May be diluted with most IV solutions except biological and colloidal fluids (blood products, protein solutions). Aseptic technique imperative. Shake vidarabine well before measuring dose. Warm diluent to 35° to 40° C (95° to 100° F) to facilitate solution. Thoroughly agitate diluted solution until completely clear by visual inspection. When completely clear and in solution, no further agitation is necessary.
Neonatal dilution: Each 1 ml of vidarabine must be diluted with 9 ml of normal saline or sterile water for injection. Provides a suspension of 20 mg/ml. Note all instructions above.

Rate of administration: Total daily dose must be infused over 12 to 24 hours at a constant rate. Use of an infusion pump is recommended to avoid accidental overdose. Use of an in-line filter (0.45 micron) is required.

Actions: An antiviral drug obtained from fermentation cultures of *Streptomyces antibioticus.* Rapidly changed to Ara-Hx, a metabolite, and distributed in the tissues. Plasma and tissue levels are maintained by slow IV infusion. Excreted in the urine.

Indications and uses: (1) Treat and reduce mortality of herpes simplex viral encephalitis; (2) treat and reduce mortality of neonatal herpes simplex viral infections (e.g., disseminated infection with visceral involvement, encephalitis, infections of the skin, eyes and mouth); (3) reduce complications of herpes zoster in immunocompromised patients.

Precautions: (1) confirm diagnosis of HSV encephalitis by cell culture from a brain biopsy. (2) Does not alter morbidity and resulting neurological problems in the comatose patient with herpes simplex viral encephalitis; early diagnosis essential. (3) For IV infusion only. Avoid rapid or bolus injection. (4) Will produce teratogenic effects on the fetus. (5) Use caution in cerebral edema or potential fluid overload. (6) Monitor blood counts frequently during therapy. (7) Probably ineffective in the immunosuppressed patient except in herpes zoster. (8) Must be initiated within 72 hours of onset of vesicular lesions. (9) Use only freshly prepared solution, stable at room temperature 48 hours. (10) Inhibited by allopurinol.

Contraindications: Vidarabine sensitivity.

Incompatible with: Blood products, protein solutions. Consider specific use.

Side effects: Incidence increases in impaired renal or hepatic function. Anorexia; ataxia; confusion; decreased hematocrit, hemoglobin, white blood cells, and platelets; diarrhea; dizziness; elevated AST and total bilirubin; fluid overload; hallucinations; hematemesis; malaise; nausea; pain at injection site; pruritus; psychosis, rash; tremor; vomiting; weight loss.

Antidote: Notify physician of all side effects. In acute overdose, monitor hematological, renal, and hepatic functions carefully. Doses over 20 mg/kg/day can produce bone marrow depression. Treat allergic reaction as indicated and resuscitate as necessary.

VINBLASTINE SULFATE pH 3.5 to 5.0

(Velban, ♣ Velbe, Velsar, VLB)

Usual dose: 3.7 mg/M^2 initially. Administered once every 7 days, increasing the dose to specific amounts (5.5, 7.4, 9.25, 11.1 mg/M^2) a single step each week until the white blood cell count is decreased to 3,000 cells/ml, remission is achieved, or a maximum dose of 18.5 mg/M^2 is reached. Maintenance dose is one step below any dose that causes leukopenia (3,000 cells/ml or less), once every 7 to 14 days. Usually 5.5 to 7.4 mg/M^2.

Pediatric dose: 2.5 mg/M^2 initially. Use same procedure as for adult dose using steps to 3.75, 5.0, 6.25, and 7.5 mg/M^2. Maximum dose is 12.5 mg/M^2. Maintenance dose is calculated by same parameters as adult dose. Usually differs with each individual.

Dilution: *Specific techniques required, see Precautions.* Each 10 mg is diluted with 10 ml of sodium chloride for injection. 1 mg equals 1 ml. Do not add to IV solutions. May be given direct IV or through Y-tube or three-way stopcock of a free-flowing IV infusion.

Rate of administration: Total desired dose, properly diluted, over 1 minute.

Actions: An alkaloid of the periwinkle plant with antitumor activity. Cell cycle specific for M phase. Thought to interfere with the metabolic pathways of amino acids. Sometimes pharmacologically effective without any noticeable improvement in symptoms of malignancy. Cell energy production and synthesis of nucleic acid may also be inhibited. Some excretion through bile and urine.

Indications and uses: To suppress or retard neoplastic growth. Remission and probable cure has been achieved with bleomycin and cisplatin in testicular malignancies. Response has been noted in Hodgkin's disease, non-Hodgkin's lymphomas, breast and renal cell malignancies.

Precautions: (1) Follow guidelines for handling cytotoxic agents. See Appendix, p. 677. (2) Administered by or under the direction of the physician specialist. (3) Store in refrigerator before and after dilution. Potency maintained for 30 days after dilution. (4) Determine absolute patency, quality of vein, and adequate circulation of extremity. Severe cellulitis may result from extravasation. Rinse syringe and needle with venous blood before withdrawal from the vein. (5) May cause corneal ulceration with accidental contact to the eye. (6) White blood cell count must be checked before each dose. Must be above 4,000 cells/ml. (7) Often used with other antineoplastic drugs and corticosteroids in reduced doses to achieve tumor remission. (8) Dosage based on average weight in presence of edema or ascites. (9) May produce teratogenic effects on the fetus. Has a mutagenic potential and must be given with caution in men and women capable of conception. (10) Inhibited by some amino acids, glutamic acid, and tryptophan. (11) Potentiates anticoagulants. (12) Potentiated by other antineoplastics. (13) Be alert for signs of bone marrow depression or infection. (14) Do not administer any vaccines or chloroquine to patients receiving antineoplastic drugs. (15) Use caution in presence of ulcerated skin areas or impaired liver function. (16) Allopurinol may prevent formation of uric acid crystals. (17) Maintain adequate hydration. (18) Prophylactic antiemetics may increase patient comfort.

Contraindications: Bacterial infection or leukopenia below 3,000 cells/ml.

Incompatible with: Limited information available. Consider incompatible with any other drug in syringe or solution because of toxicity and specific use.

Side effects: Usually dose related and not always reversible: abdominal pain, alopecia, anorexia, cellulitis, constipation, convulsions, diarrhea, dizziness, extravasation, gonadal suppression, headache, hemorrhage, ileus, leukopenia (severe), malaise, mental depression, myelosuppression, nausea, numbness, oral lesions, paresthesias, peripheral neuritis, pharyngitis, Raynaud's syndrome, reflex depression (deep tendon), skin lesions, thrombophlebitis, tumor site pain, vomiting, weakness.

Antidote: For extravasation, discontinue the drug immediately and administer into another vein. Hyaluronidase should be injected locally into extravasated area. Use a fine hypodermic needle. Elevate extremity; moist heat may be helpful. Notify the physician of all side effects; symptomatic treatment is often indicated. Glutamic acid blocks toxicity of vinblastine, but also blocks its antineoplastic activity.

VINCRISTINE SULFATE pH 3.5 to 5.5

(LCR, Oncovin, VCR, Vincasar PFS)

Usual dose: 1.4 mg/M^2 administered once every 7 days. Various dosage schedules have been used with caution. In impaired hepatic function, give initial doses of 0.05 to 1 mg/M^2. May be increased gradually based on individual response.

Pediatric dose: 2 mg/M^2. For children weighing less than 10 kg (22 lb) or with a body surface area less than 1 M^2, give 0.05 mg/kg of body weight once a week.

Dilution: *Specific techniques required, see Precautions.* Diluent provided, or each 1 mg is diluted with 10 ml of sterile water or normal saline for injection. 0.1 mg equals 1 ml (may use as little as 2 ml diluent for each 1 mg). Do not add to IV solutions. May be given direct IV or through Y-tube or three-way stopcock of a free-flowing IV infusion. Available in preservative-free solutions.

Rate of administration: Total desired dose, properly diluted, over 1 minute.

Actions: An alkaloid of the periwinkle plant with antitumor activity. Cell cycle specific for the M phase. Well absorbed except in spinal fluid, it is primarily excreted through bile and feces.

Indications and uses: To suppress or retard neoplastic growth; good response experienced in leukemia, Hodgkin's disease, lymphosarcoma, oat cell, and others.

Investigational uses: Treatment of idiopathic thrombocytopenic purpura; treatment of Kaposi's sarcoma.

Precautions: (1) Follow guidelines for handling cytotoxic agents. See Appendix, p. 677. (2) Administered by or under the direction of the physician specialist. (3) Store in refrigerator before and after dilution. Potency maintained for 14 days after dilution. Label vial pertaining to milligrams per milliliter. (4) Determine absolute patency and quality of vein and adequate circulation of extremity. Severe cellulitis may result from extravasation. (5) Usually given with other antineoplastic drugs and corticosteroids in reduced doses to achieve tumor remission. Use caution to prevent bone marrow depression. Use with asparaginase or doxorubicin not recommended. Acute pulmonary reactions can occur with mitomycin-C. Use extreme caution in combination with radiation therapy. (6) May cause corneal ulceration with accidental contact to the eye; flush eyes with water immediately. (7) Dosage based on average weight in presence of edema or ascites. (8) Inhibited by glutamic acid. (9) May produce teratogenic effects on the fetus. Has a mutagenic potential and must be given with caution in men and women capable of conception. Discontinue breast feeding. (10) Do not administer any vaccine or chloroquine to patients receiving antineoplastic drugs. (11) Potentiates anticoagulants. (12) Be alert for signs of bone marrow depression or infection. (13) Use caution in preexisting neuromuscular disease or impaired liver function. (14) Allopurinol may prevent formation of uric acid crystals. (15) Maintain adequate hydration. (16) Prophylactic antiemetics may increase patient comfort. (17) Inappropriate secretion of antidiuretic hormone (ADH) may require fluid limitation. (18) Use a stool softener and/or stimulant laxatives to prevent impaction. (19) Potentiated by calcium channel blockers (e.g., verapamil). (20) Inhibits digoxin and phentoin; increased doses of these drugs may be required.

Contraindications: There are no absolute contraindications.

Incompatible with: All solutions except normal saline or dextrose in water. pH must not be less than 3.5 or more than 5.5. Consider incompatible with any other drug in syringe or solution because of toxicity and specific use.

Side effects: Frequently dose related and not always reversible: abdominal pain, alopecia, anaphylaxis, ataxia, bronchospasm, cellulitis, constipation, convulsions, cranial nerve damage, diarrhea, dysuria, extravasation, fever, foot-drop, gonadal suppression, headache, hypertension, hypotension, leukopenia (rare), muscle wasting, nausea, neuritic pain, oral lacerations, paralytic ileus, paresthesias, polyuria, reflex changes, sensory impairment, shortness of breath, tingling and numbness of extremities, thrombocytopenia (rare), thrombophlebitis, upper colon impaction, uric acid nephropathy, vomiting, weakness, weight loss.

Antidote: For extravasation, discontinue the drug immediately and administer into another vein. Hyaluronidase should be injected locally into extravasated area. Use a fine hypodermic needle. Elevate extremity; moist heat may be helpful. Notify the physician of all side effects; symptomatic treatment is often indicated. Will probably reduce dose at earliest signs of neurological toxicity (tingling and numbness of extremities). Discontinue for inappropriate ADH secretion or hyponatremia. Glutamic acid blocks toxicity of vincristine, but also blocks its anti- neoplastic activity. Folinic acid, 100 mg IV every 3 hours for 24 hours and then every 6 hours for at least 48 hours, may be helpful in overdose. Supportive measures still required.

✤ VINDESINE SULPHATE

(✤ **Eldisine**)

Usual dose: 3 mg/M^2 administered once every 7 to 10 days. Repeat for 8 cycles. May be adjusted upward if necessary. Do not exceed 4 mg/M^2. Decrease dose in significant hepatic disease and in patients with bone marrow depression from previous treatment. May be increased gradually based on clinical response. Decreased bone marrow function induced by disease will require full doses to restore marrow function. Will require constant monitoring.

Pediatric dose: 4 mg/M^2 administered once every 7 to 10 days. Repeat for 8 cycles. 2 mg/M^2/day for 2 consecutive days may be given as an alternate regimen. Follow by 5 to 7 days without the drug and repeat for 8 cycles.

Dilution: *Specific techniques required, see Precautions.* Each 5 mg vial must be diluted with 5 ml of bacteriostatic normal saline for injection. 1 mg equals 1 ml. Do not add to IV solutions. Must be given direct IV or through Y-tube or three-way stopcock of a free-flowing IV infusion.

Rate of administration: Total desired dose, properly diluted, over 1 to 3 minutes.

Actions: An antineoplastic agent; a vinca alkaloid with properties similar to but more potent than vincristine and vinblastine. Cell cycle specific for the M phase. Can prevent invasion of normal tissue by malignant cells. Has been effective in patients who have relapsed undergoing multiple-agent treatment that included vincristine. Well distributed through plasma and body tissues, it is primarily excreted through bile and feces.

Indications and uses: Treatment of acute lymphocytic leukemia of childhood resistant to vincristine and non–oat cell lung cancer.

Precautions: (1) Follow guidelines for handling cytotoxic agents. See Appendix, p. 677. (2) Administered by or under the direction of the physician specialist. (3) Monitor blood count 1 or 2 times weekly. Temporary leukopenia is an expected effect and is directly related to the dose. Discontinue or reduce dosage if abnormal depression of the bone marrow occurs (sustained white blood cell count below 2,500/mm^3). Maximum depression usually occurs in 3 to 5 days, and recovery of bone marrow should occur 7 to 10 days after each dose. (4) Strict adherence to recommended dosage schedule is very important. Changes may result in increased side effects. (5) Determine absolute patency and quality of vein and adequate circulation of extremity. Severe cellulitis and phlebitis with sloughing can result from extravasation. (6) Use extreme caution in patients with impaired liver function, preexisting neuromuscular disease, or those taking other neurotoxic drugs (e.g., antineoplastics [cisplatin], phenothiazines [prochlorperazine]). Neurotoxicity may require dose reduction or discontinuation of vindesine.

(7) Prior radiation therapy or treatment with other anit-neoplastic agents may cause thrombocytopenia (platelets below 200,000/mm^3). Not common in patients with normal bone marrow function receiving once-a-week dosage. (8) May cause corneal ulceration with accidental contact to the eye; flush eyes with water immediately. (9) Dosage based on average weight in presence of edema or ascites; calculate carefully, overdose may be fatal. (10) Embryotoxic and may be teratogenic. Must be given with caution in men and women capable of conception. Discontinue breast feeding. (11) Do not administer any vaccine or chloroquine to patients receiving antineoplastic drugs. (12) Be alert for any sign of infection. Infections must be brought under control before beginning therapy with vindesine. (13) Maintain adequate hydration. (14) Prophylactic antiemetics may increase patient comfort. (15) Use a stool softener to prevent impaction. May also need a stimulant laxative. Monitor bowel sounds to prevent obstipation. (16) Inappropriate secretion of antidiuretic hormone (ADH) may require fluid limitation and diuretics (e.g., furosemide [Lasix]). (17) Stable after dilution at room temperature for 24 hours and up to 14 days if refrigerated (2° to 8° C [35° to 46°F). Label vial pertaining to milligrams per milliliter.

Contraindications: Drug-induced severe granulocytopenia or thrombocytopenia; serious bacterial infections.

Incompatible with: Any other drug in syringe or solution.

Side effects: Frequently dose related and not always reversible: abdominal pain; alopecia; anorexia; cellulitis; constipation; convulsions; depression; diarrhea; epilation, chills, and fever; extravasation; generalized musculoskeletal pain; granulocytopenia; headache; jaw pain; leukopenia (rare); loss of deep tendon reflexes; macular skin rash; malaise; nausea; neuritic pain; oral lacerations; pain in tumor site; paralytic ileus; peripheral neuritis; thrombocytopenia (rare); thrombophlebitis; tingling and numbness of extremities (paresthesias); upper color impaction; vomiting.

Overdose: Cardiovascular collapse, ileus, inappropriate secretion of ADH hormone, seizures, serious bone marrow depression, death.

Antidote: For extravasation, discontinue the drug immediately and administer into another vein. Hyaluronidase should be injected locally into extravasated area. Use a fine hypodermic needle. Moist heat may be helpful. Elevate extremity above the heart. Notify the physician of all side effects; symptomatic and supportive treatment is often indicated. Will probably reduce dose at earliest signs of neurological toxicity (tingling and numbness of extremities). Discontinue or reduce dose with abnormal depression of bone marrow; blood transfusion may be required. Discontinue for inappropriate ADH secretion or hyponatremia. Diuretics and fluid restriction may be required for inappropriate secretion of ADH hormone. Diazepam (Valium) or phenobarbital may be required for seizures.

WARFARIN SODIUM pH 7.2 to 8.3

(Coumadin)

Usual dose: 40 to 60 mg initially (0.75 to 1 mg/kg of body weight). Maintenance dose is 2 to 10 mg. Dosage adjusted according to PT. Maintain with oral therapy when possible. Reduce dose by one half in the elderly or debilitated.

Dilution: Diluent provided. Each 50 mg of lyophilized powder is diluted with 2 ml. Rotate vial to dissolve completely. May not be mixed with infusion fluids. Give through Y-tube or three-way stopcock of IV infusion tubing. Compatible in a syringe with sodium heparin. May be given together to accomplish immediate and long-term anticoagulation simultaneously.

Rate of administration: 25 mg (1 ml) or fraction thereof over 1 minute.

Actions: An anticoagulant that acts by depressing the formation of prothrombin and other coagulation factors in the liver. Effective anticoagulant levels are reached in 12 to 24 hours and last for about 4 days. Well-established clots are not dissolved, but growth is prevented. Does cross the placental barrier. Metabolized in the liver and excreted in changed forms in the urine. Secreted in breast milk.

Indications and uses: Prevention and/or treatment of all types of thromboses and emboli and situations and diseases predisposing to the formation of thromboses or emboli.

Precautions: (1) PT must be done before initial injection. Usually repeated daily thereafter during IV therapy. Draw blood for prothrombin just before any heparin dose being given concomitantly. Dosage adjusted daily according to prothrombin activity. 20% of normal activity is desirable (21 to 35 seconds, with a control of 14 seconds). (2) Decrease dosage gradually. Abrupt withdrawal may precipitate increased coagulability. (3) Use with caution in hepatic or renal insufficiency, trauma involving large raw surfaces, extensive surgical procedures, hypertension, diabetes, the elderly or debilitated, or a history of allergic problems. (4) Skin necrosis can occur, especially in the presence of protein C deficiency. (5) Capable of innumerable interactions. Monitor PT carefully when drugs are added or discontinued. (6) Potentiated by acidifying agents, alcohol, anabolic agents, analgesics, anesthetics, antibiotics, antineoplastics, chloral hydrate, diuretics, glucagon, hepatotoxic drugs, salicylates, skeletal muscle relaxants, thyroid preparations, vitamin B complex, and many others. Severe bleeding may result. (7) Inhibited by barbiturates, corticosteroids, benzodiazepines, digitalis, diuretics, vitamins C and K, xanthines, and many others. (8) Potentiates anticonvulsants, insulin, and others. (9) May be fatal with cinchophen and diuretics. (10) Concurrent use with streptokinase or urokinase may be hazardous.

Contraindications: Active bleeding; anesthesia (major regional block); blood dyscrasias; continuous GI suctioning; history of bleeding; inadequate laboratory facilities; pregnancy and lactation; recent surgical procedures, especially neurosurgical, ophthalmic, and extensive traumatic procedures; subacute bacterial endocarditis; threatened abortion; vitamin C deficiency.

Incompatible with: Amikacin (Amikin), ammonium chloride, ascorbic acid, dextrose (any percent solution), epinephrine (Adrenalin), metaraminol (Aramine), oxytocin, promazine (Sparine), tetracycline (Achromycin), vancomycin (Vancocin), vitamin B complex with C.

Side effects: Allergic reactions (rare), alopecia (rare), bruising, epistaxis, hematuria, PT less than 20% activity, tarry stools, any other signs of bleeding.

Antidote: Discontinue drug and notify physician of any side effects. Phytonadione (Aquamephyton) is a specific antagonist and indicated in overdose or desired warfarin sodium reversal. Will impede subsequent anticoagulant therapy.

ZIDOVUDINE

pH 5.5

(Azidothymidine, AZT, Compound S, Retrovir)

Usual dose: 1 to 2 mg/kg every 4 hours. Up to 5 mg/kg every 4 hours has been used. Initiate oral therapy as soon as possible (100 mg orally approximately equal to 1 mg/kg IV). Impaired renal or hepatic function may increase toxicity. Dosage adjustment may be required.

Dilution: Each 1 mg of the calculated dose must be diluted in at least 0.25 ml or 5% dextrose in water to a 4 mg/ml or less solution. For a 70 kg patient at 1 mg/kg, a 70 mg dose would be diluted in 17.5 ml (equals 4 mg/ml [70 mg in 35 ml equals 2 mg/ml]).

Rate of administration: Each single dose properly diluted must be delivered at a constant rate over 1 hour. Avoid rapid infusion or IV bolus.

Actions: An antiviral agent. Through a specific process this thymidine analog inhibits the in vitro replication and terminates the DNA chain of some retroviruses including HIV (HTLV III, LAV, or ARV). May also have antiviral activity against the Epstein-Barr virus. Metabolized by glucuronidation in the liver and excreted through the kidneys.

Indications and uses: Decrease the severity of symptoms in symptomatic HIV (AIDS and advanced ARC) when the patient has a history of *Pneumocystis carinii* pneumonia (PCP) or an absolute CD4 (T4 helper/inducer) lymphocyte count of less than 200/mm^3.

Precautions: (1) Specific use only, confirm history of *Pneumocystis carinii* and/or CD4 lymphocyte count of less than 200/mm^3 before beginning therapy. (2) Do not give IM. (3) Observe closely; not a cure for HIV infections. Patients may acquire illnesses associated with AIDS or ARC, including opportunistic infections. Trimethoprim-sulfamethoxazole (Bactrim), pyrimethamine (Daraprim), and acyclovir (Zovirax) may be indicated to treat opportunistic infections. (4) Zidovudine has not been shown to reduce the risk of transmission to others. (5) Use with extreme caution in patients with bone marrow compromise as indicated by a granulocyte count of less than 1000/mm^3 or hemoglobin below 9.5/dl. (6) Frequent blood counts are required. Hematologic toxicity, including granulocytopenia, severe anemia, and occasionally reversible pancytopenia are common. Anemia occurs most commonly after 4 to 6 weeks of therapy; dosage adjustments, discontinuation, and/or transfusions may be required. (7) Toxicity may be increased by nephrotoxic and/or cytotoxic drugs and/or drugs that interfere with red or white blood cell number and function (e.g., amphotericin B [Fungizone], dapsone, doxorubicin [Adriamycin], flucytosine, interferon, pentamidine [Pentam 300], vinblastin [Velban], vincristine [Oncovin], vindesine [Eldesine]). (8) Use caution with any drug metabolized by glucuronidation (e.g., acetaminophen, diazepam [Valium], morphine); toxicity of both drugs may be increased. (9) Probenicid may inhibit glucuronidation or reduce renal excretion of Zidovudine. Acetaminophen (Tylenol), aspirin, or indomethacin (Indocin) may inhibit glucuronidation. (10) Acetaminophen has increased the incidence of granulocytopenia. (11) Hematologic toxicity may be increased by ganciclovir (CyTovene) and experimental nucleoside analogs being evaluated in AIDS and ARC patients (e.g., didanosine [DDI]) because of their effect on red or white blood cell number of function. The same analogs can affect DNA replication and may antagonize effects of zidovudine. Avoid concomitant administration. (12) Use with acyclovir may cause neurotoxicity. (13) Safety for use in children under 12 years of age not established. (14) Safety for use during pregnancy and lactation not established. Discontinue breast feeding. (15) Store undiluted vials at 15° to 25° C (59° to 77° F). Protect from light. Stable after dilution for 8 hours at room temperature, 24 hours if refrigerated.

Contraindications: Life-threatening allergic reactions to any of the components.

Incompatible with: Blood products and protein solutions.

Side effects: Directly related to dose and duration and inversely related to T4 lymphocyte numbers. Anaphylaxis, anemia (severe), anorexia, asthenia, diaphoresis, diarrhea, dizziness, dyspepsia, dyspnea, fever, GI pain, granulocytopenia, headache insomnia, malaise, myalgia, nausea, pancytopenia (reversible), paresthesia, rash, somnolence, taste perversion, vomiting.

Antidote: Notify physician of all side effects; most will be treated symptomatically. Moderate anemia or granulocytopenia may respond to a reduction in dose. Discontinue zidovudine for severe anemia (less than 7.5 g/dl or a 25% reduction from baseline) or severe granulocytopenia (less that 750/mm^3 or 50% reduction from baseline). Transfusions may be required. Rash may be the first sign of anaphylaxis; notify physician and treat with diphenhydramine (Benadryl), epinephrine (Adrenalin), and corticosteroids as indicated.

PUBLICATIONS

Additional and more detailed information on all included drugs may be found in the following publications:

American Hospital Formulary Service, Bethesda, Md, 1990, American Society of Hospital Pharmacists. (Updated quarterly).

Goodman LS, Gilman A, and Goodman AG, editors: The pharmacological basis of therapeutics, ed 7, New York, 1985, Macmillan Publishing Company.

Kastrup EK, editor: Facts and comparisons, St. Louis, 1991, Facts and Comparisons Division, JB Lippincot Company. (Updated monthly.)

Manufacturer's literature.

Pagliaro AM and Pagliaro LA, editors: Pharmacologic aspects of nursing, St. Louis, 1986, The CV Mosby Company. (Updated monthly.)

Tatro, David S, Pharm D, editors: Drug Interaction Facts, St. Louis, 1991, Facts and Comparisons Division, JB Lippincot Company. (Updated quarterly.)

Trissel LA: Handbook on injectable drugs, ed 6, 1990, American Society of Hospital Pharmacists, Inc.

APPENDIX

Recommendations for the Safe Handling of Parenteral Antineoplastic Drugs

INTRODUCTION

The majority of antineoplastic drugs are toxic compounds. Many are known to cause carcinogenic, mutagenic, or teratogenic effects. On direct contact, some antineoplastic drugs may cause irritation to the skin, eyes, and mucous membranes, and ulceration and necrosis of tissue. The toxicity of parenteral antineoplastic drugs dictates that the exposure of medical personnel to these drugs should be minimized. At the same time, the requirement for maintenance of aseptic conditions during drug preparation must be satisfied.

This brochure reviews routes through which exposure may occur and presents recommendations for the safe handling of parenteral antineoplastic drugs by pharmacists, nurses, physicians, and other personnel who are involved in the preparation and administration of these drugs to patients. This brochure was prepared in response to numerous inquiries received by NIH from practicing pharmacists, nurses, and physicians requesting information on safe handling practices for the preparation and administration of parenteral antineoplastic drugs.

POTENTIAL ROUTES OF EXPOSURE

The potential routes of exposure during the preparation and administration of antineoplastic drugs are primarily through inhalation of the aerosolized drug and by direct skin contact.

During the preparation of these drugs, a variety of manipulations are used which may result in aerosol generation, spraying, and splattering. Examples of these manipulations include: the withdrawal of needles from drug vials; the use of syringes and needles or filter straws for drug transfers; the breaking open of ampules; and the expelling

From U.S. Department of Health and Human Services, Public Health Service, National Institutes of Health: NIH Publication No. 83-2621. Prepared by the Division of Safety, in collaboration with Clinical Center pharmacy and nursing staff, and the National Cancer Institute.

of air from a syringe when measuring the precise volume of a drug.

Good pharmaceutical practice calls for the use of aseptic techniques and a sterile environment when preparing parenteral drugs. Many pharmacies provide this sterile environment by using a horizontal laminar flow clean work bench. While this type of unit provides product protection, it exposes the operator, and other room occupants, to aerosols generated during drug preparation procedures. A Class II laminar flow (vertical) biological safety cabinet will provide both product and operator protection. This is accomplished by filtering cabinet incoming and exhaust air through high-efficiency particulate air (HEPA) filters. It should be noted that these filters are not effective for volatile materials, because the filters do not capture vapors and gases.

During administration, clearing air from a syringe or infusion line and leakage at tubing, syringe, or stopcock connections present obvious opportunities for accidental skin contact and aerosol generation. The practice of clipping used needles and syringes will also produce a considerable aerosol.

The disposal of antineoplastic drugs and trace contaminated materials (gloves, gowns, needles, syringes, vials, etc.), presents a possible source of exposure by these drugs to nurses, physicians, and pharmacists in addition to support and housekeeping personnel. Excreta from patients receiving certain antineoplastic drug therapy (e.g., high dose methotrexate) may contain high concentrations of the drug. Nursing personnel should be aware of this source of potential exposure to antineoplastic drugs and take appropriate precautions to avoid accidental contact.

The potential risks to nurses, physicians, and pharmacists from repeated contact with parenteral antineoplastic drugs can be effectively controlled by a combination of specific containment equipment and certain work techniques which are described in the following recommendations. For the most part, the techniques are merely an extension of good work practices by medical personnel and may be supplemented as deemed appropriate for the work being performed.

RECOMMENDED PRACTICES FOR PERSONNEL PREPARING PARENTERAL ANTINEOPLASTIC DRUGS

Professionally accepted standards concerning the aseptic preparation of parenteral products should be followed. Only properly trained personnel should handle antineoplastic drugs. Training sessions should be offered to new professionals as well as technical and housekeeping personnel who may come in contact with these agents. Safe handling should be the focus of such training.

A. All procedures involved in the preparation of parenteral antineoplastic drugs should be performed in a Class II laminar flow biological safety cabinet. Careful consideration should be given to selecting a cabinet size that will accommodate the preparation unit's work load.

B. Personnel should be familiar with the capabilities, limitatons, and proper utilization of the biological safety cabinet selected. A Class II, Type A cabinet will provide product protection and prevent exposure of the operator to aerosols. The filtered exhaust from this type of cabinet is normally discharged into the room environment. Where possible, however, it is desirable to discharge the filtered exhaust air to the outdoors. This can be accomplished by installing an exhaust canopy over the Class II, Type A cabinet or by the use of a Class II, Type B biological safety cabinet which discharges exhaust air to the outdoors.

C. The safety cabinet work surface should be covered with plastic-backed absorbent paper. This will reduce the potential for dispersion of droplets and spills and facilitate clean-up. The paper should be changed after any overt spills and after each work shift.

D. Personnel preparing the drugs should wear surgical gloves and a closed front surgical-type gown with knit cuffs. Gowns may be of washable or disposable variety. Overtly contaminated gloves or outer garments should be removed and replaced. In case of skin contact with the drug, thoroughly wash the affected area with soap and water. Flush affected eye(s) with copious amounts of water for at least 15 minutes while holding the eyelid(s) open; then seek evaluation by a physician.

E. Vials containing reconstituted drugs should be vented to reduce internal pressure. This will help to reduce the possibility of spraying and spillage when a needle is withdrawn from the septum.

F. A sterile alcohol dampened cotton pledget should be carefully wrapped around the needle and vial top during withdrawal from the vial septum. Similarly, an alcohol dampened cotton pledget should be carefully placed at the needle or syringe tip when ejecting air bubbles from a filled syringe. This practice will control the dripping and aerosol production which may occur during these procedures. *Avoid self-inoculation.* Take care when conducting any procedure that involves the use of needles.

G. The external surfaces of syringes and I.V. bottles should be wiped clean of any drug contamination.

H. When breaking the top off a glass ampule, wrap the ampule neck at the anticipated break point with a sterile alcohol dampened cotton pledget to contain the aerosol produced and also to protect fingers from being lacerated by the broken glass.

I. Syringes and I.V. bottles containing antineoplastic drugs should be properly identified and dated. When these items are delivered to a nursing ward, an additional label such as "Caution—Cancer Chemotherapy, Dispose of Properly." is recommended.

J. Wipe down the interior of the safety cabinet with 70% alcohol using a disposable towel after completing all drug preparation operations.

K. Contaminated needles and syringes should be disposed of intact, to prevent aerosol generation created by clipping needles. Place them in a leakproof and puncture resistant container. This container, was well as contaminated bottles, vials, gloves, absorbent paper, disposable gowns, gauze, etc., should be placed in an appropriately labeled plastic bag-lined box, sealed and incinerated. Washable gowns may be laundered in a normal fashion.

L. Wash hands after removing gloves. Gloves are not a substitute for handwashing.

M. Waste antineoplastic drugs should be disposed of in accordance with Federal and State requirements applicable to toxic chemical waste.

RECOMMENDED PRACTICES FOR PERSONNEL ADMINISTERING PARENTERAL ANTINEOPLASTIC

A. A protective outer garment such as a closed front surgical-type gown with knit cuffs should be worn. Gowns may be of washable or disposable variety.

B. Disposable surgical gloves should be worn during those procedures where leakage of the drugs may result, i.e., removing air bubbles from syringes and I.V. tubing, injecting of drugs, disconnecting I.V. tubing, and fixing leaking tubing or syringe connections. Discard gloves after each use.

C. When bubbles are removed from syringes or I.V. tubing, a sterile alcohol dampened cotton pledget should be carefully placed over the tips of needles, syringes, or I.V. tubing in order to collect any of the antineoplastic drugs that may be inadvertently discharged.

D. Contaminated needles and syringes should be disposed of intact, to prevent aerosol generation created by clipping needles. Place them in a leakproof and puncture resistant container. This container, as well as contaminated bottles, vials, gloves, absorbent paper, disposable gowns, gauze, etc., should be placed in an appropriately labeled plastic bag-lined box, sealed and incinerated. Washable gowns may be laundered in a normal fashion.

E. In case of skin contact with an antineoplastic drug, thoroughly wash the affected area with soap and water. Flush affected eye(s) with copious amounts of water for at least 15 minutes while holding the eyelid(s) open; then seek evaluation by a physician. Wash hands after administering any antineoplastic drug and as dictated by good medical practice.

• • •

Personnel should be knowledgeable of those antineoplastic drugs that are excreted in high concentrations from patients following administration. Care should be taken to avoid skin contact and minimize aerosol generation during disposal of the excreta. Gloves should always be worn by personnel disposing of excreta from patients treated with these types of drugs.

INDEX

Bold type indicates generic drug name.
Italic type indicates drug categories and listings.

D

N

O